Clinical Guide to the Diagnosis and Treatment of Mental Disorders

● FIRST

● TASMAN

CLINICAL GUIDE TO THE DIAGNOSIS AND TREATMENT OF MENTAL DISORDERS

Michael B. First
Associate Professor of Clinical Psychiatry
Department of Psychiatry
Columbia University College of Physicians and Surgeons
New York, NY
USA

Allan Tasman
Professor and Chair
Department of Psychiatry and Behavioral Sciences
University of Louisville School of Medicine
Louisville, KY
USA

WILEY

Telephone (+44) 1243 779777
Email (for orders and customer service enquires): cs-books@wiley.co.uk
Visit our Home Page on www.wiley.co.uk or www.wiely.com

Reprinted August 2006

This publication is designed to provide accurate and authoritative information in regard to the subject matter
covered. It is sold on the understanding that the Publisher is not engaged in rendering professional services.
If professional advice or other expert assistance is required, the services of a competent professional should
be sought.

Other Wiley Editorial Offices

John Wiley & Sons, Inc., 111 River Street,
Hoboken, NJ 07030, USA

Jossey-Bass, 989 Market Street,
San Francisco, CA 94103-1741, USA

Wiley-VCH Verlag GmbH, Boschstr. 12,
D-69469 Weinheim, Germany

John Wiley & Sons Australia Ltd, 42 McDougall Street,
Milton, Queensland 4064, Australia

John Wiley & Sons (Asia) Pte Ltd, 2 Clementi Loop #02-01,
Jin Xing Distripark, Singapore 129809

John Wiley & Sons Canada Ltd, 22 Worcester Road,
Etobicoke, Ontario, Canada, M9W 1L1

Wiley also publishes its books in a variety of electronic formats. Some content that appears in print may not
be available in electronic books.

Library of Congress Cataloging-in-Publication Data

Clinical guide to the diagnosis and treatment of mental disorders/edited by Michael B. First, Allan Tasman.
  p. ; cm.
  Includes bibliographical references and index.
  ISBN-13: 978-0-470-01915-3 (pbk. : alk. paper)
  ISBN-10: 0-470-01915-8 (pbk. : alk. paper)
  1. Mental illness. 2. Psychiatry. I. First, Michael B., 1956–
II. Tasman, Allan, 1947–
  [DNLM: 1. Mental Disorders–diagnosis. 2. Mental Disorders–therapy.
WM 140 C6405 2006]
RC469.C555 2006
616.89–dc22   2006008578

British Library cataloguing in Publication Data

A Catalogue record for this book is available from the British Library

ISBN-10: 0-470-01915-8 (P/B)
ISBN-13: 978-0-470-01915-3 (P/B)

Typeset in 9.5/11.5pt Times Roman by Thomson Press (India) Limited, New Delhi, India
Printed and bound in Great Britain by Antony Rowe Ltd, Chippenham, UK
This book is printed and acid-free paper responsibly manufactured from sustainable forestry
in which at least two trees are planted for each one used for paper production.

Dedications

To Leslee, my bashert

Michael

With love and thanks to my family, in particular to my
father, Goodman Tasman, for your support and inspiration

Allan

Table of Contents

Preface

The publication of DSM-III in 1980 revolutionized psychiatry. Among its many accomplishments (e.g., increased diagnostic reliability), it provided both a common language for naming, describing, and identifying the complete range of mental disorders seen in clinical practice, as well as an organizational plan embodied in the diagnostic groupings contained in the DSM-III classification (i.e., grouping together Organic Mental Disorders, Psychotic Disorders, Mood Disorder, Anxiety Disorders, etc.) Its appeal is several-fold: (1) it is *authoritative*; the information contained in the DSM is authored by the leading experts in psychiatry and psychology; (2) it is *comprehensive*: all disorders seen by mental health professionals are covered in the DSM; (3) it is *clinically useful*: material included in the DSM is intended to be of practical use in making psychiatric diagnoses; (4) it is *educational*: material is included also for the purpose of educating the reader about mental disorders, such as how they present, sex ratio, prevalence rates; and (5) it is *relatively concise*: all the information is contained in a single volume, of around 900 pages in length.

Although the DSM is indispensable in the evaluation and treatment of individuals with mental disorders, arriving at a psychiatric diagnosis is only the first step in the process. Once the clinician determines the diagnosis, he or she must then choose from among a range of available treatment options. Certainly the biggest limitation of the DSM-IV-TR is its omission of any information about the management and treatment of individuals with mental disorders. DSM-IV-TR users must turn elsewhere for information about which treatment to choose—either to books written specifically about the treatment of a disorder or books covering treatment in general. *DSM-IV-TR Mental Disorders: Diagnosis, Etiology, and Treatment* (edited by First and Tasman), adapted from Section 5 of the two-volume textbook *Psychiatry*, 2nd edition (edited by Tasman, Kay, and Lieberman), was published in May 2004 and combined information about the diagnosis, etiology, and treatment of mental disorders into a single volume. Unfortunately, its length and cost greatly limited its utility as a helpful guide for students and practicing clinicians. This *Clinical Guide to the Diagnosis and Treatment of Mental Disorders* arises from our efforts to create a more concise and more clinician-friendly version of the original First and Tasman book.

This book retains the breadth of the *Diagnosis, Etiology, and Treatment* book but not the depth—we will continue to have the same number of chapters which cover all of the disorders in the DSM-IV-TR but the content has been edited to meet the clinical needs of the readership. Rather than serving as a reference book about mental disorders, we see this book as an accessible clinical guide to diagnosis and treatment. As such, the "Etiology" sections from the original book have been eliminated and the "Diagnosis" and "Treatment" sections have been condensed with the goal of retaining only information which is clinically relevant. In addition, details of studies establishing the epidemiology of the disorders or the efficacy of treatments have been removed, as have all of the references. Readers interested in this information should refer to the corresponding chapters in the original book.

The organization of the chapters in this book closely parallels the layout of disorders in the DSM-IV-TR. The amount of space allocated to each disorder in this book varies according to clinical importance. Thus, unlike DSM-IV-TR, in which all of the anxiety disorders are covered in the same chapter, the book splits up the major anxiety disorders among several different chapters. Within each chapter, this book for the most part follows a consistent structure. The "Diagnosis" section for each disorder begins with introductory material describing the features of the disorder and includes information about assessment issues, comorbid conditions, associated features, epidemiology, course (which includes age at onset, prognosis, and outcome), and differential diagnosis. The "Treatment" sections summarize the available treatments for the disorders, and often are broken down into "Somatic Treatments" and "Psychosocial Treatments" for ease of reference.

The factual content of the chapters in this book has been adapted from the "Disorders" section of the 2nd edition of the two-volume Tasman, Kay, and Lieberman textbook *Psychiatry*, which was published by Wiley in 2003. We would like to acknowledge the excellent contributions made by the original contributors to these chapters, who are listed in the Acknowledgments of this book. Two new chapters, covering Amphetamine-Related Disorders by Kevin

Sevarino and Reactive Attachment Disorder by Brian Stafford and Charles Zeanah were developed for the original First and Tasman book (and thus are included in an edited form here), as no chapters covering these disorders were included in the original two-volume textbook. We would also like to express our gratitude to Deborah Russell and Andrea Baier at John Wiley & Sons for their help in the editing and production of this book.

Michael B. First
Allan Tasman

April 2006

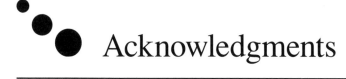

Acknowledgments

We would like to gratefully acknowledge the authors of those chapters in *Psychiatry*, 2nd edition from which material in this book was adapted.

Henry David Abraham	*Substance Abuse: Hallucinogen- and MDMA-Related Disorders*
Sonia Ancoli-Israel	*Sleep and Sleep–Wake Disorders*
Martin M. Antony	*Anxiety Disorders: Social and Specific Phobias*
Gordon J. G. Asmundson	*Anxiety Disorders: Panic Disorder with and without Agoraphobia*
Thomas F. Babor	*Substance Abuse: Alcohol Use Disorders*
Mark S. Bauer	*Mood Disorders: Bipolar (Manic–Depressive) Disorders*
Jean C. Beckham	*Anxiety Disorders: Traumatic Stress Disorders*
Olga Brawman-Mintzer	*Anxiety Disorders: Generalized Anxiety Disorder*
Alan Breier	*Schizophrenia and Other Psychoses*
Edwin H. Cook	*Childhood Disorders: The Autism Spectrum Disorders*
Jonathan R. T. Davidson	*Anxiety Disorders: Traumatic Stress Disorders*
Jane L. Eisen	*Obsessive–Compulsive Disorder*
Stuart Eisendrath	*Factitious Disorders*
Rif S. El-Mallakh	*Substance Abuse: Hallucinogen- and MDMA-Related Disorders*
Milton Erman	*Sleep and Sleep–Wake Disorders*
Susan J. Fiester	*Substance Abuse: Nicotine Dependence*
Anne Fleming	*Factitious Disorders*
Robert L. Frierson	*Delirium and Dementia*
Paul J. Fudala	*Substance Abuse: Opioid Use Disorder*
J. Christian Gillin	*Sleep and Sleep–Wake Disorders*
Reed D. Goldstein	*Mood Disorders: Depression*
Roland R. Griffiths	*Substance Abuse: Caffeine Use Disorders*
Amanda J. Gruber	*Substance Abuse: Cannabis-Related Disorders*
Alan M. Gruenberg	*Mood Disorders: Depression*
Jeffrey M. Halperin	*Childhood Disorders: Attention-Deficit and Disruptive Behavior Disorders*
John H. Halpern	*Substance Abuse: Hallucinogen- and MDMA-Related Disorders*
Carlos A. Hernandez-Avila	*Substance Abuse: Alcohol Use Disorders*
Charles Y. Jin	*Substance Abuse: Cocaine Use Disorders*
William M. Klykylo	*Childhood Disorders: Communication Disorders*
Thomas R. Kosten	*General Approaches to Substance and Polydrug Use Disorders*
Henry R. Kranzler	*Substance Abuse: Alcohol Use Disorders*
James L. Levenson	*Psychological Factors Affecting Medical Condition*
Bennett L. Leventhal	*Childhood Disorders: The Autism Spectrum Disorders*
Stephen B. Levine	*Sexual Disorders*
Walter Ling	Substance Abuse: Sedative, Hypnotic, or Anxiolytic Use Disorders
Joyce H. Lowinson	*Substance Abuse: Phencyclidine Use Disorders*

Christopher P. Lucas	*Childhood Disorders: Elimination Disorders and Childhood Anxiety Disorders*
R. Bruce Lydiard	*Anxiety Disorders: Generalized Anxiety Disorder*
José R. Maldonado	*Dissociative Disorders*
John S. March	*Anxiety Disorders: Traumatic Stress Disorders*
Randi E. McCabe	*Anxiety Disorders: Social and Specific Phobias*
Elinore F. McCance-Katz	*Substance Abuse: Cocaine Use Disorders*
Laura F. McNicholas	*Substance Abuse: Opioid Use Disorders*
Jeannine Monnier	*Anxiety Disorders: Generalized Anxiety Disorder*
David P. Moore	*Mental Disorders due to a General Medical Condition*
Stephanie Mullins	*Personality Disorders*
Jeffrey H. Newcorn	*Childhood Disorders: Attention-Deficit and Disruptive Behavior Disorder; Adjustment Disorders*
Thomas Owley	*Childhood Disorders: The Autism Spectrum Disorders*
Jayendra K. Patel	*Schizophrenia and Other Psychoses*
Michele T. Pato	*Obsessive–Compulsive Disorder*
Teri Pearlstein	*Mood Disorders: Premenstrual Dysphoric Disorder*
Katharine A. Phillips	*Obsessive–Compulsive Disorder*
Debra A. Pinals	*Schizophrenia and Other Psychoses*
Harrison G. Pope, Jr	*Substance Abuse: Cannabis-Related Disorders*
Mark A. Riddle	*Childhood Disorders: Tic Disorders*
Neil Rosenberg	*Substance Abuse: Inhalant-Related Disorders*
Kurt P. Schulz	*Childhood Disorders: Attention-Deficit and Disruptive Behavior Disorders*
David Shaffer	*Childhood Disorders: Elimination Disorders and Childhood Anxiety Disorders*
Vanshdeep Sharma	*Childhood Disorders: Attention-Deficit and Disruptive Behavior Disorders*
Charles W. Sharp	*Substance Abuse: Inhalant-Related Disorders*
Larry B. Silver	*Childhood Disorders: Learning and Motor Skills Disorders*
Daphne Simeon	*Impulse Control Disorders*
David E. Smith	*Substance Abuse: Sedative, Hypnotic, or Anxiolytic Use Disorders*
David Spiegel	*Dissociative Disorders*
Eric C. Strain	*Substance Abuse: Caffeine Use Disorders*
James J. Strain	*Adjustment Disorders*
Ludwik S. Szymanski	*Childhood Disorders: Mental Retardation*
Steven Taylor	*Anxiety Disorders: Panic Disorder with and without Agoraphobia*
Jane A. Ungemack	*Substance Abuse: Alcohol Use Disorders*
John T. Walkup	*Childhood Disorders: Tic Disorders*
B. Timothy Walsh	*Eating Disorders*
Donald R. Wesson	*Substance Abuse: Sedative, Hypnotic or Anxiolytic Use Disorders*
Thomas A. Widiger	*Personality Disorders*
Maija Wilska	*Childhood Disorders: Mental Retardation*
Ronald M. Winchel	*Impulse Control Disorders*
George E. Woody	*Substance Abuse: Opioid Use Disorder*
Yoram Yovell	*Impulse Control Disorders*
Sean H. Yutzy	*Somatoform Disorders*
Douglas Ziedonis	*Substance Abuse: Nicotine Dependence*
Stephen R. Zukin	*Substance Abuse: Phencyclidine Use Disorders*
Ilana Zylberman	*Substance Abuse: Phencyclidine Use Disorders*

1 Psychiatric Diagnosis

There is a natural human predilection to categorize and classify in order to simplify and organize the wide range of observable phenomena and experiences that one is confronted with, thus facilitating both their understanding and their predictability. Many (if not most) of the mental disorders that afflict contemporary individuals have occurred in antiquity. For example, the first recorded depiction of mental illness dates to 3000 B.C. Egypt, with a description of the syndrome senile dementia attributed to Prince Ptah-hotep. The current system for the diagnosis of mental disorders, the *Diagnostic and Statistical Manual of Mental Disorders*, Fourth Edition Text Revision (DSM-IV-TR), is just the latest example from the long and colorful history of psychiatric classification.

GOALS OF THE DSM-IV-TR

Perhaps the most important goal of the DSM-IV-TR is to allow mental health practitioners and researchers to communicate more effectively with each other by establishing a convenient shorthand for describing the mental disorders that they encounter. For example, telling a colleague that an individual whom you have just evaluated has major depressive disorder can convey a great deal of information in only a few words. First of all, it indicates that depressed mood or loss of interest is a central aspect of the presenting problem and that the depression is not the kind of "normal" mood fluctuation that lasts for only a few days but rather that it persists every day for an extended period of time, for at least 2 weeks. Furthermore, one can expect to find a number of additional symptoms occurring at the same time, like suicidal ideation and changes in appetite, sleep, energy, and psychomotor activity. Finally, information is also communicated about what is not to be found in this individual—specifically, that the depression is not caused by the direct physiological effects of alcohol, other drugs, medications, or a general medical condition; and that there is no history of schizophrenia or manic or hypomanic episodes.

DSM-IV-TR also facilitates the identification and management of mental disorders in both clinical and research settings. Most of the DSM-IV-TR diagnostic labels provide considerable and important predictive power. For example, making a diagnosis of bipolar disorder suggests the choice of treatment options (e.g., mood stabilizers), that a certain course may be likely (e.g., recurrent and episodic), and that there is an increased prevalence of this disorder in family members. By defining more or less homogeneous groups of individuals for study, DSM-IV-TR can also further efforts to understand the etiology of mental disorders. DSM-IV-TR also plays an important role in education. In its organization of disorders into major classes, the system offers a structure for teaching phenomenology and differential diagnosis. DSM-IV-TR is also useful in psychoeducation by showing individuals suffering from symptoms of a mental disorder that their pattern of symptoms is not mysterious and unique but rather has been identified and studied in others.

DSM-IV-TR OVERVIEW

The remainder of this chapter provides an overview of the DSM-IV-TR multiaxial system as well as a presentation of some of the organizational principles of the various diagnostic groupings included in the DSM-IV-TR classification. The chapters in this book are organized according to their presentation in the DSM-IV-TR classification and provide detailed information regarding the diagnosis, epidemiology, course, and treatment of these disorders.

DSM-IV-TR MULTIAXIAL SYSTEM

The multiaxial system was first introduced by DSM-III in order to encourage the clinician to focus his or her attention during the evaluation process on issues above and beyond the psychiatric diagnosis. Use of the multiaxial system requires that information be noted on each of the five different axes, each axis

Clinical Guide to the Diagnosis and Treatment of Mental Disorders. M. B. First and A. Tasman
© 2006 John Wiley & Sons, Ltd.   ISBN 0 470 019158

devoted to a different aspect of the evaluation process. Axes I, II, and III are the diagnostic axes that divide up the diagnostic pie into three separate domains. Axis I is for "clinical syndromes and disorders," an admittedly confusing name since Axis II and Axis III also include clinical disorders. The most accurate name for Axis I is "diagnoses not coded on Axis II and Axis III," since Axis II and Axis III were carved out of Axis I specifically to draw attention to certain disorders that clinicians were more likely to overlook.

That said, Axis II is designated for coding personality disorders and traits and mental retardation. There have been many recent criticisms of the coding of personality disorders on Axis II. Critics correctly point out that there is no firm conceptual basis for this division. Although disorders on Axis II tend to be lifelong and pervasive, a number of disorders on Axis I (e.g., schizophrenia, autistic disorder, dysthymic disorder) fit this description as well. Others have made the incorrect assumption that categories on Axis II are unresponsive to medication treatment, which is at odds with more recent evidence that medications are often helpful in the treatment of personality disorders. The fact is that the Axis I/Axis II division is strictly pragmatic. First introduced in DSM-III, Axis II was designed to draw attention to certain disorders that were thought to be overshadowed in the face of the more florid Axis I presentations. In DSM-III, Axis II was reserved for personality disorders in adults and specific developmental disorders in children. In DSM-III-R, all of the developmental disorders (i.e., mental retardation, pervasive developmental disorders, specific developmental disorders) were coded on Axis II along with the personality disorders. In DSM-IV-TR, Axis II was modified once again so that only personality disorders and traits and mental retardation remain on Axis II. Certainly the placement of personality disorders on a separate axis has increased both their clinical visibility and their importance as a subject for research studies. Whether the Axis I/Axis II division has finally outlived its usefulness remains a topic of heated debate and will be revisited during the DSM-V deliberations.

Axis III, like Axis II, is intended to encourage clinicians to pay special attention to conditions that they tend to overlook, in this case, clinically relevant general medical conditions. The concept of "clinically relevant" is intended to be broad. For example, it would be appropriate to list hypertension on Axis III even if its only relationship to an Axis I disorder is its

impact on the options for the choice of antidepressant medication.

Psychosocial stressors are well known to play an important role in the etiology, maintenance, and management of a number of mental disorders. Axis IV provides the clinician with the opportunity to list clinically relevant psychosocial and environmental problems (e.g., homelessness, poverty, divorce). To facilitate a comprehensive evaluation of such problems, DSM-IV-TR includes a psychosocial and environmental checklist that allows the clinician to indicate which types of problems are present and relevant (Figure 1-1).

Mental disorders differentially impact on the individual's level of functioning. For example, one individual with schizophrenia may function quite well, being able to live in the community, marry and have a family, and maintain a steady job, whereas another individual with schizophrenia may function quite poorly, requiring chronic institutionalization. Since both of these individuals have symptoms that meet the diagnostic criteria for schizophrenia, their important differences in functioning are not captured by the clinical diagnosis alone. Some of the differences in functioning may be due to different symptom profiles or symptom severities. Other differences may be related to resilience factors or different levels of psychosocial support. Whatever the reason, the DSM-IV-TR multiaxial system provides the clinician with the ability to indicate the individual's overall level of functioning in addition to the diagnosis

Check:

___ Problems with primary support group (childhood, adult, parent–child). Specify: _____

___ Problems related to the social environment. Specify: _____

___ Educational problems. Specify: _____

___ Occupational problems. Specify: _____

___ Housing problems. Specify: _____

___ Economic problems. Specify: _____

___ Problems with access to health care services. Specify: _____

___ Problems related to interaction with the legal system/crime. Specify: _____

___ Other psychosocial problems. Specify: _____

Figure 1-1 *DSM-IV-TR Axis IV: psychosocial and environmental checklist. (Reprinted with permission from the Diagnostic and Statistical Manual of Mental Disorders, Fourth Edition, Text Revision, pp36, Copyright 2000. American Psychiatric Association.)*

on Axis V, using the Global Assessment of Functioning (GAF) Scale (Figure 1-2). This GAF Scale has been criticized because it is not actually a "pure" measure of an individual's ability to function since it incorporates symptom severity into the scale; for example, level 41 to 50 is for serious symptoms (e.g., suicidal ideation,

severe obsessional rituals, frequent shoplifting) or any serious impairment in social, occupational, or school functioning (e.g., no friends, unable to keep a job). For this reason, the DSM-IV-TR includes a scale (the Social and Occupational Functioning Scale [SOFAS]) that relies exclusively on functioning in its appendix

Global Assessment of Functioning (GAF) Scale

Consider psychological, social and occupational functioning on a hypothetical continuum of mental health-illness. Do not include impairment in functioning due to physical (or environmental) limitations.

Code	(Note: Use intermediate codes when appropriate, e.g., 45,68,72.)
100 – 91	**Superior functioning in a wide range of activities, life's problems never seem to get out of hand, is sought out by others because of many positive qualities. No symptoms.**
90 – 81	**Absent or minimal symptoms** (e.g., mild anxiety before an examination), **good functioning in all areas, interested and involved in a wide range of activities, socially effective, generally satisfied with life, no more than everyday problems or concerns** (e.g., an occasional argument with family members).
80 – 71	**If symptoms are present, they are transient and expectable reactions to psychosocial stressors** (e.g., difficulty concentrating after family argument); **no more than slight impairment in social, occupational, or school functioning** (e.g., temporarily falling behind in school work).
70 – 61	**Some mild symptoms** (e.g., depressed mood and mild insomnia) **OR some difficulty in social, occupational, or school functioning** (e.g., occasional truancy, or theft within the household), **but generally functioning pretty well, has some meaningful interpersonal relationships.**
60 – 51	**Moderate symptoms** (e.g., flat affect and circumstantial speech, occasional panic attacks) **OR moderate difficulty in social, occupational, or school functioning** (e.g., few friends, conflicts with peers or coworkers).
50 – 41	**Serious symptoms** (e.g., suicidal ideation, severe obsessional rituals, frequent shoplifting) **OR any serious impairment in social, occupational, or school functioning** (e.g., no friends, unable to keep a job).
40 – 31	**Some impairment in reality testing or communication** (e.g., speech is at times illogical, obscure, or irrelevant) **OR major impairment in several areas, such as work or school, family relations, judgment, thinking, or mood** (e.g., depressed man avoids friends, neglects family, and is unable to work; child frequently beats up younger children, is defiant at home, and is failing at school).
30 – 21	**Behavior is considerably influenced by delusions or hallucinations OR serious impairment in communication or judgment** (e.g., sometimes incoherent, acts grossly inappropriately, suicidal preoccupation) **OR inability to function in almost all areas** (e.g., stays in bed all day; no job, home or friends).
20 – 11	**Some danger of hurting self or others** (e.g., suicide attempts without clear expectation of death, frequently violent, manic excitement) **OR occasionally fails to maintain minimal personal hygiene** (e.g., smears feces) **OR gross impairment in communication** (e.g., largely incoherent or mute).
10 – 1	**Persistent danger of severely hurting self or others** (e.g., recurrent violence) **OR persistent inability to maintain minimal personal hygiene OR serious suicidal act with clear expectation of death.**
0	Inadequate information

Figure 1-2 *DSM-IV-TR Axis V: Global Assessment Functioning Scale. (Reprinted with permission from the Diagnostic and Statistical Manual of Mental Disorders, Fourth Edition, Text Revision, pp34, Copyright 2000. American Psychiatric Association.)*

Table 1-1	Example of DSM-IV-TR Multiaxial Evaluation
Axis I	296.23 Major depressive disorder, single episode, severe but without psychotic features, with postpartum onset. 307.51 Bulimia nervosa
Axis II	301.6 Dependent personality disorder Frequent use of denial
Axis III	Rheumatoid arthritis
Axis IV	Partner relational problem
Axis V	GAF = 35 (current)

of Criteria Sets and Axes Provided for Further Study. An example of a DSM-IV-TR multiaxial evaluation for a hypothetical individual with depression is shown in Table 1.1.

DSM-IV-TR CLASSIFICATION AND DIAGNOSTIC CODES

The "DSM-IV-TR Classification of Mental Disorders" refers to the comprehensive listing of the official diagnostic codes, categories, subtypes, and specifiers (see below). It is divided into various "diagnostic classes" that group disorders together on the basis of common presenting symptoms (e.g., mood disorders, anxiety disorders), typical age at onset (e.g., disorders usually first diagnosed in infancy, childhood, and adolescence), and etiology (e.g., substance-related disorders, mental disorders due to a general medical condition).

The diagnostic codes listed in the DSM-IV-TR are derived from the *International Classification of Diseases*, Ninth Revision, Clinical Modification (ICD-9-CM), the official coding system for reporting morbidity and mortality in the United States. That is the reason the codes go from 290.00 to 319.00; they are actually derived from the mental disorders section of a much larger coding system for all medical disorders that extend from 001 to 999. Clinicians working in the United States are required to use ICD-9-CM in order to get reimbursement from both government agencies (e.g., Medicare and Medicaid) and private insurers. To insure that users of the DSM-IV-TR are able to meet this requirement without doing any cumbersome code conversions, the DSM-IV-TR contains the current ICD-9-CM codes. Because the ICD-9-CM codes are updated on a yearly basis (i.e., every October 1), the DSM-IV-TR codes have to be similarly updated as changes to the codes in the ICD-9-CM mental disorder section occur. Successive printings of DSM-IV-TR have been modified to include these updated codes. In addition, updated diagnostic codes are available on the DSM-IV-TR web site (www.dsm4tr.org)

DSM-IV-TR Classification

NOS = Not Otherwise Specified.

An x appearing in a diagnostic code indicates that a specific code number is required.

An ellipsis (...) is used in the names of certain disorders to indicate that the name of a specific mental disorder or general medical condition should be inserted when recording the name (e.g., 293.0 Delirium Due to Hypothyroidism).

If criteria are currently met, one of the following severity specifiers may be noted after the diagnosis:

Mild
Moderate
Severe

If criteria are no longer met, one of the following specifiers may be noted:

In Partial Remission
In Full Remission
Prior History

Disorders Usually First Diagnosed in Infancy, Childhood, or Adolescence

MENTAL RETARDATION

Note: *These are coded on Axis II.*
317   Mild Mental Retardation
318.0   Moderate Mental Retardation
318.1   Severe Mental Retardation
318.2   Profound Mental Retardation
319   Mental Retardation, Severity Unspecified

LEARNING DISORDERS

315.00   Reading Disorder
315.1   Mathematics Disorder
315.2   Disorder of Written Expression
315.9   Learning Disorder NOS

MOTOR SKILLS DISORDER

315.4   Developmental Coordination Disorder

COMMUNICATION DISORDERS

315.31   Expressive Language Disorder
315.32   Mixed Receptive–Expressive Language Disorder
315.39   Phonological Disorder
307.0   Stuttering
307.9   Communication Disorder NOS

PERVASIVE DEVELOPMENTAL DISORDERS

299.00   Autistic Disorder
299.80   Rett's Disorder
299.10   Childhood Disintegrative Disorder
299.80   Asperger's Disorder
299.80   Pervasive Developmental Disorder NOS

ATTENTION-DEFICIT AND DISRUPTIVE BEHAVIOR DISORDERS

314.xx   Attention-Deficit/Hyperactivity Disorder
  .01   Combined Type
  .00   Predominantly Inattentive Type
  .01   Predominantly Hyperactive-Impulsive Type
314.9   Attention-Deficit/Hyperactivity Disorder NOS
312.xx   Conduct Disorder
  .81   Childhood-Onset Type
  .82   Adolescent-Onset Type
  .89   Unspecified Onset
313.81   Oppositional-Defiant Disorder
312.9   Disruptive Behavior Disorder NOS

FEEDING AND EATING DISORDERS OF INFANCY OR EARLY CHILDHOOD

307.52   Pica
307.53   Rumination Disorder
307.59   Feeding Disorder of Infancy or Early Childhood

TIC DISORDERS

307.23   Tourette's Disorder
307.22   Chronic Motor or Vocal Tic Disorder
307.21   Transient Tic Disorder
         Specify if: Single Episode/Recurrent
307.20   Tic Disorder NOS

ELIMINATION DISORDERS

—.—   Encopresis
787.6   With Constipation and Overflow Incontinence
307.7   Without Constipation and Overflow Incontinence
307.6   Enuresis (Not Due to a General Medical Condition)
         Specify type: Nocturnal Only/Diurnal Only/ Nocturnal and Diurnal

OTHER DISORDERS OF INFANCY, CHILDHOOD, OR ADOLESCENCE

309.21   Separation Anxiety Disorder
         Specify if: Early Onset
313.23   Selective Mutism
313.89   Reactive Attachment Disorder of Infancy or Early Childhood
         Specify type: Inhibited Type/Disinhibited Type
307.3   Stereotypic Movement Disorder
         Specify if: With Self-Injurious Behavior
313.9   Disorder of Infancy, Childhood, or Adolescence NOS

Delirium, Dementia, and Amnestic and Other Cognitive Disorders

DELIRIUM

293.0   Delirium Due to … [*Indicate the General Medical Condition*]
—.—   Substance Intoxication Delirium (*refer to Substance-Related Disorders for substance-specific codes*)
—.—   Substance Withdrawal Delirium (*refer to Substance-Related Disorders for substance-specific codes*)
—.—   Delirium Due to Multiple Etiologies (*code each of the specific etiologies*)
780.09   Delirium NOS

DEMENTIA

294.xx   Dementia of the Alzheimer's Type, With Early Onset (*also code 331.0 Alzheimer's disease on Axis III*)
  .10   Without Behavioral Disturbance
  .11   With Behavioral Disturbance
294.xx   Dementia of the Alzheimer's Type, With Late Onset (*also code 331.0 Alzheimer's disease on Axis III*)
  .10   Without Behavioral Disturbance
  .11   With Behavioral Disturbance
290.xx   Vascular Dementia
  .40   Uncomplicated
  .41   With Delirium
  .42   With Delusions
  .43   With Depressed Mood
         Specify if: With Behavioral Disturbance

Code presence or absence of a behavioral disturbance in the fifth digit for Dementia Due to a General Medical Condition:

294.10 =	Without Behavioral Disturbance
294.11 =	With Behavioral Disturbance
294.1x	Dementia Due to HIV Disease (*also code 042 HIV on Axis III*)
294.1x	Dementia Due to Head Trauma (*also code 854.00 head injury on Axis III*)
294.1x	Dementia Due to Parkinson's Disease (*also code 331.82 Dementia with Lewy Bodies on Axis III*)
294.1x	Dementia Due to Huntington's Disease (*also code 333.4 Huntington's disease on Axis III*)
294.1x	Dementia Due to Pick's Disease (*also code 331.11 Pick's disease on Axis III*)
294.1x	Dementia Due to Creutzfeldt–Jakob Disease (*also code 046.1 Creutzfeldt–Jakob disease on Axis III*)
294.1x	Dementia Due to ... [*Indicate the General Medical Condition not listed above*] (*also code the general medical condition on Axis III*)
—.—	Substance-Induced Persisting Dementia (*refer to Substance-Related Disorders for substance-specific codes*)
—.—	Dementia Due to Multiple Etiologies (*code each of the specific etiologies*)
294.8	Dementia NOS

AMNESTIC DISORDERS

294.0	Amnestic Disorder Due to ... [*Indicate the General Medical Condition*] *Specify if*: Transient/Chronic
—.—	Substance-Induced Persisting Amnestic Disorder (*refer to Substance-Related Disorders for substance-specific codes*)
294.8	Amnestic Disorder NOS

OTHER COGNITIVE DISORDERS

294.9	Cognitive Disorder NOS

Mental Disorders Due to a General Medical Condition Not Elsewhere Classified

293.89	Catatonic Disorder Due to ... [*Indicate the General Medical Condition*]
310.1	Personality Change Due to ... [*Indicate the General Medical Condition*] *Specify type*: Labile Type/Disinhibited Type/Aggressive Type/Apathetic Type/Paranoid Type/Other Type/Combined Type/Unspecified Type

293.9	Mental Disorder NOS Due to ... [*Indicate the General Medical Condition*]

Substance-Related Disorders

The following specifiers apply to Substance Dependence as noted:
[a]With Physiological Dependence/Without Physiological Dependence
[b]Early Full Remission/Early Partial Remission/Sustained Full Remission/Sustained Partial Remission
[c]In a Controlled Environment
[d]On Agonist Therapy
The following specifiers apply to Substance-Induced Disorders as noted:
[I]With Onset During Intoxication/[W]With Onset During Withdrawal

ALCOHOL-RELATED DISORDERS

Alcohol Use Disorders

303.90	Alcohol Dependence[a,b,c]
305.00	Alcohol Abuse

Alcohol-Induced Disorders

303.00	Alcohol Intoxication
291.81	Alcohol Withdrawal *Specify if*: With Perceptual Disturbances
291.0	Alcohol Intoxication Delirium
291.0	Alcohol Withdrawal Delirium
291.2	Alcohol-Induced Persisting Dementia
291.1	Alcohol-Induced Persisting Amnestic Disorder
291.x	Alcohol-Induced Psychotic Disorder
.5	With Delusions[I,W]
.3	With Hallucinations[I,W]
291.89	Alcohol-Induced Mood Disorder[I,W]
291.89	Alcohol-Induced Anxiety Disorder[I,W]
291.89	Alcohol-Induced Sexual Dysfunction[I]
291.82	Alcohol-Induced Sleep Disorder[I,W]
291.9	Alcohol-Related Disorder NOS

AMPHETAMINE (OR AMPHETAMINE-LIKE)-RELATED DISORDERS

Amphetamine Use Disorders

304.40	Amphetamine Dependence[a,b,c]
305.70	Amphetamine Abuse

Amphetamine-Induced Disorders

292.89	Amphetamine Intoxication
	Specify if: With Perceptual Disturbances
292.0	Amphetamine Withdrawal
292.81	Amphetamine Intoxication Delirium
292.xx	Amphetamine-Induced Psychotic Disorder
.11	With Delusions[I]
.12	With Hallucinations[I]
292.84	Amphetamine-Induced Mood Disorder[I,W]
292.89	Amphetamine-Induced Anxiety Disorder[I]
292.89	Amphetamine-Induced Sexual Dysfunction[I]
292.85	Amphetamine-Induced Sleep Disorder[I,W]
292.9	Amphetamine-Related Disorder NOS

CAFFEINE-RELATED DISORDERS

Caffeine-Induced Disorders

305.90	Caffeine Intoxication
292.89	Caffeine-Induced Anxiety Disorder[I]
292.85	Caffeine-Induced Sleep Disorder[I]
292.9	Caffeine-Related Disorder NOS

CANNABIS-RELATED DISORDERS

Cannabis Use Disorders

304.30	Cannabis Dependence[a,b,c]
305.20	Cannabis Abuse

Cannabis-Induced Disorders

292.89	Cannabis Intoxication
	Specify if: With Perceptual Disturbances
292.81	Cannabis Intoxication Delirium
292.xx	Cannabis-Induced Psychotic Disorder
.11	With Delusions[I]
.12	With Hallucinations[I]
292.89	Cannabis-Induced Anxiety Disorder[I]
292.9	Cannabis-Related Disorder NOS

COCAINE-RELATED DISORDERS

Cocaine Use Disorders

304.20	Cocaine Dependence[a,b,c]
305.60	Cocaine Abuse

Cocaine-Induced Disorders

292.89	Cocaine Intoxication
	Specify if: With Perceptual Disturbances
292.0	Cocaine Withdrawal
292.81	Cocaine Intoxication Delirium

292.xx	Cocaine-Induced Psychotic Disorder
.11	With Delusions[I]
.12	With Hallucinations[I]
292.84	Cocaine-Induced Mood Disorder[I,W]
292.89	Cocaine-Induced Anxiety Disorder[I,W]
292.89	Cocaine-Induced Sexual Dysfunction[I]
292.85	Cocaine-Induced Sleep Disorder[I,W]
292.9	Cocaine-Related Disorder NOS

HALLUCINOGEN-RELATED DISORDERS

Hallucinogen Use Disorders

304.50	Hallucinogen Dependence[b,c]
305.30	Hallucinogen Abuse

Hallucinogen-Induced Disorders

292.89	Hallucinogen Intoxication
292.89	Hallucinogen Persisting Perception Disorder (Flashbacks)
292.81	Hallucinogen Intoxication Delirium
292.xx	Hallucinogen-Induced Psychotic Disorder
.11	With Delusions[I]
.12	With Hallucinations[I]
292.84	Hallucinogen-Induced Mood Disorder[I]
292.89	Hallucinogen-Induced Anxiety Disorder[I]
292.9	Hallucinogen-Related Disorder NOS

INHALANT-RELATED DISORDERS

Inhalant Use Disorders

304.60	Inhalant Dependence[b,c]
305.90	Inhalant Abuse

Inhalant-Induced Disorders

292.89	Inhalant Intoxication
292.81	Inhalant Intoxication Delirium
292.82	Inhalant-Induced Persisting Dementia
292.xx	Inhalant-Induced Psychotic Disorder
.11	With Delusions[I]
.12	With Hallucinations[I]
292.84	Inhalant-Induced Mood Disorder[I]
292.89	Inhalant-Induced Anxiety Disorder[I]
292.9	Inhalant-Related Disorder NOS

NICOTINE-RELATED DISORDERS

Nicotine Use Disorder

305.1	Nicotine Dependence[a,b]

Nicotine-Induced Disorder

292.0   Nicotine Withdrawal
292.9   Nicotine-Related Disorder NOS

OPIOID-RELATED DISORDERS

Opioid Use Disorders

304.00   Opioid Dependence[a,b,c,d]
305.50   Opioid Abuse

Opioid-Induced Disorders

292.89   Opioid Intoxication
            Specify if: With Perceptual Disturbances
292.0   Opioid Withdrawal
292.81   Opioid Intoxication Delirium
292.xx   Opioid-Induced Psychotic Disorder
   .11   With Delusions[I]
   .12   With Hallucinations[I]
292.84   Opioid-Induced Mood Disorder[I]
292.89   Opioid-Induced Sexual Dysfunction[I]
292.85   Opioid-Induced Sleep Disorder[I,W]
292.9   Opioid-Related Disorder NOS

PHENCYCLIDINE (OR PHENCYCLIDINE-LIKE)-RELATED DISORDERS

Phencyclidine Use Disorders

304.60   Phencyclidine Dependence[b,c]
305.90   Phencyclidine Abuse

Phencyclidine-Induced Disorders

292.89   Phencyclidine Intoxication
            Specify if: With Perceptual Disturbances
292.81   Phencyclidine Intoxication Delirium
292.xx   Phencyclidine-Induced Psychotic Disorder
   .11   With Delusions[I]
   .12   With Hallucinations[I]
292.84   Phencyclidine-Induced Mood Disorder[I]
292.89   Phencyclidine-Induced Anxiety Disorder[I]
292.9   Phencyclidine-Related Disorder NOS

SEDATIVE-, HYPNOTIC-, OR ANXIOLYTIC-RELATED DISORDERS

Sedative, Hypnotic, or Anxiolytic Use Disorders

304.10   Sedative, Hypnotic, or Anxiolytic Dependence[a,b,c]
305.40   Sedative, Hypnotic, or Anxiolytic Abuse

Sedative-, Hypnotic-, or Anxiolytic-Induced Disorders

292.89   Sedative, Hypnotic, or Anxiolytic Intoxication
292.0   Sedative, Hypnotic, or Anxiolytic Withdrawal
            Specify if: With Perceptual Disturbances
292.81   Sedative, Hypnotic, or Anxiolytic Intoxication Delirium
292.81   Sedative, Hypnotic, or Anxiolytic Withdrawal Delirium
292.82   Sedative-, Hypnotic-, or Anxiolytic-Induced Persisting Dementia
292.83   Sedative-, Hypnotic-, or Anxiolytic-Induced Persisting Amnestic Disorder
292.xx   Sedative-, Hypnotic-, or Anxiolytic-Induced Psychotic Disorder
   .11   With Delusions[I,W]
   .12   With Hallucinations[I,W]
292.84   Sedative-, Hypnotic-, or Anxiolytic-Induced Mood Disorder[I,W]
292.89   Sedative-, Hypnotic-, or Anxiolytic-Induced Anxiety Disorder[W]
292.89   Sedative-, Hypnotic-, or Anxiolytic-Induced Sexual Dysfunction[I]
292.85   Sedative-, Hypnotic-, or Anxiolytic-Induced Sleep Disorder[I,W]
292.9   Sedative-, Hypnotic-, or Anxiolytic-Related Disorder NOS

POLYSUBSTANCE-RELATED DISORDER

304.80   Polysubstance Dependence[a,b,c,d]

OTHER (OR UNKNOWN) SUBSTANCE-RELATED DISORDERS

Other (or Unknown) Substance Use Disorders

304.90   Other (or Unknown) Substance Dependence[a,b,c,d]
305.90   Other (or Unknown) Substance Abuse

Other (or Unknown) Substance-Induced Disorders

292.89   Other (or Unknown) Substance Intoxication
            Specify if: With Perceptual Disturbances
292.0   Other (or Unknown) Substance Withdrawal
            Specify if: With Perceptual Disturbances
292.81   Other (or Unknown) Substance-Induced Delirium

292.82	Other (or Unknown) Substance-Induced Persisting Dementia
292.83	Other (or Unknown) Substance-Induced Persisting Amnestic Disorder
292.xx	Other (or Unknown) Substance-Induced Psychotic Disorder
.11	With Delusions[I,W]
.12	With Hallucinations[I,W]
292.84	Other (or Unknown) Substance-Induced Mood Disorder[I,W]
292.89	Other (or Unknown) Substance-Induced Anxiety Disorder[I,W]
292.89	Other (or Unknown) Substance-Induced Sexual Dysfunction[I]
292.85	Other (or Unknown) Substance-Induced Sleep Disorder[I,W]
292.9	Other (or Unknown) Substance-Related Disorder NOS

Schizophrenia and Other Psychotic Disorders

295.xx   Schizophrenia

The following Classification of Longitudinal Course applies to all subtypes of Schizophrenia.

Episodic With Interepisode Residual Symptoms (*specify if*: With Prominent Negative Symptoms)/ Episodic With No Interepisode Residual Symptoms/ Continuous (*specify if*: With Prominent Negative Symptoms)

Single Episode In Partial Remission (*specify if*: With Prominent Negative Symptoms)/Single Episode In Full Remission

Other or Unspecified Pattern
- .30 Paranoid Type
- .10 Disorganized Type
- .20 Catatonic Type
- .90 Undifferentiated Type
- .60 Residual Type

295.40   Schizophreniform Disorder
Specify if: Without Good Prognostic Features/With Good Prognostic Features

295.70   Schizoaffective Disorder
Specify type: Bipolar Type/Depressive Type

297.1   Delusional Disorder
Specify type: Erotomanic Type/ Grandiose Type/Jealous Type/ Persecutory Type/Somatic Type/ Mixed Type/Unspecified Type

298.8   Brief Psychotic Disorder
Specify if: With Marked Stressor(s)/Without Marked Stressor(s)/With Postpartum Onset

297.3	Shared Psychotic Disorder
293.xx	Psychotic Disorder Due to… [*Indicate the General Medical Condition*]
.81	With Delusions
.82	With Hallucinations
—.—	Substance-Induced Psychotic Disorder (*refer to Substance-Related Disorders for substance-specific codes*) *Specify if*: With Onset During Intoxication/With Onset During Withdrawal
298.9	Psychotic Disorder NOS

Mood Disorders

Code current state of Major Depressive Disorder or Bipolar I Disorder in fifth digit:

1 = Mild
2 = Moderate
3 = Severe Without Psychotic Features
4 = Severe With Psychotic Features
   Specify: Mood-Congruent Psychotic Features/ Mood-Incongruent Psychotic Features
5 = In Partial Remission
6 = In Full Remission
0 = Unspecified

The following specifiers apply (for current or most recent episode) to Mood Disorders as noted:

[a]Severity/Psychotic/Remission Specifiers/[b]Chronic/[c]With Catatonic Features/[d]With Melancholic Features/[e]With Atypical Features/[f]With Postpartum Onset

The following specifiers apply to Mood Disorders as noted:

[g]With or Without Full Interepisode Recovery/[h]With Seasonal Pattern/[i]With Rapid Cycling

DEPRESSIVE DISORDERS

296.xx	Major Depressive Disorder,
.2x	Single Episode[a,b,c,d,e,f]
.3x	Recurrent[a,b,c,d,e,f,g,h]
300.4	Dysthymic Disorder *Specify if*: Early Onset/Late Onset *Specify*: With Atypical Features
311	Depressive Disorder NOS

BIPOLAR DISORDERS

296.xx	Bipolar I Disorder,
.0x	Single Manic Episode[a,c,f]

Specify if: Mixed
.40 Most Recent Episode Hypomanic[g,h,i]
.4x Most Recent Episode Manic[a,c,f,g,h,i]
.6x Most Recent Episode Mixed[a,c,f,g,h,i]
.5x Most Recent Episode Depressed[a,b,c,d,e,f,g,h,i]
.7 Most Recent Episode Unspecified[g,h,i]
296.89 Bipolar II Disorder[a,b,c,d,e,f,g,h,i]
Specify (current or most recent episode):
Hypomanic/Depressed
301.13 Cyclothymic Disorder
296.80 Bipolar Disorder NOS
293.83 Mood Disorder Due to … [*Indicate the General Medical Condition*]
Specify type: With Depressive Features/With Major Depressive-like Episode/With Manic Features/With Mixed Features
—.— Substance-Induced Mood Disorder (*refer to Substance-Related Disorders for substance-specific codes*)
Specify type: With Depressive Features/With Manic Features/With Mixed Features
Specify if: With Onset During Intoxication/ With Onset During Withdrawal
296.90 Mood Disorder NOS

Anxiety Disorders

300.01 Panic Disorder Without Agoraphobia
300.21 Panic Disorder With Agoraphobia
300.22 Agoraphobia Without History of Panic Disorder
300.29 Specific Phobia
Specify type: Animal Type/Natural Environment Type/Blood–Injection–Injury Type/Situational Type/Other Type
300.23 Social Phobia
Specify if: Generalized
300.3 Obsessive–Compulsive Disorder
Specify if: With Poor Insight
309.81 Posttraumatic Stress Disorder
Specify if: Acute/Chronic
Specify if: With Delayed Onset
308.3 Acute Stress Disorder
300.02 Generalized Anxiety Disorder
293.89 Anxiety Disorder Due to … [*Indicate the General Medical Condition*]
Specify if: With Generalized Anxiety/ With Panic Attacks/With Obsessive–Compulsive Symptoms
—.— Substance-Induced Anxiety Disorder (*refer to Substance-Related Disorders for substance-specific codes*)

Specify if: With Generalized Anxiety/With Panic Attacks/With Obsessive–Compulsive Symptoms/With Phobic Symptoms
Specify if: With Onset During Intoxication/ With Onset During Withdrawal
300.00 Anxiety Disorder NOS

Somatoform Disorders

300.81 Somatization Disorder
300.82 Undifferentiated Somatoform Disorder
300.11 Conversion Disorder
Specify type: With Motor Symptom or Deficit/With Sensory Symptom or Deficit/ With Seizures or Convulsions/With Mixed Presentation
307.xx Pain Disorder
.80 Associated With Psychological Factors
.89 Associated With Both Psychological Factors and a General Medical Condition
Specify if: Acute/Chronic
300.7 Hypochondriasis
Specify if: With Poor Insight
300.7 Body Dysmorphic Disorder
300.82 Somatoform Disorder NOS

Factitious Disorders

300.xx Factitious Disorder
.16 With Predominantly Psychological Signs and Symptoms
.19 With Predominantly Physical Signs and Symptoms
.19 With Combined Psychological and Physical Signs and Symptoms
300.19 Factitious Disorder NOS

Dissociative Disorders

300.12 Dissociative Amnesia
300.13 Dissociative Fugue
300.14 Dissociative Identity Disorder
300.6 Depersonalization Disorder
300.15 Dissociative Disorder NOS

Sexual and Gender Identity Disorders

SEXUAL DYSFUNCTIONS

The following specifiers apply to all primary Sexual Dysfunctions:

Lifelong Type/Acquired Type/Generalized Type/ Situational Type Due to Psychological Factors/Due to Combined Factors

SEXUAL DESIRE DISORDERS

302.71 Hypoactive Sexual Desire Disorder
302.79 Sexual Aversion Disorder

SEXUAL AROUSAL DISORDERS

302.72 Female Sexual Arousal Disorder
302.72 Male Erectile Disorder

ORGASMIC DISORDERS

302.73 Female Orgasmic Disorder
302.74 Male Orgasmic Disorder
302.75 Premature Ejaculation

SEXUAL PAIN DISORDERS

302.76 Dyspareunia (Not Due to a General Medical Condition)
306.51 Vaginismus (Not Due to a General Medical Condition)

SEXUAL DYSFUNCTION DUE TO A GENERAL MEDICAL CONDITION

625.8 Female Hypoactive Sexual Desire Disorder Due to … [*Indicate the General Medical Condition*]
608.89 Male Hypoactive Sexual Desire Disorder Due to … [*Indicate the General Medical Condition*]
607.84 Male Erectile Disorder Due to … [*Indicate the General Medical Condition*]
625.0 Female Dyspareunia Due to … [*Indicate the General Medical Condition*]
608.89 Male Dyspareunia Due to … [*Indicate the General Medical Condition*]
625.8 Other Female Sexual Dysfunction Due to … [*Indicate the General Medical Condition*]
608.89 Other Male Sexual Dysfunction Due to … [*Indicate the General Medical Condition*]
—.— Substance-Induced Sexual Dysfunction (*refer to Substance-Related Disorders for substance-specific codes*)
Specify if: With Impaired Desire/With Impaired Arousal/With Impaired Orgasm/ With Sexual Pain

Specify if: With Onset During Intoxication
302.70 Sexual Dysfunction NOS

PARAPHILIAS

302.4 Exhibitionism
302.81 Fetishism
302.89 Frotteurism
302.2 Pedophilia
Specify if: Sexually Attracted to Males/ Sexually Attracted to Females/Sexually Attracted to Both
Specify if: Limited to Incest
Specify type: Exclusive Type/Nonexclusive Type
302.83 Sexual Masochism
302.84 Sexual Sadism
302.3 Transvestic Fetishism
Specify if: With Gender Dysphoria
302.82 Voyeurism
302.9 Paraphilia NOS

GENDER IDENTITY DISORDERS

302.xx Gender Identity Disorder
.6 in Children
.85 in Adolescents or Adults
Specify if: Sexually Attracted to Males/ Sexually Attracted to Females/Sexually Attracted to Both/Sexually Attracted to Neither
302.6 Gender Identity Disorder NOS
302.9 Sexual Disorder NOS

EATING DISORDERS

307.1 Anorexia Nervosa
Specify type: Restricting Type; Binge-Eating/Purging Type
307.51 Bulimia Nervosa
Specify type: Purging Type/Nonpurging Type
307.50 Eating Disorder NOS

Sleep Disorders

PRIMARY SLEEP DISORDERS

Dyssomnias

307.42 Primary Insomnia
307.44 Primary Hypersomnia
Specify if: Recurrent
347.00 Narcolepsy
780.57 Breathing-Related Sleep Disorder

327.xx   Circadian Rhythm Sleep Disorder
.31   Delayed Sleep Phase Type
.35   Jet Lag Type
.36   Shift Work Type
.30   Unspecified Type
307.47   Dyssomnia NOS

Parasomnias

307.47   Nightmare Disorder
307.46   Sleep Terror Disorder
307.46   Sleepwalking Disorder
307.47   Parasomnia NOS

SLEEP DISORDERS RELATED TO ANOTHER MENTAL DISORDER

327.02   Insomnia Related to ... [Indicate the Axis I or Axis II Disorder]
327.15   Hypersomnia Related to ... [Indicate the Axis I or Axis II Disorder]

OTHER SLEEP DISORDERS

327.xx   Sleep Disorder Due to ... [Indicate the General Medical Condition]
.01   Insomnia Type
.14   Hypersomnia Type
.44   Parasomnia Type
.8   Mixed Type
—.—   Substance-Induced Sleep Disorder (refer to Substance-Related Disorders for substance-specific codes)
Specify type: Insomnia Type/Hypersomnia Type/Parasomnia Type/ Mixed Type
Specify if: With Onset During Intoxication/ With Onset During Withdrawal

Impulse Control Disorders Not Elsewhere Classified

312.34   Intermittent Explosive Disorder
312.32   Kleptomania
312.33   Pyromania
312.31   Pathological Gambling
312.39   Trichotillomania
312.30   Impulse-Control Disorder NOS

Adjustment Disorders

309.xx   Adjustment Disorder
.0   With Depressed Mood

.24   With Anxiety
.28   With Mixed Anxiety and Depressed Mood
.3   With Disturbance of Conduct
.4   With Mixed Disturbance of Emotions and Conduct
.9   Unspecified
Specify if: Acute/Chronic

Personality Disorders

Note: These are coded on Axis II
301.0   Paranoid Personality Disorder
301.20   Schizoid Personality Disorder
301.22   Schizotypal Personality Disorder
301.7   Antisocial Personality Disorder
301.83   Borderline Personality Disorder
301.50   Histrionic Personality Disorder
301.81   Narcissistic Personality Disorder
301.82   Avoidant Personality Disorder
301.6   Dependent Personality Disorder
301.4   Obsessive–Compulsive Personality Disorder
301.9   Personality Disorder NOS

Other Conditions that May Be a Focus of Clinical Attention

PSYCHOLOGICAL FACTORS AFFECTING MEDICAL CONDITION

316   ... [Specified Psychological Factor] Affecting ... [Indicate the General Medical Condition]
Choose name based on nature of factors:
Mental Disorder Affecting Medical Condition
Psychological Symptoms Affecting Medical Condition
Personality Traits or Coping Style Affecting Medical Condition
Maladaptive Health Behaviors Affecting Medical Condition
Stress-Related Physiological Response Affecting Medical Condition
Other or Unspecified Psychological Factors Affecting Medical Condition

MEDICATION-INDUCED MOVEMENT DISORDERS

332.1   Neuroleptic-Induced Parkinsonism
333.92   Neuroleptic Malignant Syndrome
333.7   Neuroleptic-Induced Acute Dystonia

333.99   Neuroleptic-Induced Acute Akathisia
333.82   Neuroleptic-Induced Tardive Dyskinesia
333.1   Medication-Induced Postural Tremor
333.90   Medication-Induced Movement Disorder
          NOS

OTHER MEDICATION-INDUCED DISORDER

995.2   Adverse Effects of Medication NOS

RELATIONAL PROBLEMS

V61.9   Relational Problem Related to a Mental
          Disorder or General Medical Condition
V61.20   Parent–Child Relational Problem
V61.10   Partner Relational Problem
V61.8   Sibling Relational Problem
V62.81   Relational Problem NOS

PROBLEMS RELATED TO ABUSE OR NEGLECT

V61.21   Physical Abuse of Child (*code 995.54 if
          focus of attention is on victim*)
V61.21   Sexual Abuse of Child (*code 995.53 if focus
          of attention is on victim*)
V61.21   Neglect of Child (*code 995.52 if focus of
          attention is on victim*)
—.—   Physical Abuse of Adult
V61.12   (if by partner)
V62.83   (if by person other than partner) (*code
          995.83 if focus of attention is on victim*)
—.—   Sexual Abuse of Adult
V61.12   (if by partner)
V62.83   (if by person other than partner) (*code
          995.83 if focus of attention is on victim*)

ADDITIONAL CONDITIONS THAT MAY BE A FOCUS OF CLINICAL ATTENTION

V15.81   Noncompliance With Treatment
V65.2   Malingering
V71.01   Adult Antisocial Behavior
V71.02   Child or Adolescent Antisocial Behavior
V62.89   Borderline Intellectual Functioning

Note: *This is coded on Axis II*
780.93   Age-Related Cognitive Decline
V62.82   Bereavement
V62.3   Academic Problem
V62.2   Occupational Problem
313.82   Identity Problem
V62.89   Religious or Spiritual Problem
V62.4   Acculturation Problem
V62.89   Phase of Life Problem

ADDITIONAL CODES

300.9   Unspecified Mental Disorder (nonpsychotic)
V71.09   No Diagnosis or Condition on Axis I
799.9   Diagnosis or Condition Deferred on Axis I
V71.09   No Diagnosis on Axis II
799.9   Diagnosis Deferred on Axis II

MULTIAXIAL SYSTEM

Axis I   Clinical Disorders
          Other Conditions that May Be a Focus of
          Clinical Attention
Axis II   Personality Disorders
          Mental Retardation
Axis III General Medical Conditions
Axis IV   Psychosocial and Environmental Problems
Axis V   Global Assessment of Functioning

DISORDERS USUALLY FIRST DIAGNOSED IN INFANCY, CHILDHOOD, OR ADOLESCENCE

The classification begins with disorders usually first diagnosed in infancy, childhood, or adolescence. The provision for a separate section for so-called childhood disorders is only for convenience. Although most individuals with these disorders present for clinical attention during childhood or adolescence, it is not uncommon for some of these conditions to be diagnosed for the first time in adulthood (e.g., attention-deficit/hyperactivity disorder). Moreover, many disorders included in other sections of the DSM-IV-TR have an onset during childhood (e.g., major depressive disorder). Thus, a clinician evaluating a child or adolescent should not only focus on those disorders listed in this section but also consider disorders from throughout the DSM-IV-TR. Similarly, when evaluating an adult, the clinician should also consider the disorders in this section since many of them persist into adulthood (e.g., stuttering, learning disorders, tic disorders).

The first set of disorders included in this diagnostic class—mental retardation, learning and motor skills disorders, and communication disorders—are covered in detail in Chapters 2, 3, and 4, respectively. While these are not, strictly speaking, regarded as mental disorders, they are included in the DSM-IV-TR to facilitate differential diagnosis and to increase recognition of these conditions among mental health professionals. Autism and other pervasive developmental disorders are discussed in Chapter 5 and are characterized by gross qualitative impairment in social relatedness, in language, and in repertoire of interests and activities.

Disorders covered include autistic disorder, Asperger's disorder, Rett's disorder, and childhood disintegrative disorder. Attention-deficit/hyperactivity disorder and other disruptive behavior disorders (Chapter 6) are grouped together because they are all characterized (at least in their childhood presentations) by disruptive behavior. The chapter on feeding disorders (Chapter 7) includes both the DSM-IV-TR categories of pica, rumination disorder, and feeding disorder of infancy and early childhood (also known as *failure to thrive*). Tic disorders (Chapter 8) and elimination and other disorders of infancy and early childhood (Chapters 9 and 10) conclude the childhood section.

DELIRIUM, DEMENTIA, AMNESTIC DISORDER, AND OTHER COGNITIVE DISORDERS

In DSM-III-R, delirium, dementia, amnestic disorder, and other cognitive disorders were included in a section called *organic mental disorders*, which contained disorders that were due to either a general medical condition or substance use. In DSM-IV, the term organic was eliminated because of the implication that disorders not included in that section (e.g., schizophrenia, bipolar disorder) did not have an organic component. In fact, virtually all mental disorders have both psychological and biological components, and to designate some disorders as organic and the remaining disorders as nonorganic reflected a reductionistic mind–body dualism that is at odds with our understanding of the multifactorial nature of the etiological underpinnings of disorders.

DSM-IV replaced each unitary organic mental disorder (e.g., organic mood disorder) with its two component parts: mood disorder due to a general medical condition and substance-induced mood disorder. Because of their central roles in the differential diagnosis of cognitive impairment, delirium, dementia, and amnestic disorder are contained within the same diagnostic class in DSM-IV-TR and are discussed in Chapter 11.

Whereas both delirium and dementia are characterized by multiple cognitive impairments, delirium is distinguished by the presence of clouding of consciousness, which is manifested by an inability to appropriately maintain or shift attention. DSM-IV-TR includes three types of delirium: delirium due to a general medical condition, substance-induced delirium, and delirium due to multiple etiologies.

Dementia is characterized by clinically significant cognitive impairment in memory that is accompanied by impairment in one or more other areas of cognitive functioning (e.g., language, executive functioning). DSM-IV-TR includes several types of dementia based on etiology, including dementia of the Alzheimer's type, vascular dementia, a variety of dementia due to general medical and neurological conditions (e.g., human immunodeficiency virus infection, Parkinson's disease), substance-induced persisting dementia, and dementia due to multiple etiologies.

In contrast to dementia, amnestic disorder is characterized by clinically significant memory impairment occurring in the absence of other significant impairments in cognitive functioning. DSM-IV-TR includes amnestic disorder due to a general medical condition and substance-induced persisting amnestic disease.

MENTAL DISORDERS DUE TO A GENERAL MEDICAL CONDITION NOT ELSEWHERE CLASSIFIED

This diagnostic class includes all of the specific mental disorders due to a general medical condition and is discussed in Chapter 12. In DSM-IV-TR, most of the mental disorders due to a general medical condition have been distributed throughout the various diagnostic classes alongside their "nonorganic" counterparts in the classification. For example, mood disorder due to a general medical condition and substance-induced mood disorder are included in the mood disorders section of DSM-IV-TR. Two specific types of mental disorders due to a general medical condition (i.e., catatonic disorder due to a general medical condition and personality change due to a general medical condition) are physically included in this diagnostic class.

SUBSTANCE-RELATED DISORDERS

Substance-related disorders in DSM-IV-TR are more than just disorders related to taking drugs of abuse. They also include medication side effects and the consequences of toxin exposure. Two types of substance-related disorders are included in DSM-IV-TR: substance use disorders (dependence and abuse), which describe the maladaptive nature of the pattern of substance use; and substance-induced disorders, which cover psychopathological processes caused by the direct effects of substances on the central nervous system. Criteria sets for substance dependence, substance abuse, substance intoxication, and substance withdrawal that apply across all drug classes are included before the substance-specific sections of DSM-IV-TR. A discussion of these so-called generic criteria that apply to all substance-related disorders is covered in Chapter 13. Detailed discussions of each of the DSM-IV-TR drug classes are covered in Chapters 14 to 24.

SCHIZOPHRENIA AND OTHER PSYCHOTIC DISORDERS

The title of this diagnostic class is potentially misleading for two reasons: (1) there are other disorders that have psychotic features that are not included in this diagnostic class (e.g., mood disorders with psychotic features, delirium) and (2) it may incorrectly imply that the other psychotic disorders included in this section are related in some way to schizophrenia (which is only true for schizophreniform disorder and possibly schizoaffective disorder). Instead, what ties together all of the disorders in this diagnostic class is the presence of prominent psychotic symptoms. Included here are schizophrenia, schizophreniform disorder, schizoaffective disorder, delusional disorder, shared psychotic disorder, and brief psychotic disorder, each of which is discussed in varying detail in Chapter 25.

It should be noted that the definition of the term *psychosis* has been used in different ways historically and is not even used consistently across the various categories in the DSM-IV-TR. The most restrictive definition of psychosis (used in substance-induced psychotic disorder) requires a break in reality testing such that the person has delusions or hallucinations with no insight into the fact that the delusions or hallucinations are caused by taking drugs. A somewhat less restrictive definition of psychosis (not used in DSM-IV-TR but advocated by some members of the DSM-IV Psychotic Disorders Workgroup as more appropriate for substance-induced psychosis) includes hallucinations or delusions even if the person has insight into their origin (e.g., it would include an individual who was hallucinating after taking phencyclidine [PCP] even if he were aware that the hallucinations were due to the PCP). A much broader definition of psychosis (utilized in the definition of schizophrenia, schizophreniform, and brief psychotic disorder) goes beyond delusions and hallucinations to include grossly disorganized speech and catatonic or grossly disorganized behavior as evidence for psychosis. Finally, the term psychosis was in the past used most broadly to refer to any condition that caused serious functional impairment (e.g., "affective psychosis" is used in ICD-9 to refer to major mood disorders). This definition is not used in DSM-IV-TR.

MOOD DISORDERS

This diagnostic class includes disorders in which the predominant disturbance is in the individual's mood.

Although the term *mood* is broadly defined to include depression, euphoria, anger, and anxiety, the DSM-IV-TR generally restricts mood disturbances to depressed, elevated, or irritable mood.

The mood disorders section begins with the criteria for mood episodes (major depressive episode, manic episode, hypomanic episode, mixed episode), which are the building blocks for the episodic mood disorders. The codable mood disorders come next and are divided into the depressive disorders (i.e., major depressive disorder and dysthymic disorder, described in Chapter 26) and the bipolar disorders (i.e., bipolar I disorder, bipolar II disorder, and cyclothymic disorder, described in Chapter 28). Finally, the many specifiers that provide important treatment-relevant information close this section. Several so-called *subthreshold mood disorders* (i.e., they are characterized by depression but fall short of meeting the diagnostic criteria for either major depressive disorder or dysthymic disorder) are included in DSM-IV-TR appendix B, for Criteria Sets and Axes Provided for Further Study. These include minor depressive disorder, brief recurrent depressive disorder, mixed anxiety depressive disorder, postpsychotic depressive disorder of schizophrenia (all briefly described in Chapter 26), and premenstrual dysphoric disorder (described in detail in Chapter 27).

ANXIETY DISORDERS

The common element joining these disparate categories together is the fact that the anxiety is a prominent part of their clinical presentation. This grouping has been criticized because of evidence suggesting that at least some of the disorders are likely to be etiologically distinct from the others. Most particularly, obsessive–compulsive disorder and posttraumatic stress disorder seem to share little in common with the other anxiety disorders. In fact, separate diagnostic classes for stress-related disorders (that would also include adjustment disorders and perhaps dissociative disorders) and for obsessive–compulsive spectrum disorders (which might also include trichotillomania, tic disorders, hypochondriasis, body dysmorphic disorder, and other disorders characterized by compulsive behavior) have been proposed.

Detailed discussions of the various anxiety disorders are covered in Chapters 29 to 33 in this section of the textbook.

SOMATOFORM DISORDERS

This diagnostic class includes disorders in which the defining feature is a physical complaint or bodily concern that is not better accounted for by a general medical condition or another mental disorder. These disorders (which are discussed in detail in Chapter 34) can be divided into three groups on the basis of the focus of the individual's concerns: (1) focus on the physical symptoms themselves (somatization disorder, undifferentiated somatoform disorder, pain disorder, and conversion disorder); (2) focus on the belief that one has a serious physical illness (hypochondriasis); and (3) focus on the belief that one has a defect in physical appearance (body dysmorphic disorder).

FACTITIOUS DISORDERS

This diagnostic class contains only one disorder: factitious disorder, which describes presentations in which the individual intentionally produces or feigns physical or psychological symptoms in order to fulfill a psychological need to assume the sick role. It is discussed in detail in Chapter 35. Factitious disorder should always be distinguished from malingering, in which the individual similarly pretends to have physical or psychological symptoms. The difference is that in malingering, the person's motivation is to achieve some external gain (e.g., disability benefits, lessening of criminal responsibility, shelter for the night). For this reason, unlike factitious disorder, malingering is not considered a mental disorder.

DISSOCIATIVE DISORDERS

The common element in this group of disorders is the symptom of dissociation that is defined as a disruption in the usually integrated functions of consciousness, memory, identity, and perception. Four specific disorders are included (dissociative amnesia, dissociative fugue, dissociative identity disorder, and depersonalization disorder) and are discussed in detail in Chapter 36.

SEXUAL AND GENDER IDENTITY DISORDERS

This diagnostic class contains three relatively disparate types of disorders, linked together only by virtue of their involvement in human sexuality. Sexual dysfunctions refer to disturbances in sexual desire or functioning, paraphilias refer to unusual sexual preferences that interfere with functioning (or in the case of preferences that involve harm to others like pedophilia, merely acting on those preferences), and gender identity disorder refers to a serious conflict between one's internal identity of maleness and femaleness (gender identity) and one's anatomical sexual characteristics. These categories are discussed in detail in Chapter 37.

EATING DISORDERS

Although the name of this diagnostic class focuses on the fact that the disorders in this section are characterized by abnormal eating behavior (refusal to maintain adequate body weight in the case of anorexia nervosa and discrete episodes of uncontrolled eating of excessively large amounts of food in the case of bulimia nervosa), of near equal importance is the individual's pathological overemphasis on body image. A third category, which is being actively researched but has not been officially added to the DSM-IV-TR, is binge-eating disorder (included in the appendix of Criteria Sets and Axes Provided for Further Study). Like bulimia nervosa, individuals with binge-eating disorder have frequent episodes of binge-eating. However, unlike bulimia nervosa, these individuals do not do anything significant to counteract the effects of their binge-eating (i.e., they do not purge, use laxatives or diet pills, or excessively exercise). All three disorders are described in Chapter 38.

SLEEP DISORDERS

Sleep disorders are grouped into four sections on the basis of presumed etiology (primary, related to another mental disorder, due to a general medical condition, and substance induced). Two types of primary sleep disorders are included in DSM-IV-TR: dyssomnias (problems in regulation of amount and quality of sleep) and parasomnias (events that occur during sleep). The dyssomnias include primary insomnia, primary hypersomnia, circadian rhythm sleep disorder, narcolepsy, and breathing-related sleep disorder, whereas the parasomnias include nightmare disorder, sleep terror disorder, and sleepwalking disorder. Sleep disorders are described in detail in Chapter 39.

IMPULSE CONTROL DISORDERS NOT ELSEWHERE CLASSIFIED

As is suggested by the title of this diagnostic grouping, no one diagnostic class in DSM-IV-TR comprehensively includes all of the impulse control disorders. A number of disorders characterized by impulse control problems are classified elsewhere (e.g., conduct disorder, attention-deficit/hyperactivity disorder, oppositional-defiant disorder, delirium, dementia, substance-related disorders, schizophrenia and other psychotic disorders, mood disorders, antisocial and borderline personality disorders). What ties together the disorders in this class is that they present with clinically significant impulsive behavior and that they are not better accounted for by one of the mental disorders included in other parts of DSM-IV-TR. Five such disorders are included here: intermittent explosive disorder, pathological gambling, pyromania, kleptomania, and trichotillomania. These are discussed in Chapter 40.

ADJUSTMENT DISORDERS

All DSM-IV-TR categories (except NOS categories) take priority over adjustment disorder. This category is intended to apply to maladaptive reactions to psychosocial stressors that do not meet the criteria for any specific DSM-IV-TR disorder. These are discussed in Chapter 41.

PERSONALITY DISORDERS

This diagnostic class is for personality patterns that significantly deviate from the expectations of the person's culture, are pervasive, and lead to significant impairment or distress. Ten specific personality disorders are included in DSM-IV-TR: paranoid personality disorder (pervasive distrust and suspiciousness of others), schizoid personality disorder (detachment from social relationships and a restricted expression of emotions), schizotypal personality disorder (acute discomfort with close relationships, perceptual distortions, and eccentricities of behavior), antisocial personality disorder (disregard for the rights of others), borderline personality disorder (instability of personal relationships, instability of self-image, and marked impulsivity), histrionic personality disorder (extensive emotionality and attention seeking), narcissistic personality disorder (grandiosity, need for admiration, and lack of empathy), avoidant personality disorder (social inhibition, feelings of inadequacy, and hypersensitivity to negative evaluation), dependent personality disorder (excessive need to be taken care of), and obsessive–compulsive personality disorder (preoccupation with orderliness, perfectionism, and mental and personal control at the expense of flexibility, openness, and efficiency). These are discussed in detail in Chapter 42.

OTHER CONDITIONS THAT MAY BE A FOCUS OF CLINICAL ATTENTION

This section of DSM-IV-TR is for problems that are not mental disorders but that may be a focus of attention for treatment by a mental health professional. *Psychological factors affecting medical condition* are intended to allow the clinician to note the presence of psychological factors (e.g., Axis I or II disorder) that adversely affect the course of a general medical condition, including factors that interfere with treatment and factors that constitute health risks to the individual. This condition is described in Chapter 43.

APPENDIX CATEGORIES

DSM-IV-TR aims to be on the trailing edge rather than the cutting edge of research. A new category was considered for inclusion only if there was a substantial research literature behind it. Although there were proposals for more than 100 new categories to be introduced into DSM-IV, only a handful of new categories were added. Text and criteria for another 17 proposed categories have been included in a DSM-IV-TR appendix, Criteria Sets and Axes Provided for Further Study (Table 1-2). These criteria sets have been included to provide a common language for researchers and psychiatrists who are interested in further investigating their potential utility and validity.

Table 1-2	Criteria Sets and Axes Provided for Further Study

Postconcussional disorder
Mild cognitive disorder
Caffeine withdrawal
Postpsychotic depression of schizophrenia
Simple deteriorative disorder
Minor depressive disorder
Recurrent brief depressive disorder
Premenstrual dysphoric disorder
Mixed anxiety–depressive disorder
Factitious disorder by proxy
Dissociative trance disorder
Binge-eating disorder
Depressive personality disorder
Passive–aggressive personality disorder (negativistic personality disorder)
Defensive Functioning Scale
Global Assessment of Relational Functioning Scale
Social and Occupational Functioning Assessment Scale

Source: Data from American Psychiatric Association (1994) *Diagnostic and Statistical Manual of Mental Disorders*, 4th ed. APA, Washington, DC.

2 Childhood Disorders: Mental Retardation

DIAGNOSIS

Some common misconceptions about mental retardation are that it is a specific and lifelong disorder with a unique personality pattern and that comorbid mental disorders existing with mental retardation are different from those encountered in other individuals. Although mental retardation is listed as a mental disorder in the DSM-IV-TR, it is not a unique nosological entity. Instead, a diagnosis of mental retardation refers to the level of a person's intellectual and adaptive functioning below a cutoff point that is not even natural but is arbitrarily chosen in relation to the average level of functioning of the population at large. Its chief function is administrative, defining a group of persons who are in need of support and educational services. Thus, mental retardation does not have a single cause, mechanism, course, or prognosis. It has to be differentiated from the diagnosis (if known) of the underlying medical condition.

The American Association on Mental Retardation (AAMR) has published over the years 10 definitions of mental retardation. The most recent definition published in 2002 in the 10th edition of the manual on definition, classification, and system of supports of the American Association on Mental Retardation is as follows: "Mental retardation is a disability characterized by significant limitations both in intellectual functioning and in adaptive behavior as expressed in conceptual, social, and practical adaptive skills. This disability originates before age 18 years." Significant limitation in intellectual functioning is defined as at least 2 standard deviations below the mean for the assessment instrument. The standard error of measurement for the instrument (usually between 3 and 5 points) should be taken into consideration. Persons with mental retardation can be classified in various ways, such as by IQ levels, or by the intensity of supports required by them, depending on the purpose for which the diagnosis is used. Significant limitation in adaptive behavior is defined as performance of at least 2 standard deviations below the mean on an instrument normed on the general population. The AAMR manual emphasizes the requirement for detailed assessment of individuals and their needs in all relevant domains, including psychological and emotional, and is by far the most modern and comprehensive available.

DSM-IV-TR defines mental retardation in a manner generally compatible with the AAMR definition. Mental retardation is coded on Axis II, as conceptually, it fits more with personality disorders listed on this axis than with the other mental illnesses listed on Axis I. It was also expected that placement on Axis II would encourage clinicians to diagnose both mental retardation and mental disorders when faced with a person who has

---

DSM-IV-TR Criteria

317–319 MENTAL RETARDATION

A. Significantly subaverage intellectual functioning: an IQ of approximately 70 or below on an individually administered IQ test (for infants, a clinical judgment of significantly subaverage intellectual functioning).
B. Concurrent deficits or impairments in present adaptive functioning (i.e., the person's effectiveness in meeting the standards expected for his or her cultural group) in at least two of the following areas: communication, self-care, home living, social/interpersonal skills, use of community resources, self-direction, functional academic skills, work, leisure, health, and safety.
C. The onset is before age 18 years.

Severity	Approximate IQ Range	Code
Mild	50–55 to approx. 70	317
Moderate	35–40 to approx. 50–55	318
Severe	20–25 to approx. 35–40	318.1
Profound	Below 20–25	318.2
Unspecified		319

Reprinted with permission from the *Diagnostic and Statistical Manual of Mental Disorders*, 4th ed., Text Rev. Copyright 2000 American Psychiatric Association.

---

such comorbidity, rather than subsume both under the diagnosis of mental retardation.

The clinical presentation of persons with mental retardation is influenced by multiple factors, which can be grossly divided into biological (such as syndromes underlying the retardation), psychological (the level of the person's intellectual and adaptive functioning), and environmental (such as cultural expectations and services received).

The more severe the mental retardation, the earlier the child will come to medical attention, because the developmental delay will be obvious earlier, and associated physical impairments will be more prevalent. Conversely, children with mild mental retardation may not be diagnosed until they reach school age, when they fail in academic learning. If the sociocultural environment does not value and stress early academic learning and early education is not available, mild mental retardation might go undetected, especially if the person has relatively good adaptive skills. A false-positive diagnosis of mental retardation can also occur, especially if psychological tests are not sensitive to cultural background, and there is a language barrier between the child and the tester.

The importance of the earliest diagnosis possible cannot be overstated because the prognosis will be much better if the intervention that results from the diagnostic knowledge is begun as early as possible.

The AAMR published in 2002 a new edition of its manual *Mental Retardation: Definition, Classification and Systems of Supports.* Several dimensions of mental retardation are described, which might also serve as an outline for its assessment:

- **Dimension I:** Intellectual abilities.
- **Dimension II:** Adaptive behavior (Conceptual, social, and practical skills).

Assessment of the above dimensions is essentially ascertaining that the respective criteria for the diagnosis of mental retardation are met. The intellectual functioning is assessed in individual testing with one of the standardized intelligence tests appropriate for the person's cultural, linguistic, and social background, and communication skills. Standardized tests and scales, such as the Vineland Adaptive Behavior Scales and the AAMR Adaptive Behavior Scales as well as history and direct observations are used.

- **Dimension III:** Participation, interactions, and social roles.
- **Dimension IV:** Health (physical health, mental health, etiological factors).

This is described in the following section of this chapter.

- **Dimension V:** Context (environments and culture).

This is a comprehensive description of the person's current environment: its nature, strengths, and weaknesses, and supports for the person's development and well-being (including factors such as poverty, family and its attitudes, availability of education, and other services). In all aspects of the assessment, attention should be paid both to the strengths as well as to the weaknesses and the impairments.

Elements of Biomedical Assessment

First Stage Workup. The scheme for assessing the etiology of mental retardation is summarized in Figure 2.1.

History. Obtaining a detailed history is most important. The family history, especially occurrence in the family of similar cases, congenital anomalies, severe mental illness, and consanguinity should be explored. The risk of recessively inherited diseases increases if there has been intermarriage between the parents' families in earlier generations. Drawing the family tree is helpful. The gestational, birth and neonatal, as well as developmental history is also most important. The presence of an appropriate relationship between weight, length, and head circumference at birth must be assessed as well as their relationship to the gestational age to evaluate possible intrauterine growth retardation, microcephaly, and so on. All events that may have affected CNS development during childhood as well as developmental milestones must be recorded.

Physical Examination. This is essential and should also focus on searching for physical phenotypical manifestations of various mental retardation-associated syndromes and dysmorphic features different from familial phenotype. Neurological examination and growth measurements are part of physical examination.

Diagnostic Studies. The Consensus Conference for Evaluation of Mental Retardation recommended, in addition to previously mentioned history taking and physical examination, the following: banded karyotype and fragile X studies by DNA method for both males and females with unexplained mental retardation. These studies are essential if the family history is positive or if the physical and behavioral phenotypes are without major findings. Neuroimaging, preferably MRI, is to be performed if the individual has neurologic symptoms, cranial abnormalities, microcephaly, or macrocephaly.

After this basic workup, the probable cause or at least timing of the injury should become apparent, thus

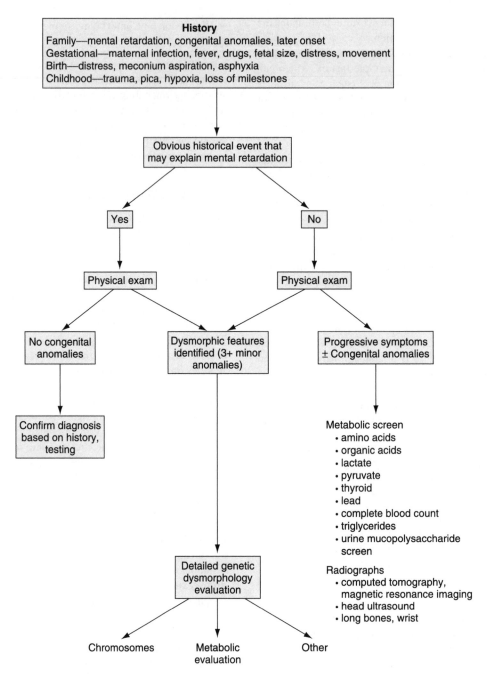

Figure 2-1 *Diagnostic approach to mental retardation of all ages. (Source: Szymanski LS and Kaplan LC (1991) Mental retardation. (Reprinted with permission from the Textbook of Child & Adolescent Psychiatry. Copyright 1991, American Psychiatric Press.)*

allowing discussion with the family concerning possible inheritance. Sometimes the history alone might provide this information, but even then a detailed physical examination for signs indicative of abnormal prenatal development is necessary.

Prenatal Diagnosis. Prenatal diagnostic methods are increasingly available. Amniocentesis with chromosomal studies is usually recommended for women 35 years or older. Prenatal diagnostic studies should be made available to everyone requesting them and should be used if there is a known risk for a genetic or congenital problem. Even if the parents do not plan a therapeutic abortion, if the results are positive for a certain disorder, they will be able to prepare for the birth of a child with special needs and to marshal support.

The currently available techniques include amniocentesis (useful in diagnosing chromosomal and metabolic disorders), chorionic villus sampling (for chromosomal and molecular genetic studies), and maternal serum alpha-fetoprotein screening (for neural tube defects). Ultrasound scanning is often performed around the 20th week of gestation to screen for major malformations. Carrier screening, which is increasingly available for certain recessive disorders, should be offered to all persons in high-risk populations, such as Ashkenazi Jews (for Tay–Sachs disease). Careful counseling is necessary to help the prospective parents decide on all available options if they are found to be positive for the particular trait.

Differential Diagnosis

The diagnosis of mental retardation itself should be relatively straightforward as it reflects the current level of intellectual and adaptive functioning. Some persons with learning disorders or communication disorders might appear to have a low level of functioning, but appropriate psychological and communication testing will demonstrate that the impairment is in the development of specific skills and is not generalized. Dementia can be diagnosed at any age, whereas mental retardation is diagnosed only if the onset is before age 18 years. However, both disorders might be diagnosed in persons younger than age 18. It is often asked how one differentiates between mental retardation and autistic disorder. Actually, such a question is erroneous because these disorders are not mutually exclusive; in fact, most persons with autism also have mental retardation. An uncomplicated mental retardation is not associated with qualitative impairment in social interaction and communication, which is diagnostic of autistic disorder.

TREATMENT

Mental retardation is a functional disability: thus, the goal of treatment should be to reduce or eliminate the disability. There are three aspects to the treatment:

1. Treatment of the underlying disorder that is causative of mental retardation (e.g., phenylketonuria [PKU]).
2. Treatment of the comorbid disorders that add to the functional disability, whether physical or mental.
3. Interventions targeted at the functional disability of the mental retardation itself: educational, habilitative, and supportive approaches depending on the person's individualized needs.

The current approach to the services for persons with mental retardation is based on the following principles:

- The *normalization principle*, which refers to making available to individuals with mental retardation patterns and conditions of everyday life that are as close as possible to the norms and patterns of the mainstream of society. This has largely evolved into the *principle of inclusion*, which is usually interpreted as an active effort to include persons with mental retardation in all normal aspects and opportunities of society's life, through providing them with supports necessary for success. The ultimate goal is to eventually end segregated services and education and provide persons with mental retardation with the necessary, specialized support services in regular educational, living, and work settings.
- The *right to community living*, which confers the right to live with a family, preferably one's own or a substitute one if necessary (foster or adoptive). This includes moving individuals living in large residential facilities to as normal a setting as possible, for example, community residences, supervised apartments, and foster homes. Furthermore, children are not to be institutionalized, regardless of the level of retardation, and, generally, neither are adults. However, some children are still placed in special residential schools (usually private) for specific reasons, typically medical or behavioral needs that require specialized treatment. Historically, a majority of persons with mental retardation lived at home and no more than 10% were in institutions at any point. However, institutions played a disproportionate role in attitudes to their care. At their peak in 1967, there were 194,650 persons living in them: this number dropped to 52,801 in 1998. In 2000, there were eight states that closed all their large residential facilities. In contrast, the number of persons living in small (less than six persons) residences in the community increased dramatically.
- *Education and training for all children* to a maximum possible extent, regardless of their disability and the degree of the disability, by including them full time in an age-appropriate regular classroom. This educational program is individualized according to the child's needs. Services of special educators and therapists, as necessary, are also provided in these programs. This has to be distinguished from

mainstreaming, which refers to placement in special classes in regular schools but with participation in some activities of regular classes.

- *Employment of adults in the community* according to their abilities is another aspect of inclusion. The current trend is to employ them in competitive job markets with supports, such as vocational training and supports by job coaches. However, many individuals, especially those with severe degrees of disability, are still placed in sheltered workshops or occupational–recreational day programs.
- *Use of normal community services and facilities* (shopping, banking, transportation, recreation) through training and ongoing supports.
- *Advocacy and appropriate protective measures*, for example, against inappropriate use of pharmacological and behavioral measures as substitutes for active education and treatment, inclusion in research programs without proper, truly informed consent, and general exploitation and abuse.

Overall Goals of Psychiatric Treatment of Persons with Mental Retardation

The most common mistake made by mental health clinicians treating persons with mental retardation is to consider suppression (usually with medications) of single problems (as a rule disruptive behaviors) as the only goal of treatment. This approach used to be the rule in the past when people with mental retardation were not expected to achieve any measure of independence and keeping them docile was the goal. Lately, such approaches are reemerging, partly related to the pressure from insurers to achieve a fast and inexpensive symptomatic improvement, even if short lived. Fortunately, in the past three decades, the quality of life (QOL) has been assuming a central role as the goal of treatment in the mental retardation field. More recently, the importance of the subjective aspects of QOL have been stressed: the individual's subjective feeling of contentment, well-being, and satisfaction with his or her own life as opposed to the caregiver's satisfaction. In other words, personal happiness of the person with mental retardation is now stressed as a goal of habilitation as well as specific treatment.

The goal of any form of psychiatric treatment of persons with mental retardation is to contribute to this sense of satisfaction with one's own life, or happiness, in the context of a comprehensive treatment program. Suppression of behaviors inconvenient to caregivers is not enough, especially if they are a response to an inadequate habilitation program and the treatment (usually medications) is used in lieu of such a program. Furthermore, medications may suppress a person's functioning through side effects such as drowsiness.

Psychotropic medications are used to treat a diagnosed mental disorder toward the goal of maximizing a person's quality of life. They should not be used merely to suppress a single, objectionable behavior without regard to the effect on a person's global adjustment, functioning, and quality of life. They cannot be used as punishment, for staff convenience (such as in understaffed facilities), in lieu of appropriate habilitative programs (if such is unavailable), or in dosages that interfere with such programs and with a person's quality of life.

These drugs are always used as part of a comprehensive, treatment/habilitation program designed and supervised by an interdisciplinary team of which the psychiatric clinician is an integral part. They should not be prescribed merely in brief "psychopharmacology consultation" or "medication review," in isolation from other aspects of the treatment.

Review of Classes of Psychotropic Drugs

Only issues specific to persons with mental retardation are discussed here.

Neuroleptics (*Antipsychotics*). The use of antipsychotic drugs in persons with mental retardation is the same as that for the general population—primarily for the treatment of psychosis, sometimes for Tourette's disorder, and as an emergency treatment of dangerous behavior. The problem with persons with mental retardation is in making the correct diagnosis of psychosis, especially schizophrenia. Perhaps because of the difficulty (or ignorance) of making a more specific diagnosis, antipsychotic agents have been used for "off-label" indications, such as aggression, destructiveness, Self-injurious behaviour (SIB), and any disruptive behavior. While these medications may sometimes be effective in these cases, success cannot be reliably predicted. If the drug is effective in alleviating such behaviors, it does not necessarily mean that the individual had a psychotic disorder.

The recognition of side effects might be difficult in persons with limited language, and extended observation by trained staff may be necessary. Drowsiness might have an adverse effect on learning and on general level of activity. A common mistake is to confuse akathisia, especially upon withdrawal, with reemergence of behavior problems and to make the disorder worse by increasing the dose. Many adults with mental retardation have been on older antipsychotics for years, often for no clear reason. Many of these individuals have side effects such as Parkinsonian symptoms, and tardive dyskinesia (that might appear only upon discontinuation trial). Because of a higher tendency to cause adverse effects (to which this population might be more susceptible), these drugs (thioridazine in particular) are being discontinued and, if necessary, changed to newer, second generation antipsychotics. The latter are, of course, not free from side effects. Weight gain, especially from olanzapine and clozapine, might be particularly severe and troublesome. The discontinuation of antipsychotic medications should be gradual and slow to minimize side effects from withdrawal, including behavior problems such as irritability, insomnia, SIB, and aggression. Clonidine might be helpful for these symptoms.

There are case reports of successful use of clozapine in persons with mental retardation and schizophrenia or bipolar disorder who did not respond to other agents. The need for weekly blood tests may be a problem in less than cooperative persons.

Antidepressants. The principal uses of antidepressant medications, as in the general population, include treatment of depression as well as anxiety, panic, and obsessive–compulsive disorder (OCD). Selective serotonin reuptake inhibitors (SSRIs) are now first-line drugs because of favorable effectiveness/side effect profile. Tricyclic antidepressants, principally desipramine, were used in the treatment of ADHD if stimulants and clonidine were not effective, but there has been concern about cardiotoxic side effects. Precipitation of excitement, mania, and seizures by antidepressants might be a problem, and careful prior diagnostic assessment and follow-up are necessary. There are a few studies, mostly case reports, that have suggested that SSRIs might be helpful in reducing self-stimulatory, ritualistic, and self-injurious behaviors, although the improvement might be short lived. In some cases where antidepressants are effective in reducing aggressive behavior, there is the possibility that they actually might help the underlying depression that has led to the aggression.

Antianxiety Drugs. Benzodiazepines have been used for alleviation of anxiety, but their side effects, such as paradoxical rage reactions, adverse effects on cognition, and serious withdrawal symptoms, argue against their chronic use, and a trial of an SSRI might be preferable. Occasional use might be helpful in emergency situations in which extreme anxiety is present as well as in preparation for anxiety-inducing medical procedures. The usefulness of buspirone, a nonsedating anxiolytic, with short half-life, in persons with combined anxiety and aggression or SIB, has been suggested by one study. Benzodiazepines are still used for the treatment of generalized anxiety and panic disorders, but usually only when there is no response to antidepressants. There is still a fair amount of combined use of neuroleptics and anxiolytics, especially in institutionalized persons with a history of aggression. However, this may lead to significant CNS depression, and benzodiazepine use might actually lead to disinhibition. Therefore, prolonged use of anxiolytics to control undesirable behaviors is generally not recommended.

As with other medications, comprehensive diagnostic assessment is a prerequisite to the use of anxiolytics. In particular, environmental anxiety-provoking factors have to be ruled out and, if present, have to be dealt with in addition to pharmacological means if these are used.

Mood Stabilizers. The use of these agents in persons with and without mental retardation is similar. Lithium carbonate, the original mood stabilizer, was shown to be effective for bipolar disorders in persons with mental retardation during the 1970s. However, it has considerable side effects and managing them may be difficult in persons who might be less than cooperative. It has been supplanted increasingly by anticonvulsants, including carbamazepine and valproic acid, as well as newer ones, like gabapentin and lamotrigine. Currently, the primary use is in the treatment of mania and for augmentation of antidepressants. These drugs may also be used in a therapeutic trial in some individuals with implusive aggressive behavior. Some clinical experiences indicate that the prognosis might be better in the presence of mood lability and an abnormal electroencephalogram. As seizures are frequently associated with mental retardation, these drugs offer a parsimonious way of managing both seizures and behavioral symptoms.

Stimulants. As in persons without mental retardation, drugs such as methylphenidate and dextroamphetamine are effective in the treatment of ADHD. They have been studied primarily in children and adolescents with mild mental retardation or PDD. Their effectiveness in persons with significant retardation is less certain. Tics are one side effect of methylphenidate: if the individual is engaging in self-stimulatory behaviors, videotaping might provide a record for later reference regarding whether additional tics have emerged. The diagnosis of ADHD in this population may not be easy, especially in persons with significant mental retardation, as the symptoms have to be assessed in the context of the developmental level.

Other Psychotropic Agents. Propranolol and other beta-adrenergic blockers have been tried extensively in all kinds of aggressive behavior, often with mixed or poor results. Depression might be a side effect of these agents, leading to reduction in the person's functioning, even if the aggressive behaviors might appear to improve, because of apathy induced by the drug. They may be also effective in the treatment of anxiety, especially its somatic symptoms, and for akathisia related to neuroleptic drugs.

Clonidine, a presynaptic alpha-2-adrenergic agonist also used as an antihypertensive, is commonly used in the treatment of ADHD in children without mental retardation, and more recently for children with pervasive developmental disorder (PDD); there have been case reports of its effectiveness in persons with fragile X. While tics are not a side effect, drowsiness, hypotension, bradycardia, and skin rash (from patch) might be troublesome. It has also been reported to be effective in some cases of akathisia related to neuroleptic drug withdrawal.

Naltrexone, an oral antagonist of endogenous opioid receptors, has been tried in a number of studies in cases of severe SIB, following some case reports of earlier successes with a similar agent, naloxone, which had to be administered parenterally. It appears that it is effective in 35–70% of cases, at least for a short time.

Other Treatments. For many years, there have been reports of beneficial effects of a variety of treatments, especially in children with PDDs, Down syndrome, and fragile X syndrome. These treatments include various nutritional supplements, vitamin supplements (such as megavitamins, various combinations of vitamins, minerals and enzymes, B_6, B_6 with magnesium, folic acid, etc.), restriction diets (such as diets without certain food additives, gluten, casein, yeast), and so on. Often, these approaches generate considerable excitement both in families and researchers. However, as a rule, they are based on anecdotal reports or studies with methodological problems, results of which are not replicated in well-designed studies. One should bear in mind that persons with developmental disabilities, especially PDDs, may have very unusual eating habits resulting in restricted diets. Therefore, in such cases a nutritional consultation is advisable. If a deficiency is found, an appropriate supplementation and correction of dietary habits is, of course, needed. One example is zinc deficiency associated with pica, which was shown to disappear or decrease after treatment with 100 mg of chelated zinc for 2 weeks.

Electroconvulsive therapy has fallen into disuse in this population as the result of past inappropriate uses and strict, current regulations. Occasional case reports of its successful use can still be found in the literature.

Psychosocial Interventions

Programmatic and Educational Approaches. The goal of these interventions is to provide a proper living and programmatic environment. For instance, certain persons easily become overstimulated, anxious, and disruptive in noisy and confused large workshops; arranging for a smaller and quieter workroom is preferable to a prescription for a neuroleptic. The vocational and educational program should be individualized and should focus on developing the person's strengths and providing an opportunity for success. In turn, this will lead to results such as an improvement in self-image. Many persons with severe mental retardation are placed in prevocational training indefinitely, for example, screwing or unscrewing nuts and bolts, although no one expects them to ever be employed on an assembly line. They often engage in a struggle with caregivers because of their noncompliance and may resort to aggression, which leads to removal for a "time out" and thus avoidance of a boring task. Creating a more suitable task—even such as making rounds of the workshop to collect or deliver materials—might be more interesting and appropriate. Functional analysis of behavior is an invaluable guide to these interventions. As discussed previously, such approaches should be explored prior to resorting to the use of medications for disruptive behaviors.

Psychotherapies. Psychotherapy in this population is not different in nature from psychotherapy in persons with average intelligence and is similar to treating children, inasmuch as in both cases, the techniques and the therapist have to adapt to the developmental needs of the individual. The treatment should be driven by the individual's needs and responses and not by the therapist's theoretical orientation. The indications are the presence of concerns and conflicts, especially about oneself; impairments in interpersonal skills; or other mental disturbances that are known to improve through psychotherapy. The prerequisites include communication skills permitting a meaningful interchange with the therapist, an ability to develop even a minimal relationship, and the availability of a trained, experienced, and unprejudiced therapist who is comfortable working in a team setting.

Guidelines for psychotherapy in this population include the following:

1. Appropriate goals should be set and should be reconciled with the expectations of the caregivers, the

therapist, and the individual with mental retardation. Common goals include improvement in self-image and impulse control, learning to express feelings in a socially appropriate manner, and understanding in a constructive manner one's own disabilities and strengths.

2. Verbal techniques should be adapted to the individual's language and cognitive level, and nonverbal ones should be age-appropriate.

3. Limits and directiveness should be used as needed: nondirective therapy might lead to the individual's confusion.

4. The therapist has to be active (supportive but not paternalistic), has to use herself or himself liberally as a treatment tool, and has to be able to focus on the immediate reality rather than just intellectualize. A mix of techniques, for example, cognitive psychotherapy and behavior modification, may be required.

5. As in all treatment modalities, the therapist should be involved in all aspects of the individual's program and should collaborate with other providers and with the family.

Group psychotherapy might be particularly effective in helping individuals with mental retardation handle issues related to the understanding of their own disability and learn social skills because of the peer support the group offers. In general, therapy should be seen as a cognitive learning process, using the therapist's support and leading individuals to the acquisition of understanding and necessary skills, both of concrete behaviors and of handling one's own emotions. Group psychotherapy should be differentiated from group counseling, which is usually educational in nature, focused on a specific subject (e.g., sexuality education), and does not have to be conducted by a mental health professional with a therapeutic goal and plan.

Behavioral Treatment. Detailed functional analysis is a prerequisite. This treatment should optimally use rewards that should be age-appropriate, preferably social, and the frequency of rewarding should be adapted to a person's cognitive level, so that he or she can understand why they are given. Consistency and generalization among different settings are essential. Thus, if such techniques are successfully used at the school, the family or other caregivers should be trained to use them at home as well. The focus should not be on elimination of objectionable behaviors only, but on teaching appropriate replacement behaviors. Aversive techniques involving active punishment (electric shocks, spraying of noxious substances into a person's face) are not used except in a few controversial settings. There is a professional consensus that these techniques should not be used at all, or used only when all other techniques have failed and the individual's behavior poses severe danger to herself or himself or to others (such as intractable SIB). Even then, these techniques should be used only if proved effective and for a limited time.

COMPARISON OF DSM-IV-TR AND ICD-10 DIAGNOSTIC CRITERIA

The method of defining the levels of severity differ slightly between the two systems. The ICD-10 Diagnostic Criteria for Research define the levels using exact cutoff scores: Mild is defined as 50 to 69, Moderate is defined as 35 to 49, Severe is defined as 20 to 34, and Profound is defined as below 20. In contrast, DSM-IV-TR provides somewhat greater flexibility in relating severity to a given IQ score by defining severity levels using overlapping scores (i.e., mild is 50 to 55, moderate is from 35–40 to 50–55, severe is from 20–25 to 35–40, and profound is below 20–25). Within the overlapping range, the severity is determined by the level of adaptive functioning.

CHAPTER

3

Childhood Disorders: Learning and Motor Skills Disorders

DIAGNOSIS

It is important not only to understand the diagnostic criteria used in DSM-IV-TR but also the criteria used by school systems. In clinical practice, the clinician usually needs to help the family in getting the school system to identify the child or adolescent as having a disability and to provide the necessary services. Thus, the clinician must know and understand the educational criteria.

The research of the past 30 years on neurologically based learning disorders stressed not the specific skill disorder but the underlying processing problems. The psychological and educational diagnostic tests used clarify areas of learning abilities and learning disabilities covering the four phases of processing (Table 3-1). Thus, although one assesses for problems with reading, mathematics, or writing, it is important in the diagnostic process also to explore the underlying processing problems that result in these skill disorders.

The DSM-IV-TR criteria for each of the learning disorders require that the child's achievement in reading, mathematics, or writing, as measured by individually administered standardized tests, is substantially below those expected given the individual's chronological age and measured intelligence, and age-appropriate education (criterion A). Developmental coordination disorder similarly requires that performance of daily activities involving motor coordination be substantially below that expected given the child's chronological age and

measured intelligence. Thus, these conditions can be given to children with mental retardation (MR) so long as the learning or motor skills problem is substantially out of proportion to other developmental deficits associated with the MR. The problem must significantly interfere with the child's academic achievement in order to qualify for a disorder (criterion B) and, if a sensory deficit is present (e.g., hearing loss), the difficulties are in excess of those usually associated with it. For the learning disorders, the presence of a general medical condition (e.g., neurological conditions) or sensory deficit is noted on Axis III. In contrast, the definition of developmental coordination disorder specifically excludes the diagnosis if the coordination problems are due to a general medical condition or if the criteria are met for a pervasive developmental disorder.

Federal guidelines for determining whether a student in a public school is eligible for special programs for learning disabilities list four criteria:

1. Documented evidence indicating that general education has been attempted and found to be ineffective in meeting the student's educational needs.
2. Evidence of a disorder in one or more of the basic psychological processes required for learning. A psychological process is a set of mental operations that transform, access, or manipulate information. The disorder is relatively enduring and limits ability to perform specific academic or developmental learning tasks. It may be manifested differently at different developmental levels.
3. Evidence of academic achievement significantly below the student's level of intellectual function (a difference of 1.5 to 1.75 standard deviations between achievement and intellectual functioning is considered significant) on basic reading skills, reading comprehension, mathematical calculation, mathematical reasoning, or written expression.
4. Evidence that the learning problems are not due primarily to other handicapping conditions (i.e.,

Table 3-1	Areas of Psychological Processing that Affect Learning	
Area of Processing	**Examples**	
Input	Visual or auditory perception	
Integration	Sequencing, abstracting, organization	
Memory	Short-term, rote, long-term	
Output	Language, motor	

Clinical Guide to the Diagnosis and Treatment of Mental Disorders. M. B. First and A. Tasman
© 2006 John Wiley & Sons, Ltd.   ISBN 0 470 019158

impairment of visual acuity or auditory acuity, physical impairment, emotional handicap, mental retardation, cultural differences, or environmental deprivation).

The presence of a central nervous system processing deficit is essential for the diagnosis of a learning disability. A child might meet the discrepancy criteria, but without central processing deficits in functions required for learning, he or she is not considered to have a learning disability. The question of the significant discrepancy between potential and actual achievement determines eligibility for services.

If a child or adolescent is experiencing academic difficulty, she or he would normally be referred to the special education professionals within the school system. However, the student with academic difficulties often presents with emotional or behavior problems and is more likely to be referred to a mental health professional. It is critical to understand this potential referral bias. This mental health professional must clarify whether the observed emotional, social, or family problems are causing the academic difficulties or whether they are a consequence of the academic difficulties and the resulting frustrations and failures experienced by the individual, the teacher, and the parents.

The evaluation of a child or adolescent with academic difficulties and emotional or behavior problems includes a comprehensive assessment of the presenting emotional, behavior, social, or family problems as well as a mental status examination. The clinician should obtain information from the child or adolescent, parents, teachers, and other education professionals to help clarify whether there might be a learning disorder or a motor skills disorder and whether further psychological or educational studies are needed.

Children who experience problems in reading typically have difficulty in decoding the letter–sound associations involved in phonic analysis. As a result, they may read in a disjointed manner, knowing a few words on sight and stumbling across other unfamiliar words. If they have difficulty with visual tracking, they may skip words or lines. If comprehension is a problem, they report that they have to read material over and over before they understand.

Children with mathematical difficulties may have problems learning math concepts or retaining this information. They may make careless mistakes when doing calculations. Problems with visual–spatial tasks or with sequencing might interfere with producing on paper what is known. A problem may not be completed or steps skipped. They might have difficulty shifting from one operation to the next and, as a result, add when they should subtract. A visual–spatial difficulty might result

in misaligned columns or rows, or decimals put in the wrong place.

Children who have difficulties with writing also may have a problem with handwriting. They grasp the pencil or pen differently and tightly. They write slowly, and their hands get tired. Often, they prefer printing rather than cursive writing. Most also have problems with the language of writing. They have difficulty with spelling, often spelling phonetically. They may have difficulty with grammar, punctuation, and capitalization.

Many if not most students with a learning disorder also have difficulties with memory or organization. The child or adolescent with a memory problem has difficulty following multistep directions or reads a chapter in a book but forgets what was read. Others might have sequencing problems, performing instructions out of order. In speaking or writing, the facts may come out but in the wrong sequence. Students with organizational difficulties may not be able to organize their life (notebook, locker, desk, bedroom); they forget things or lose things; they have difficulty with time planning; or they have difficulty using parts of information from a whole concept or putting parts of information together into a whole concept.

Children and adolescents with a developmental coordination disorder may show evidence of gross motor or fine motor difficulties. The gross motor problems might result in difficulty with walking, running, jumping, or climbing. The fine motor problems may result in difficulty with buttoning, zipping, tying, holding a pencil or pen or crayon, arts and crafts activities, or handwriting. Both gross and fine motor difficulties may result in the individual performing poorly in certain sports activities.

The evaluation of cognitive, academic, and neuropsychological functioning is critical to any assessment of learning problems. Results of this psychoeducational assessment will indicate the parameters of the individual's academic and cognitive liabilities while identifying her or his assets. If any of the clinical evaluations yield results suggestive of a learning disorder, a more involved psychoeducational assessment is needed. An appropriate psychoeducational evaluation will reveal the magnitude of the child's learning difficulties as well as the nature of the child's cognitive assets and deficits.

A family evaluation must include an assessment of the parents and of the entire family. A judgment is made on the order in which these assessments are best done. The first clinical question is whether the family is functional or dysfunctional. If the family is largely functional, there may be normal parenting issues that may be contributing to the child's difficulty. If there is no evidence of a psychopathological process within the family, alternative explanations should be considered for the learning disorder, which do not relate to family issues.

Learning problems are attributed to cognitive deficits or behavior problems in the child or adolescent. Environmental factors involving the school or community, however, can also contribute to academic difficulties. Thus, the clinician should be aware of how social, cultural, or institutional structures can influence learning. Data collection within this context is accomplished through formal and informal observations of the system and the cultural milieu. With this understanding as a backdrop, one can conduct a more direct assessment of how specific environmental or school considerations can affect a given individual.

Individuals with a learning disorder or a motor skills disorder might have other mental disorders or a related neurological disorder. They might also have social problems. It is not uncommon for children and adolescents with learning disorders or a motor skills disorder to also have a diagnosable mental disorder. For many, these psychological problems are secondary to the frustrations and failures experienced because these disabilities were not identified or were inadequately treated. For others, these conditions may be another reflection of a dysfunctional nervous system. The presenting behavioral or emotional issues might be the individual's characterological style for coping with a dysfunctional nervous system.

About one-third of youths diagnosed as having a conduct disorder or young adults diagnosed as having a personality disorder, especially the borderline type, have unrecognized or recognized and poorly treated learning disabilities (learning disorders).

The learning disabilities that result in learning disorders or motor skills disorder may directly contribute to peer problems by interfering with success in doing activities required to interact with certain age groups (e.g., visual perception and visual–motor problems interfering with ability to quickly do such eye–hand activities as catching, hitting, or throwing a ball).

Many children and adolescents with learning disorders have difficulty learning social skills and being socially competent. These individuals do not pick up such social cues as facial expressions, tone of voice, or body language and therefore do not adapt their behaviors appropriately.

The first neurologically based disorder recognized as frequently associated with a learning disability (learning disorder) was attention-deficit/hyperactivity disorder (ADHD). Since there is a continuum of disorders associated with neurological dysfunction that are often

found together, when one is diagnosed, the others must be considered in the diagnostic process.

Differential Diagnosis

The presenting problem is academic difficulty. The differential diagnostic process must clarify the reason for the academic difficulty. A *decision tree* for academic difficulties is useful for exploring all of the possible reasons for such difficulties (see Figure 3-1). Three principal areas of inquiry concerning the factors contributing to the student's learning difficulties are explored. The first involves considerations that are related to the child's or adolescent's psychiatric, medical, or psychoeducational status. The second area of inquiry is family functioning. The third area to explore involves the environmental and cultural context in which the student functions.

Difficulties in academic performance of children or adolescents can be related to a range of psychiatric, medical, or cognitive factors. To best determine the primary source of academic difficulties, the evaluation should involve a comprehensive examination of these areas. The psychiatric evaluation should clarify whether there is a psychopathological process. If one is present, it is useful first to determine whether the problems relate to a disruptive behavior disorder or to another mental disorder. In particular, the disruptive behavior disorders have high comorbidity with academic difficulties. A full assessment should clarify whether a disruptive behavior disorder is causing the difficulty with academic performance or is secondary to this difficulty. Disruptive behavior disorders can result in the student being unavailable for learning or being so disruptive as to require his/her removal from traditional learning environments. The frustration and failures caused by a learning disorder can be manifested by a disruptive behavior disorder. In some cases, the disruptive behavior disorder coexists with the learning disorder and the relation is less clear. Children and adolescents with ADHD have particular difficulty maintaining attention, and possibly with processing information. As a result, the same variables that have an impact on their attention also have an impact on their ability to learn. In such instances, they may have a learning disorder and ADHD.

Internalizing disorders such as depression or anxiety may result in an uncharacteristic disinterest in or avoidance of school expectations. If one of the internalizing disorders is present, it is important to clarify whether it is secondary or primary to the academic difficulty. Cognitive and language deficits as well as social skills deficits are often associated with learning

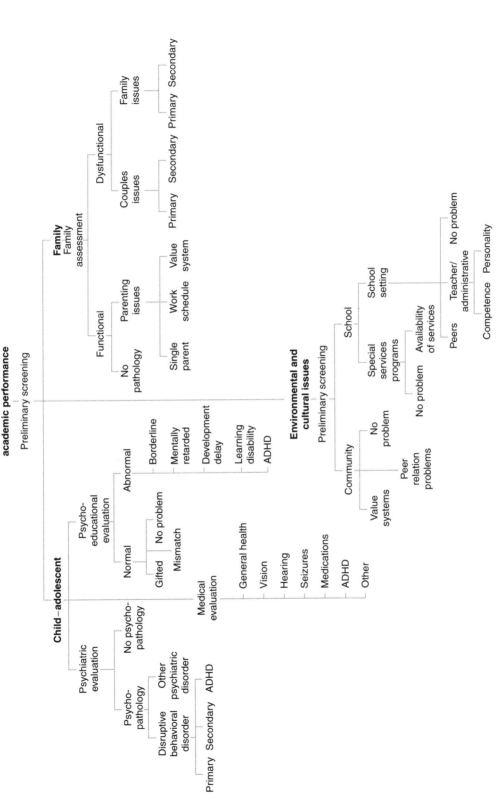

Figure 3-1 *Academic underachievement and the clinical decision-making process. ADHD, Attention-deficit/hyperactivity disorder. (Source: Reprinted from Child Adolesc Psychiatr Clin N Am 2, Ostrander Clinical observations suggesting a learning disability, 249–263, Copyright 1993 with permission from Elsevier.)*

disorders and can contribute to a dysphoric or anxious presentation.

The medical evaluation is necessary to explore the influence of health factors on the individual's availability and ability to learn. Problems in acquiring academic content can be significantly affected by most visual or hearing deficits. Generally poor health can influence the stamina, motivation, and concentration needed to focus adequately on academic demands. Medications used for any purpose might cause sedation or other side effects that may affect the child's ability to learn. Early developmental insults can result in global or focal deficits in neurological development. Undiagnosed seizures, especially *petit mal* and partial complex seizures, can result in difficulties in general cognitive functioning, specific deficits in memory, and problems with attention.

TREATMENT

Treatment is directed at the underlying disabilities by use of educational interventions. Psychological interventions are also directed at any existing emotional, social, or family difficulties. In addition, social skills training may be helpful.

Somatic Treatments

No medication has been found to be effective for treating the learning disorders or motor skills disorder. If the individual with these disorders also has ADHD, it is important that medication be used to minimize the hyperactivity, distractibility, or impulsivity so that the student can be available for learning.

Educational Interventions

The goal of special educational interventions is to help children and adolescents overcome or compensate for their learning disorders or motor skills disorder so that they can succeed in school. These efforts involve remedial and compensatory approaches and use a multisensory approach that facilitates building on all areas of strength while compensating for any areas of weakness. These efforts are to be provided in as close to a regular classroom setting as possible. It is essential that the classroom teacher knows how to adapt the classroom, curriculum, and teaching style to best accommodate each student's areas of difficulty.

Learning disorders such as reading, mathematics, or writing disorders, are not cured. With appropriate interventions, children and adolescents with reading disorders learn to read and spell at a slower rate than do normally developing individuals. It is essential for these students to learn compensatory skills and for the classroom teachers to provide essential accommodations.

Educational Interventions for Developmental Coordination Disorders. The approaches for helping children and adolescents with this disorder focus on academic skills, life skills, or athletic skills. That is, the focus of intervention might be on specific skills needed for school (e.g., handwriting), on dressing and other life skills (e.g., buttoning, zipping, tying, eating), or on skills needed to do better in sports (e.g., catching, hitting, throwing, running).

Psychotherapeutic Interventions

Learning disorders affect all aspects of the child's or adolescent's life. The same processing problems that interfere with reading, writing, mathematics, and language may interfere with communicating with peers and family, with success in sports and activities, and with such daily life skills as dressing oneself or cutting food.

Lack of success in school can lead to a poor self-image and low self-esteem. Some individuals may become anxious or depressed, or a disruptive behavior disorder may develop.

Genetic and family studies show that in about 40% of children and adolescents with learning disabilities (learning disorders), there is a familial pattern. Thus, from an early identification perspective, each sibling must be considered as possibly having a learning disorder. Also, there is a 40% likelihood that one of the parents may also have a learning disorder. This parent may not have known of this problem. If this is true, the parent, for the first time, may be able to understand a lifetime of difficulties or underachievement. Further, when the psychiatrist offers suggestions for this parent, the parent's areas of difficulty must be considered. Do not ask a mother to be more organized when she has been just as disorganized as her child all her life.

Some children or adolescents may need specific individual, behavioral, group, or family therapy. If so, it is critical that the therapist understands the impact that the learning disorder has had on the individual and how these disabilities might affect the process of therapy. As noted earlier, many students with a learning disorder have difficulties with peers and social skills problems. Social skills training might be helpful.

Once the diagnosis is established, it is critical that the clinician explains to the individual and to the parents what the problems are, focusing not only on the areas of learning difficulties but also on the areas of learning strengths.

If the presenting behavior problems are not serious, it may be best first to provide family education and to give some time to see how this new knowledge affects the family. Concurrently, the parents are taught how to advocate for the necessary services within the school system. It may be that once the academic issues are addressed and the family begins to change, the behavior problems will diminish and no further help will be needed.

The next step is family counseling. Parents are taught how to use their knowledge of their son's or daughter's strengths and weaknesses to modify family patterns; select appropriate chores; choose appropriate activities, sports, and camps; and address stresses within the family. Once taught the necessary knowledge about the child or adolescent and the concepts of intervention, families can often move ahead, creatively working out their own problems.

For some children and adolescents, individual behavioral therapy or psychotherapy may be indicated to help them develop new strategies for interacting with peers, parents, and teachers.

Because this form of therapy requires listening and talking, it is important for the therapist to know whether the individual has a disability in these areas. If so, the therapist has to develop ways of accommodating these problems if therapy is to progress. If a speech and language therapist is working with the individual, she or he might offer suggestions.

The initial phases of family therapy might focus on helping the identified individual regain control over his or her behavior and helping the parents retake control of the family. A behavioral management approach is often the first intervention.

Useful interventions attempt to enhance social–cognitive skills and are directed at altering specific behavior patterns. Social–cognitive approaches are based on those cognitive processes that are related to competent, prosocial behavior. Targets of intervention are directed toward the underlying cognitive variables that are linked to positive peer acceptance.

The enhancement of social–cognitive skills typically involves three kinds of skill development: (1) accurate interpretation of social situations; (2) effective use of social behaviors in interactions with others; and (3) the evaluation of one's own performance and the ability to make adjustments, depending on the environmental context.

The first step in developing these skills typically requires the clinician to provide verbal instructions concerning the relevant skills (e.g., conversational skills). The skills are then modeled by the clinician. It is also important to discuss and emphasize positive outcomes associated with these skills. In the process, the clinician must confront and restructure thoughts that may inhibit the desired behaviors. The child is then required to rehearse the skills in simulated conditions, with the clinician providing reinforcement and corrective feedback as warranted. Generalization is stressed through homework assignments whereby skills are attempted in the natural environment and classroom.

COMPARISON OF DSM-IV-TR AND ICD-10 DIAGNOSTIC CRITERIA

In ICD-10, DSM-IV-TR Reading Disorder is referred to as "Specific Reading Disorder" and DSM-IV-TR Mathematics Disorders as "Specific Disorder of Arithmetic Skills." For both of these learning skills disorders, the ICD-10 Diagnostic Criteria for Research suggest that the cutoff be 2 standard deviations below the expected level of reading achievement and mathematics achievement, respectively. In contrast, DSM-IV-TR does not specify a score cutoff, instead recommending that the score be "substantially below that expected, given the person's chronological age, measured intelligence, and age-appropriate education." Furthermore, in contrast to DSM-IV-TR, which permits both to be diagnosed if present, ICD-10 Reading Disorder takes precedence over Mathematics Disorder so that if criteria are met for both, only Reading Disorder is diagnosed.

ICD-10 does not include a Disorder of Written Expression (as in DSM-IV-TR), but instead includes a Specific Spelling Disorder. DSM-IV-TR includes spelling problems as part of the definition of Disorder of Written Expression but requires writing problems in addition to spelling in order to warrant this diagnosis.

Finally, DSM-IV-TR Coordination Disorder is referred to as "Specific Developmental Disorder of motor function" in ICD-10. Furthermore, the ICD-10 Diagnostic Criteria for Research suggest that the cutoff be two standard deviations below the expected level on a standardized test of fine or gross motor coordination.

4

Childhood Disorders: Communication Disorders

The disorders of communication have traditionally been insufficiently familiar to mental health professionals despite the fact that clinical practice is founded upon communication. A knowledge of these disorders is especially of crucial importance in the care of children, since they are deeply interwoven in all aspects of normal development, psychopathology, and the functions of daily life. These disorders share many common features, as noted in Table 4-1. Selective mutism is not regarded as a disorder of communication *per se*, and is included among other disorders of childhood. (Refer to Chapter 9, on childhood anxiety disorders.)

DIAGNOSIS OF COMMUNICATION DISORDERS

It is essential that the mental health professional seeing children is familiar with the expected milestones of speech and language development. This knowledge forms the basis for effective observation in a clinical

Table 4-1	Features Common to All Communication Disorders

Inadequate development of some aspect of communication
Absence (in developmental types) of any demonstrable causes of physical disorder, neurological disorder, global mental retardation, or severe environmental deprivation
Onset in childhood
Long duration
Clinical features resembling the functional levels of younger normal children
Impairments in adaptive functioning, especially in school
Tendency to occur in families
Predisposition toward boys
Multiple presumed etiological factors
Increased prevalence in younger age range
Diagnosis requiring a range of standardized techniques
Tendency toward certain specific associated problems, such as attention-deficit/hyperactivity disorder
Wide range of subtypes and severity

Source: Reprinted from *Psychiatric Disorders in Children and Adolescents*, Baker L, Specific communication disorders, 257–270, Copyright 1990 with permission from Elsevier.

setting (see Figure 4-1 for diagnostic decision tree). The clinician should ask the parents or guardians about the child's speech and language, both in terms of development and in terms of current function. Much can be learned from even a few questions: Does the child seem to hear and understand what is being said? Does the child require visual prompts? Does the child in fact use spoken language to communicate? How long and complicated are his/her sentences? Does the child "make sense" to outsiders? Can he/she be clearly understood even by strangers? Which sounds does the child find difficult? Does the child use unusual volume, pitch, or nasality? Does he/she observe the rules of conversation? Parent–child communication should also be observed.

Children must be assessed in an environment that fosters verbal communication and observed in a variety of interactions because their speech and language vary so much over time in quantity and quality. For younger children, this may best be done in the context of a play situation. The clinician should note how well a child can follow and draw inferences from a conversation. "Production" refers to speech, its fluency, and intelligibility. "Phonation" refers to the utterance of vocal sounds produced by the larynx. "Pragmatics" are those aspects of language that render it useful for social communication beyond the most concrete level. Does the child appreciate the nuances of his/her partner's conversation, as for example, when they signal beginnings and endings of conversations, topic changes, or the child's turn to talk?

Pragmatic language involves nonverbal elements. Deficiencies in this area impair abstraction and may render the individual almost "robotlike." In all cases, observations should be made in as relaxed a fashion as possible, avoiding interrogation or rote exercises. If a child fails to communicate a given item, necessary help including nonverbal prompts should be offered, so that the child has the experience of success. A sense of failure will stifle communication.

Clinical Guide to the Diagnosis and Treatment of Mental Disorders. M. B. First and A. Tasman
© 2006 John Wiley & Sons, Ltd.   ISBN 0 470 019158

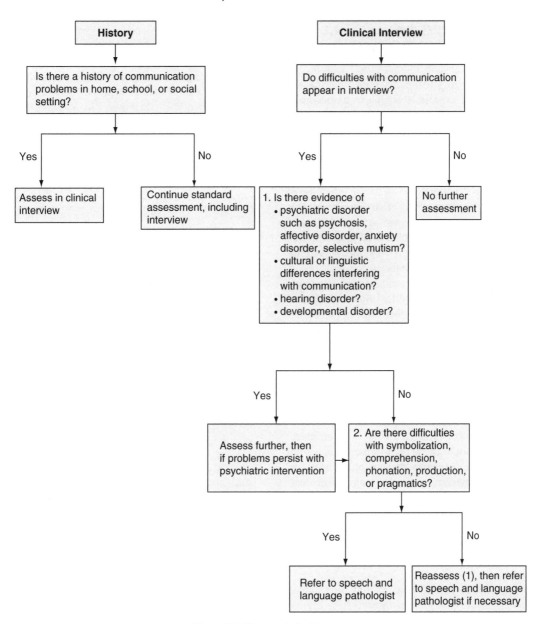

Figure 4-1 *Diagnostic decision tree.*

In school settings, all of the phenomena seen in a clinical interview may also be pursued. Children with communication disorders often feel challenged by the demands of the classroom and may limit or withdraw from conversation entirely. Thus, the task-oriented group setting of the classroom may not elicit a child's best communication. It may, however, demonstrate the practical effectiveness of the child's everyday efforts. At the same time, teachers sometimes have more individual conversations with children than even their parents do, and their experiences may make them the first adults to detect communication problems. In many areas, young children receive some type of formal communication screening in school. Therefore, teacher input is essential in the evaluation of these children.

Clinician should be acutely concerned with the comorbidity of all communication disorders with many mental disorders. Approximately half of the children with a speech or language disorder have some other definable Axis I clinical disorder. Similarly, among children with a psychiatric diagnosis made first, there is a remarkably increased likelihood of speech and language disorders, which often go undetected.

DIAGNOSIS OF EXPRESSIVE LANGUAGE DISORDER AND MIXED RECEPTIVE–EXPRESSIVE LANGUAGE DISORDER

Expressive language disorder denotes an impairment in the development of expressive language. Its diagnosis requires the use of one or more standardized assessment measures that are individually administered. When appropriate instruments are unavailable, as for example, in the case of a member of a population for which no instrument has been standardized, this diagnosis may be made through a thorough functional investigation of an individual's language ability. Individuals with this disorder have expressive language scores well below those obtained from measures of nonverbal intelligence and of receptive language. DSM-IV-TR does not require any particular degree of discrepancy in scores.

The presence of a test score by itself does not define the condition: the affected individual must have clinical symptoms that might include disturbances of vocabulary, grammar (e.g., tenses), or syntax (e.g., sentence length or complexity). The diagnosis of this condition also requires that the individual having it experiences social, academic, or occupational difficulties directly related to the condition. The presence of a mixed receptive–expressive language disorder (MRELD) or a pervasive developmental disorder (PDD) supersedes this diagnosis, and it is not made in their presence. Similarly, it may not be made in the presence of mental retardation, motor or sensory deficits, or environmental observation, unless the expressive language difficulties experienced are beyond what would be expected for individuals with these conditions. This condition may be acquired, as from a medical condition affecting the central nervous system (CNS), or it may be developmental, in the sense of arising early in life without known origin.

The inclusion of MRELD in DSM-IV represented the most significant change from previous classification systems, which posited the existence of receptive language disorders in a solitary form. The existence of this category reflects the clinical observation that receptive language disorders in children seldom, if ever, can occur without concurrent (and perhaps resultant) problems with expression. DSM-IV-TR notes that this is in direct contrast with such entities as Wernicke's aphasia in adults, which affects reception alone. Children with these conditions have significant measurable deficits in standardized individual assessments, of both receptive and expressive language, compared to their similarly assessed nonverbal intelligence.

Children with MRELD may have all the problems of ELD. In addition, they do not understand all that they hear. The deficits may be mild or severe, and at times deceptively subtle, since children with this disorder may conceal them or avoid interaction. All areas and levels of language comprehension may be disturbed. Phonological disorder is especially common among children with these disorders. In addition, many of these children may present at least some manifestations of learning disorders. Other conditions that are broadly considered as neurodevelopmental are also noted in these children, such as motor delays, coordination disorders, and enuresis. The extent of these associations, while apparently considerable, is difficult to quantify because of methodologic variations in the literature. The combination of these disorders and the stress they create frequently lead to adjustment disorders and social withdrawal.

Differential Diagnosis

These disorders are distinguished from each other by the presence or absence of receptive problems. Children with autism may have any or all of the characteristics of the language disorders. However, they have many additional problems including the use of language in a restricted and often stereotypic fashion rather than for communicative purposes. They also have difficulties with a wider range of interactions with persons and objects in their environment, and exhibit a restricted range of behaviors. The language impairments of mental retardation, oral-motor deficits, or environmental deprivation are not diagnosed in this category unless they are well in excess of what is expected. Language impairment due to environmental deprivation tends to improve dramatically with environmental improvement. Sensory deficits, especially hearing impairment, may restrict language development. Any indication of potential hearing impairment, no matter how tenuous, should prompt a referral for an audiologic evaluation. Obviously, hearing and language disorders can and do coexist. Some children develop an acquired aphasia as a complication of general medical illness. This condition is usually temporary; only if it persists beyond the acute course of the medical illness is a language disorder diagnosed.

DIAGNOSIS OF PHONOLOGICAL DISORDER AND STUTTERING

Phonological disorder was formerly known as articulation or developmental articulation disorder. It is characterized by an individual's failure to use speech sounds appropriate for their developmental level and dialect. The affected individual may substitute one sound for another (e.g., /l/ for /r/), omit certain sounds entirely, or exhibit other errors in organization, use, or production of sounds. By definition in DSM-IV-TR these difficulties interfere with social, academic, or occupational functions. The symptoms may occur during development without discernible cause or they may be related to CNS, motor, or sensory dysfunction, or to environmental deprivation. In the latter cases, speech difficulties must be in excess of those usually associated with the particular problem for the diagnosis to be made. This condition ranges in severity from very mild problems to severe disorders, which render speech totally unintelligible.

Stuttering is one of the most commonly recognized disorders of speech. Some occurrence of the symptoms of stuttering is normal in the earlier stages of development, and the condition is properly diagnosed only when the symptoms are perceived to be in excess of what is developmentally expected. Similarly, since occasional symptoms appear in the speech of nearly all persons, the diagnosis is not made unless the disturbances interfere with social, academic, or occupational functioning. The condition may be associated with motoric or sensory deficits; when this is the case, the diagnosis is made only when symptoms exceed those expected with these problems. The characteristic symptoms of stuttering are disturbances in fluency (such as repetitions of sounds, syllables or words, interjections, and circumlocutions) and in time patterning (sound prolongations, broken words, and blocking). "Cluttering," the disturbance in rate and length of speech noted in DSM-III-R, is subsumed in DSM-IV-TR under CD-NOS, or ELD.

Course

The course of PD is much more encouraging than those of other communication disorders. Milder cases may not be discovered until the child starts school. These cases often recover spontaneously, especially if the child does not encounter adverse psychosocial consequences because of his speech. Severe cases associated with anatomic malformations may at times require surgical intervention, and its course and outcome depend upon the results of the surgery. Between these two extremes are children who gradually improve, often to the point of total remission, and whose improvement may be accelerated by speech therapy.

Stuttering usually appears in early childhood, as early as 2 years of age and frequently has its onset around age 5. The onset of stuttering is typically regarded as gradual, with repetition of initial consonants or first words or phrases heard in the beginning. The

disorder can wax and wane during childhood. By early adolescence it abates spontaneously in some cases, and from 60% to 80% of individuals eventually recover totally or to a major extent. Stuttering may persist into adulthood, often leading to adverse social and occupational consequences.

Differential Diagnosis

These conditions should be distinguished from the normal dysfluencies that occur among young children. For example, misarticulation of some sounds, such as /l/, /r/, /s/, /z/, /th/, and /ch/, is common among preschoolers and resolves with age. As with the language disorders, these diagnoses are given in the case of motor or sensory deficit, mental retardation, or environmental deprivation only if the disorder is much more severe than expected in these conditions. Problems limited to voice alone are included under CDNOS.

DIAGNOSIS OF COMMUNICATION DISORDER NOT OTHERWISE SPECIFIED

This category includes disorders that do not meet criteria for other specific communication disorders or do so incompletely. DSM-IV-TR cites voice disorders of pitch, loudness, quality, tone, or resonance, as an example. It is used to describe disorders that do not fit the criteria for any of the other communication disorders and is generally used only to describe voice disorders. These are disorders of pitch, intonation, volume, or resonance. Hyponasality is one example of a voice disorder as characterized by the "adenoidal" speech that brought many children to surgery in an earlier era. Hypernasality, secondary to velopharyngeal insufficiency, may be associated with serious voice problems. Air escapes into the nasal cavity resulting in nasal air emission, snorting, or a nasal grimace during speech.

TREATMENT OF COMMUNICATION DISORDERS

Speech and language therapy, the most important approach for these disorders, typically has three major goals: the development and improvement of communication skills with concurrent remediation of deficits, the development of alternative or augmentative communication strategies where required, and the social habilitation of the individual in regard to communication. Thus, a very great range of approaches and components must be employed in treating children with communication disorders. The speech and language pathologist (SLP) plays the most direct role in

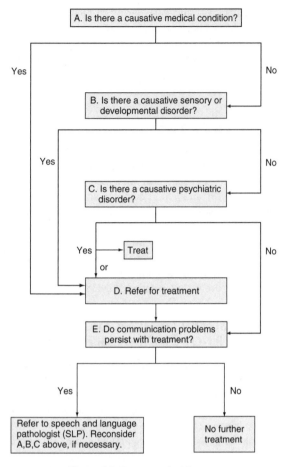

Figure 4-2 *Treatment decision tree.*

treatment of these conditions: this role is illustrated by the diagnostic treatment tree (Figure 4-2).

The mental health professional may have a major role in the treatment of communication disorders. These children and their families may present for psychotherapy or other treatment for disorders based on or related to communication problems. Thus, the clinician may, in the first place, be a case finder or a case manager, facilitating the evaluation and treatment of these disorders by a multidisciplinary team. The demonstrated psychiatric comorbidity of these disorders will necessitate the clinician's involvement on many levels, both as a clinician primarily treating a child, and as a therapist, counselor, and agent of advice and support for the entire family. Psychotherapy does not directly address language disorders, although older literature has cited improvement in stuttering following family and individual treatment. The psychotherapist must, in any event, be sensitive to the manner in which communication disorders can affect or interfere

with the therapeutic process. Nonverbal augments or prompts should be sensitively provided to children who need them.

The role of psychotropic medication in the management of communication disorders is mainly limited to the treatment of comorbid psychiatric problems according to standard practices. Outcome studies of communication therapy, especially for the language disorders, have often been complicated by multiple theories of language development, diagnostic and methodologic variations, lack of standardization of therapeutic techniques, and comorbidity. Thus, the literature in this area is relatively sparse and not always conclusive. Nonresponse to initial treatment may be common, requiring patience and persistence. It is important to note in assessing these issues that, even when communication therapy does not lead to apparent improvements in language beyond developmental improvements, it may still facilitate the child's use of extant language for environmental- and self-control.

COMPARISON OF DSM-IV-TR AND ICD-10 DIAGNOSTIC CRITERIA

Regarding expressive language disorder, the ICD-10 Diagnostic Criteria for Research suggest specific cutoffs for the expressive language scores: 2 standard deviations below the expected level and 1 standard deviation below nonverbal IQ. Furthermore, in contrast to DSM-IV-TR, the diagnosis cannot be made if there are any neurological, sensory, or physical impairments that directly affect the use of spoken language or if there is mental retardation.

For DSM-IV-TR mixed receptive–expressive language disorder, the corresponding ICD-10 disorder is "receptive language disorder." In contrast to DSM-IV-TR, which specifies both expressive and receptive language difficulties because these generally occur together, the ICD-10 definition only mentions deviations in language comprehension. Like with expressive language disorder, the ICD-10 Diagnostic Criteria for Research suggest a cutoff of receptive language scores of 2 standard deviations below the expected level and 1 standard deviation below nonverbal IQ. Furthermore, in contrast to DSM-IV-TR, the diagnosis cannot be made if there are any neurological, sensory, or physical impairments that directly affect receptive language or if there is mental retardation.

As compared to DSM-IV-TR phonological disorder, in which no mention is made of assessment using standardized tests, the ICD-10 Diagnostic Criteria for Research suggest that articulation skills, as assessed on standardized tests, are 2 standard deviations below the expected level and 1 standard deviation below nonverbal IQ. Furthermore, in contrast to DSM-IV-TR, the diagnosis cannot be made if there are any neurological, sensory, or physical impairments that directly affect receptive language or if there is mental retardation.

Regarding stuttering, in contrast to DSM-IV-TR, which establishes clinical significance based on interference with academic or occupational achievement or with social communication, the ICD-10 Diagnostic Criteria for Research establish clinical significance by requiring a minimum duration of at least three months.

CHAPTER

5 Childhood Disorders: Pervasive Developmental Disorders

The pervasive developmental disorders (PDDs) have been more recently conceptualized as the autism spectrum disorders (ASDs) in order to recognize the commonality of these conditions with the paradigmatic disorder, autistic disorder. The ASDs are a group of neurodevelopmental syndromes characterized by disturbances in social interactions, language and communication, and the presence of stereotyped behaviors and interests. Diagnoses subsumed under the category of the ASDs (and PDDs) include Autistic Disorder, Rett's Disorder, Childhood Disintegrative Disorder, Asperger's Disorder, and Pervasive Developmental Disorder Not Otherwise Specified (PDDNOS). A comparison of the definitions of the ASDs is shown in Table 5-1.

More recently, the ASDs have been conceptualized as a spectrum of conditions that are related by the common features of the disorders: difficulties in social interactions and use of language, and restricted interests and repetitive behaviors. The term spectrum implies that there are phenomenological commonalities to these disorders that justify that they are grouped, but that component symptoms in each syndrome vary in severity. Despite the enormous heterogeneity evident in this area, there is increasing evidence that conceptualizing these disorders as a spectrum is useful and valid.

DIAGNOSIS

ASDs are notoriously heterogeneous in their presentation: there may be variability in the particular symptoms manifested in any individual at a given point in time and there may be significant levels of comorbidity. Nonetheless, autism has been consistently one of the most reliably diagnosed disorders of childhood. Accurate diagnosis requires that the clinician looks for the particular symptoms and signs that characterize it: peculiar and deficient modes of social interaction,

---

DSM-IV-TR Diagnostic Criteria

299.00 AUTISTIC DISORDER

A. A total of six (or more) items from (1), (2), and (3), with at least two from (1) and one each from (2) and (3):
  (1) qualitative impairment in social interaction as manifested by at least two of the following:
    (a) marked impairment in the use of multiple nonverbal behaviors such as eye-to-eye gaze, facial expression, body postures, and gestures to regulate social interaction
    (b) failure to develop peer relationships appropriate to developmental level
    (c) a lack of spontaneous seeking to share enjoyment, interests, or achievements with other people (e.g., by a lack of showing, bringing, or pointing out objects of interest)
    (d) lack of social or emotional reciprocity
  (2) qualitative impairments in communication manifested by at least one of the following:
    (a) delay in, or total lack of, the development of spoken language (not accompanied by an attempt to compensate through alternative modes of communication such as gesture or mime)
    (b) in individuals with adequate speech, marked impairment in the ability to initiate or sustain a conversation with others
    (c) stereotyped and repetitive use of language or idiosyncratic language
    (d) lack of varied, spontaneous make-believe play or social imitative play appropriate to developmental level
  (3) restricted repetitive and stereotyped patterns of behavior, interests, and activities, as manifested by at least one of the following:
    (a) encompassing preoccupation with one or more stereotyped and restricted patterns of interest that is abnormal in either intensity or focus
    (b) apparently inflexible adherence to specific, nonfunctional routines or rituals
    (c) stereotyped and repetitive motor mannerisms (e.g., hand or finger flapping or twisting, or complex whole-body movements)
    (d) persistent preoccupation with parts of objects

B. Delays or abnormal functioning in at least one of the following areas, with onset before age 3 years: (1) social interaction, (2) language as used in social communication, or (3) symbolic or imaginative play.
C. The disturbance is not better accounted for by Rett's disorder or childhood disintegrative disorder.

Reprinted with permission from the *Diagnostic and Statistical Manual of Mental Disorders*, 4th ed., Text Rev. Copyright 2000 American Psychiatric Association.

Clinical Guide to the Diagnosis and Treatment of Mental Disorders. M. B. First and A. Tasman
© 2006 John Wiley & Sons, Ltd. ISBN 0 470 019158

DSM-IV-TR Diagnostic Criteria

299.80 Asperger's Disorder

A. Qualitative impairment in social interaction, as manifested by at least two of the following:

   (1) marked impairment in the use of multiple nonverbal behaviors such as eye-to-eye gaze, facial expression, body postures, and gestures to regulate social interaction

   (2) failure to develop peer relationships appropriate to developmental level

   (3) a lack of spontaneous seeking to share enjoyment, interests, or achievements with other people (e.g., by a lack of showing, bringing, or pointing out objects of interest to other people)

   (4) lack of social or emotional reciprocity

B. Restricted repetitive and stereotyped patterns of behavior, interests, and activities, as manifested by at least one of the following:

   (1) encompassing preoccupation with one or more stereotyped and restricted patterns of interest that is abnormal in either intensity or focus

   (2) apparently inflexible adherence to specific, nonfunctional routines or rituals

   (3) stereotyped and repetitive motor mannerisms (e.g., hand or finger flapping or twisting, or complex whole-body movements)

   (4) persistent preoccupation with parts of objects

C. The disturbance causes clinically significant impairment in social, occupational, or other important areas of functioning.

D. There is no clinically significant general delay in language (e.g., single words used by age 2 years, communicative phrases used by age 3 years).

E. There is no clinically significant delay in cognitive development or in the development of age-appropriate self-help skills, adaptive behavior (other than in social interaction), and curiosity about the environment in childhood.

F. Criteria are not met for another specific pervasive developmental disorder or schizophrenia.

Reprinted with permission from the *Diagnostic and Statistical Manual of Mental Disorders*, 4th ed., Text Rev. Copyright 2000 American Psychiatric Association.

deficits in communication, and the focused behaviors and interests.

Many consider the disturbance of social development, including difficulty in developing meaningful attachments and interpersonal reciprocity, to be the central impairment in ASD. There is definitely variation in the clinical presentation. For instance, while many children with ASD will seem aloof and unattached to their parents, many will display age-appropriate separation anxiety. Typically, a child with autistic disorder has abnormal patterns of eye contact and facial expression. When compared with normal children, children with autism fail to consistently maintain eye contact or vary facial expression to establish social contact. These children seem to have considerable difficulty in effectively coordinating social cues. They have difficulty

demonstrating empathy or perceiving or anticipating others' moods or responses. The child with ASD often acts in a socially inappropriate manner or lacks the social responsiveness needed to succeed in social settings, leading to difficulty in the development of close, meaningful relationships. Some children with ASD eventually develop warm, friendly relationships with family while their relationships with peers lag behind considerably, and these deficits typically persist across time.

Another area of difficulty is in the acquisition and proper use of language for communication. It is estimated that only about half of the children with autistic disorder develop functional speech. This is not merely a delay in development of speech; speech patterns may be deviant and idiosyncratic compared with normal children. If autistic children do begin to speak, their babble is frequently decreased in quantity and lacking in vocal experimentation. When children with autistic disorder do acquire some speech, it is often peculiar and lacking in social perspective. Some children with autistic disorder are even loquacious, although their speech tends to be repetitious and self-directed rather than aimed at maintaining a reciprocal dialogue. People with autistic disorder commonly make use of stereotyped speech, including immediate and delayed echolalia, pronoun reversal, and neologisms. Speech usage is often idiosyncratic, may consist of concrete and poorly constructed grammar, may not be used to convey social meaning, and is often literal, lacking in inference, and lacking in imagination. The delivery of speech is frequently abnormal with atypical tone, pitch, and cadence. Paradoxically, children with autistic disorder often have echolalia, in which prosody and other aspects of speech are frequently imitated verbatim.

Individuals with autistic disorder routinely engage in unusual patterns of behavior. Most people with ASD also resist or have significant difficulty with new experiences or transitions. They are commonly resistant to changes in their environment. They often repeatedly perform stereotyped motor acts such as hand clapping or flapping, or peculiar finger movements. These movements frequently occur at the periphery of their vision near their own face. Some children with autistic disorder engage in self-injurious behaviors including biting or striking themselves or banging their heads. This is most likely to occur with severe or profound mental retardation but is also seen in children with autistic disorder without mental retardation. Their play only occasionally involves traditional toys, and objects may be used in ways other than intended (for instance, a doll is used as a hammer), and there is a paucity of make-believe play. Individuals with autistic disorder seem to have unusual sensitivity to some sensory experiences, particularly, specific sounds.

Table 5-1	Comparison of Domains of Diagnostic Criteria for Pervasive Developmental Disorders				
	Autistic Disorder	**Rett's Disorder**	**Childhood Disintegrative Disorder**	**Asperger's Disorder**	**Pervasive Developmental Disorder NOS**
Age at onset	Delays or abnormal functioning in social interaction, language, or play by age 3 years	Apparently normal prenatal development Apparently normal motor development for first 5 months Deceleration of head growth between ages 5 and 48 months	Apparently normal development for at least the first 2 years Clinically significant loss of previously acquired skills before 10 years of age	No clinically significant delay in language, cognitive development, or development of age-appropriate self-help skills, adaptive behavior, and curiosity about the environment in childhood	Category used in cases of pervasive impairment in social interaction and communication, with presence of stereotyped behaviors or interests when criteria are not met for a specific disorder
Social interaction	Qualitative impairment in social interaction, as manifested by at least two of the following: • Marked impairment in the use of multiple nonverbal behaviors (e.g., eye-to-eye gaze) • Failure to develop peer relationships appropriate to developmental level • Lack of spontaneous seeking to share enjoyment with other people • Lack of social or emotional reciprocity	Loss of social engagement early in the course (although often social interaction develops later)	Same as autistic disorder along with loss of social skills (previously acquired)	Same as autistic disorder	
Communication	Qualitative impairments of communication as manifested by at least one of the following: • Delay in, or total lack of, the development of spoken language • Marked impairment in initiating or sustaining a conversation with others, in individuals with adequate speech • Stereotyped and repetitive use of language or idiosyncratic language • Lack of varied, spontaneous make-believe, or imitative play	Severely impaired expressive and receptive language development and severe psychomotor retardation	Same as autistic disorder along with loss of expressive or receptive language previously acquired	No clinically significant delay in language	
Behavior	Restricted, repetitive, and stereotyped patterns of behavior, as manifested by one of the following: • Preoccupation with one or more stereotyped or restricted patterns of interest • Adherence to nonfunctional routines or rituals • Stereotyped and repetitive motor mannerisms • Persistent preoccupation with parts of objects	Loss of previously acquired purposeful hand movement. Appearance of poorly coordinated gait or trunk movements	Same as autistic disorder along with loss of bowel or bladder control, play, motor skills previously acquired	Same as autistic disorder	
Exclusions	Disturbance not better accounted for by Rett's disorder or childhood disintegrative disorder		Disturbance not better accounted for by another PDD or schizophrenia	Criteria are not met for another PDD or schizophrenia	

Source: Reprinted with permission from the *Diagnostic and Statistical Manual of Mental Disorders*, Fourth Edition, Text Revision, Copyright 2000. American Psychiatric Association.

Other problems in autistic disorder and other PDDs include impairment in "joint attention," the sharing or mutual focus on an object or event by two or more people, and the ability to shift attention when the social situation calls for it. Many children with ASD also have symptoms of hyperactivity and difficulty sustaining attention, but these should be distinguished from the joint attentional dysfunction found in all individuals with autistic disorder. Examples of joint attention include social exchanges that require pointing, referential gaze, and gestures showing interest.

Asperger's disorder and autistic disorder, as classically described, share many common features, including an unusual use of pronouns, continuous repetition of certain words or phrases, exhaustive focus of speech on particular topics, difficulty in social reciprocity, engaging in repetitive play, and an excessive focus on certain interests. However, children with Asperger's disorder speak at about the same time as other children do and eventually gain a full complement of language and syntax. Thus, the predominant differentiating feature between autistic disorder and Asperger's disorder is that those with Asperger's disorder do not have a delay in general (i.e., nonsocial) language development.

Rett's disorder is a developmental disorder that preferentially strikes girls and differs substantially from autistic disorder past the toddler stage. Typically, a child with Rett's disorder has an uneventful prenatal and perinatal course that continues through at least the first 6 months. With the onset of the classic form of the disease, there is deceleration of head growth, usually between 5 months and 4 years of age. In toddlerhood, the manifestations can be similar to autistic disorder in which there is frequently impairment in language and social development, along with presence of stereotyped motor movements. In particular, there is a loss of acquired language, restricted interest in social contact or interactions, and the start of hand-wringing, clapping, or tapping in the midline of the body. This type of activity begins after purposeful hand movement is lost. Serious psychomotor retardation as well as receptive and expressive language impairments sets in. Between the ages of 1 and 4 years, truncal apraxia and gait apraxia typically ensue.

Childhood disintegrative disorder and autistic disorder have some similarities in that they both involve deficits in social interaction and communication as well as repetitive behaviors. However, the symptoms of childhood disintegrative disorder appear abruptly or in the period of a few months' time after 2 years or more of normal development. There is generally no prior serious illness or insult, although a few cases have been linked to certain brain ailments such as measles,

encephalitis, leukodystrophies, or other diseases. With the onset of childhood disintegrative disorder, the child loses previously mastered cognitive, language, and motor skills and regresses to such a degree that there is loss of bowel and bladder control. Children with childhood disintegrative disorder tend to lose abilities that would normally allow them to take care of themselves, and their motor activity contains fewer complex, repetitive behaviors than autistic disorder. Some children with this disorder experience regression that occurs for a time and then becomes stable. The majority of children with this disorder deteriorate to a severe level of mental retardation; a few retain selected abilities in specific areas. Differential diagnosis of childhood disintegrative disorder requires obtaining a particularly thorough developmental history, history of course of illness, and an extensive neurological evaluation and testing.

PDDNOS (also known as atypical autism) should be reserved for cases in which there are qualitative impairments in reciprocal social development, and either communication or imaginative and flexible interests are met, but not the full criteria for a specific PDD. It is important in the education of parents, teachers, and colleagues to be clear that PDDNOS is closely related to autistic disorder, because many families have been given diagnoses of both autistic disorder and PDDNOS and have the mistaken impression that this represents strong diagnostic disagreement between clinicians.

The diagnosis of ASD first involves completing a comprehensive psychiatric examination (Table 5-2). The clinician should obtain a full developmental history,

Table 5-2	Suggested Workup for Children and Adults with Autistic Disorder or Other Pervasive Developmental Disorders

History

Particular attention to:
    Developmental phases of language, social interactions, play
    Family history of psychiatric and neurological disease

Physical examination
Thorough physical examination including a search for:
    Neurological problems
    Cardiac problems
    Congenital anomalies
    Skin lesions or abnormalities
    Dysmorphology

Psychological evaluation
    Autism Diagnostic Interview—Revised
    Autism Diagnostic Observation Schedule
    Cognitive testing (e.g., Differential Abilities Scales)
    Vineland Adaptive Behavior Scales

Speech and language evaluation

Audiological evaluation

Visual acuity evaluation

including all information regarding pregnancy and delivery.

In terms of direct observation, the child with ASD poses some unique challenges. Because of his or her dislike of novelty, the first visit to the clinician's office is sometimes an anxiety-provoking undertaking. If the child is having difficulty, it is usually preferable, especially on the first visit, to allow the parents to intervene. This will allow the clinician to see how (effectively) the family responds to this distress, and how the child responds to the efforts of caregivers to soothe the child. During observation, the clinician needs to assess social interaction, communication, unusual behaviors, and all other information in the context of developmental level.

A full physical examination should be undertaken. In addition to the standard comprehensive examination, the clinician should observe for dysmorphic features and unusual dermatologic lesions. The clinician must maintain a high suspicion for seizures in this population, both when taking the history and during the examination. A full neurological examination should be done with an emphasis on looking at motor impairments like hypotonia and apraxia.

There are no diagnostic laboratory tests for ASD. What laboratory tests are ordered as a part of an initial workup is dependent on history and examination results.

All children with autism require a careful language assessment that may include hearing testing and assessment of expressive and receptive, verbal and nonverbal language. Speech and language therapists trained to work with this population are an essential part of the assessment team.

Children with ASD should have a neuropsychological assessment at the time of initial assessment and at periodic intervals thereafter. The initial evaluation helps establish the diagnosis and a baseline level of functioning. Additionally, it can be utilized to make the appropriate adjustments in the child's educational plan. The later evaluations serve to chart progress, evaluate the success of (pharmacological, behavioral, and academic) interventions, and assess for possible regression in particular areas.

Differential Diagnosis

Although there may initially be some difficulty in differentiating ASD from other syndromes (Table 5-3), especially in the context of considerable comorbidity, the diagnosis usually becomes clear with careful differentiation. Mental retardation commonly occurs in ASD,

Table 5-3	Differential Diagnosis of Autistic Disorder and Other Pervasive Developmental Disorders

Developmental language disorder
Mental retardation
Acquired epileptic aphasia (Landau–Kleffner's syndrome)
Fragile X syndrome
Schizophrenia
Selective mutism
Psychosocial deprivation
Hearing impairment
Visual impairment
Traumatic brain injury
Dementia
Metabolic disorders (inborn errors of metabolism, e.g., phenylketonuria)

and children with mental retardation may present with stereotyped movements or obsessiveness. However, the child with mental retardation and not with ASD will have social and communicative skills commensurate with their level of overall development.

Differentiating ASD from childhood schizophrenia is not usually difficult. The onset of psychosis in childhood is extraordinarily rare, and hallucinations and delusions are not a part of the ASD picture. It is important not to diagnose some of the atypical features in ASD as psychotic and equally important to recognize that verbal individuals with ASD have impaired language that should not be confused with schizophrenia. One should also recognize that onset of symptoms before age 3 is almost never consistent with schizophrenia. Selective mutism can be differentiated by the child's ability to interact normally in some environments.

Children exposed to severe neglect can sometimes present with symptoms that look like ASD, but these symptoms will usually show dramatic improvement when the child is in a more appropriate environment.

Perhaps the most difficult differentiation is in a child with severe obsessive–compulsive disorder (OCD) who also has unusual interests and is somewhat rigid in terms of being inflexible to changes in routines or transitions to a new activity. It is even further complicated if attentional problems coexist. In these cases, it is important to emphasize the social difficulties of children with ASD; even if the child with OCD is difficult interpersonally, his or her ability to maintain eye contact, interpret social situations and emotions, and otherwise interact socially is relatively preserved.

TREATMENT

Developing a comprehensive individual intervention program for a child with ASD is a daunting task for the child's parents (Figure 5-1). Each child is unique, with

Identification of developmental delay by caretaker

Evaluation by pediatrician

↓↓
↓↓ Referral for specialty testing
↓↓

ADOS, ADI, measures of intellectual functioning and daily functioning, full physical, history, and labs

↓↓
↓↓ Autism spectrum disorder established
↓↓

Initiation of treatment includes:

1. Implementing changes in the child's academic program including relevant changes in the curriculum in order to tailor it to the child's specific needs, as well as probable speech, occupational, and physical therapy.

2. The use of behavioral programs in order to improve social and communication difficulties as well as address negative behaviors.

3. Examination of any symptoms that may be potential target symptoms for a pharmacological intervention.

Figure 5-1 *An example of the typical progression from identification, to evaluation, to treatment of a child with ASD (ADOS, Autism Diagnostic Observation Schedule; ADI, Autism Diagnostic Inventory).*

a different set of difficulties as well as strengths. The child's primary physician must work with the parents to help make this task less overwhelming. This usually means maintaining a tempered optimism about the future and providing encouragement without being unrealistic. The physician can anticipate being asked about a wide array of alternative treatments being offered in the community, which vary enormously in their claims, in the integrity of those making the claims, and in their ultimate safety and utility. It is helpful to listen and then educate the family, at a level commensurate with their sophistication, about how to analyze and interpret claims and the science underlying these treatments. Most parents are able to incorporate information about the need for controlled studies, replication, and the importance of information being published in peer-reviewed journals.

Autistic disorder is recognized as a chronic disorder with a changing course requiring a long-term course of treatment that includes the necessity of intervention with various treatments at different times (Table 5-4). At the present time, most treatments for the ASDs are symptom directed. Thus, treatments of the other ASDs are the same as those used in autistic disorder because similar types of symptoms are targeted for treatment in each of these disorders. Given that there is no cur-

Table 5-4	Summary of Treatment Principles
Psychosocial Interventions	
Educational	
Curricula that target communication	
Behavioral techniques	
Structured milieu	
Vocational training and placement: other specialized interventions such as speech and language therapy, physical therapy, and occupational therapy	
Social skills training	
Individual psychotherapy	
for high-functioning	
individuals	
Medical Interventions	
Cohesive physician–patient relationship	
Supportive measures with families coping with autistic disorder	
Behavioral treatment	
Pharmacotherapy to address problem signs and symptoms	

rent cure for autistic disorder or the other ASDs goals of treatment should encompass the short-term and long-term needs of the individual and his or her family (Table 5-5). Goals for treatment, in terms of four quintessential aims, include:

1. the advancement of normal development, particularly regarding cognition, language, and socialization;

Table 5-5	Goals for Treatment

Advancement of normal development, particularly regarding cognition, language, and socialization
Promotion of learning and problem solving
Reduction of behaviors that impede learning
Assistance of families coping with autistic disorder
Treatment of comorbid psychiatric disorders

2. the promotion of learning and problem solving;
3. the reduction of behaviors that impede the learning process;
4. the assistance of families coping with autism.

These goals are broad in nature; therefore, it is key to separate these goals into immediate and long-term needs for each individual with ASD. Each goal requires a distinct scheme of its own.

Every attempt should be made to achieve treatment goals in a community-based environment since institutionalization may hinder a child's ability to learn means of functioning and adapting in typical social settings. Community-based treatment can usually be maintained, except in times of extreme stress or need, during which time a child (and family) might benefit from respite care or brief hospitalization. Effective treatment often entails setting appropriate expectations for the child and adjusting the child's environment to foster success.

Psychological Treatments

Because the autistic individual often requires diverse treatments and services simultaneously, the role of the primary physician is to be the coordinator of services. Frequent visits with the child and the child's caretakers initially allow the physician to assess the individual needs of the child while establishing a therapeutic alliance. An effective approach often calls for the services of a number of professionals working in a multidisciplinary fashion. This group may include psychiatrists, pediatricians, pediatric neurologists, psychologists, special educators, speech and language therapists, social workers, and other specialized therapists.

There is significant controversy over what particular forms of therapy are best for children with ASD. Some of this controversy is a result of claims of children making dramatic improvements with some of these therapies.

A prerequisite to putting a behavioral plan in place with a child with ASD is to identify the problem behaviors. These behaviors often include interfering repetitive actions, self-injurious behaviors, or aggression. While there is little difficulty in identifying these highly visible behaviors, what is much more difficult is (1) determining the antecedents to these behaviors and (2) knowing what constitutes an appropriate reaction to these behaviors on the part of the caregiver. To determine the antecedent is often extraordinarily difficult, since it is often not apparent as to what exactly happened in the environment that stimulated the behavior. This is particularly true if the behavior is chronic and has developed some autonomous function (i.e., no longer a stimulus–response event). To make things more complicated, it could be internal perception or the meaning of what happened in a child with autism (poor language and socially nonresponsive) that may have initiated the behavior.

The key to success is a gradual shaping of the behavior rather than dramatic expectations and harsh consequences. One should begin intervention by evaluating possible underlying stimuli or predisposing factors for the behavior. Strategies include determining when, where, and for how long an activity can take place. Additional strategies include making environmental changes that reduce anxiety and even ignoring behaviors that do not create undue problems.

Up to 50% of children with ASD will not acquire useful language. For those with some but not fully intact language skills, speech therapy is an important part of therapeutic and academic planning. An emphasis on the social use of language is often helpful, and when the child can articulate some of his or her needs, there is often a reduction in problem behaviors.

Longitudinal studies indicate that children who have not acquired useful language by the age of 7 usually have long-standing verbal communication difficulties. For these children, it is often helpful to devise an alternative means of communication. Some children can learn sign language, although there is great variability in how much each child is able to learn, difficulties with generalizing to environments other than where signs are learned, and the fact that signs continue to be used mostly to satisfy needs rather than being utilized in a spontaneous social sense. Additionally, it seems to be best to continue to pair signs with appropriate vocalizations, however limited. Alternatively (or additionally), the use of augmentative communication systems may be helpful. Irrespective of the technique used, establishing a consistent method of communication is central to the treatment of individuals with ASD.

Problems with social interactions, especially reciprocal social interactions, are common to every person with ASD. Helping individuals with ASDs address these challenges is difficult but also critical for enhancing overall functioning.

Three primary techniques can be effectively utilized:

1. **Establish proximity**. Proximity refers to the fact that it is very helpful to have the child with ASD near other children in the environment. The mere proximity increases the likelihood of interaction and imitation as well as positive social reinforcement.
2. **Use prompts and reinforcement**. The use of prompts relates to having specific cues to use previously learned behaviors in social settings (e.g., "Raise your hand if you have a question"). Attention to reinforcement means that even a less than fully competent attempt at appropriate social behavior, even if it is a response to a prompt, gets clear and effective reinforcement when it occurs (e.g., calling on the child promptly when he raises his hand to ask a question and also saying "You did a good job when you raised your hand to ask the question"). Teaching such prompting and reinforcement should be for everyone who interacts with the individual with ASD.
3. **Encourage peer initiation**. It is helpful to train peers who are likely to interact with the child or adult with ASD in techniques for initiating social contact. For many individuals, this means explaining the disability and dealing with fears or biases. For others, it may mean encouraging them to persist in their attempts at engagement, even in the face of limited, inappropriate, or inadequate responses. Persistence usually leads to familiarity and eventually to some level of social engagement.

Considering the many needs of the child with ASD, academic resources and placement naturally emerge as important components to the child's overall treatment. The reasons for this are manifold. First and foremost, schools are where children go to acquire social skills and acquaintances, as well as academic skills. Second, schools often have a variety of skilled professionals who are trained to provide necessary services for the individual with ASD. And, finally, in the United States, all public schools have a statutory obligation to provide all children (even those with disabilities) with a free and appropriate education in the least restrictive environment. Thus, schools often become the base and the requisite individualized educational plan (IEP)

becomes the road map of interventions for children with ASD.

Somatic Treatments

At this time, there are no pharmacological agents with US Food and Drug Administration (FDA) approved labeling specific for the treatment of autistic disorder or other PDDs in either children or adults. This is all the more problematic because many of the symptoms commonly seen in autistic disorder and other PDDs (rituals, aggressive behavior, and hyperactivity) are also commonly seen in children, adolescents, and adults with mental retardation but without a PDD. Some of the pharmacological strategies for the treatment of autistic disorder have been extrapolated from studies of related conditions, largely in adults, including attention-deficit/hyperactivity disorder and OCD. While there may not be FDA-approved treatments, there are treatment options available. However, clinicians and families should be reminded before any treatment is initiated that (1) current treatments target symptoms, (2) current treatments do not target a specific etiological mechanism for ASD, (3) anecdotal reports do not establish efficacy, effectiveness, or safety for any treatment, (4) controlled, double-blind trials (preferably with replication) are the contemporary standard for determining if a treatment is safe and appropriate, and (5) all treatments have side effects.

Before specific pharmacological agents are discussed, it must be stressed that one should not use psychopharmacological agents with the expectation that they will cure children with autistic disorder. Although this seems obvious, one should realize that many parents and teachers of children with autistic disorder expect medication to eliminate core social, cognitive, and communication dysfunction. There is no pharmacological substitute for appropriate educational, behavioral, psychotherapeutic, vocational, and recreational programming. It is essential to remember and to remind parents, teachers, and others that medication should always be seen as an adjunct to these core interventions that address the developmental challenges associated with these disorders. The clinician providing the medication should reiterate this message to the parents and others involved in the child's treatment by consistently reminding them of the specific behavioral targets of the medication, and assessing the effectiveness of the medication in the context of change in these behavioral symptoms, and how the pharmacotherapy facilitates the other interventions.

Table 5-6	Psychopharmacological Approach to Presenting Symptoms in Pervasive Developmental Disorders

Rituals, Compulsions, Irritability

Potent serotonin transporter inhibitors
   Selective serotonin reuptake inhibitor
      Fluoxetine 5–80 mg/d in a single dose
      Paroxetine 2.5–50 mg/d in one or two divided doses
      Sertraline 25–200 mg/d in one or two divided doses
      Fluvoxamine 25–300 mg/d in two or three divided doses
      Citalopram 5–40 mg/d in a single or two divided doses
   Tricyclic antidepressants
      Clomipramine 25–250 mg/d in one or two divided doses

Hyperactivity, Distractibility, Impulsivity

Stimulant medications
   Methylphenidate 5–60 mg/d in three to five divided doses
   Dextroamphetamine 5–60 mg/d in three to five divided doses
Clonidine 0.05–0.3 mg/d in one to three divided doses or by transdermal skin patch
Naltrexone 0.5–2.0 mg/kg/d in a single dose

Aggression, Irritability

Sympatholytics
   Propranolol 20–400 mg/d in three to four divided doses
   Nadolol 40–400 mg/d in a single dose
Anticonvulsants
   Carbamazepine to a blood level of 4–12 ng/mL
   Valproate to a blood level of 50–100 ng/mL
Lithium to a serum level of 0.8–1.2 mEq/L
Neuroleptics
Naltrexone 0.5–2.0 mg/kg/d in a single dose

The use of medications to treat autistic disorder and other ASDs appears to have significant potential as an adjunct to educational, environmental, and social interventions. It is a reasonable goal for the pharmacotherapist to adopt the judicious use of psychopharmacological agents, such as SSRIs or Clomipramine (Table 5-6) to assist in alleviating symptoms that have been found to respond to pharmacological intervention. This focus on facilitating adaptation requires attention to five important principles:

1. Environmental manipulations, including behavioral treatment, may be as effective as, if not more effective than, medication for selected symptomatic treatment.
2. It is essential that the living arrangement for the individual must ensure safe and consistent administration and monitoring of the medication to be used.
3. Individuals with autistic disorder and other ASDs often have other DSM-IV-TR Axis I disorders. If a comorbid DSM-IV-TR Axis I disorder is present, standard treatment for that disorder should be initiated first.
4. Medication should be selected on the basis of potential effects on target symptoms and there should be an established way of specifically monitoring the response to the treatment over time.
5. A careful assessment of the risk/benefit ratio must be made before initiating treatment and, to the extent possible, the individual's caretakers and the individual must understand the risks and benefits of the treatment.

Antidepressants. SSRI medications are most effective when insistence on routines or rituals are present to the point of manifest anxiety or aggression in response to interruption of the routines or rituals, or after the onset of another disorder such as major depressive disorder or OCD. The common side effects associated with SSRIs are motor restlessness, insomnia, elation, irritability, and decreased appetite, each of which may occur alone or, more often, together. Because many of these symptoms may be present in the often cyclical natural course of ASD before the medication is initiated, the emergence of new symptoms, a different quality of the symptoms, and occurrence of these symptoms in a new cluster are clues that the symptoms are side effects of medication rather than part of the natural course of the disorder.

Stimulants. Small but significant reductions in inattention and hyperactivity ratings may be seen in children with autistic disorder in response to stimulants such as methylphenidate and dextroamphetamine. However, stereotypies may worsen, so drug trials must always be assessed to determine whether the therapeutic effects outweigh side effects. A key distinction in assessing attentional problems of children with ASD is the distinction between poor sustained attention (characteristic of children with attention-deficit/hyperactivity disorder) and poor joint attention (characteristic of children with autistic disorder). Problems in joint attention require educational and behavioral interventions or treatment of rituals with a potent serotonin transporter inhibitor. Problems in maintenance of attention of the type seen in attention-deficit/hyperactivity disorder are more likely to respond to stimulants.

Sympatholytics. The α2-adrenergic receptor agonist clonidine may reduce irritability as well as hyperactivity and impulsivity; however, tolerance developed several months after initiation of the treatment in each child who was treated long-term. Tolerance was not prevented by transdermal skin patch administration of the drug. However, tolerance may have been reduced in several cases by administering clonidine in the morning and then 6 to 8 hours later with a 16- to 18-hour interval between the last dose of one day and the first dose of the next day. If tolerance does develop, the dose should not be increased because tolerance to sedation does not occur, and sedation may lead to increased aggression due to disinhibition or decreased cognitive control of impulses. Adrenergic receptor antagonists, such as propranolol and nadolol, have not been tested in double-blind trials in ASD. However, open trials have reported the use of these medications in the treatment of aggression and impulsivity in developmental disorders.

Typical Neuroleptics. Reduction of fidgetiness, interpersonal withdrawal, speech deviance, and stereotypies has been documented in response to Trifluoperazine, thioridazine, haloperidol, and pimozide. However, individuals with autistic disorder are as vulnerable to potentially irreversible tardive dyskinesia as any other group of young children with a mental disorder. Owing to the often earlier age at initiation of pharmacotherapy, individuals with ASD treated with typical neuroleptics may be at higher risk because of the potential increased lifetime exposure of medication. These medications also have significant additional side effects of varying sorts and severity that should significantly limit their routine use in the care of individuals with ASD, especially as first-line treatments.

Atypical Neuroleptics. Because of the positive response of many children with autistic disorder to typical neuroleptics, similar medications with reduced risk of tardive dyskinesia must be considered. In addition, atypical neuroleptics are often effective in treating the negative symptoms of schizophrenia, which seem similar to several of the social deficits in autistic disorder. Both risperidone and olanzapine have shown promise in reducing hyperactivity, impulsivity, aggressiveness, and obsessive preoccupations. It seems clear that atypical neuroleptics will likely play a role for the treatment of carefully selected individuals with severe symptoms of ASD.

Anticonvulsants. Because 25–33% of individuals with autistic disorder have seizures, the psychopharmacological management of individuals with autistic disorder or other ASD must take into consideration the past or current history of epilepsy and the potential role of anticonvulsants. Unfortunately, very few studies have been undertaken in this area. In a small open trial of divalproex in 2001, 10 of 14 individuals responded favorably, showing improvements in affective stability,

impulsivity, and aggression. The anticonvulsant class to be avoided, when possible, is the category comprising barbiturates (e.g., phenobarbital). Because barbiturates have been associated with hyperactivity, depression, and cognitive impairment, they should be changed to an alternative drug, depending on the seizure type. In addition, phenytoin (Dilantin) is sedating and causes hypertrophy of the gums and hirsutism, which may contribute to the social challenges for people with autistic disorder. Carbamazepine and valproate may have positive psychotropic effects, particularly when cyclical irritability, insomnia, and hyperactivity are present. Several children with autistic disorder were treated with valproic acid after electroencephalographical abnormalities were found. These children had an improvement in behavioral symptoms associated with autistic disorder after valproate treatment.

Naltrexone. Naltrexone has little efficacy in treating the core social and cognitive symptoms of autistic disorder. It may have, however, a role in the treatment of self-injurious behavior, although the controlled data are equivocal. Potential side effects include nausea and vomiting. Controlled trials in autistic disorder have not shown liver dysfunction or other physical side effects. Naltrexone may have an adverse effect on the outcome of Rett's disorder.

Lithium. Adolescents and adults with autistic disorder often exhibit symptoms in a cyclic manner and so there is much interest in how these individuals might respond to agents typically used in bipolar disorder. A single open trial of lithium revealed no significant improvement in symptoms in individuals with autistic disorder without bipolar disorder.

Anxiolytics. Benzodiazepines have not been studied systematically in children and adolescents with autistic disorder. However, their use in reducing anxiety in short-term treatment, such as before dental procedures, is similar to their use in management of anxiety in people without a PDD.

COMPARISON OF DSM-IV-TR AND ICD-10 DIAGNOSTIC CRITERIA

The DSM-IV-TR and ICD-10 item sets and diagnostic algorithms for autistic disorder are almost identical. However, the ICD-10 exclusion criterion is considerably more broad, requiring that a number of other disorders should be considered instead (e.g., early onset schizophrenia, mental retardation with an associated emotional or behavioral disorder). In ICD-10, this disorder is referred to as childhood autism.

The DSM-IV-TR and ICD-10 item sets and diagnostic algorithms for Rett's disorder and Asperger's disorder are almost identical. In ICD-10, these disorders are referred to as Rett's syndrome and Asperger's syndrome, respectively.

Regarding childhood disintegrative disorder, the DSM-IV-TR and ICD-10 item sets and diagnostic algorithms are identical except for the C criterion, in which ICD-10 also allows for a "general loss of interest in objects and the environment." In ICD-10, this disorder is referred to as other childhood disintegrative disorder.

Childhood Disorders: Attention-Deficit and Disruptive Behavior Disorders

DIAGNOSIS

Attention-deficit/hyperactivity disorder (ADHD), conduct disorder (CD), and oppositional-defiant disorder (ODD) form the attention-deficit and disruptive behavior disorders (AD-DBDs) in DSM-IV-TR. As a group, these are the most common disorders of childhood. There is also an increasing recognition that these disorders continue into adulthood. In DSM-IV-TR, ADHD is defined as a persistent pattern of inattention and/or hyperactivity–impulsivity that is more frequently displayed and more severe than is typically observed in individuals at a comparable level of development. Three subtypes of ADHD are identified: (1) a predominantly hyperactive–impulsive type, (2) a predominantly inattentive type, and (3) a combined type. In order to qualify for the diagnosis, at least some of the symptoms must have been present and caused impairment before age 7 years. Additionally, some symptoms causing impairment in social or academic/occupational functioning must be evident in more than one setting. ADHD can be diagnosed in individuals of all ages, although it is sometimes difficult to establish the childhood onset of symptoms in older individuals.

The essential feature of CD is a repetitive and persistent pattern of behavior in which the basic rights of others or major age-appropriate societal norms or rules are violated. Similar to ADHD, symptoms of CD are seen in multiple settings and cause significant impairment in functioning. Adults with conduct problems, whose behavior does not meet criteria for antisocial personality disorder, may have symptoms that meet criteria for CD and thus qualify for the diagnosis. Subtypes of CD are determined on the basis of age of onset. The childhood-onset subtype is diagnosed in children who show at least one of the behaviors before the age of 10 years, while the adolescent-onset subtype is characterized by the absence of any CD behaviors before 10 years of age.

The essential feature of ODD is a recurrent pattern of negativistic, defiant, disobedient, and hostile behavior toward authority figures that persists for at least 6 months.

The rationale for grouping ADHD, CD, and ODD is that similar areas of difficulty are present in children with these disorders. Academic difficulties, poor social skills, and overrepresentation of boys are among the shared characteristics. Further, the three disorders demonstrate a commonality of core symptoms, with impulsivity being prominent in all three conditions. Not surprisingly, there is a high degree of comorbidity among the three disorders.

The clinical evaluation of a child with possible AD-DBD requires a multisource, multimethod approach. In addition to clinical interviews of parents and children, supplemental information may be obtained from school reports, rating scales completed by teachers and parents, neuropsychological test data and direct observations of the child. In addition, several structured and semistructured interviews are available, although these tend to be used primarily in research settings. Generally, adults are considered to be the best informants of disruptive behaviors, although children and adolescents may provide important data regarding internalizing symptoms and some infrequent behavior problems, such as antisocial acts.

Rating scales facilitate the systematic acquisition of information about the child's behavior in different settings in a cost-effective manner. Most are standardized and provide scores that are norm referenced by age and gender. The systematic use of these instruments ensures that a complete set of specific behaviors is assessed at different points in time, enabling comparisons over the course of treatment.

Clinical Guide to the Diagnosis and Treatment of Mental Disorders. M. B. First and A. Tasman
© 2006 John Wiley & Sons, Ltd.   ISBN 0 470 019158

DSM-IV-TR Diagnostic Criteria

314.0x ATTENTION-DEFICIT/HYPERACTIVITY DISORDER

A. Either (1) or (2)

(1) Six (or more) of the following symptoms of "inattention" have persisted for at least 6 months to a degree that is maladaptive and inconsistent with developmental level:

Inattention
(a) often fails to give close attention to details or makes careless mistakes in schoolwork, work, or other activities.
(b) often has difficulty sustaining attention in tasks or play activities.
(c) often does not seem to listen when spoken to directly.
(d) often does not follow through on instructions and fails to finish schoolwork, chores, or duties in the workplace.
(e) often has difficulty organizing tasks and activities.
(f) often avoids, dislikes, or is reluctant to engage in tasks that require sustained mental effort.
(g) often loses things necessary for tasks or activities.
(h) is often easily distracted by extraneous stimuli.
(i) is often forgetful in daily activities.

(2) Six (or more) of the following symptoms of "hyperactivity–impulsivity" have persisted for at least 6 months to a degree that is maladaptive and inconsistent with developmental level:

Hyperactivity
(a) often fidgets with hands or feet or squirms in seat.
(b) often leaves seat in classroom or in other situations in which remaining seated is expected.
(c) often runs about or climbs excessively in situations in which it is inappropriate (in adolescents or adults, may be limited to subjective feelings of restlessness).
(d) often has difficulty playing or engaging in leisure activities quietly.
(e) is often "on the go" or often acts as if "driven by a motor."
(f) often talks excessively.

Impulsivity
(g) often blurts out answers before questions have been completed.
(h) often has difficulty awaiting turn.
(i) often interrupts or intrudes on others.

B. Some hyperactive–impulsive or inattentive symptoms that caused impairment were present before age 7 years.
C. Some impairment from the symptoms is present in two or more settings (e.g., at school [work] and at home).
D. There must be clear evidence of clinically significant impairment in social, academic, or occupational functioning.
E. The symptoms do not occur exclusively during the course of a Pervasive Developmental Disorder, Schizophrenia, or other Psychotic Disorder and are not better accounted for by another mental disorder (e.g., Mood Disorder, Anxiety Disorder, Dissociative Disorder, or a Personality Disorder).

Code based on type:
314.01 Attention-Deficit/Hyperactivity Disorder, Combined Type: if both Criteria A1 and A2 are met for the past 6 months;
314.00 Attention-Deficit/Hyperactivity Disorder, Predominantly Inattentive Type: if Criterion A1 is met but Criterion A2 is not met for the past 6 months;
314.01 Attention-Deficit/Hyperactivity Disorder, Predominantly Hyperactive-Impulsive Type: if Criterion A2 is met but Criterion A1 is not met for the past 6 months.
Coding note: For individuals (especially adolescents and adults) who currently have symptoms that no longer meet full criteria, "In Partial Remission" should be specified.

Reprinted with permission from the *Diagnostic and Statistical Manual of Mental Disorders*, 4th ed., Text Rev. Copyright 2000 American Psychiatric Association.

There is an ever-growing number of rating scales, but the most commonly used are the Conners Teachers Rating Scale—Revised (CTRS-R) and the Child Behavior Checklist (CBCL), which are available in parent and teacher versions and possess solid normative bases. Rating scales have several limitations, and diagnoses should not be made on the bases of these data alone. Interviews with children and their parents form the core of the clinical evaluation. In clinical practice, interviews usually follow a loosely structured format with a flexible approach that allows for the in-depth exploration of relevant clinical information. It is essential that the interviewer directly enquires about

all symptoms of ADHD and common comorbidities, and therefore some structured questioning is usually required.

Psychological and cognitive test performance is generally not required to determine the presence of an AD-DBD. Nevertheless, because the AD-DBDs are frequently associated with learning problems, neuropsychological testing may be indicated, particularly when assessment of cognitive functioning is required. Information from a neuropsychological and/or educational evaluation can often be used to supplement the clinical evaluation by providing an understanding of the individual child's level of cognitive and attentional

DSM-IV-TR Diagnostic Criteria

312.8x CONDUCT DISORDER

A. A repetitive and persistent pattern of behavior in which the basic rights of others or major age-appropriate societal norms or rules are violated, as manifested by the presence of three (or more) of the following criteria in the past 12 months, with at least one criterion present in the past 6 months.

Aggression to people and animals

    (1) often bullies, threatens, or intimidates others.
    (2) often initiates physical fights.
    (3) has used a weapon that can cause serious physical harm to others.
    (4) has been physically cruel to people.
    (5) has been physically cruel to animals.
    (6) has stolen while confronting a victim.
    (7) has forced someone into sexual activity.

Destruction of property

    (1) has deliberately engaged in fire setting with the intention of causing serious damage.
    (2) has deliberately destroyed others' property.

Deceitfulness or theft

    (1) has broken into someone else's house, building or car.
    (2) often lies to obtain goods or favors or to avoid obligations.
    (3) has stolen items of nontrival value without confronting a victim.

Serious violations of rules

    (1) often stays out at night despite parental prohibitions, beginning before age 13 years.
    (2) has run away from home overnight at least twice while living in parental or parental surrogate home.
    (3) is often truant from school, beginning before age 13 years.

B. The disturbance in behavior causes clinically significant impairment in social, academic or occupational functioning.
C. If the individual is age 18 years or older, criteria are not met for Antisocial Personality Disorder.

Code based on age at onset:
312.81 Conduct Disorder, Childhood-Onset Type: onset of at least one criterion characteristic of Conduct Disorder prior to age 10 years
312.82 Conduct Disorder, Adolescent-Onset Type: absence of any criteria characteristic of Conduct Disorder prior to age 10 years
312.89 Conduct Disorder, Unspecified Onset: age at onset is not known

Specify severity:
Mild: few if any conduct problems in excess of those required to make the diagnosis and conduct problems cause only minor harm to others (e.g., lying, truancy, staying out after dark without permission)
Moderate: number of conduct problems and effect on others intermediate between "mild" and "severe" (e.g., stealing without confronting a victim, vandalism)
Severe: many conduct problems in excess of those required to make the diagnosis or conduct problems cause considerable harm to others (e.g., forced sex, physical cruelty, use of a weapon, stealing while confronting a victim, breaking and entering)

Reprinted with permission from the *Diagnostic and Statistical Manual of Mental Disorders*, 4th ed., Text Rev. Copyright 2000 American Psychiatric Association.

functioning, as well as screening for suspected mental retardation or learning disabilities.

At the present time, there are no laboratory measures that can serve as diagnostic tools for AD-DBDs. Similarly, findings from neuroimaging studies have neither been consistent enough nor specific enough to warrant their use as diagnostic tools.

Many children with AD-DBDs have impaired social skills and consequently experience difficulties with peer relationships. Information regarding social adjustment is crucial in treatment planning, since increased impairment in social and school function is predictive of poor outcome. Parent–child interactions also play a role in the maintenance of disruptive behaviors, poor

social skills, the presence of internalizing symptoms, and response to treatment.

There is a high rate of comorbidity among the three disorders that comprise the AD-DBD group and several other diagnostic categories Among the AD-DBDs, approximately 90% of children with CD would also meet the criteria for ODD. Furthermore, 40% of children with ADHD also have ODD and 40% of children with ODD have ADHD. In terms of the comorbidity of the AD-DBD group with other diagnostic categories, it has been estimated that 15–20% of children with ADHD have comorbid mood disorders, 20–25% have anxiety disorders and 6–20% have learning disabilities. Other conditions which may occur comorbidly with the

---

DSM-IV-TR Diagnostic Criteria

313.81 Oppositional-Defiant Disorder

A. A pattern of negativistic, hostile, and defiant behavior lasting at least 6 months, during which four (or more) of the following are present:

(1) often loses temper.
(2) often argues with adults.
(3) often actively defies or refuses to comply with adults' requests or rules.
(4) often deliberately annoys people.
(5) often blames others for his or her mistakes or misbehavior.
(6) is often touchy or easily annoyed by others.
(7) is often angry and resentful.
(8) is often spiteful or vindictive.

Note: Consider a criterion met only if the behavior occurs more frequently than is typically observed in individuals of comparable age and developmental level.

B. The disturbance in behavior causes clinically significant impairment in social, academic, or occupational functioning.
C. The behaviors do not occur exclusively during the course of a Psychotic or Mood Disorder.
D. Criteria are not met for Conduct Disorder, and, if the individual is age 18 years or older, criteria are not met for Antisocial Personality Disorder

Reprinted with permission from the *Diagnostic and Statistical Manual of Mental Disorders,* 4th ed., Text Rev. Copyright 2000 American Psychiatric Association.

AD-DBDs include Tourette's disorder (TD), drug and alcohol abuse or dependence, and mental retardation.

Studies examining prevalence rates of the AD-DBDs in community samples are characterized by considerable variability, although rates are generally high. While DSM-IV-TR estimates the prevalence rates for ADHD to range from 2% to 7% in school-age children, rates as high as 17.1% have been reported in community surveys. Rates for CD have been estimated to be as low as 0.9% for school-age children but as high as 8.7% in adolescents. The overall prevalence of ODD varies across studies from 5.7% to 9.9%.

In school-age children, boys have higher rates than girls for all three disorders. In clinic settings, the ratio of boys to girls is about 9:1, but in community samples, this decreases to approximately 3:1. Furthermore, teachers tend to identify fewer girls than boys as having ADHD symptoms. The combined type of ADHD is the most common subtype in both genders. However, in the predominantly hyperactive–impulsive subtype of ADHD, the male-to-female ratio is approximately 4:1, while in the predominantly inattentive subtype the ratio falls to 2:1. In general, prevalence declines with age, but follow-up studies of children and adolescents indicate that the disorder frequently persists into adulthood. Longitudinal studies have reported rates of

childhood cases that persist into adulthood to range from 4% to 75%. These highly variable rates may be accounted for by methodological differences. Factors that appear to predict the persistence of ADHD into adulthood include a positive family history for ADHD and the presence of psychiatric comorbidity, particularly aggression.

Course

Some behaviors characteristic of the AD-DBDs are observable as early as the preschool years. Hyperactivity and attentional problems emerge gradually and may overlap with the emergence of oppositional behaviors, giving the appearance of a simultaneous, rather than a sequential, onset. It is now recognized that while hyperactivity and, to a lesser extent, attentional problems show a gradual decline through adolescence and adulthood, many individuals with ADHD continue to have attentional, behavioral and emotional problems well into adolescence and adulthood. Typically, adults with ADHD are less overtly overactive, although they may retain a subjective sense of restlessness. Impairment in these adults is more often a result of inattention, disorganization, and impulsive behavior.

The developmental course of oppositional behaviors shows greater variability. When the oppositionality is of a persistent nature and lasts beyond the preschool years, the escalation to more disruptive behaviors is more likely. In most oppositional children, who are usually not physically aggressive, oppositional behaviors peak around age 8 years and decline beyond that. In a second group of children, delinquent behaviors follow the onset of oppositional behaviors. Early physical aggression is a key predictor of this latter trajectory.

Generally, conduct problems first appear in middle childhood. In males, the progression to more serious forms of conduct problems, such as rape or mugging, generally emerge after age 13 years. When CD is seen in adolescence for the first time, the problems tend to diminish by adulthood.

Considerable data indicate that a subgroup of hyperactive children show high rates of delinquency and substance abuse during adolescence, and this continues into adulthood. However, it is likely because of the comorbidity with CD or bipolar disorder that higher rates of substance abuse are found in adolescents with ADHD

Differential Diagnosis

Proper differential diagnosis of ADHD, CD, and ODD requires not only discrimination among the three disorders but also from a wide range of other psychiatric, developmental, and medical conditions. Among the AD-DBDs, the relationship between ADHD and CD has been the most studied. It is now generally accepted that the two disorders can be differentiated despite the high degree of overlap, both in terms of symptom presentation and co-occurrence within individuals. ADHD can be conceptualized as a cognitive/developmental disorder, with an earlier age of onset than CD. ADHD children more frequently show deficits on measures of attentional and cognitive function, and have increased motor activity and greater neurodevelopmental abnormalities. In contrast, CD children tend to be characterized by higher levels of aggression and greater familial dysfunction.

A significant proportion of children present with symptoms of both ADHD and CD, and both conditions should be diagnosed when this occurs. Comorbid ADHD and CD are consistently reported to be more disabling than either disorder alone. These children retain the difficulties found in both disorders and tend to show increased levels of aggressive behaviors at an early age, which remain remarkably persistent. This is in contrast to the more typical episodic course seen in children who have CD alone. Finally, children with comorbid ADHD and CD appear to have a poorer long-term outcome than those with either disorder alone.

The relationship of ADHD to ODD is less well studied. However, it does appear that among children with ADHD, those who are most hyperactive/impulsive are at greatest risk for developing ODD. Despite the high degree of comorbidity, it is possible to distinguish between the two disorders. ODD symptoms, such as "loses temper," "actively defies," and "swears," are less characteristic of children with ADHD. In general, the onset of ODD symptoms peaks by age 8 years and shows a declining course thereafter. On the other hand, hyperactivity and attentional problems appear at a much earlier age and often persist, although the levels of inattentiveness and/or hyperactivity often decrease with age.

The relationship of ODD and CD is more complex. The question has been raised as to whether these diagnoses constitute different levels of severity of a single phenomenon, or whether they should be viewed as distinct. A diagnosis of CD supersedes ODD since approximately 90% of children with CD would also meet the criteria for ODD. Although the majority of ODD children will not develop CD, in some cases ODD appears to represent a developmental precursor of CD. In cases where ODD precedes CD, the onset of CD is typically before age 10 years (childhood-onset CD). In children who have the onset of CD after age 10 years,

symptoms of ODD and ADHD are usually not present during early childhood. It has been shown that children with ODD demonstrate lower degrees of impairment and are more socially competent as compared to children with CD. Furthermore, children with CD come from less-advantaged families, and have greater conflict with school and judicial systems as compared to children with ODD. Family adversity scores in children with ODD are usually intermediate between those of children with CD and normal children.

Mood and anxiety disorders, learning disorders, mental retardation, pervasive developmental disorders, organic mental disorders, and psychotic disorders may all present with impairment of attention, as well as hyperactive/impulsive behaviors. The diagnosis of ADHD in DSM-IV-TR requires that the symptoms of inattention/cognitive disorganization and impulsivity/hyperactivity are not better accounted for by one of the above conditions. Differentiating ADHD from bipolar disorder in childhood is complicated by the low base rate of bipolar disorder and the variability in clinical presentation. Even though there are phenomenological similarities between the two disorders, there is little evidence to suggest that most children with externalizing symptoms are at risk for bipolar disorder. A positive family history of bipolar disorder is especially helpful in diagnosing bipolar disorder in children. In addition, a variety of medical conditions such as epilepsy, Tourette's disorder, thyroid disease, postinfectious and/or posttraumatic encephalopathy, and sensory impairments can present with symptoms similar to ADHD and must also be considered. Finally, many medications that are prescribed to children can mimic ADHD symptomatology. Examples include anticonvulsants (e.g., phenobarbital), antihistamines, decongestants, bronchodilators (e.g., theophylline), and systemic steroids.

TREATMENT

Successful treatment planning in children with AD-DBDs requires consideration of not only the core symptomatology but also of family and social factors and comorbidity with other disorders. Given the heterogeneity of the three disorders that make up the AD-DBDs, the wide-ranging effects of the disruptive behaviors, the high rates of comorbidity, and the presence of associated features such as learning disabilities, multimodal treatments (i.e., psychopharmacologic and psychosocial) are almost always warranted. Nevertheless, good response can be achieved with either treatment alone in certain instances (e.g., medication treatment for uncomplicated ADHD or ADHD + ODD; psychosocial treatment for ADHD + anxiety disorder). A diagnosis of ODD without any comorbid condition will usually be responsive to behavioral intervention without medication. One should always attempt, however, to rule out the possibility that ADHD is also present. Similarly, treatment of children with CD without comorbidity usually involves psychosocial interventions with the possibility of augmenting treatment with one of several pharmacological agents. In contrast, comorbid ADHD + CD almost always requires medication, and medication response is augmented if psychosocial treatment is offered concomitantly.

Somatic Treatments

Psychostimulants. It is well established that psychostimulants are extremely effective in treating a wide range of disruptive behaviors above and beyond their effects on ADHD. Nevertheless, ADHD remains the primary indication for the use of these medications. Methylphenidate (MPH), dextroamphetamine (DEX), and mixture of amphetamine salts (MAS) (which is a mixture of several amphetamine compounds, 75% of which is DEX) have all been shown to be effective in treating ADHD.

The stimulants produce significant improvement in attention, hyperactivity, impulse control, and aggressiveness, leading to better organization of behavior, task completion, and self-regulation. There is a fairly robust improvement in social skills, as evidenced by peer ratings and parent and teacher ratings of social function. There is also improvement in academic productivity, although change in actual academic performance has been more difficult to demonstrate. Although most data with stimulants have been obtained in samples of school-age children with ADHD, there is increasing recognition that stimulants can be used successfully across the lifespan.

The decision to prescribe psychostimulant medication is best undertaken following a comprehensive assessment, with full consideration given to the range of pharmacologic and nonpharmacologic treatment options that are available. Several of the rating scales used in assessment (e.g., the Conners questionnaires) are sensitive to medication effects and can be used to monitor adequacy of dose and maintenance of medication effects. Prior to a trial with any of the stimulants, baseline data should be obtained, including general medical status, and more specific evaluations of height, weight, blood pressure, and a complete blood count.

The decision regarding which stimulant to select is best determined by considering properties intrinsic to the different medications—such as duration of activity and adverse effect profile—as well as the circumstances of the individual (e.g., when is peak medication level needed most, what is the individual's lifestyle, etc.).

Regardless of one's view regarding the first choice stimulant, and although the different stimulants work on average about as well as one another, nonresponders to one medication may respond well to another, since their mechanisms of action are not identical.

Adverse effects (AE) of stimulants are generally mild, but occasionally can become problematic. The most commonly observed AEs include headache, abdominal pain, decreased appetite (with or without weight loss), and initial insomnia. There are slight increases in pulse and BP, which are not very meaningful at the group level, but can take on greater significance for particular individuals. Affective changes, including blunted affect, irritability, and mood lability can also be seen, either at peak dose or when the dose wears off. Use of longer-acting psychostimulants tends to minimize mood lability and other AEs that are often considered to be a reflection of the on–off effects that are more frequently seen with IR preparations. Motor or vocal tics can develop or, more often, can be exacerbated, but there has been a convergence of evidence that stimulant treatment does not necessarily exacerbate tics. There has been some concern that stimulants can precipitate psychotic symptoms such as hallucinations, although this is very rare and almost always seen as a reflection of excessive dosing or use in individuals with disorders other than ADHD (e.g., psychotic disorders). The FDA has recently added a warning about the potential for psychotic symptoms emerging with stimulant treatment.

Atomoxetine. Atomoxetine (Strattera) is a medication with highly potent and selective activity to block the noradrenergic transporter. It is structurally distinct from both the stimulants and the tricyclic antidepressants and is the first nonstimulant medication labeled for the treatment of ADHD.

Atomoxetine can be administered on either a twice-daily or once-daily schedule, despite the fact that its half-life in the overwhelming majority of individuals is 4 hours. Despite this fact, therapeutic benefit seems to be maintained over the full day. Adverse effects with atomoxetine have been relatively mild, with decreased appetite and a small increase in pulse and blood pressure being the two most consistent findings. Because it is not a stimulant, and because its effects are highly selective for NA and not DA, atomoxetine is thought to not have abuse potential.

Tricylic Antidepressants. The noradrenergic tricyclic antidepressants, principally imipramine and desipramine, have been the most extensively studied and, until the mid-1990s, were the most often prescribed nonstimulant medication for individuals with

ADHD. In the case of both of these medications, cardiac side effects are of concern and premedication workup must include at least an EKG. Tachycardia and postural hypotension are commonly seen but are not often problematic. Prolongation of the PR and QT intervals may be a greater source of concern and should be reviewed with a pediatric cardiologist. The decision to prescribe tricyclics for ADHD children must be made with the knowledge that several sudden deaths have been reported in children taking desipramine. Although it has been argued that data do not support the conclusion that tricyclics have a high degree of cardiovascular toxicity in children, proper informed consent should be obtained. It should also be noted that neither imipramine nor desipramine is FDA approved for the treatment of ADHD children.

Other Antidepressants. Bupropion and venlafaxine are chemically unrelated to other known antidepressants. Both have been studied for their potential utility in the AD-DBDs. Bupropion in ADHD is not generally believed to be effective as stimulants. There are similar but more preliminary data indicating that venlafaxine might be useful for ADHD.

Serotonin Reuptake Inhibitors. Clomipramine, a mixed noradrenergic and serotonergic agonist, and fluoxetine, a selective serotonin reuptake inhibitor (SSRI), have been used occasionally in the treatment of children with ADHD. Although there have been no studies using SSRIs in ADHD and comorbid CD/ODD, these medications are of some interest in light of recent findings implicating serotonergic mechanisms in aggression and reported utility of fluoxetine in treating adults with impulsive aggression. At present, there are no controlled trials to support the efficacy of the SSRIs for the core symptoms of ADHD, and their role in treating comorbid ADHD and CD/ODD is inferential only.

Alpha-2-adrenergic Agonists. Because of their role in treating overarousal and aggression, the alpha-2 agonists seem to be suited for use in children with comorbid ODD/CD/aggression. They have been effective in treating individuals suffering from ADHD who either have diagnosed tic disorders, or are at increased risk to develop them, such as those children with a positive family history of tics. This is particularly important since as many as 40–60% of individuals with Tourette's syndrome seen in psychiatric settings also have ADHD, and many of these individuals have significant behavior problems. Although the alpha-2 agonists may be less effective than stimulants in the treatment of ADHD,

they may be particularly useful in individuals whose tics worsen on a stimulant medication. These agonists have also been used in combination with a stimulant. There have been, however, safety considerations involving this combination. These primarily involve the possibility of additive risk of rebound hypertension of alpha-2 agonists with the mild increase in pulse and blood pressure from stimulants.

Clonidine has been the most often studied of the alpha-2s, although the empirical database for both clonidine and guanfacine remains quite small.

The most common side effect of the alpha-2 medications is sedation, although this tends to decrease after several weeks. Dry mouth, nausea, and photophobia are among the other adverse effects reported. At high doses, hypotension and dizziness are also possible. Glucose tolerance may decrease, especially in those at risk for diabetes. It is important to carefully evaluate cardiovascular function when using the alpha-2 agonists, especially when used in combination with stimulant treatment as noted earlier. Additionally, there have been reports of sudden death in three cases treated with the combination of clonidine and methylphenidate, although a review of this situation by the FDA concluded that these unfortunate events were not attributable to the combination. However, careful monitoring is required. Since clonidine is not FDA approved for use in ADHD, informed consent should clearly indicate that this is an "off-label" treatment.

Other Agents. A variety of other pharmacotherapeutic agents have been utilized in the treatment of aggression and episodic dyscontrol, although efficacy in children with comorbid ADHD and CD has not yet been demonstrated. Among these medications, lithium has been the best studied.

Neuroleptic medications have also been used in treatment of the AD-DBDs, principally to treat children with severe behavioral problems characterized by aggression and combativeness. Although older neuroleptics such as chlorpromazine, thioridazine, and halperidol are FDA approved for the treatment of severe behavior problems in children, they are infrequently used at present. Recently, there has been more interest in the atypical neuroleptics, such as risperidone, because of their low risk of TD and other side effects.

During the course of the last few years, there has been a remarkable increase in the number of medications that are used in the treatment of ADHD and CD. It is important to keep in mind that the majority of the medications are not approved by the FDA for specific use in ADHD and/or CD and as such their use for these two disorders continues to be "off-label". An additional complication is that, in general, prescribing practices tend to vary among different settings and even among different physicians in the same setting. Consequently, less than optimal treatment is likely to result in inadequate or partial improvement.

Psychosocial Treatments. A variety of psychosocial therapies, such as behavior therapy, contingency management, and cognitive behavioral therapy (CBT), have been found to be useful for treating children with AD-DBD. Among the systematically studied psychosocial interventions are home-based interventions/parent training, classroom-based behavior modifications, social skills training, and intensive summer treatment programs. Since family, peer, and school interactions are important in the morbidity and maintenance of these disorders, it is important to utilize psychosocial treatments to target each of these areas. In contrast to these more structured techniques, individual play therapy with children is generally ineffective in decreasing problem behaviors of the AD-DBDs.

Despite their potential benefits, difficulties encountered with psychosocial interventions are that short-term gains are often limited to the period that the programs are actually in effect. Furthermore, a substantial number of children, particularly those with the most severe presentation and with greatest psychosocial adversity, fail to show improvement. Additional problems in implementation include the unwillingness of many teachers to use behavioral programs and the fact that as many as half the parents discontinue parent training. Finally, the fact that these interventions are labor-intensive and reported long-term improvements have been modest, makes these therapies of limited value when used alone. These interventions are often more efficacious than medication alone in children with ADHD who also have symptoms of anxiety.

Combined Treatments

The 1997 multimodal treatment study of children with ADHD (MTA) was a landmark multisite clinical trial,

conducted at six performance sites across the US and Canada, that examined the comparative response to 14 months of medication and psychosocial treatments, administered alone or together, in 579 seven- to nine-year-old children with combined subtype ADHD. The principal objectives of the study were to determine the relative effectiveness of the three active treatments in comparison to one another, and in comparison with community standard care. The study indicated that, for ADHD symptoms, treatments that included medication performed better than other treatments in reducing ADHD symptoms. For non-ADHD symptoms, only combined treatment was statistically superior to the community standard care, although it was not different from the medication group.

COMPARISON OF DSM-IV-TR AND ICD-10 DIAGNOSTIC CRITERIA

For attention-deficit/hyperactivity disorder, the item set chosen for the ICD-10 Diagnostic Criteria for Research is almost identical to the items in the DSM-IV-TR criteria set but the algorithm is quite different, resulting in a more narrowly defined ICD-10 category. Specifically, whereas the DSM-IV-TR algorithm requires either six inattention items or six hyperactive/impulsive items, the ICD-10 Diagnostic Criteria for Research requires at least six inattention items, at least three hyperactive items, and at least one impulsive item. Instead of subtyping the disorder on the basis of the predominant type, ICD-10 subspecifies the condition whether criteria are also met for a CD.

Although formatted quite differently, the DSM-IV-TR and ICD-10 item sets and diagnostic algorithms for CD are almost identical. Although ICD-10 provides a list of 23 items (in contrast with the 15 included in the DSM-IV-TR criteria for CD), only the last 15 items count towards a diagnosis of CD. Although the first 8 items on the CD list are identical to the DSM-IV-TR items for OD, ICD-10 ODD can be considerably more severe because up to 2 of the items can be drawn from the 15 items that comprise the CD item set.

Childhood Disorders: Feeding and Eating Disorders of Infancy or Early Childhood

Feeding Disorder of Infancy or Early Childhood

DIAGNOSIS

Feeding Disorder of Infancy or Early Childhood is defined in the DSM-IV-TR as a persistent failure to eat adequately with significant failure to gain weight or a significant loss of weight over a period of at least 1 month. However, this general definition of feeding disorder in DSM-IV-TR does not take into account the heterogeneity of feeding and growth problems in infants and its implication for treatment. Several authors have used various diagnostic methods and assigned different labels to address the heterogeneity of feeding problems associated with failure to thrive. Because of the diversity of feeding disorders associated with failure to thrive and the lack of a subclassification of feeding disorder as defined in DSM-IV-TR, this chapter focuses on a classification of feeding disorders proposed by Chatoor. Three developmental feeding disorders are described as (1) feeding disorder of state regulation, (2) feeding disorder of poor mother–infant reciprocity, and (3) feeding disorder of separation (infantile anorexia). In addition, two feeding disorders are described that are not linked to specific developmental stages: (1) sensory food aversions, a common feeding disorder that becomes evident during the introduction of different milks, baby food, or table food with various tastes and consistencies, and (2) posttraumatic feeding disorder, which is characterized by an acute disruption in the regulation of eating and can occur at various ages and stages of feeding development.

Feeding Disorder of State Regulation

In this condition, the infant has difficulty reaching and maintaining a calm state of alertness for feeding, either being too sleepy or too agitated or distressed to feed.

Young infants who present with feeding difficulties and growth failure dating to the postnatal period need to be considered for the diagnosis of a feeding disorder of state regulation. In addition to the usual history, the mother and her infant should be observed during feeding and during play to assess the infant's special characteristics, the infant's regulation of state and feeding behavior, and the mother's ability to read the infant's signals and to respond to them in a contingent way.

The information from the infant's and the mother's histories and the observation of the mother–infant dyad will determine which factors contribute to the difficulties in the infant's regulation of feeding. Because medical problems (e.g., cardiac or pulmonary disease) may contribute to the feeding problems, their impact on the feeding relationship of mother and infant needs to be considered.

Feeding Disorder of Poor Caregiver–Infant Reciprocity

Children with this condition show a lack of developmentally appropriate signs of social reciprocity with the primary caregiver during feeding, leading to significant growth deficiency. However, because of the difficulty of assessing attachment in infants under 1 year of age, feeding disorder of poor caregiver–infant reciprocity was chosen as diagnostic label to capture the lack of engagement between mother and infant in this feeding disorder.

Most of these infants are not brought for pediatric well-baby care but present to the emergency department because of an acute illness, when their poor nutritional state draws the attention of pediatricians. Because of their severe failure to thrive, these infants frequently require hospitalization. During the hospitalization, the psychiatric consultant is usually called in to assist in the diagnosis and treatment of the infant's growth and developmental problems.

Many of the mothers of affected children are elusive and avoidant of any contact with professionals. Consequently, the observation of mother–infant interactions may have to be obtained indirectly, through the report of other professionals who admitted the infant to the hospital.

Another important part of the assessment involves the direct observation and examination of these infants. Infants with feeding disorders of poor mother–infant reciprocity characteristically feed poorly, avoid eye contact, and are weak in the first few days of hospitalization. When picked up, they might scissor their legs and hold up their arms in a surrender posture to balance their heads, which seem too heavy for their weak bodies. They usually do not cuddle like healthy well-fed infants, rather they keep their legs drawn up or appear hypotonic, like rag dolls. These infants, however, appear to blossom under the care of a primary care nurse who engages with them during feeding and plays with them. They become increasingly responsive, begin to smile, feed hungrily, and gain weight. These striking changes in behavior of these young infants when they are fed and attended to by a nurturing caretaker are characteristic of a feeding disorder of poor mother–infant reciprocity and differentiate these infants from infants with organic problems that have resulted in growth failure and developmental delays. The infants with organic failure to thrive usually respond best to their mothers and do not show the avoidance of eye contact and general withdrawal so characteristic of infants with this feeding disorder.

Infantile Anorexia

In this condition, the infant refuses to eat adequate amounts of food for at least 1 month, leading to significant growth deficiency. The onset of the food refusal under 3 years of age is most commonly during the transition to spoon- and self-feeding. Furthermore, the infant does not communicate hunger signals, lacks interest in food, but shows strong interest in exploration and/or interaction with the caregiver. Infants with this infantile anorexia are usually referred for a psychiatric evaluation due to food refusal and growth failure. The infants' food refusal usually becomes of concern between 6 months and 3 years, most commonly between 9 and 18 months of age, during the transition to spoon- and self-feeding.

The diagnostic evaluation of this feeding disorder should include the infant's feeding, developmental, and health history, and the observation of mother and infant during feeding. In addition to the infant's history, the mother's perception of her infant's temperament, her family situation, her childhood background, and her own eating habits and attitude toward limit setting need to be explored.

Sensory Food Aversions

In this disorder, the infant consistently refuses to eat specific foods with specific tastes, textures, and/or smells. Sensory food aversions occur along a spectrum of severity. Some children refuse to eat only a few types of food, making it possible for the parents to accommodate the child's food preferences. Others may refuse most foods, disrupt family meals, and cause serious parental concern about the children's nutrition. The diagnosis of a feeding disorder should only be made if the food selectivity results in nutritional deficiencies, and/or has led to oral motor delay.

The evaluation of infants and young children with sensory food aversions should address how many foods the child consistently refuses and how many foods he or she usually accepts. A nutritional assessment needs to look not only at the anthropometric measures of the child to rule out acute and/or chronic malnutrition, but needs to address whether the child may lack adequate intake of vitamins, zinc, iron, and/or protein. In addition, an oral motor assessment needs to determine whether the child has fallen behind in this area of development. Delayed oral motor development will limit the kind of foods the child should be offered in order to prevent choking, and may be associated with a delay in speech development. In addition, the parents' food preferences during childhood and adulthood should be explored to assess whether the parents may be limited in the variety of foods they offer their child.

Posttraumatic Feeding Disorder

These children refuse to eat any solid food after they have experienced an episode of choking. This disorder is characterized by the infant's consistent refusal to either drink from the bottle or to eat any solid foods, and in most severe cases, by the infant's refusal to eat at all. Depending on the mode of feeding that the infants appear to associate with the traumatic event(s), some refuse to eat solids, but will continue to drink from the bottle; whereas others may refuse to drink from the bottle, but are willing to eat solids. Some infants may put baby food in their mouths, but then spit out any food that has any little lumps in it. Most infants get stuck in these food patterns and may lose weight or lack certain nutrients because of their limited diet.

Reminders of the traumatic event(s) (e.g., the bottle, the bib, or the high chair) may cause intense distress for some infants, whereby they become fearful when they are positioned for feedings and/or presented with feeding utensils and food. They resist being fed by crying, arching, and refusing to open their mouths. If food is placed in their mouths, they intensely resist swallowing. They may gag or vomit, let the food drop out, actively spit the food out, or store the food in their cheeks and spit it out later. The fear of eating seems to override any awareness of hunger. Therefore, infants who refuse all foods, including liquids and solids, require acute intervention due to dehydration and starvation.

In addition to a thorough history about the onset of the infant's food refusal and the medical and developmental history, the observation of the infant and mother during feeding is critical for understanding this feeding disorder and differentiating it from infantile anorexia and from sensory food aversions. It is helpful to ask the mother to bring a variety of foods, including those that the infant refuses and those that he or she accepts. Infants with a posttraumatic feeding disorder characteristically appear engaged and comfortable with their mothers as long as the feared food is out of sight.

TREATMENT

Treatment begins with the first contact with the infant and his or her caregivers. The establishment of a therapeutic alliance with the caregivers is critical to any successful treatment.

Feeding Disorder of State Regulation

Treatment needs to take maternal as well as infant factors that have interfered with feeding into consideration. Treatment can be directed toward the infant, toward the mother, and toward the mother–infant interaction.

Videotaping the feeding and observing the tape together with the mother can heighten her awareness of the infant's reactions during feeding and enhance her ability to read the infant's cues. The therapist can then engage the mother in a dialogue on how to respond to the infant's cues most effectively. Because of the complexity of the factors that may contribute to this feeding disorder, the therapist needs to use a flexible approach when addressing both partners in the feeding relationship.

Feeding Disorder of Poor Caregiver–Infant Reciprocity

Because of the complexity of the issues involved in the etiology of nonorganic failure to thrive, most psychiatrists and researchers suggest that multiple and case-specific interventions may be required.

During a hospitalization, a number of infant-directed interventions can be carried out while a more in-depth evaluation of the mother and the mother–infant relationship takes place. Improvement of the infant's health and affective availability can then be used to engage the mother with her infant and in the treatment process. The mother's ability to engage her infant and to participate in the treatment process has to be at the core of the treatment plan.

Because the mothers frequently present with a variety of psychological and social disturbances, including a history of abuse or neglect, their problems need to be explored while nutritional, emotional, and developmental rehabilitation goes on with the infant. In some situations of severe neglect or associated abuse, the case needs to be reported to protective services, which at times can be instrumental in mobilizing the family or in finding foster care.

Discharge from the hospital is a critical time when all services need to be in place to ensure appropriate follow-through of the treatment plan for these vulnerable infants. Because of the complexity of the problems involved in the etiology of this feeding disorder, a flexible multidisciplinary approach that is coordinated by the primary therapist is usually most effective for both partners in the feeding relationship.

Infantile Anorexia

The major goal of the treatment is to facilitate internal regulation of eating by the infant. The intervention consists of three components:

1. Assess and then explain the infant's special temperamental characteristics and developmental conflicts to the mother to help her understand the lack of expected hunger cues and the infant's struggle for control during the feeding situation.
2. Explore the mother's upbringing and the effect it has had on the parenting of her infant to help the mother understand her conflicts and difficulties in regard to limit setting.
3. Explain the concept of internal versus external regulation of eating. Help the mother to develop mealtime routines that facilitate the infant's awareness of hunger, leading to internal regulation of eating, improved food intake, and growth. In addition, coach the parents to set limits to the infant's behaviors that interfere with eating. These feeding guidelines include:

   a. Schedule meals and snacks at regular 3- to 4-hour intervals and do not allow the infant to snack or drink from the bottle or breast in between.

b. Limit meal duration to 30 minutes.
c. Praise the infant for self-feeding but stay emotionally neutral whether the infant eats little or a lot.
d. Do not use distracting toys or television during feedings.
e. Eliminate desserts or sweets as a reward at the end of the meal; rather integrate them into regular meals and snacks.
f. Put the infant in "time-out" for inappropriate behaviors during feeding (e.g., throwing the spoon or food, climbing out of the high chair).

These three steps in the treatment are best accomplished in three sessions lasting two to three hours each and grouped close together within a two- to three-week period. The intensity of this brief intervention facilitates a close therapeutic alliance between the therapist and the mother and gives the mother the opportunity to experience the support she needs to make major changes in her interactions with her infant.

This initial intensive phase of the intervention can be followed up by a telephone call and by a few visits spaced three to four weeks apart. The intervention focuses primarily on the mother because in infantile anorexia, the mother's feeding relationship with the infant is seen as central. Nevertheless, the other relationships, such as with the father, should not be overlooked.

Giving the mother the choice as to who in the family (or anyone else) should be included in the therapeutic process, and at what point, is part of putting the mother in control. Because many of the mothers have felt helpless as children and ineffective as parents, the empowerment of the mother is critical to the success of the treatment.

Sensory Food Aversion

In young infants (4–7 months of age), a few repeated exposures to new foods enhance the infants' acceptance not only of that food but also of other similar foods. However, this changes in the second year of life, when the acceptance of new foods only increased significantly after 10 or more exposures to those same foods.

If infants show strong aversive reactions (e.g., gagging or vomiting) early on when offered a certain food, it is advisable to give up on that particular food and not offer it again. If the infant shows a less severe reaction (e.g., grimaces or wants to spit out a new food), it is also best to stop offering the new food during that feeding, but introduce it again after a few days in a small amount and paired with some other food that the infant likes. It is important to increase the amounts of the new food very gradually until the infant appears comfortable with it.

Posttraumatic Feeding Disorder

Because of the complexity of many of these cases, a multidisciplinary team is best equipped to meet all the needs of these infants and their parents.

Before any psychiatric treatment can be successfully initiated, the medical and nutritional needs of the infant need to be addressed. In severe cases of total food refusal, it is important to act quickly to maintain the infant's hydration.

The psychiatric treatment of this feeding disorder involves a desensitization of the infant to overcome the anticipatory anxiety about eating and return to internal regulation of eating in response to hunger and satiety. It is most important to help the parents understand the dynamics of a posttraumatic feeding disorder so that they can recognize the infant's anticipatory anxiety and become active participants in the treatment. After identification of triggers of anticipatory anxiety (e.g., the sight of the high chair, the bottle, or certain types of food), a desensitization by gradual exposure can be initiated or a more rapid desensitization through more intensive behavioral techniques can be implemented.

With both techniques, it is important to have a professional assess the infant's oral motor coordination because many infants who refuse to eat for extended periods fall behind in their oral motor development due to lack of practice. Consequently, a 2-year-old may have the oral motor skills of a 1-year-old and will not be able to handle the chunky foods that require chewing. The rapid introduction of table food to a child who has delayed oral motor skills may lead to choking, thereby creating a setback to the desensitization process.

As summarized in Figure 7-1, each of these five feeding disorders presents with specific symptom patterns and characteristic mother–infant interactions that help diagnose and differentiate the various feeding disorders. The correct diagnosis is critical because a treatment that is helpful for one feeding disorder may be ineffective or may even worsen another feeding disorder. These treatments are based primarily on clinical experience, and further empirical research is needed to establish which treatments are most effective for each feeding disorder.

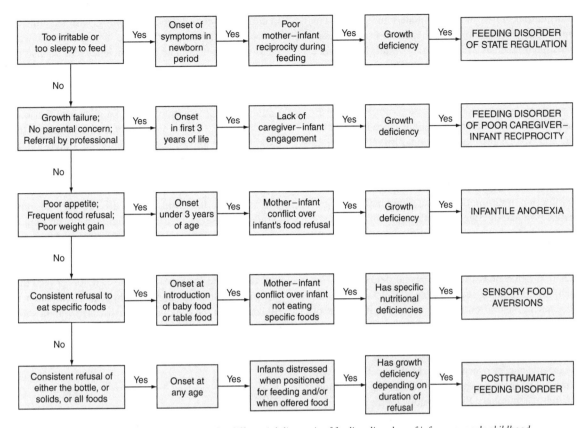

Figure 7-1 *Diagnostic decision tree for differential diagnosis of feeding disorders of infancy or early childhood.*

Rumination Disorder

DIAGNOSIS

Infants with rumination disorder repeatedly regurgitate and rechew food for a period of at least 1 month following a period of normal functioning. Most frequently, infants who ruminate come to the attention of professionals because of "frequent vomiting" and weight loss. Some infants ruminate primarily during the transition to sleep when left alone, and their ruminatory activity might not be readily observed. However, these infants are frequently found in a puddle of vomitus, which should raise suspicion of rumination. Other infants can be observed to posture with the back arched, to put the thumb or whole hand into the mouth, or to suck on the tongue rhythmically to initiate the regurgitation of food. Most of the regurgitated food is initially vomited, but gradually the infant appears to learn to hold more of the food in the mouth to rechew and reswallow. "Experienced" ruminators appear to be able to bring up food through repeated tongue movements. They learn to rechew and reswallow the food without losing any

of it. Their rumination can be inferred only from the movements of their cheeks and foul oral odor because of the frequent regurgitation.

In addition to taking a thorough medical history, it is important to explore the onset of vomiting and the social context under which the symptoms developed. An acute medical illness or a stressor in the parents' life is frequently associated with the onset of vomiting.

Some infants ruminate only when left alone or when stressed in a relationship; others appear so "addicted" to the rumination that they ruminate continuously after being fed, and they become distressed if interrupted in their ruminatory activity. In addition to assessing the rumination in the infant, the mother–infant relationship and the mother's life circumstances need to be evaluated because the mother's ability to soothe and to stimulate her infant is critical for successful intervention.

TREATMENT

On the basis of the assumption that rumination is a learned habit reinforced by increased attention for regurgitation, unlearning by counterconditioning has been suggested. A number of alternative procedures of punishment, such as aversive taste stimuli (lemon juice or hot sauce), have been developed. There are a number of difficulties, however, with the use of aversive taste stimuli as punishment. Frequently, the infants are out of reach of the caretakers when they ruminate; consequently, the use of lemon juice or hot sauce is inconsistent, and this delays learning. Some infants appear to become adapted to these aversive taste stimuli. Scolding the infant by shouting "No," placing the infant down, and leaving the room for 2 minutes immediately on initiation of rumination by the infant have been suggested as more effective alternatives. If the infant is not ruminating on the caretaker's return, he or she is to be picked up, washed, and played with as a reward.

It has been postulated that for some infants, the rumination behavior is related to social deprivation. For such infants, holding the child for 10 to 15 minutes before, during, and after meals may be the treatment of choice. Psychodynamic approaches are based on the assumption that rumination results from a disturbance in the mother–infant relationship. Mothers of ruminating infants may be overwhelmed by their personal lives, which make them unavailable or tense in their relationship with their infants. Psychotherapy for the mother and environmental changes that produce enhanced mothering have been proposed to address these problems.

Before embarking on treatment, both the child and the child's mother should be looked at individually. The diagnostic evaluation needs to determine whether the infant's rumination is situational or pervasive, whether the infant has learned to ruminate because of little stimulation and gratification from the mother, or whether the rumination serves the infant as a way of relieving tension in a stressed mother–infant relationship. After an understanding of the mother's situation has been gained, treatment is best individualized by use of a combination of psychodynamic and behavioral interventions to enhance the mother–infant relationship in general, and to address the symptom of rumination in particular.

Pica

DIAGNOSIS

Young children with this disorder typically eat plaster, paper, paint, cloth, hair, insects, animal droppings, sand, pebbles, and dirt. Because mouthing of objects is still common in toddlers between 1 and 2 years, the diagnosis of pica should be made only if the behavior is persistent and inappropriate for the child's developmental level. The diagnosis of pica should be explored

in children with accidental poisoning, with lead intoxication, or with worm infestation. Young children with signs of malnutrition or iron deficiency should also be considered for the diagnosis of pica.

The assessment should include the history of the child's development, in general, and feeding in particular. Special attention should be given to other oral activities (e.g., thumb sucking or nail biting) that the child may use for self-soothing and relief of tension. In addition, the home environment and the parents' relationship with each other and with the child need to be explored to assess the parents' availability to nurture and supervise the child. Above all, mother and child should be observed during a meal and during play to gain a better understanding of their relationship and how the symptoms of pica can be understood in the context of that relationship.

If the diagnosis of pica is established, it is critical that the child undergo a thorough physical examination to rule out any of the complications associated with this disorder, such as nutritional deficiencies (especially iron deficiency), lead poisoning, intestinal infections (toxoplasmosis or intestinal parasites), or gastrointestinal bezoars.

Course

In many instances, the disorder is believed to be self-limited and to remit spontaneously after a few months. Some children, however, are somewhat retarded in the use of their speech and show conflicts about their dependency needs and aggressive feelings. Half of the adolescents in this group may show depression or personality disorders, or engage in other forms of disturbed oral activities (e.g., thumb sucking, nail biting), and use tobacco, alcohol, or drugs. There may be a relationship between pica in childhood and symptoms of bulimia nervosa in adolescence.

TREATMENT

In treating pica, one must consider the various factors that appear to contribute to the development of pica as well as its complications. It is important to treat the child medically while addressing the psychosocial needs of the child's family as well. The mothers need to be made aware of the dangers of pica and should be enlisted in providing a childproof environment. This might include removing lead from paint in old substandard housing units or instituting anthelmintic therapy for family pets. A psychoeducational treatment approach teaching the mothers the dangers of pica would also provide social support to help them become more available to their children. Other investigators have used aversive and nonaversive behavioral therapy, physical restraints, environmental enrichment with group or individual play, and time-out and overcorrection to treat this disorder.

COMPARISON OF DSM-IV-TR AND ICD-10 DIAGNOSTIC CRITERIA

In contrast to DSM-IV-TR, which allows the diagnosis of pica to be made in the presence of other mental disorders, if it is sufficiently severe to warrant independent clinical attention, the ICD-10 Diagnostic Criteria for Research for pica exclude this diagnosis in the presence of any other mental disorder (except mental retardation). ICD-10 does not have a separate category for rumination disorder. Instead, it includes this DSM-IV-TR category within its definition of Feeding Disorder of Infancy and Childhood, which combines rumination with the persistent failure to eat adequately.

8 Childhood Disorders: Tic Disorders

DIAGNOSIS

Tourette's disorder is the most notable of the tic disorders. The cardinal features of Tourette's disorder and the other tic disorders are motor and vocal tics. Motor tics are usually brief, rapid, and stereotyped movements, but can also be slower, more rhythmical, or even dystonic in nature. Simple motor tics are movements of individual muscle groups and include brief movements such as eye blinking, head shaking, and shoulder shrugging. Complex motor tics involve multiple muscle groups, such as a simultaneous eye deviation, head turn, and shoulder shrug. Some complex tics appear more purposeful, such as stereotyped hopping, touching, rubbing, or obscene gestures (copropraxia). Vocal tics are usually brief, staccato-like sounds, but can also be words or phrases. Simple vocal tics, often caused by the forceful movement of air through the nose and mouth, include sniffing, throat clearing, grunting, or barking-type sounds. Complex vocal tics usually include words, phrases, or the rep-

etition of one's own words (palilalia) or the words of others (echolalia). Coprolalia (repetition of obscene phrases), often incorrectly considered essential for the diagnosis of Tourette's disorder, is an uncommon symptom with only 2–6% of Tourette's disorder cases so affected.

Tics most often begin early in childhood, wax and wane in severity, and change in character and quality over time. Tics are exacerbated by excitement and tension, and can attenuate during periods of focused, productive activity and sleep. Tics are involuntary, yet because they are briefly suppressible or can be triggered by environmental stimuli (e.g., mimicking another person's movement, speech, or behavior), they may appear as volitional acts. Individuals with a tic disorder describe tension developing if a tic is resisted, which only subsides by completion of the tic. In some individuals, tics are preceded or provoked by a thought or physical sensation referred to as a premonitory urge.

There are four diagnostic categories included in the tic disorders section in DSM-IV-TR: Tourette's Disorder, Chronic Motor or Vocal Tic Disorder (CT), Transient Tic Disorder and Tic Disorder Not Otherwise Specified, which is a residual category for tic disorders not meeting the duration or age criteria of the other categories. In general, diagnostic decisions are based on whether both motor and phonic tics are present (i.e., if both are present, the diagnosis is Tourette's), duration of time affected with tics (Tourette's and CT persist for at least a year whereas Transient Tic Disorder lasts at least 4 weeks but no more than 12 months), age at onset (age of onset is before age 18 for all three of the specific tic disorders), and the lack of another medical cause for the tics.

Clinical assessment of the tic disorders begins with identification of the specific movements and sounds. It is also important to identify the severity of and impairment caused by the tics. Questioning individuals with tics and their families about the presence of simple and complex movements in muscle groups from head to toe

---

DSM-IV-TR Diagnostic Criteria

307.23 TOURETTES' DISORDER

A. Both multiple motor and one or more vocal tics have been present at some time during the illness, although not necessarily concurrently. (A tic is a sudden, rapid, recurrent, nonrhythmic, stereotyped motor movement or vocalization.)
B. The tics occur many times a day (usually in bouts) nearly every day or intermittently throughout a period of more than 1 year, and during this period there was never a tic-free period of more than 3 consecutive months.
C. The onset is before age 18 years.
D. The disturbance is not due to the direct physiological effects of a substance (e.g., stimulants) or a general medical condition (e.g., Huntington's disease or postviral encephalitis).

Reprinted with permission from the *Diagnostic and Statistical Manual Disorders*, 4th Ed., Test Rev. Copyright 2000 American Psychiatric Association

---

is a good beginning. Because vocal tics usually follow the development of motor tics, questions about the presence of simple sounds are next. Inquiring about the presence of complex vocal tics completes the tic inventory. It is helpful to elucidate other aspects of tic severity, such as the absolute number of tics, the frequency, forcefulness, and intrusiveness of the symptoms, the ability of the individual to successfully suppress the tics, and how noticeable the tics are to others. It is also important to know whether premonitory sensory or cognitive experiences are a component of specific tics because these intrusive experiences may disrupt functioning more than the tics themselves. Although the waxing and waning nature of the tics and the replacement of one tic with another do not directly affect severity, identifying the characteristic course of illness is important for diagnostic confidence.

Last, it is important to assess the impairment due to the tics themselves. Whereas tic severity is frequently correlated with overall impairment, it is not uncommon to identify individuals in whom tic severity and impairment are not correlated. Individuals who experience more impairment than their tic symptoms apparently warrant are a particular clinical challenge. A number of clinical features of tics are associated with impairment:

- Large, disruptive, or painful motor movements
- Vocalizations that call attention to the individual
- Premonitory sensations or cognitions that intrude into consciousness
- Tics that are socially unacceptable.

Whereas tic severity and impairment are often correlated, many individuals with mild tics are most impaired by the comorbid conditions attention-deficit/hyperactivity disorder (ADHD), obsessive–compulsive disorder (OCD), and learning disorders (see next section). An adequate assessment of these conditions is part of any comprehensive evaluation.

It is standard for any evaluation to rule out all other mental disorders. In complex cases of Tourette's disorder, the multitude of behavioral and emotional symptoms can be formulated in a number of different ways. Behavioral and emotional problems can be seen as components of the Tourette's disorder diathesis, as a reaction to having a chronic disorder, or as part of an independent psychiatric disorder that is complicating the clinical picture. Clinical formulations that oversimplify and do not consider the presence of multiple independent disorders may lead to incorrectly attributing unrelated symptoms to Tourette's disorder and may result in diagnostic imprecision and treatment failures. It is important to identify all possible mental disorders in individuals with Tourette's disorder so that the hierarchy of disabling conditions can be identified and treatment initiated accordingly. Positive family history of another mental disorder (e.g., major depressive disorder or panic disorder) may provide clues to the possible mental disorder complicating the presentation of an individual with Tourette's disorder.

Psychosocial issues can play a role in tic severity and in overall adaptation and impairment. Assessment of family, peer, and school support for the youngster (adequate protection) along with assessment for the presence of opportunities to be intellectually, physically, and socially challenged is important. The balance between protection and challenge in children is critical for long-term development. An environment that is too protective decreases opportunities for building skills. An environment that is too challenging can lead to frustration, anger, and maladaptive coping.

Tic assessment requires a careful evaluation of observable tic symptoms. Interestingly, the absence of tic symptoms during an evaluation, in spite of the parent's or child's report, is not uncommon and should not necessarily lead to clinical doubt. Occasionally, an additional clinical observer (e.g., nurse or medical student) may identify tics more readily than the psychiatrist conducting the evaluation. Other than the observation of tics in the interview, there are no pathognomonic physical examination findings. Individuals with Tourette's disorder have been noted to have nonfocal and nonspecific subtle neurological findings ("soft" signs). If tic suppression with neuroleptic agents is considered, a more structured method of documenting the complex movements that are part of the pretreatment baseline evaluation is useful for following the progression of the disease and for subsequent assessment for neuroleptic-induced movements.

No specific laboratory or imaging tests are helpful in making the diagnosis or in assessing an individual with Tourette's disorder. Laboratory assessment is most often done as part of a routine health screen or in anticipation of medication interventions. Currently, laboratory testing for Pediatric Autoimmune Neuropsychiatric Disorders Associated with Streptococcal Infection (PANDAS) and group A beta-hemolytic streptococcal infections (e.g., throat culture, antistreptolysin titer, and screening for antineuronal antibodies) is experimental unless there are clinical signs and symptoms of acute infection.

Frequently Co-occurring Symptoms and Disorders

There is considerable evidence that there is a broad array of co-occurring clinical problems in clinically ascertained subjects with Tourette's disorder. These co-occurring problems can be more disabling than tics and are often the reason people with tics come to clinical attention. The nature and range of these problems is broad and includes problems with mood, impulse control, obsessive–compulsive behaviors, anxiety, attention and learning problems, and conduct problems. In some individuals, these problems reach diagnosable proportions, but in many others, they are less severe and do not fulfill diagnostic criteria. The most common co-occurring disorders are ADHD (50–60%) and OCD (30–70%). The exact relationship of these problems to Tourette's disorder is unclear.

Differences in clinical phenomenology have been noted in studies of obsessions and compulsions in individuals with Tourette's disorder compared with individuals with OCD (without Tourette's disorder) (Table 8-1). Individuals with Tourette's disorder have greater concern with physical symmetry, evenness, and exactness, which are often described as "just right" phenomena, and concerns with impulse control. In contrast, individuals with OCD have more frequent concerns regarding contamination and more cleaning and grooming rituals than do individuals with Tourette's disorder.

Whereas most cases of Tourette's disorder currently presenting for care are children, there are adults who seek a clinical evaluation as a result of having a child diagnosed with Tourette's disorder or learning about Tourette's disorder in the media. Often, these adults have been able to function in spite of their tics. Others may have been given an incorrect diagnosis for their tic disorder or may have been in treatment for co-occurring psychiatric problems without any awareness of the relationship of those problems to the tic disorder. Even though these adults have not previously been diagnosed with a tic disorder, most are aware of their tics and may have experienced the psychosocial stigma commonly associated with a tic disorder. For these adults, a new diagnosis of Tourette's disorder may be psychologically complicated. The relief provided by knowing their diagnosis may be mixed with new questions about Tourette's disorder and its potential impact on their lives.

Tic disorders appear to be common ($>1:100$), whereas Tourette's disorder is less common ($5:10,000$), but perhaps not as rare as previously thought. In general, tic disorders are more common in children than adults, and people with mild tic disorders are much more common than those with severe, complex symptoms. Also, people with tic disorders may present for clinical attention with tics, but tics may not end up as the focus of clinical attention, as comorbid conditions are often more impairing than the tics themselves. Given these realities, the number of adults with persistent and severely impairing tics that warrant tic-suppressing medication is probably very small and these cases may still be considered rare. A similar pattern is seen in children, with fewer children presenting with severe tics warranting tic suppression than children with mild to moderate tics and comorbid psychiatric disorders. Perhaps the most common are those children with transient tics that are not impairing and without comorbid conditions. This last group of children may never come to clinical attention.

Course

In Tourette's disorder, tic symptoms usually begin in childhood; mean age at onset is 7 years. The first tic may develop during the teenage years, but this is unusual. Motor tics of the eyes and face are the most common and the earliest presenting symptoms. Vocal tics tend to follow the development of motor tics. Complex tics of both types tend to follow the development of simple tics. Longitudinal studies suggest that tic severity is greatest in most individuals during the latency and early teenage years. Most individuals experience a decline in tic severity as they get older and only a small percentage of individuals (10%) experience a severe or deteriorating course.

Table 8-1	Obsessions and Compulsions Characteristic of Obsessive–Compulsive Disorder and Tourette's Disorder	
	Obsessive–Compulsive Disorder	**Tourette's Disorder**
Obsessions	Contamination	"Just right" phenomena
	Dirt and germs	Symmetry
	Body wastes	Blurting out obscenity
	Environmental	Saying the right thing
		Violent images
		Sexual thoughts
		Embarrassment
Compulsions	Cleaning	Touching
		Blinking
		Repeating
		Self-injurious behavior
		Hoarding
		Counting
		Ordering

Source: Adapted from George MS, Trimble MR, Ring HA, et al. (1993) Obsessions in obsessive–compulsive disorder with and without Gilles de la Tourette's syndrome. *Am J Psychiatr* **150**, 93–97. Copyright 1993 American Psychiatric Association.

The course of ADHD symptoms in persons with Tourette's disorder is similar to that in children without Tourette's disorder. ADHD symptoms usually begin earlier than the tic symptoms.

Obsessive–compulsive symptoms in persons with Tourette's disorder generally begin somewhat later than ADHD and tics, and may actually progress differentially from tic symptoms. Tic symptoms tend to improve into adulthood; obsessive–compulsive symptoms may actually increase in severity.

Differential Diagnosis

Tics have many characteristics that differentiate them from the other movement disorders (Table 8-2). Perhaps most important to "ruling in" tics as a diagnostic possibility is the childhood history of simple motor tics in the face. Other movement disorders do not have a similar pattern of movement onset or location. There are atypical presentations of tic disorders that may resemble other movement disorders, but these would be unusual and would probably require a consultation with a movement disorders expert.

Movement disorders such as chorea and dystonia are continuous movements and can be distinguished from tics, which are intermittent. Paroxysmal dyskinesias, although episodic, are more often characterized by choreiform and dystonic movements, which are different from tics. Myoclonic movements and exaggerated startle responses are also intermittent movements but are usually large-muscle movements that occur in response to a person-specific stimulus. Complex tics can be more difficult to differentiate from other complex movements such as mannerisms, gestures, or stereotypies. In a person with clear-cut motor tics, it may be difficult to differentiate a complex motor tic from a "camouflaged" tic (making a simple tic appear to be a purposeful action, e.g., an upward hand movement that

Table 8-2	Differential Diagnosis of Tics
Simple, rapid movements	
Myoclonus	
Chorea	
Seizures	
Simple, sustained movements	
Dystonia	
Athetosis	
Complex or sustained movements	
Mannerisms	
Stereotypies	
Restless legs	

Source: Jankovic J (1992) Diagnosis and classification of tics and Tourette syndrome. *Adv Neurol* **58**, 7–14, copyright, Lipincott, Williams & Wilkins.

the person turns into a hair smoothing gesture), mannerism, gesture, or stereotypy. Mannerisms or gestures are often not impairing; stereotypies tend to occur exclusively in children and adults with developmental disabilities and mental retardation.

It is also possible to have a tic disorder and another movement disorder. For example, tic movements can co-occur with dystonia. Similarly, it is not uncommon in tertiary referral centers to see developmentally disabled children and adults with both tics and stereotypies.

TREATMENT

The initiation of treatment can be a delicate process, given the difficulties individuals with tics and their families experience before finding appropriate care. Most families are frightened about their child's having a neuropsychiatric disorder and envision a grim prognosis. After the evaluation is completed, often in the first session, general education of the individual and family about the course of the tic disorder is essential. Most children and families are relieved to hear that the majority of persons with tics have consistent improvement in tic severity as they move through their teenage years and into adulthood. They are also pleased to hear that tic symptoms are not inherently impairing. In this regard, it is often helpful to cite examples of sports personalities or other public figures who have identified themselves as having Tourette's disorder and are doing well both personally and professionally.

Once issues regarding the tics are discussed and clarified, the focus shifts to the presence of comorbid conditions. Identifying whether ADHD, LD, and OCD are present is especially important because they are often the more common impairing conditions in these children. Yet the transition to addressing the co-occurring problems is often not easy. Individuals, families, and mental health professionals are usually focused on the tic symptoms. Tics are more readily apparent and relatively easy to suppress with medications, whereas the co-occurring conditions, especially if they are internalizing disorders, are easy to overlook. One of the major pitfalls of treatment of individuals with Tourette's disorder is to pursue tic suppression to the exclusion of the treatment of other co-occurring conditions that are present and possibly more impairing.

Creating the hierarchy of the most impairing conditions is the next major step in treatment. Most clinicians, as part of their formulation, create some clinical hierarchy; yet in Tourette's disorder, with the multitude of often complex problems, it is essential that a conscious effort be made to formulate, organize, and create hierarchies for treatment. For example, children with moderate tics and separation anxiety with school refusal should be considered for treatment with a selective serotonin reuptake inhibitor (SSRI) for their separation anxiety rather than neuroleptics for tic suppression. It is possible that with successful treatment of the anxiety disorder, the individual may also experience a reduction in tic severity.

Somatic Treatments

The goal of pharmacological treatment is the reduction of tic severity, not necessarily the elimination of tics. Haloperidol has been used effectively to suppress motor and phonic tics for more than 30 years. Since that time, a number of other neuroleptic agents have also been identified as useful in tic suppression, including fluphenazine and pimozide. In Europe, the substituted benzamides, sulpiride and tiapride, and the non-neuroleptic tetrabenazine have also been shown to be useful. Preliminary results with risperidone have been mixed, whereas trials with clozapine are more uniformly negative. The major drawback with neuroleptic agents is the frequent and significant side effects, which often preclude continued use of the medication.

There are continuing efforts to identify tic-suppressing agents with tolerable side effects. Most frequently cited in this regard are the alpha-adrenergic agonists clonidine and guanfacine. Both of these agents were developed as antihypertensives. These agents do not appear to be uniformly effective in tic suppression, but they can be effective for some individuals without significant side effects. Both clonidine and guanfacine also appear to be useful for some of the symptoms of ADHD, which makes these agents a reasonable first choice for those individuals with both Tourette's disorder and ADHD.

Antipsychotics. Side effects with all neuroleptics are common and are the reason that neuroleptics are not used by the majority of individuals with Tourette's disorder. Side effects include those traditionally seen with neuroleptics, such as sedation, acute dystonic reactions, extrapyramidal symptoms including akathisia, weight gain, cognitive dulling, and the common anticholinergic side effects. There have also been reports of subtle, difficult-to-recognize side effects with neuroleptics, including clinical depression, separation anxiety, panic attacks, and school avoidance.

Dosage reduction is the most prudent response to side effects, although the addition of medications such as benztropine for the extrapyramidal symptoms can be useful. Dosage reduction in those children with Tourette's disorder who have been administered neuroleptics long-term may be complicated by withdrawal dyskinesias and significant tic worsening or rebound. Withdrawal dyskinesias are choreoathetoid movements of the orofacial region, trunk, and extremities that appear after neuroleptic discontinuation or dosage reduction and tend to resolve in 1 to 3 months. Tic worsening even above pretreatment baseline level (i.e., rebound) can last up to 1 to 3 months after discontinuation or dosage reduction. Tardive dyskinesia, which is similar in character to withdrawal dyskinesia, most often develops during the course of treatment or is "unmasked" with dosage reductions. Rarely have cases of tardive dyskinesia been reported to occur in individuals with Tourette's disorder.

The atypical neuroleptics appear to have replaced the standard neuroleptics as the mainstay of treatment for the psychotic disorders. Given the potentially lower risk for tardive dyskinesia with these agents, their efficacy has been assessed for tic suppression in individuals with Tourette's disorder. To date, there are only small controlled or open trials to guide the clinician in the use of these agents. Clozapine does not appear to be effective as a tic-suppressing agent and its hematological side effects preclude its use. Risperidone has been effective in reducing tic symptom severity in one controlled trial and may have the added benefit of augmenting SSRIs in treating tic-related OCD.

Olanzapine in low doses does not appear to have the same tic-suppressing power as the typical neuroleptics. The side effects, especially weight gain, have dampened the enthusiasm for the atypicals risperidone, olanzapine, and quetiapine.

Clonidine and Guanfacine. There is a long history of the use of the alpha-adrenergic agonist clonidine for suppression of tics and ADHD symptoms. Whereas controlled trials have shown that some individuals benefit with symptom reduction, the overall effect of clonidine for tic suppression and ADHD is more modest than that achieved with the "gold standards" (haloperidol and the stimulants, respectively) for these conditions. Given clonidine's mild side effect profile, it is often the first drug used for tic suppression, especially in those children with Tourette's disorder and ADHD. The onset of action is slower for tic suppression (3–6 weeks) than for ADHD symptoms. Side effects, in addition to sedation, include irritability, headaches, decreased salivation, and hypotension and dizziness at higher doses. Interestingly, owing to clonidine's short half-life, some individuals experience mild withdrawal symptoms between doses. More severe rebound in autonomic activity and tics can occur if the medication is discontinued abruptly.

Guanfacine is an alpha-2-adrenergic agonist that potentially offers greater benefit than clonidine because of differences in site of action, side effects, and duration of action. Guanfacine may have a greater impact on attention without the significant sedation associated with the nonselective alpha-2-adrenergic agonist clonidine. Guanfacine's long half-life offers the advantage of twice-a-day dosing, which is more convenient than the multiple dosing required with clonidine. Clinically, the effect on tics is less than would be expected with neuroleptics.

Benzodiazepines. Benzodiazepines can be useful in decreasing comorbid anxiety in individuals with Tourette's disorder. In addition, clonazepam appears also to be useful in selected individuals for tic reduction. Often, doses of 3 to 6 mg/day may be necessary for tic reduction. Because sedation is a significant side effect at these dosages, an extended titration phase of 3 to 6 months may be necessary. Similarly, a slow taper is required to avoid withdrawal symptoms.

Pergolide. Agonist activity on presynaptic dopamine neurons results in decreased dopamine release and may therefore result in decreased tic severity in people with Tourette's disorder. Pergolide, a mixed D_1–D_2–D_3 dopamine agonist often used for restless leg syndrome, may be superior to placebo in reducing tic severity and was associated with few adverse events. Doses used are low, as higher doses may be associated with dopamine agonist effects postsynaptically.

Psychosocial Treatments

Published studies of behavioral approaches to tic suppression are few but show some promise. The behavioral technique shown to be most effective is habit reversal training. For Tourette's disorder, habit reversal training is the use of a competing muscle contraction or behavioral response that opposes the tic movement. This method is usually combined with relaxation training, self-monitoring, awareness training, and positive reinforcement. In the few published studies of habit reversal training, there were marked overall reductions in tic frequency. Treatment averaged 20 training sessions during an 8- to 11-month period. Marked tic reduction was noted at 3 to 4 months. Interestingly, urges or sensations experienced before the tic movements also decreased with behavioral treatment.

There are no published systematic studies of psychosocial interventions for individuals with Tourette's disorder. Most treatment efforts are based on a combination of traditional psychosocial interventions and clinical judgment.

Perhaps the most useful psychosocial and educational intervention is to make the individual aware of the Tourette Syndrome Association, both national and local chapters. This and other self-help groups can be useful as a source of support and education for individuals with tics, families, and mental health professionals.

Individual psychotherapy can be useful for support, development of awareness, or for addressing personal and interpersonal problems more effectively. Family therapy can be useful when families have problems adjusting, functioning, and communicating. Although most families do well, some families have difficulties understanding the involuntary nature of tics and may punish their children for their tics, even after diagnosis and education. Alternatively, some families have more behavior difficulties with their children after diagnosis than before. Many parents of children with Tourette's disorder inadvertently lower general behavior expectations because of confusion about what behaviors are tics and what behaviors are not tics. Sometimes parents decrease behavior expectations for their children because of the parents' desire not to add any additional stress to the youngster's life. Also, with confusion in the field regarding the scope of problems in Tourette's disorder, some parents see all maladaptive behaviors as involuntary and do not hold their children responsible for their behaviors. For children with Tourette's disorder to do well, they need support from their family to develop effective self-control in areas not affected by Tourette's disorder so that optimal adaptation can occur.

For children, active intervention at school is essential to create a supportive yet challenging academic and social environment. Efforts to educate teachers, principals, and other students can result in increased awareness of Tourette's disorder and tolerance for the child's symptoms.

Many young adults are finding Tourette's disorder support and social groups important for interpersonal contact and continued adult development. Efforts to keep people with Tourette's disorder working are important, as are rehabilitation efforts for those who are not working. Finding housing and obtaining disability or public assistance may be necessary for the most disabled individuals with Tourette's disorder.

Treatment-Refractory Cases

Perhaps the most important "treatment" in individuals with severe incapacitating tics is a full clinical reevaluation to assess the adequacy of previous evaluations and treatment efforts. It is not uncommon for treatment-refractory individuals to have had inadequate evaluations and treatment trials.

When a single tic or a few tics are refractory and impairing, the injection of botulinum toxin into the specific muscle group can be helpful. This strategy is most useful for painful, dystonic tics. Treatment has a long duration of action, but the effect does decrease in 2 to 4 months, and repeated injections may be necessary. Specific side effects are few, other than weakness in the affected muscle. Some individuals reported the loss of the premonitory sensation with their botulinum toxin treatment. For the mental health clinician it is essential to work with a neurologist experienced in using botulinum toxin.

There have been reports in the literature and the media concerning the use of neurosurgical approaches for the treatment of refractory tics. To date, the optimal size and location of the surgical treatment lesions are not known, results are variable, and thus such approaches cannot be recommended at present.

COMPARISON OF DSM-IV-TR AND ICD-10 DIAGNOSTIC CRITERIA

The ICD-10 and DSM-IV-TR criteria sets for the tic disorders are almost identical.

9 Childhood Disorders: Elimination Disorders and Childhood Anxiety Disorders

Enuresis

DIAGNOSIS

Functional enuresis is defined as the intentional or involuntary passage of urine in bed or clothes in the absence of any identified physical abnormality in children older than 4 years of age. Although there is no good evidence that the condition is primarily psychogenic, it is often associated with a mental disorder, and enuretic children are frequently referred to mental health services for treatment. The DSM-IV-TR diagnosis of Enuresis (Not Due to a General Medical Condition) is made if there is repeated voiding of urine that is clinically significant, as defined by either occurring at a frequency of twice a week for at least 3 consecutive months, or else causing clinically significant impairment in social, academic, or other important areas of functioning. Furthermore, the diagnosis is only given if the individual's chronological age is at least 5 years (or equivalent developmental level).

Information on the frequency, periodicity, and duration of symptoms is needed to make the diagnosis and distinguish functional enuresis from sporadic seizure-associated enuresis. If there is diurnal enuresis, an additional treatment plan is required. A family history of enuresis increases the likelihood of a diagnosis of functional enuresis and may explain the later age at which the children are presented for treatment. Projective identification by the affected parent—whereby the parent does not separate their own feelings about having had the diagnosis with the current experience of their affected child—may further hinder treatment. For subjects with secondary enuresis, the precipitating factors should be elicited, although such efforts often represent an attempt to assign a meaning after the event.

The child's views and any misconceptions that he or she may have about the enuresis, its causes, and its treatment should be fully explored. Asking the child for three wishes may help determine whether the enuresis is a concern to the child. This may unmask marked embarrassment or guilt from behind a facade of denial about the problem, and can be educational for parents who believe their children could stop wetting "if only they wanted to or tried harder." Pictures drawn by the child that describe how the child views himself or herself when enuresis is a problem and when it is not are appropriate for younger children, and can graphically illustrate the misery experienced by children with enuresis.

All children should have a routine physical examination, with particular emphasis placed on the detection of congenital malformations that are possibly indicative of urogenital abnormalities. A midstream specimen of urine should be examined for the presence of infection. Radiological or further medical investigation is indicated only in the presence of infected urine, enuresis with symptoms suggestive of recurrent urinary tract infection (UTI) (frequency, urgency, and dysuria), or polyuria.

Course

Nocturnal enuresis is as common in boys as in girls until the age of 5 years, but by age 11 years, boys outnumber girls 2 : 1. Not until the age of 8 years do boys achieve the same levels of nighttime continence that are seen in girls by the age of 5 years. This appears to be due to slower physiological maturation in boys. In addition, the increased incidence of secondary enuresis (occurring after an initial 1-year period of acquired continence) in boys further affects the sex ratio seen in later childhood. Daytime enuresis occurs more commonly in girls.

Differential Diagnosis

The presence or absence of conditions often seen in association with enuresis, such as developmental delay,

Clinical Guide to the Diagnosis and Treatment of Mental Disorders. M. B. First and A. Tasman
© 2006 John Wiley & Sons, Ltd.   ISBN 0 470 019158

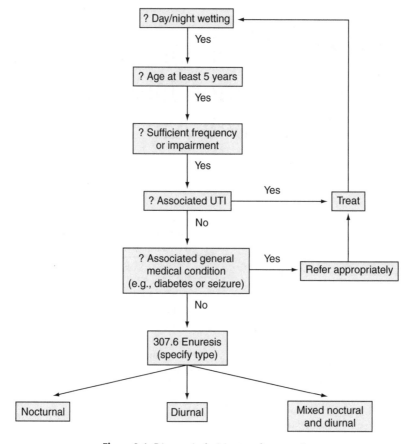

Figure 9-1 *Diagnostic decision tree for enuresis.*

UTI, constipation, and comorbid psychiatric disorder, should be assessed and ruled out as appropriate (Figure 9-1). Other causes of nocturnal incontinence should be excluded, for example, those leading to polyuria (diabetes mellitus, renal disease, diabetes insipidus) and, rarely, nocturnal epilepsy.

TREATMENT OF NOCTURNAL ENURESIS

Questions that are useful in obtaining information for treatment planning include "Why is this a problem?" and "Why does this need treatment now?" because these factors may influence the choice of treatment (is a rapid effect needed?) or point to other pressures or restrictions on therapy. It is important to inquire about previous management strategies—for example, fluid restriction, night lifting (getting the child out of bed to take to the toilet, in an often semiasleep state), rewards, and punishments—used at home. Parents often come with the assertion that they have tried everything and that nothing has helped. Examining the reasons for the failure of simple strategies is useful for ensuring that more sophisticated treatments do not befall the same

fate. Practical management for nocturnal enuresis is presented in Table 9-1.

About 10% of children have a reduction in the number of wet nights after a single visit to a clinician in which the only intervention was the recording of baseline wetting frequency and simple reassurance. Such reassurance should make clear that enuresis is a biological condition that is made worse by stress and that may be associated in a noncausal way with other psychiatric disorders. Younger children can be told that their problem is shared by many others of the same age. The excellent prognosis for individuals who comply with therapy should be stressed. Recording the frequency of enuresis can be achieved by using a simple star chart. This is most effective if performed by the child, who records each dry night with a star. The completed chart is then shown to the parents on a daily basis, and they can provide appropriate praise and reinforcement.

Waking and Fluid Restriction

Although systematic studies have failed to show any effect of these interventions with enuretic inpatients, it may

Table 9-1	Practical Management of Nocturnal Enuresis
Stage 1	**Assessment** Obtain history: frequency, periodicity, and duration of wetting. Why is this a problem? Why now? Mental status: views and misconceptions (parent and child). Discover reasons for previous failure or failures. Perform routine physical examination (any minor congenital abnormalities?). Midstream specimen of urine must be obtained. Radiology and further physical investigation is needed only if symptoms or evidence of urinary tract infection (dysuria and frequency or positive culture results) or polyuria.
Stage 2	**Advice** Education that enuresis is common and not deliberate. Aim to reduce punitive behavior. Transmit optimism: however, anticipate disappointment at no instant cure. Preview the stepwise recovery and warn of the possibility of relapse.
Stage 3	**Baseline** Use star chart. Focus on positive achievements (be creative). Examine the effect of simple interventions (e.g., lifting)
Stage 4	**Night Alarm** First-line management unless important to obtain rapid short-term effect. Demonstrate night-alarm equipment in the office. Telephone follow-up within a few days of commencing therapy. *Or* **Drug Therapy** If rapid suppression of wetting is needed (e.g., before vacation or camp, to defuse aggressive or hostile situation between child and parents and siblings). When family has proved incapable of using the equipment. After failure or multiple relapses. Medication of choice: DDAVP, (Desmopressin) 20–40 μg at night

be that these strategies work for the majority of enuretic children who are not referred for treatment. If waking does appear to reduce the number of wet nights from baseline, a more systematic application may be indicated.

Surgery

On the basis of the premise that enuresis is causally associated with outflow-tract obstruction, various surgical procedures have been advocated. Reported positive treatment effects are slight (no controlled studies exist), and there remains a significant potential for adverse effects (urinary incontinence, epididymitis, and aspermia).

Pharmacotherapy

Although it has been repeatedly demonstrated that temporary suppression rather than cure of enuresis is the usual outcome of drug therapy, it remains the most widely prescribed treatment in the United States. Four classes of drugs have principally been employed: synthetic antidiuretic hormones, tricyclic antidepressants, stimulants, and anticholinergic agents. There is no evidence that stimulants or anticholinergic agents are effective.

Synthetic Antidiuretic Hormone. The drug is usually administered intranasally, although oral preparations of equal efficacy have been developed (equivalent oral dose is 10 times the intranasal dose). It has been shown that almost 50% of children are able to stop wetting completely with a single nightly dose of 20–40 mcg of DDAVP given intranasally. A further 40% are afforded a significant reduction in the frequency of enuresis with this treatment. As with tricyclic antidepressants, however, when treatment is stopped, the vast majority of individuals relapse. Side effects of this medication include nasal pain and congestion, headache, nausea, and abdominal pain. Serious problems of water intoxication, hyponatremia, and seizures are rare. It is important to be aware that intranasal absorption is reduced when the child has a cold or allergic rhinitis. The mode of action of desmopressin is unknown.

Tricyclic Antidepressants. The short-term effectiveness of imipramine and other related antidepressants has also been demonstrated via many randomized double-blind placebo-controlled trials For example imipramine reduces the frequency of enuresis in about 85% of bed wetters and eliminates enuresis in about 30% of these individuals. Nighttime doses of 1–2.5 mg/kg are usually effective, and a therapeutic effect is usually evident in the first week of treatment. Relapse after withdrawal of medication is almost inevitable, so that 3 months after the cessation of tricyclic antidepressants, nearly all children will again have enuresis at pretreatment levels. Side effects are common and include dry mouth, dizziness, postural hypotension, headache, and constipation. Toxicity after accidental ingestion or overdose is a serious consideration, causing cardiac effects, including arrhythmias and conduction defects, convulsions, hallucinations, and ataxia. Concern has been expressed about the possibility of sudden death (presumably caused by arrhythmia) in children taking tricyclic drugs. The mode of action for tricyclic antidepressants is unclear.

Stimulant Medication. Sympathomimetic stimulants such as dexamphetamine have been used to reduce the depth of sleep in children with enuresis but because there is no evidence that enuresis is related to abnormally deep sleep, their lack of effectiveness in stopping bed-wetting is no surprise.

Anticholinergic Drugs. Drugs such as propantheline, oxybutynin, and terodiline can reduce the frequency of voiding in individuals with neurogenic bladders, reduce urgency, and increase functional bladder capacity. There is no evidence, however, that these anticholinergic drugs are effective in bed-wetting, although they may have a role in diurnal enuresis. Side effects are frequent and include dry mouth, blurred vision, headache, nausea, and constipation.

Psychosocial Treatments

The original night alarm used two electrodes separated by a device (e.g., bedding) connected to an alarm. When the child wet the bed, the urine completed the electrical circuit, sounded the alarm, and the child awoke. All current night-alarm systems are merely refinements on this original design. A vibrating pad beneath the pillow can be used instead of a bell or buzzer, or the electrodes can be incorporated into a single unit or can be miniaturized so that they can be attached to night (or day) clothing. With treatment, full cessation of enuresis can be expected in 80% of cases. Reported cure rates (defined as a minimum of 14 consecutive dry nights) have ranged from 50% to 100%.

The main problem with this form of enuretic treatment, however, is that cure is usually achieved only within the second month of treatment. This factor may influence clinicians to prescribe pharmacological treatments that, although are more immediately gratifying, do not offer any real prospect of cure. A further consequence of the delayed response to a night alarm is that families fail to persist with the treatment and may abandon the treatment too soon. Relapse after successful treatment, if it occurs, will usually take place within the first 6 months after cessation of treatment. It is reported that approximately one-third of children relapse; however, no clear predictors of relapse have been identified.

Table 9-2 presents various remedies for night-alarm problems.

Ultrasonic Bladder Volume Alarm. The traditional enuresis alarm has good potential for a permanent cure, but the child is mostly wet during treatment. Furthermore, the moisture alarm requires that the child make

Table 9-2	Problem Solving for the Night Alarm
Bell "does not work"	Check position, connections, and batteries.
	If using separating sheet, check that it is porous.
	Check that child is not turning off equipment.
	Place alarm out of easy reach.
Child does not wake	Make alarm louder.
	Parent should wake child.
Child does not become dry	Ensure compliance. Ensure that child responds promptly.
	Use adjuvant DDAVP or dextroamphetamine.
	Ensure that child has role (e.g., change own bedsheets) after alarm.
False alarms	Ensure that separating sheet is big enough, not soiled, and will insulate.
	Use thicker nightclothes.
Relapse	Repeat treatment.
	Consider overlearning after response to re-treatment.

the somewhat remote association between the alarm event and a full bladder after the bladder has emptied. Bladder-volume tracking seems to be a promising treatment for nocturnal enuresis in that it prevents the enuretic event, appears to facilitate a permanent cure, and is noninvasive. This approach uses a miniature bladder-volume measurement instrument during sleep.

TREATMENT OF DIURNAL ENURESIS

Daytime enuresis, although it can occur together with nighttime enuresis, has a different pattern of associations, and responds to different methods of treatment. It is much more likely to be associated with urinary tract abnormalities, including UTI, and to be comorbid with other psychiatric disorders. As a result, a more detailed and focused medical and psychiatric evaluation is indicated. Urine should be checked repeatedly for infection, and the threshold for ordering ultrasonographical visualization of the urological system should be low. The history may make it apparent that the daytime wetting is situation specific. For example, school-based enuresis in a child who is too timid to ask to use the bathroom could be alleviated by the teacher tactfully reminding the child to go to the bathroom at regular intervals.

Observation of children with diurnal enuresis has established that they do experience an urge to pass urine before micturition but that either this urge is ignored or the warning comes too late to be of any use because of an "irritable bladder." Therefore, treatment strategies are based on establishing a pattern of toileting before the times that diurnal enuresis is likely to occur (usually between 12 noon and 5 PM), and using positive reinforcement to promote regular use of the bathroom.

Unlike nocturnal enuresis, drug treatment with tricyclic antidepressants, such as imipramine, is ineffective, whereas the use of anticholinergic agents such as oxybutynin and terodiline shows a therapeutic impact on the frequency of daytime enuresis.

Encopresis

DIAGNOSIS

Encopresis is usually defined as the intentional or involuntary passage of stool in inappropriate places in the absence of any identified physical abnormality in children older than 4 years. The distinction is drawn between encopresis with constipation (retention with overflow) and encopresis without constipation. Other classification schemes include making a primary–secondary distinction (based on having a 1-year period of continence), or soiling with fluid or normal feces.

Less than one-third of children in the United States have completed toilet training by the age of 2 years. Bowel control is usually achieved before bladder control. The age cutoff for "normality" is set at 4 years, the age at which 95% of children have acquired fecal

continence. As with urinary continence, girls achieve bowel control earlier than boys do.

The main efforts during the diagnostic process are to establish the presence or absence of constipation and, to a lesser extent, distinguish continuous (primary) from discontinuous (secondary) soiling (Figure 9-2). Three types of identifiable encopresis in children have been identified: (1) it is known that the child can control defecation, but she or he chooses to defecate in inappropriate places; (2) there is true failure to gain bowel control, and the child is unaware of or unable to control soiling; and (3) soiling is due to excessively fluid feces, whether from constipation and overflow, physical disease, or anxiety. In practice, there is frequently an overlap among types or progression from one to another. Unlike enuresis, fecal soiling rarely occurs at night or during sleep, and if present, is indicative of a poor prognosis.

In the first group, in which bowel control has been established, the stool may be soft or normal (but different from fluid-type feces seen in overflow). Soiling due to acute stress events (e.g., the birth of a sibling, a change of school, or parental separation) is usually brief once the stress has abated, given a stable home environment and sensible management. In more severe pathological family situations, including punitive management

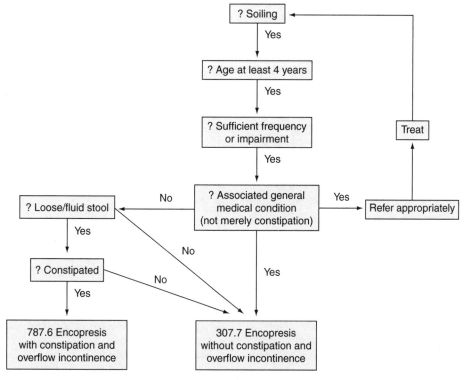

Figure 9-2 *Diagnostic decision for encopresis.*

or frank physical or sexual abuse, the feces may be deposited in places designed to cause anger or irritation or there may be associated smearing of feces on furniture and walls. Other covert aggressive antisocial acts may be evident, with considerable denial by the child of the magnitude or seriousness of the problem.

In the second group, in which there is failure to learn bowel control, a nonfluid stool is deposited fairly randomly in clothes, at home, and at school. There may be conditions such as mental retardation or specific developmental delay, spina bifida, or cerebral palsy that impair the ability to recognize the need to defecate, and the appropriate skills needed to defer this function until a socially appropriate time and location. In the absence of low IQ or pathological physical condition, individuals with encopresis have been reported as having associated enuresis, academic skills problems, and antisocial behavior. They present to pediatricians primarily, and are usually younger (age 4 to 6 years) than other encopretic individuals.

In the third group, excessively fluid feces are passed, which may result from conditions that cause true diarrhea (e.g., ulcerative colitis) or, much more frequently, from constipation with overflow causing spurious diarrhea. A history of retention, either willful or in response to pain, is prominent in the early days of this form of encopresis, although later it may be less apparent because of fecal overflow. Behavior such as squatting on the heels to prevent defecation or marked anxiety about the prospect of using the toilet (although rarely amounting to true phobic avoidance) may be described.

Having identified the presence of encopretic behavior and formed some idea of the type of encopresis (primary, secondary, retentive, or a combination), the remaining task is to discover the presence and extent of any associated conditions, both medical and psychological. The comprehensive assessment process should include a medical evaluation, psychiatric and family interviews, and a systematic behavioral recording.

The overall prevalence of encopresis in 7- and 8-year-old children has been shown to be 1.5%, with boys (2.3%) affected more commonly than girls (0.7%). There was a steadily increasing likelihood of continence with increasing age, until by age 16 years the reported prevalence was almost zero. A retrospective study of clinic-referred encopretic children has shown that 40% of cases are primary (true failure to gain control), with a mean age of 6.7 years, and 60% of cases are secondary, with a mean age of 8 years. Eighty percent of the children were constipated, with no difference in this feature seen between primary and secondary subtypes.

TREATMENT

Practical management for encopresis is presented in Table 9-3. The principal approach to treatment is predicated on the results of the evaluation and the clinical category assigned. This differentiates between the need to establish a regular toileting procedure in children in whom there has been a failure to learn this social behavior and the need to address a psychiatric disorder, parent–child relationship difficulties, or other stresses in the child who exhibits loss of this previously acquired skill in association with these factors. In both cases, analysis of the soiling behavior may identify reinforcing factors important in maintaining

Table 9-3	Practical Management of Encopresis
Stage 1	**Assessment** Whether primary or secondary. Is there physical cause? Presence or absence of constipation. Presence or absence of acute stress. Presence or absence of psychiatric disorder including phobic symptoms or smearing. ABC (antecedents, behavior, consequences) of encopresis including secondary gain. Discover reasons for previous failure or failures.
Stage 2	**Advice** Education regarding diet, constipation, and toileting. Aim to reduce punitive or coercive behavior. Transmit optimism; however, anticipate disappointment at no instant cure. Preview the stepwise recovery and warn of the possibility of relapse.
Stage 3	**Toileting** Baseline observation using star chart. Focus on positive achievements, e.g., toileting, rather than soiling. High-fiber diet (try bran in soup, milk shakes). Toilet after meals, 15 minutes maximum. Check that adequately rising intra-abdominal pressure is present. Graded exposure scheme if "pot phobic." *with* **Laxatives** Indicated if physical examination or abdominal radiograph shows fecal loading. Medication of choice: Senokot syrup (senna) up to 10 mL b.i.d., lactulose syrup up to 30 mL (20 mg) b.i.d. Dosage will be reduced over time; titrate with bowel frequency. **Enemas** Microenema (e.g., bisacodyl, 30 mL) if the bowel is excessively loaded with rock-like feces.
Stage 4	**Biofeedback** Consider after relapse or failure to respond to toileting or laxatives.

dysfunction. Detection of significant constipation will, in addition, provide an indication for adjuvant laxative therapy.

Behavioral Treatments

Behavioral therapy is the mainstay of treatment for encopresis. In the younger child who has been toilet trained, this focuses on practical elimination skills, for example, visiting the toilet after each meal, staying there for a maximum of 15 minutes, using muscles to increase intra-abdominal pressure, and cleaning oneself adequately afterward. Parents or caretakers, or both, need to be educated in making the toilet a pleasant place to visit and should stay with the younger child, giving encouragement and praise for appropriate effort. Systematic recording of positive toileting behavior, not necessarily being clean (depending on the level of baseline behavior), should be performed with a personal star chart.

Removing the child's and family's attention from the encopresis alone and onto noticing, recording, and rewarding positive behavior often defuses tension and hostility and provides the opportunity for therapeutic improvement. Identifying and eliminating sources of secondary gain, whereby soiling is reinforced by parental (or other individuals') actions and attention, even if negative or punitive, make positive efforts more fruitful. Formal therapy, either individual or family based, is indicated in only a minority of individuals with an associated mental disorder, marked behavioral disturbance (e.g., smearing, other aggressive soiling), or clear remediable family or social stresses.

Physical Treatments

In children with retention, leading to constipation and overflow, medical management is nearly always required, although it is usually done with oral laxatives or microenemas alone. The use of more intrusive and invasive colonic and rectal washout or surgical disimpaction procedures is nearly always the result of the clinician's impatience rather than the true clinical need.

Biofeedback Therapy

The finding that some children with treatment-resistant retentive encopresis involuntarily contract the muscles of the pelvic floor and the external anal sphincter, effectively impeding passage of stool has led to efforts to use biofeedback in such instances. Benefits are unclear.

Separation Anxiety Disorder

DIAGNOSIS

Separation anxiety disorder (SAD) is typified by developmentally inappropriate and excessive anxiety concerning separation from home or attachment figures.

The assessment strategy will depend upon the child's age, symptom profile, the sources of available information, and the purpose of the assessment. Separation anxiety is normal at some ages, and is maximal around 14 months of age. The most prevalent symptoms in

DSM-IV-TR Diagnostic Criteria

309.21 SEPARATION ANXIETY DISORDER

A. Developmentally inappropriate and excessive anxiety concerning separation from home or from those to whom the individual is attached, as evidenced by three (or more) of the following:
  (1) recurrent excessive distress when separation from home or major attachment figures occurs or is anticipated
  (2) persistent and excessive worry about losing, or about possible harm befalling major attachment figures
  (3) persistent and excessive worry that an untoward event will lead to separation from a major attachment figure (e.g., getting lost or being kidnapped)
  (4) persistent reluctance or refusal to go to school or elsewhere because of fear of separation
  (5) persistently and excessively fearful or reluctant to be alone, or without major attachment figures at home, or without significant adults in other settings
  (6) persistent reluctance or refusal to go to sleep without being near a major attachment figure or to sleep away from home
  (7) repeated nightmares involving the theme of separation
  (8) repeated complaints of physical symptoms (such as headaches, stomach aches, nausea, or vomiting) when separation from major attachment figures occurs or is anticipated
B. The duration of the disturbance is at least 4 weeks.
C. The onset is before age 18 years.
D. The disturbance causes clinically significant distress or impairment in social, academic (occupational), or other important areas of functioning.
E. The disturbance does not occur exclusively during the course of a pervasive developmental disorder, schizophrenia, or other psychotic disorder and, in adolescents and adults, is not better accounted for by panic disorder with agoraphobia.

Specify if:

Early Onset: if onset occurs before age 6 years.

Reprinted with permission from the *Diagnostic and Statistical Manual of Mental Disorders*, 4th ed., Text Rev. Copyright 2000 American Psychiatric Association.

young children (aged 5–8) are worry about losing, or about possible harm to an attachment figure, and reluctance or refusal to go to school. Children aged 9–12 most frequently reported recurrent excessive distress when separated from home or attachment figures, whereas adolescents (aged 13–16 years) had physical symptoms on school days. More symptoms were reported with decreasing age.

Other anxiety disorders must be distinguished from separation anxiety disorder. In contrast to SAD, where the anxiety is focused on separation issues, in generalized anxiety disorder (GAD) the anxiety is more free floating, less situation specific, and occurs independent of separation from the primary attachment figure. Children with social phobia will display a fear of social situations in which they may be the object of public scrutiny. This anxiety may be ameliorated by the presence of a familiar person but will not occur exclusively when the attachment figure is absent, as with separation anxiety.

School refusal has long been associated with separation anxiety disorder, though this relationship holds mainly for younger children when school nonattendance is most closely linked to fear of separation, whereas in adolescents fear of school and social-evaluative situations is more typical. It is important in the assessment of school nonattendance, a frequent impairment associated with SAD, to distinguish anxiety-related school refusal from conduct disorder-related truancy. Typically the school-refusing child will stay at home or with parents, whereas the truanting child will go off with peers. In the presence of school refusal, a useful approach is to attempt to categorize the behavior as fulfilling one of the following four functions: (1) avoidance of stimuli provoking specific fearfulness or anxiety (e.g., separation); (2) escape from aversive social or evaluative situations (e.g., social phobia); (3) attention-getting behavior (e.g., physical complaints/tantrums); or (4) positive tangible reinforcement (e.g., parental collusion).

The community prevalence of SAD is generally estimated to be around 4% in children and young adolescents; it decreases in prevalence from childhood through adolescence. Among clinically referred subjects (aged 5–18) with anxiety disorders, separation anxiety disorder was found to be the most frequently occurring disorder, with a lifetime prevalence of 44.7%. Separation anxiety, particularly in younger samples, is found more frequently in girls than in boys—ratio as high as 2.5 : 1.

Course

The age of onset has been reported to be 4–7 years, with earlier onset being associated with clinical status

and comorbidity. In a 3–4-year prospective study of subjects with anxiety disorders, 29% of children had separation anxiety disorder (21% had SAD as their primary diagnosis at baseline). On follow-up, 92% of children previously diagnosed with SAD no longer had symptoms that met full criteria for SAD, although 25% had developed a new disorder, most frequently a depressive disorder. Finding that 50% of adult individuals with panic disorder had experienced separation anxiety during childhood, it has been hypothesized that separation anxiety may be a childhood precursor to adult panic disorder and agoraphobia. Evidence supporting this link is uneven since most studies are retrospective, focus on separation anxiety symptoms rather than the full disorder and/or fail to include an appropriate control group.

TREATMENT

Following a good behavioral and functional analysis, the most frequently employed clinical approach to the treatment of separation anxiety and school refusal is behavioral. The principles of systematic desensitization to feared objects or situations will be employed, gradually increasing the amount of separation that can be tolerated in a graduated fashion. Systematic desensitization usually has three components. First, a response, incompatible with anxiety (often progressive muscular relaxation, but can be imagery or breathing exercises) is taught. The second component is the collaborative construction of a hierarchy of feared situations. These will range from the very mild (producing mild disquiet) to the most anxiety provoking (avoided at all costs!). It is important to include a great deal of specificity in describing these situations, including the duration spent in the feared situation, the degree to which others are present, the distance from home/attachment figure etc. After ranking these feared situations, the final component of treatment is the regular progression of exposure to feared situations while employing anxiety management techniques. It is important that the child is allowed to exercise some control over the speed with which the new settings are experienced. The avoidance of reinforcement of unwanted behaviors and the promotion of fear-coping strategies is similarly important.

In the particular example of school refusal associated with separation anxiety, it is important to encourage an early return to school so that secondary impairments (academic failure and social isolation) are minimized. Generally, if the period of absence has been less than 2 months then return is very often successful; longer than this is frequently associated with much greater difficulty negotiating adequate attendance.

In older subjects, cognitive approaches may be more successful than the primary behavior strategies usually employed with younger children. Cognitive approaches postulate that the child's maladaptive thoughts, beliefs, and attitudes (schema) cause or maintain the experience of anxiety. Treatment consists of identifying negative self-statements ("I can't ever do this"), or external beliefs ("If I'm not there my mom won't be able to cope") and replacing them with more adaptive beliefs.

Pharmacological treatment studies of separation anxiety have tended to focus on samples with school-refusal behavior and various comorbidities. Considering safety and efficacy, the SSRIs appear to be the first-line treatment for separation anxiety disorder, but more studies are needed to confirm the presently preliminary results. Tricyclic antidepressants and benzodiazepines may be considered when the child has not responded to SSRIs or when adverse effects have exceeded benefits.

In practice, however, clinicians often combine drug and psychosocial treatments, capitalizing on differences in dose–response and time–response parameters. There is some evidence that treatments can be additive (each treatment having unique benefits) or synergistic (the benefit of the combination is greater that the additive combination). Alternatively, when combining drug and psychosocial treatments, a lower dose of one or both may be possible, with a resultant decrease in expense, inconvenience, or adverse events. Drug effects are often seen sooner than those due to exposure-based therapy, though it is hoped that the slower to emerge benefits of therapy may be more long lasting.

Selective Mutism

DIAGNOSIS

The essential feature of selective mutism is the persistent failure to speak in specific social situations (e.g., school, or with peers) where speaking is expected, despite speaking in other situations (e.g., home). Previously referred to as Elective Mutism, in DSM-III the condition was renamed Selective Mutism, so as to be less judgmental (doesn't speak rather than chooses not to speak).

Prior to making a diagnosis of selective mutism, a comprehensive evaluation should be conducted to rule out other explanations for mutism and to assess important comorbid factors. For obvious reasons, the parental interview will form the mainstay of evaluation, but as discussed below, direct observation (and interview if possible) of the child can afford important diagnostic information.

It is important to obtain information about the nature of the onset (insidious or sudden), any uncharacteristic features (i.e., not talking to family members, abrupt cessation of speech in one setting, absence of communication in all settings) suggestive of other neurological or psychiatric disorders (e.g., pervasive developmental disorders, acquired aphasias), and any history of neurological insult/injury, developmental delays or atypical language and/or speech. The assessment should also include the degree to which nonverbal communication or non-face-to-face communication is possible, the presence of anxiety symptoms in areas other than speaking, social and behavioral inhibition, medical history including ear infections, and hearing deficiencies. Parents will be able to give information on where and to whom the child will speak, the child's speech and language complexity at home, articulation problems, use of nonverbal communication (gestures etc.), any history of speech and language delays, and the possible importance of bilingualism (where primary language is not English). It can be useful to have the parents provide an audiotape of the child speaking at home.

The child evaluation can assess the presence of anxiety and social inhibition (willingness to communicate through gesture or drawing). Physical examination of oral sensory and motor ability may provide evidence of neurological problems (i.e., drooling, asymmetry, orofacial weakness, abnormal gag reflex, impaired sucking or swallowing). Specialist audiometry (pure tone and speech stimuli as well as tympanometry and acoustic reflex testing) may provide evidence of hearing and/or middle ear problems that can have a significant effect on speech and language development. Cognitive abilities may be difficult to assess, but the performance section of the WISC-R or Raven's Progressive Matrices as well as the Peabody Picture Vocabulary Test may be useful in the nonverbal child.

The prevalence of selective mutism is usually reported as 0.6 to 7 per 1000, with higher incidence in females rather than males. When subjects failing to speak in the first few weeks of school (a DSM-IV-TR requirement) are excluded rates do not exceed 2 per 1000. Onset is usually in the preschool years, but the peak age of presentation and diagnosis is between 6 and 8 years. A high incidence of insidious onset of refusal to speak with anyone except family members is reported. The other typical picture is one of acute onset of mutism on starting school.

TREATMENT

Treatment has long been regarded as difficult and prognosis poor. Approaches have included behavioral therapy, family therapy, speech therapy, and more recently pharmacological agents. Unfortunately, most published studies are single case reports, with very few controlled studies. Results of pharmacotherapy use are disappointing.

Behavioral treatment focuses on mutism as a means of getting attention and/or escaping from anxiety. The goal of a treatment program should be to decrease the anxiety associated with speaking while encouraging the child to interact verbally.

COMPARISON OF DSM-IV AND ICD-10 DIAGNOSTIC CRITERIA

In contrast to DSM-IV-TR, which establishes a minimum duration of 3 months for encopresis, the ICD-10 Diagnostic Criteria for Research has set a minimum duration of 6 months. In ICD-10, this disorder is referred to as "Nonorganic Encopresis."

For enuresis, the ICD-10 Diagnostic Criteria for Research have a different frequency threshold: at least twice a month in children aged under 7 years and at least once a month in children aged 7 years or more. In contrast, DSM-IV-TR requires either a frequency of twice a week for at least 3 consecutive months (regardless of age) or else the presence of clinically significant distress or impairment. Furthermore, ICD-10 includes a very strict exclusion criterion, preventing a diagnosis of enuresis to be made if there is any evidence of another mental disorder. In ICD-10, this disorder is referred to as "Nonorganic Enuresis."

For separation anxiety disorder, the DSM-IV-TR and ICD-10 symptom items are almost identical. The ICD-10 Diagnostic Criteria for Research are narrower in that the age of onset must be before age 6 and the diagnosis cannot be made if the presentation is "part of a broader disturbance of emotions, conduct, or personality." The DSM-IV-TR criteria and ICD-10 Diagnostic Criteria for Research for selective mutism are almost identical. In ICD-10, the disorder is referred to as "elective mutism."

10

Childhood Disorders: Reactive Attachment Disorder of Infancy or Early Childhood

DIAGNOSIS

DSM-IV-TR defines Reactive Attachment Disorder (RAD) as markedly disturbed and developmentally inappropriate social relatedness in most contexts, beginning before age 5 years, as evidenced by either restricted or indiscriminate social interaction. The abnormal relatedness cannot strictly be accounted for by developmental delay or by autism. In addition, evidence of pathogenic care such as institutionalization, emotional or physical neglect, or multiple changes in primary caregivers is evident. The diagnosis means to imply that the child's attachment relationships are impaired in reaction to "pathogenic caregiving." The socially aberrant behaviors are evident across social contexts.

Reactive Attachment Disorder has two subtypes: the inhibited/emotionally withdrawn subtype and the disinhibited/indiscriminately social subtype. The inhibited subtype is marked by emotional withdrawal, failure of social and emotional reciprocity, and lack of seeking or responding to comforting when distressed. Attachment behaviors, such as seeking and accepting comfort, showing and responding to affection, relying on caregivers for help, and cooperating with caregivers are absent or markedly restricted. In addition, exploratory behavior is limited owing to the absence of a preferred attachment figure. These children may also demonstrate problems of emotion regulation that range from affective blunting to withdrawal, to "frozen watchfulness." This subtype has been described in institutionalized children and in abused or neglected children.

The disinhibited/indiscriminately social subtype is characterized by more interaction with caregivers; however, there is failure to demonstrate selectivity in interacting with others. Stranger wariness, which appears as early as 7 months of age and remains apparent

DSM-IV-TR Diagnostic Criteria

313.89 REACTIVE ATTACHMENT DISORDER OF INFANCY OR EARLY CHILDHOOD

A. Markedly disturbed and developmentally inappropriate social relatedness in most contexts, beginning before age 5 years, as evidenced by either (1) or (2)

  (1) persistent failure to initiate or respond in a developmentally appropriate fashion to most social interactions, as manifested by excessive inhibited, hypervigilant, or highly ambivalent and contradictory responses (e.g., the child may respond to caregivers with a mixture of approach, avoidance, and resistance to comforting, or may exhibit frozen watchfulness).

  (2) diffuse attachments as manifest by indiscriminate sociability with marked inability to exhibit appropriate selective attachments (e.g., excessive familiarity with strangers or lack of selectivity in choice of attachment figures).

B. The disturbance in Criterion A is not accounted for solely by developmental delay (as in Mental Retardation) and does not meet current criteria for a Pervasive Developmental Disorder.

C. Pathogenic care as evidenced by at least one of the following:

  (1) persistent disregard of the child's basic emotional needs for comfort, stimulation, and affection

  (2) persistent disregard of the child's basic physical needs

  (3) repeated changes of primary caregiver that prevent formation of stable attachments (e.g., frequent changes in foster care).

D. There is a presumption that the care in Criterion C is responsible for the disturbed behavior in Criterion A (e.g., the disturbance in Criterion A began following the pathogenic care in Criterion C).

Reprinted with permission from the *Diagnostic and Statistical Manual of Mental Disorders*, 4th ed., Text Rev. Copyright 2000 American Psychiatric Association.

Clinical Guide to the Diagnosis and Treatment of Mental Disorders. M. B. First and A. Tasman
© 2006 John Wiley & Sons, Ltd.   ISBN 0 470 019158

for several years, is absent. Children with this subtype may approach strangers without expected social wariness around unfamiliar adults, may seek comfort or help from a stranger, and may demonstrate a variety of social relatedness problems that depend upon accurately reading social cues and understanding interpersonal boundaries. This subtype has been demonstrated in maltreated children, institutionalized children, and children adopted out of institutions.

The disturbed social behavior that characterizes RAD should be evident by report or observation across most social contexts and relationships. Obviously, self-report in young children is less likely to be obtained or elicit relevant clinical information; therefore, caregiver report is essential. Observation of the child in the clinic interacting with relative strangers as well as in naturalistic settings is quite valuable. Specialized structured clinical interviews and semistructured observational assessments may be helpful in eliciting disturbances in sociability related to attachment.

The current diagnostic requirement is that marked disturbances in social behavior are apparent before the age of 5 years. There is no research evidence to support this upper limit, although the literature on maternal deprivation, maltreatment, and institutionalization suggests that earlier insults to social development and attachment result in persistent and pervasive defects in social competence.

A variety of impairments are associated with RAD. By definition, children with the disorder are socially impaired, either withdrawn and detached or socially disinhibited and indiscriminating. Long-term impairments in peer relationships are associated with indiscriminate behavior at age 4 and 8 years. In addition, cognitive delays often arise in the same contexts of deprivation that give rise to signs of RAD.

Other behavioral abnormalities that may mimic mental disorders include a quasi-autistic syndrome that appears to arise as a result of institutionalization rather than genetic or intrinsic neurobiological abnormalities. Although symptomatically virtually indistinguishable from classic autism, this institutional syndrome does not show male predominance, is not associated with enlarged head circumference, and generally shows marked improvement after the child is placed with a family.

Differential Diagnosis

Several conditions of early childhood may have symptoms that overlap with RAD and cause diagnostic confusion.

Mental Retardation (***MR***). Young children with RAD often have significant developmental delays, and the same deprivation that causes RAD also increases risk for developmental delays. Infants and toddlers with mental retardation may not develop attachments that are consistent with their age, but they should be consistent with their developmental level. Thus, it is important to assess the cognitive level of children who appear indiscriminate to be sure that they are not merely delayed in the development of selectivity as evidenced by the absence of stranger wariness and separation anxiety. A developmental screen and adjustment for the child's overall mental age should suffice.

Pervasive Developmental Disorders (***PDD***). Although deficits in reciprocal social interaction are at the core of autism and Pervasive Developmental Disorders (PDD) and are observed early in life, children with these disorders do form selective attachments, although they may be deviant. Also complicating this picture is that these children also have cognitive delay and stereotypies, conditions that are frequently associated with institutionalization or profound neglect (see below). If the psychosocial and caregiving environment is deemed adequate and there is no history of pathologic caregiving, the social disturbance is likely a social deficit in the child rather than reactive to the caregiving environment. In this case, PDD will be the most likely diagnosis. Changes in the caregiving environment will not result in improved social or attachment behaviors and may worsen the child's condition because of loss of an attachment figure.

In addition, in most cases, although cognitive and language delays may be apparent in both socially deprived children and children with PDD, there is no reason to expect the pattern of restricted interest and activities associated with PDD in children with RAD. Instead, one may expect children with the inhibited/emotionally withdrawn pattern to exhibit a pervasive social and emotional withdrawal. Furthermore, there is no reason to expect a selective deficit in symbolization in RAD; instead, one would expect expressive and receptive language and pretend play to be roughly at the same level as overall cognitive level (e.g., as assessed by developmental tests such as the Bayley scores).

Posttraumatic Stress Disorder (***PTSD***). Children who have been abused or witnessed violence may show fear, clinging, or withdrawal from caregivers, symptoms that may be consistent with the hyperarousal and avoidant clusters of a toddler's posttraumatic symptomatology. These symptoms overlap with the inhibited, hypervigilant, or highly ambivalent and contradictory responses defined by DSM-IV-TR criteria. To be certain, abuse and exposure to domestic violence is "pathogenic caregiving," but it is uncertain whether these symptoms should primarily be considered as Posttraumatic Stress Disorder (PTSD) or RAD, inhibited/emotionally withdrawn type. If in question, the clinician should inquire into and observe for reexperiencing symptoms (posttraumatic play, play reenactment, nightmares, dissociation, distress on exposure), and increased arousal (sleep disturbances, impaired concentration, hypervigilance, and exaggerated startle). At this point, however, there is no reason not to diagnose both conditions if evidence for both exists.

***Failure to Thrive* (*FTT*).** The DSM-III conceptualization of RAD included growth failure and lack of social responsivity as central features, and confusion about this initial overlap continues in the literature. In early infancy, lack of eye tracking or responsive smiling by 2 months of age, and failure to reach out to be picked up by 6 months of age should be noted as aberrant social behaviors but not diagnosed as RAD, inhibited type. If the child demonstrates psychosocial dwarfism and social inhibition or indiscriminateness, both diagnoses would be appropriate.

Conduct Disorder. There has been much confusion in older children and adolescents about RAD and psychopathy. In fact, it is unclear if RAD is identifiable in middle childhood and adolescence, and if so, what its manifestations are. The possibilities are as follows: (1) RAD resolves itself in early childhood or soon after transition to middle childhood, (2) RAD has different and yet-to-be-defined characteristics in middle childhood and adolescence, or (3) RAD is a pathway into another kind of disorder, such as disruptive behavior disorders. Some of the confusion appears to derive from the problem that children with disruptive behavior disorders often have troubled relationships with their caregivers, thus leading to an assumption that symptoms and signs of aggression, oppositionality, and anger are, in fact, disorders of attachment. In many cases, the emphasis on oppositionality, aggression, and lack of empathy suggests something other than RAD, perhaps a unique developmental path to oppositional defiant disorder or early conduct disorder.

Attention-Deficit/Hyperactivity Disorder. Young children with RAD, disinhibited type, demonstrate a persistent pattern of socially impulsive behavior. These behaviors must be distinguished from the impulsivity that characterizes ADHD. Complicating the distinction is evidence that a syndrome of inattention and overactivity may develop in the context of institutionalization.

Although ADHD and the disinhibited type of RAD may be associated with social impulsivity, there is no reason to expect children with disinhibited RAD to manifest inattention or hyperactivity. If, on the other hand, the child meets criteria for both disorders, both diagnoses should be assigned.

TREATMENT

By definition, attachment disorders are encountered in children who have not experienced an opportunity to form lasting secure relationships. Common scenarios include children raised in institutions, placed in multiple foster care homes, or who have had extremely disturbed experiences of care with a single caregiver. Intervention, therefore, should take into account the totality of the child's prior experience, current placement, and other significant relationships.

The first consideration is the child's current health and safety. Maltreatment of children under 4 years of age is associated with significant morbidity and mortality; therefore, involvement of child protective services is frequently warranted. The child should be assessed by a pediatrician for sequelae of malnutrition, substandard health care, and abuse. Given the extreme comorbidity with cognitive and speech delay, the child should also be referred to early intervention services.

Once these issues have been addressed, the nurturing environment should be evaluated and supported to help the current caregivers provide an appropriately nurturing and stimulating environment. If the child currently resides in a dangerous or destructive caregiving environment, an assessment of parental fitness may be warranted. Removal of the child is mandated if the child has sustained life-threatening injuries or is in imminent jeopardy. While the placement of the child in foster care necessarily disrupts the child's relationship with the primary caregiver, safety must be the first priority.

After placement in care, approaches to determining whether reunification is possible, or whether the child should be freed for adoption should be implemented. These approaches emphasize building new attachment relationships and helping the child transition from one setting to the next gradually. Throughout, it is necessary to maintain a focus on the child's best interest while determining whether reunification or termination of parental rights and adoption is indicated.

Owing to the multiple needs of children in foster care and their caregivers, coordination and integration of services for the child, biological parents, and foster parents is critical. Appropriate mental health, substance use, and other supportive services programs should be made available to the caregivers. Critical for all caregivers is the desire to value the baby as an individual and the ability to appropriately respond to the child's bids for comfort, safety, and autonomy.

Educational instruction about developmental capacities, temperamental characteristics, and appropriate interpretations and responses to a child's negative emotion may be indicated. Focusing on improving the parent's ability to respond as a "secure base" from which the child can explore his environment and a "safe-haven" to return to when distressed can be accomplished through focusing on the parent's behavioral interaction with the child, the parent's perception of the child's intentional bids, or a combination of the two. Barriers to the caregiver's emotional availability may be addressed in individual therapy focused on the parent's own experience of care and its influence on their own provision of care.

Long-term intervention is frequently necessary and a successful intervention should address crisis intervention, developmental guidance, and infant/toddler–parent psychotherapy in which the child is present. If working with parents who are providing the improved nurturing environment—foster parents and adoptive parents—the clinician should focus on similar aspects as above and also on "goodness-of-fit" and should assess the parents' motivation to care for this child, the parents' perceptions of the child and their derivations, and the parent's fears about the impact of the child's early environment.

Pharmacotherapy

There are no reported case reports of psychopharmacological management of either the inhibited/emotionally withdrawn or disinhibited/indiscriminately social subtypes of RAD, nor is there reason to expect these signs and symptoms to respond to psychopharmacological intervention.

Alternative Coercive Psychosocial Treatments

Several alternative treatments of attachment, such as "coercive holding therapies," "rebirthing therapies," and similar "rage reduction therapies," have resulted in the well-publicized deaths of several children. Parents of these children were following the advice of holding therapists, or allowing the therapists to coerce their children into rageful outbursts, followed by tragically misguided or frankly sadistic parental responses. It is more than likely that these cases represent early onset conduct disorders with a history of early pathologic caregiving rather than RAD. These nonconventional and not recommended treatments may be called *attachment therapies*, but are not drawn from either attachment theory or research and appear to run the risk of retraumatizing already traumatized children

COMPARISON OF DSM-IV-TR AND ICD-10 DIAGNOSTIC CRITERIA

The DSM-IV-TR Reactive Attachment Disorder has two subtypes (inhibited type and disinhibited type) that roughly correspond to the two ICD-10 categories, reactive attachment disorder of childhood and disinhibited attachment disorder of childhood. The ICD-10 categories are probably much more inclusive because they do not specify that disturbed behavior be the result of pathogenic care.

Delirium, Dementia, and Amnestic Disorders

This chapter reviews delirium, dementia, and amnestic disorders. Traditionally, these conditions have been classified as organic brain disorders to distinguish them from such diseases as schizophrenia, mania, and major depressive disorder, the so-called functional disorders. With the publication of the DSM-IV, the distinction between functional and organic disorders was eliminated. Significant research into the neurobiological aspects of mental disorders and the utilization of sophisticated neurodiagnostic tests such as positron emission tomographic scanning in individuals with schizophrenia led to the inescapable conclusion that every psychiatric condition has a biological component. Thus, the term functional became obsolete and even misleading.

The conditions formerly called organic are classified in DSM-IV-TR into three groups: (1) delirium, dementia, and amnestic and other cognitive disorders; (2) mental disorders due to a general medical condition (covered in Chapter 12 of this book); and (3) substance-related disorders (covered in Chapters 13–24 in this book). Delirium, dementia, and amnestic disorders are classified as cognitive because they feature impairment in such parameters as memory, language, or attention as a cardinal symptom. Each of these three major cognitive disorders is subdivided into categories that ascribe the etiology of the disorder to a general medical condition, the persisting effects of a substance, or multiple etiologies. A "not otherwise specified" category is included for each disorder.

Delirium

The disorders in this section share a common symptom presentation of a disturbance in consciousness and cognition, but are differentiated (as in DSM-IV-TR) on the basis of etiology (i.e., Delirium Due to a General Medical Condition, Substance-Induced Delirium, and Delirium Due to Multiple Etiologies). Information regarding the diagnosis, and treatment of delirium regardless of

its specific etiology is presented first, followed by brief sections on Delirium Due to a General Medical Condition, Medication-induced Delirium, Substance Intoxication Delirium, Substance-Withdrawal Delirium, and Delirium Due to Multiple Etiologies.

DIAGNOSIS

Delirium (also known as *acute confusional state, toxic metabolic encephalopathy*) is the behavioral response to widespread disturbances in cerebral metabolism. Like dementia, delirium is not a disease but a syndrome with many possible causes that result in a similar constellation of symptoms (the diagnostic criteria for the "syndrome" of delirium are listed as Criteria A, B, and C).

According to DSM-IV-TR, the primary feature of delirium is a diminished clarity of awareness of the environment. Symptoms of delirium are characteristically global, of acute onset, fluctuating, and of relatively brief duration. In most cases of delirium, an often overlooked prodrome of altered sleep patterns, unex-

---

DSM-IV-TR Diagnostic Criteria

DSM-IV-TR DIAGNOSTIC CRITERIA FOR DELIRIUM

A. Disturbance of consciousness (i.e., reduced clarity of awareness of the environment) with reduced ability to focus, sustain, or shift attention.
B. A change in cognition (such as memory deficit, disorientation, language disturbance) or the development of a perceptual disturbance that is not better accounted for by a preexisting, established or evolving dementia.
C. The disturbance develops over a short period of time (usually hours to days) and tends to fluctuate during the course of the day.
D. [Varies based on etiology—see specific disorders for discussion.]

Reprinted with permission from *DSM-IV-TR Guidebook*. Copyright 2004, Michael B First, Allen Frances, and Harold Alan Pincus.

Clinical Guide to the Diagnosis and Treatment of Mental Disorders. M. B. First and A. Tasman
© 2006 John Wiley & Sons, Ltd.   ISBN 0 470 019158

plained fatigue, fluctuating mood, sleep phobia, restlessness, anxiety, and nightmares occur. A review of nursing notes for the days before the recognized onset of delirium often illustrates early warning signs of the condition.

The clinical features of delirium can be divided into abnormalities of (1) arousal, (2) language and cognition, (3) perception, (4) orientation, (5) mood, (6) sleep and wakefulness, and (7) neurological functioning.

The state of arousal in individuals who are delirious may be increased or decreased. Some individuals exhibit marked restlessness, heightened startle, hypervigilance, and increased alertness. This pattern is often seen in states of withdrawal from depressive substances (e.g., alcohol) or intoxication by stimulants and hallucinogens (e.g., phencyclidine, amphetamine, lysergic acid diethylamide). Individuals with increased arousal often have such concomitant autonomic signs as pallor, sweating, tachycardia, mydriasis, hyperthermia, piloerection, and gastrointestinal distress. These individuals often require sedation with neuroleptics or benzodiazepines. Hypoactive arousal states such as those occasionally seen in hepatic encephalopathy and hypercapnia are often initially perceived as depressed or demented states. The clinical course of delirium in any particular individual may include both increased and decreased arousal states. Many such individuals display daytime sedation with nocturnal agitation and behavioral problems (sundowning).

Individuals with delirium frequently have abnormal production and comprehension of speech. Nonsensical rambling and incoherent speech may occur. Other individuals may be completely mute. Memory may be impaired, especially primary and secondary memory. Remote memory may be preserved, although the individual may have difficulty distinguishing the present from the distant past.

Perceptual abnormalities in delirium represent an inability to discriminate sensory stimuli and to integrate current perceptions with past experiences. Consequently, individuals tend to personalize events, conversations, and so forth that do not directly pertain to them, become obsessed with irrelevant stimuli, and misinterpret objects in their environment. The misinterpretations generally take the form of auditory and visual illusions. Individuals with auditory illusions, for example, might hear the sound of leaves rustling and perceive it as someone whispering about them. This interpretation may result in paranoia and sleep phobia. Typical visual illusions are that intravenous tubing is a snake or worm crawling into the skin, or that a respirator is a truck or farm vehicle about to collide with the individual. Although auditory illusions may lead to tactile hallucinations, the most common hallucinations in delirium are visual and auditory.

Orientation is often abnormal in delirium. Disorientation, in particular, seems to follow a fluctuating course, with individuals being unable to answer questions about orientation in the morning, yet be fully oriented by the afternoon. Orientation to time, place, person, and situation should be evaluated in the individual who is delirious. Generally, orientation to time is the sphere most likely impaired, with orientation to person usually preserved. Orientation to significant people (parents, children) should also be tested. Disorientation to self is rare and indicates significant impairment. The examiner should always reorient individuals who do not perform well in any portion of the orientation testing of the mental status examination, and serial testing of orientation on subsequent days is important.

Individuals with delirium are susceptible to rapid fluctuations in mood. Unprovoked anger and rage reactions occasionally occur and may lead to attacks on hospital staff. Fear is a common emotion and may lead to increased vigilance and an unwillingness to sleep because of increased vulnerability during somnolence. Apathy, such as that seen in hepatic encephalopathy, depression, use of certain medications (e.g., sulfamethoxazole [Bactrim]), and frontal lobe syndromes, is common, as is euphoria secondary to medications (e.g., corticosteroids, DDC, zidovudine) and drugs of abuse (phencyclidine, inhalants).

Sleeping patterns of individuals who are delirious are usually abnormal. During the day, they can be hypersomnolent, often falling asleep in midsentence, whereas at night they are combative and restless. Sleep is generally fragmented, and vivid nightmares are common.

Neurological symptoms often occur in delirium. These include dysphagia as seen after a cerebrovascular accident (CVA), tremor, asterixis (hepatic encephalopathy, hypoxia, uremia), poor coordination, gait apraxia, frontal release signs (grasp, suck), choreiform movements, seizures, Babinski's sign, and dysarthria. Focal neurological signs occur less frequently.

The appropriate workup of individuals who are delirious includes a complete physical status, mental status, and neurological examination. History taking from the individual, any available family, previous physicians, an old chart, and the individual's current nurse is essential. Previous delirious states, etiologies identified in the past, and interventions that proved effective should be elucidated. Appropriate evaluation of the delirious individual is reviewed in Figure 11-1.

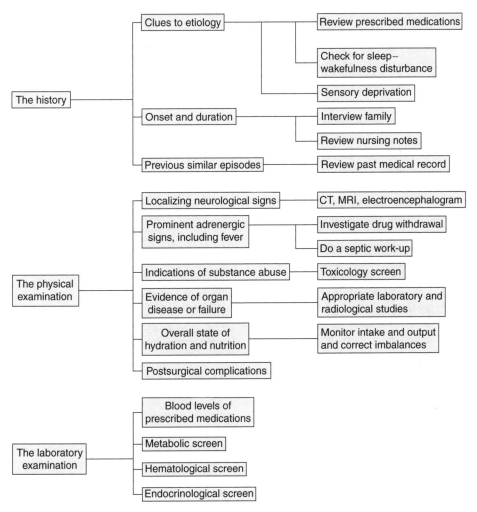

Figure 11-1 *Evaluation of delirium.*

The overall prevalence of delirium in the community is low, but delirium is common among individuals who are hospitalized. Studies of elderly patients suggest that about 40% of them admitted to general medical wards showed signs of delirium at some point during the hospitalization. Because of the increasing numbers of elderly in the US and the influence of life-extending technology, the population of hospitalized elderly is rising, and so is the prevalence of delirium. The intensive care unit, geriatric psychiatry ward, emergency department, alcohol treatment units, and oncology wards have particularly high rates of delirium.

Course

After elimination of the cause of the delirium, the symptoms gradually recede within 3 to 7 days. Some symptoms in certain populations may take weeks to resolve. The age of the individual and the period of time during which the individual was delirious affect the symptom resolution time. In general, the individual has a spotty memory for events that occurred during delirium. These remembrances are reinforced by comments from the staff ("You're not as confused today"), or the presence of a sitter, or use of wrist restraints. Such individuals should be reassured that they were not responsible for their behavior while delirious, and that no one hates or resents them for the behavior they may have exhibited. Individuals with underlying dementia show residual cognitive impairment after resolution of delirium, and it has been suggested that a delirium may merge into a dementia.

In general, the mortality and morbidity of any serious disease are doubled if delirium ensues. The risk of dying after a delirious episode is greatest in the first 2 years after the illness, with a higher risk of death from heart disease and cancer in women and from pneumonia in men. Overall, the 3-month mortality rate for persons who have an episode of delirium is about 28%, and the 1-year mortality rate for such individuals may be as high as 50%.

Differential Diagnosis

Delirium must be differentiated from dementia because the two conditions may have different prognoses. In contrast with the changes in dementia, those in delirium have an acute onset. The symptoms in dementia tend to be relatively stable over time, whereas clinical features of delirium display wide fluctuation with periods of relative lucidity. Clouding of consciousness is an essential feature of delirium, but demented individuals are usually alert. Attention and orientation are more commonly disturbed in delirium, although the latter can become impaired in advanced dementia. Perception abnormalities, alterations in the sleep–wakefulness cycle, and abnormalities of speech are more common in delirium. Most important, a delirium is more likely to be reversible than is a dementia. Delirium and dementia can occur simultaneously; in fact, the presence of dementia is a risk factor for delirium. Some studies suggest that about 30% of individuals who are hospitalized with dementia have a superimposed delirium.

Delirium must be differentiated from psychotic states related to such conditions as schizophrenia or mania and factitious disorders with psychological symptoms or malingering. Generally, the psychotic features of schizophrenia are more constant and better organized than are those in delirium, and individuals with schizophrenia seldom have the clouding of consciousness seen in delirium. The "psychosis" of individuals with factitious disorder or malingering is inconsistent, and these persons do not exhibit many of the associated features of delirium. Apathetic and lethargic individuals with delirium may occasionally resemble depressed individuals, but tests such as electroencephalogram (EEG) distinguish between the two. The EEG demonstrates diffuse slowing in most delirious states, except for the low-amplitude, fast activity EEG pattern seen in alcohol withdrawal. In contrast, the EEG in a functional depression or psychosis is normal.

Predisposing factors in the development of delirium include old age, young age (children), previous brain damage, prior episodes of delirium, malnutrition, sensory impairment (especially vision), and alcohol dependence.

The specific causes of delirium are summarized in Table 11-1. Information regarding the specific causes of delirium is included in the next sections.

Table 11-1	Causes of Delirium

Medication effect or interaction
Substance intoxication or withdrawal
Infection
Head injury
Metabolic disarray
   Acid–base imbalance
   Dehydration
   Malnutrition
   Electrolyte imbalance
   Blood glucose abnormality
   Carbon dioxide narcosis
   Uremic encephalopathy
   Hepatic encephalopathy
Cerebrovascular insufficiency
   Congestive heart failure
   Hypovolemia
   Arrhythmias
   Severe anemia
   Transient ischemia
   Acute CVA
Endocrine dysfunction
Postoperative states
   Postcardiotomy delirium
Environmental factors
   Intensive care unit psychosis
Sleep deprivation

Delirium Due to a General Medical Condition

The causes of Delirium Due to a General Medical Condition may lie in intracranial processes, extracranial ones, or a combination of the two. The most common etiological factors are described in the following subsections.

Infection Induced. Infection is a common cause of delirium among individuals who are hospitalized and typically, infected patients will display abnormalities in hematology and serology. Bacteremic septicemia (especially that caused by gram-negative bacteria), pneumonia, encephalitis, and meningitis are common offenders. The elderly are particularly susceptible to delirium secondary to urinary tract infections.

Metabolic and Endocrine Disturbances. Metabolic causes of delirium include hypoglycemia, electrolyte disturbances, and vitamin deficiency states. The most common endocrine causes are hyperfunction and hypofunction of the thyroid, adrenal, pancreas, pituitary, and parathyroid. Metabolic causes may involve consequences of diseases of particular organs, such as hepatic encephalopathy resulting from liver disease, uremic encephalopathy and postdialysis delirium resulting from kidney dysfunction, and carbon dioxide macrosis and hypoxia resulting from lung disease. The metabolic disturbance or endocrinopathy must be known to induce changes in mental status and must be confirmed by laboratory determinations or physical examination, and the temporal course of the confusion should coincide with the disturbance. In some individuals, particularly the elderly, the brain injured, and the demented, there may be a significant lag time between correction of metabolic parameters and improvement in mental state.

Low-Perfusion States. Any condition that decreases effective cerebral perfusion can cause delirium. Common offenders are hypovolemia, congestive heart failure and other causes of decreased stroke volume such as arrhythmias, and anemia, which decreases oxygen binding. Maintenance of fluid balance and strict measuring of intake and output are essential in delirious states.

Intracranial Causes. Intracranial causes of delirium include head trauma, especially involving loss of consciousness, postconcussive states, and hemorrhage; brain infections; neoplasms; and such vascular abnormalities as CVAs, subarachnoid hemorrhage, transient ischemic attacks, and hypertensive encephalopathy.

Postoperative States. Postoperative causes of delirium may include infection, atelectasis, lingering effects of anesthesia, thrombotic and embolic phenomena, and adverse reactions to postoperative analgesia. General surgery in an elderly patient has been reported to be followed by delirium in 10–14% of cases and may reach 50% after surgery for hip fracture.

Sensory and Environmental Changes. Many clinicians underestimate the disorienting potential of an unfamiliar environment. The elderly are especially prone to develop environment-related confusion in the hospital. Individuals with preexisting dementia, who may have learned to compensate for cognitive deficits at home, often become delirious once hospitalized. In addition, the nature of the intensive care unit often lends itself to periods of high sensory stimulation (as during a "code") or low sensory input, as occurs at night. Often, individuals use external events such as dispensing medication, mealtimes, presence of housekeeping staff, and physicians' rounds to mark the passage of time. These parameters are often absent at night, leading to increased rates of confusion during nighttime hours. Often, manipulating the individual's environment (see section on treatment) or removing the individual from the intensive care unit can be therapeutic.

Medication-Induced Delirium

The list of medications that can produce the delirious state is extensive (Table 11-2). The more common ones

Table 11-2	Selected Drugs Associated with Delirium
Antihypertensives	Indomethacin
Amphotericin B	Ketamine
Antispasmodics	Levodopa
Antituberculous agents	Lidocaine
Baclofen	Lithium
Barbiturates	Meperidine
Cimetidine	Morphine
Corticosteroids	Procainamide
Colchicine	Pentamidine
Contrast media	Tricyclic antidepressants
Digitalis	Zalcitabine (DDC)
Ephedrine	Zidovudine (AZT)

include such antihypertensives as methyldopa and reserpine, histamine (H_2) receptor antagonists (cimetidine), corticosteroids, antidepressants, narcotic (especially opioid) and nonsteroidal analgesics, lithium carbonate, digitalis, baclofen (Lioresal), anticonvulsants, antiarrhythmics, colchicine, bronchodilators, benzodiazepines, sedative-hypnotics, and anticholinergics. Of the narcotic analgesics, meperidine can produce an agitated delirium with tremors, seizures, and myoclonus. These features are attributed to its active metabolite normeperidine, which has potent stimulant and anticholinergic properties and accumulates with repeated intravenous dosing. In general, adverse effects of narcotics are more common in those who have never received such agents before (the narcotically naive) or who have a history of a similar response to narcotics.

Lithium-induced delirium occurs at blood levels greater than 1.5 mEq/L and is associated with early features of lethargy, stuttering, and muscle fasciculations. The delirium may take as long as 2 weeks to resolve even after lithium has been discontinued, and other neurological signs such as stupor and seizures commonly occur. Maintenance of fluid and electrolyte balance is essential in lithium-induced delirium. Facilitation of excretion with such agents as aminophylline and acetazolamide helps, but hemodialysis is often required.

Principles to remember in cases of drug-induced delirium include the facts that (1) blood levels of possibly offending agents are helpful and should be obtained, but many persons can become delirious at therapeutic levels of the drug, (2) drug-induced delirium may be the result of drug interactions and polypharmacy and not the result of a single agent, (3) over-the-counter medications and preparations (e.g., agents containing caffeine or phenylpropanolamine) should also be considered, and (4) delirium can be caused by the combination of drugs of abuse and prescribed medications (e.g., cocaine and dopaminergic antidepressants).

Substance Intoxication Delirium

The list of drugs of abuse that can produce delirium is extensive. Some such agents have enjoyed a resurgence after years of declining usage. These include lysergic acid diethylamide, psilocybin (hallucinogenic mushrooms), heroin, and amphetamines. Other agents include barbiturates, cannabis (especially dependent on setting, experience of the user, and whether it is laced with phencyclidine ["superweed"] or heroin), jimsonweed (highly anticholingeric), and mescaline. In cases in which intravenous use of drugs is suspected, HIV spectrum illness must be ruled out as an etiological agent for delirium.

The physical examination of an individual with suspected illicit drug-induced delirium may reveal sclerosed veins, "pop" scars caused by subcutaneous injection of agents, pale and atrophic nasal mucosa resulting from intranasal use of cocaine, injected conjunctiva, and pupillary changes. Toxicological screens are helpful but may not be available on an emergency basis.

Substance-Withdrawal Delirium

Alcohol and certain sedating drugs can produce a withdrawal delirium when their use is abruptly discontinued or significantly reduced. Withdrawal delirium requires a history of use of a potentially addicting agent for a sufficient amount of time to produce dependence. It is associated with such typical physical findings as abnormal vital signs, pupillary changes, tremor, diaphoresis, nausea and vomiting, and diarrhea. Individuals generally complain of abdominal and leg cramps, insomnia, nightmares, chills, hallucinations (especially visual), and a general feeling of "wanting to jump out of my skin."

Some varieties of drug withdrawal, although uncomfortable, are not life threatening (e.g., opioid withdrawal). Others such as alcohol withdrawal delirium are potentially fatal. Withdrawal delirium is much more common among individuals who are hospitalized than among individuals living in the community. The incidence of delirium tremens, for example, is found in 1% of all alcoholics, but in 5% of hospitalized alcohol abusers. Improvement of the delirium occurs when the offending agent is reintroduced or a cross-sensitive drug (e.g., a benzodiazepine for alcohol withdrawal) is employed.

Delirium Due to Multiple Etiologies

In many individuals with delirium, there are often multiple simultaneous causal factors involved. In some cases, multiple general medical conditions may impact the central nervous system (CNS) in such a way as to lead to a delirium. For example, an individual with hepatic encephalopathy who falls and hits his head may develop a delirium attributable to the combined effects of both general medical conditions. Similarly, the combined effects of a medical condition coupled with the effects of medications used to treat that condition may cause a delirium. In such situations, the diagnosis Delirium Due to Multiple Etiologies is given.

TREATMENT

Once delirium has been diagnosed, the etiological agent must be identified and treated. For the elderly, the first step generally involves discontinuing or reducing the dosage of potentially offending medications. Some delirious states can be immediately reversed with medication, as in the case of physostigmine administration for anticholinergic delirium. However, most responses are not as immediate, and attention must be directed toward protecting the individual from unintentional self-harm, managing agitated and psychotic behavior, and manipulating the environment to minimize additional impairment. Supportive therapy should include fluid and electrolyte maintenance and provision of adequate nutrition. Reorienting the individual is essential and is best accomplished in a well-lit room with a window, a clock, and a visible wall calendar. Familiar objects from home such as a stuffed animal, a favorite blanket, or a few photographs are helpful. Individuals who respond incorrectly to questions of orientation should be provided with the correct answers. Because these individuals often see many consultants, physicians should introduce themselves and state their purpose for coming at every visit. Physicians must take into account that impairments of vision and hearing can produce confusional states, and the provision of appropriate prosthetic devices may be beneficial. Around-the-clock accompaniment by hospital-provided "sitters" or family members may be required (see Table 11-3).

Table 11-3	Managing the Delirious Individual

Identify and correct the underlying cause.
Protect the patient from unintentional self-harm.
Stabilize the level of sensory input.
Reorient patient as often as possible.
Employ objects from the patient's home environment.
Provide supportive therapy (fever control, hydration).
Streamline medications.
Correct sleep deprivation.
Manage behavior with appropriate pharmacotherapy.
Address postdelirium guilt and shame for behavior that occurred during confusion.

Despite these conservative interventions, the delirious individual often requires pharmacological intervention. The liaison psychiatrist is the most appropriate person to recommend such treatment in hospital settings. The drug of choice for agitated delirious individuals has traditionally been haloperidol (Haldol). It is particularly beneficial when given by the intravenous route, and dosages as high as 260 mg/day have been used without adverse effect. Extrapyramidal symptoms may be less common with haloperidol administered intravenously as opposed to oral and intramuscular administration. In general, doses in the range of 0.5 to 5 mg intravenously are used, with the frequency of administration depending on a variety of factors, including the individual's age. An electrocardiogram should be obtained before administering haloperidol. If the QT interval is greater than 450, use of intravenous haloperidol can precipitate an abnormal cardiac rhythm known as *Torsades des pointes*. Lorazepam has also been proven effective in doses of 0.5 to 2 mg intravenously. It has been suggested that haloperidol and lorazepam act synergistically when given to the agitated individual who is delirious. If the delirium is secondary to drug or alcohol abuse, benzodiazepines or clonidine should be used. For individuals who are mildly agitated or amenable to taking medications by mouth, oral haloperidol or lorazepam is appropriate. Recent studies have advocated the use of newer atypical antipsychotics for management of behavior and psychotic features in delirium. Such agents as quetiapine, olanzapine, risperdal, and ziprasidone have been used successfully to treat delirium. Newer agents may have lower incidences of dystonias and dyskinesias, but still carry the risk of QT interval prolongation, particularly in individuals with electrolyte abnormalities. Quetiapine and olanzapine are quite sedating, and occasionally a combination of bedtime olanzapine and "as needed" haloperidol is utilized. Olanzapine may raise blood glucose levels and precipitate weight gain, and is available as a Zydis preparation, which is absorbed through the oral mucosa and can therefore be given to individuals who are unable to take medications by mouth. Parenteral forms of olanzapine and ziprasidone are also available. Whatever antipsychotic is chosen, the individual should be carefully monitored for muscle rigidity, unexplained fever, tremor, and other warning signs of neuroleptic side effects.

Dementia

The disorders in this section are characterized by the development of multiple cognitive deficits (including memory impairment) but are differentiated (as in DSM-IV-TR) on the basis of etiology (i.e., Dementia of the Alzheimer's Type, Dementia Due to Pick's Disease, Dementia Due to Parkinson's Disease, Dementia Due to Huntington's Disease, Vascular Dementia, Dementia Due to HIV Disease, Dementia Due to Head Trauma, Dementia Due to Other General Medical Conditions, Substance-Induced Persisting Dementia, and Dementia Due to Multiple Etiologies). Information regarding the diagnosis of dementia regardless of its specific etiology is presented first, followed by sections on the various specific causes of dementia.

DIAGNOSIS

Dementia is defined in DSM-IV-TR as a series of disorders characterized by the development of multiple cognitive deficits (including memory impairment) that are due to the direct physiological effects of a general medical condition, the persisting effects of a substance, or multiple etiologies (e.g., the combined effects of a metabolic and a degenerative disorder). (See DSM-IV-TR diagnostic criteria A and B, page 98.) The disorders constituting the dementias share a common symptom presentation and are identified and classified on the basis of etiology. The cognitive deficits exhibited in these disorders must be of sufficient severity to interfere with either occupational functioning or the individual's usual social activities or relationships. In addition, the observed deficits must represent a decline from a higher level of function and not be the consequence of a delirium. A delirium can be superimposed on a dementia, however, and both can be diagnosed if the dementia is observed when the delirium is not in evidence. Dementia is typically chronic and occurs in the presence of a clear sensorium. If clouding of consciousness occurs, the diagnosis of delirium should be considered. Essential to the diagnosis of dementia is the presence of cognitive deficits that include memory impairment and at least one of the following abnormalities of cognition: aphasia, agnosia, apraxia, or a disturbance in executive function.

Memory function is divided into three compartments that can easily be evaluated during a mental status examination. These are immediate recall (primary memory), recent (secondary) memory, and remote (tertiary) memory. Primary memory is characterized by a limited capacity, rapid accessibility, and a duration of seconds to a minute. The anatomic site of destruction of primary memory is the reticular activating system, and the principal activity of the primary memory is the registration of new information. Primary memory is generally tested by asking the individual to repeat immediately a series of numbers in the order given. For instance, if the examiner mentions the numbers 1-2-3, the individual should be able to repeat them in the same order. This loss of ability to register new information accounts in part for the confusion and frustration the demented individual feels when confronted with unexpected changes in daily routine.

Secondary memory has a much larger capacity than primary memory, a duration of minutes to years, and relatively slow accessibility. The anatomic site of dysfunction for secondary memory is the limbic system, and individuals with a lesion in this area may have little difficulty repeating digits immediately, but show rapid decay of these new memories. In minutes, the individual with limbic involvement may be totally unable to recall the digits or even remember that a test has been administered. Thus, secondary memory represents the retention and recall of information that has been previously registered by primary memory. Clinically, secondary memory is tested by having the individual repeat three objects after having been distracted (usually by the examiner's continuation of the Mental Status Examination) for 3 to 5 minutes. Like primary memory, secondary recall is often impaired in dementia. Often, if the examiner gives the demented individual a clue (such as "one of the objects you missed was a color"), the individual correctly identifies the object. If this occurs, the memory testing should be scored as "3 out of 3 with a clue," which is considered to be a slight impairment. Giving clues to the demented individual with a primary memory loss is pointless, because the memories were never registered. Wernicke–Korsakoff syndrome is an example of a condition in which primary memory may be intact while secondary recall is impaired.

Tertiary (remote) memory has a capacity that is probably unlimited, and such memories are often permanently retained. Access to tertiary memories is slow, and the anatomical dysfunction in tertiary memory loss is in the association cortex. In the early stages of dementia, tertiary memory is generally intact. It is tested by instructing the individual to remember personal information or past material. The personal significance of the information often influences the individual's ability to remember it. For example, a woman who worked for many years as a seamstress might remember many details related to that occupation, but could not recall the names of past presidents or three large cities in the United States. Thus, an individual's inability to remember highly significant past material is an ominous finding. Collateral data from informants is essential in the proper assessment of memory function. In summary, primary and secondary memories are most likely to be impaired in dementia, with tertiary memory often spared until late in the course of the disease.

In addition to defects in memory, individuals with dementia often exhibit impairments in language, recognition, object naming, and motor skills. Aphasia is an abnormality of language that often occurs in vascular dementias involving the dominant hemisphere. Because this hemisphere controls verbal, written, and sign language, these individuals may have significant problems interacting with people in their environment. Individuals with dementia and aphasia may exhibit paucity of speech, poor articulation, and a telegraphic pattern of speech (nonfluent, Broca's aphasia). This form of aphasia generally involves the middle cerebral artery with resultant paresis of the right arm and lower face. Despite faulty communication skills, individuals having dementia with nonfluent aphasia have normal comprehension and awareness of their language impairment. As a result, such individuals often present with significant depression, anxiety, and frustration.

By contrast, individuals having dementia with fluent (Wernicke's) aphasia may be quite verbose and articulate, but much of the language is nonsensical and rife with such paraphasias as neologisms and clang (rhyming) associations. Whereas nonfluent aphasias are usually associated with discrete lesions, fluent aphasia can result from such diffuse conditions as dementia of the Alzheimer type. More commonly, fluent aphasias occur in conjunction with vascular dementia secondary to temporal or parietal lobe CVA. Because the demented individuals with fluent aphasia have impaired comprehension, they may seem apathetic and unconcerned with their language deficits if they are, in fact, aware of them at all. They do not generally display the emotional distress of individuals with dementia and nonfluent aphasia (Table 11-4).

Individuals with dementia may also lose their ability to recognize. Agnosia is a feature of a dominant hemisphere lesion and involves altered perception in which, despite normal sensations, intellect, and language, the

Table 11-4	Classification of Aphasias		
Type	**Language**	**Comprehension**	**Motor**
Wernicke's (receptive)	Impaired Articulate Paraphasias	Impaired	Normal
Broca's (expressive)	Nonfluent Sparse Telegraphic Inarticulate	Intact	Right hemiparesis
Global	Nonfluent Mute	Impaired	Variable right hemiplegia

individual cannot recognize objects. This is in contrast to aphasia, in which the individual with dementia may not be able to name objects, but can recognize them. The type of agnosia depends on the area of the sensory cortex that is involved. Some demented individuals with severe visual agnosia cannot name objects presented, match them to samples, or point to objects named by the examiner. Other individuals may present with auditory agnosia and may be unable to localize or distinguish such sounds as the ringing of a telephone. A minority of demented individuals may exhibit astereognosis, or the inability to identify an object by palpation.

Demented individuals may also lose their ability to carry out selected motor activities despite intact motor abilities, sensory function, and comprehension of the assigned task (apraxia). Affected individuals cannot perform such activities as brushing their teeth, chewing food, or waving goodbye when asked to do so. The two most common forms of apraxia in demented individuals are ideational and gait apraxia. Ideational apraxia is the inability to perform motor activities that require sequential steps and results from a lesion involving both frontal lobes or the complete cerebrum. Gait apraxia, often seen in such conditions as normal-pressure hydrocephalus, is the inability to perform various motions of ambulation. It also results from conditions that diffusely affect the cerebrum.

Impairment of executive function affects the ability to think abstractly, plan, initiate, and end complex behavior. On Mental Status Examination, individuals with dementia display problems coping with new tasks. Activities such as subtracting serial sevens may be impaired.

In addition to the diagnostic features already mentioned, individuals with dementia display other identifying features that often prove problematic. Poor insight and judgment are common in dementia and often cause individuals to engage in potentially dangerous activities or make unrealistic and grandiose plans for the future. Visual–spatial functioning may be impaired, and if individuals have the ability to construct a plan and carry it out, suicide attempts can occur. More common is unintentional self-harm resulting from carelessness, undue familiarity with strangers, and disregard for the accepted rules of conduct. Emotional lability, as seen in pseudobulbar palsy after cerebral injury, can be particularly frustrating for caregivers, as are occasional psychotic features such as delusions and hallucinations. Changes in their environment and daily routine can be particularly distressing for demented individuals, and their frustration can be manifested by violent behavior.

Table 11-5	Evaluation of Dementia

Medical history and physical examination
Family interview
Routine laboratory
   Chemistry (SMA 20)
   Urinalysis
   Hematology (complete blood count)
Other routine tests
   Chest radiography
   Electrocardiography
Specialized laboratory
   Thyroid functions
   VDRL (fluorescent treponemal antibody screen if indicated)
   Drug screen
   Vitamin B_{12} and folate levels
   Cerebrospinal fluid analysis (if indicated)
   HIV testing (if indicated)
Other studies
   Computed tomography or magnetic resonance imaging
   Electroencephalography

The Mental Status Examination, in conjunction with a complete medical history from the individual and informants and an adequate physical examination, is essential in the evaluation and differential diagnosis of dementia (Table 11-5). The findings on the Mental Status Examination vary depending on the etiology of the dementia. In general, symptoms seen on the Mental Status Examination, whatever the etiology, are related to the location and extent of brain injury, individual adaptation to the dysfunction, premorbid coping skills and psychopathology, and concurrent medical illness.

Disturbance of memory, especially primary and secondary memory, is the most significant abnormality. Confabulation may be present as the individual attempts to minimize the memory impairment. Disorientation and altered levels of consciousness may occur, but are generally not seen in the early stages of dementia uncomplicated by delirium. Affect may be altered as in the masked facies of Parkinson's disease and the expansive affect and labile mood of pseudobulbar palsy after cerebral injury. The affect of individuals with hepatic encephalopathy is often described as blunted and apathetic. Lack of inhibition leading to such behavior as exposing oneself is common, and some conditions such as tertiary syphilis and untoward effects of some medication can precipitate mania.

The physical examination may offer clues to the etiology of the dementia; however, in the elderly, one must be aware of the normal changes associated with aging and differentiate them from signs of dementia. Often, the specific physical examination findings indicate the area of the central nervous system affected by the etiological process. Parietal lobe dysfunction is suggested by such symptoms as astereognosis, constructional apraxia, anosognosia, and problems with two-point discrimination. The dominant hemisphere parietal lobe is also involved in Gerstmann's syndrome, which includes agraphia, acalculia, finger agnosia, and right–left confusion.

Reflex changes such as hyperactive deep tendon reflexes, Babinski's reflex, and hyperactive jaw jerk are indicative of cerebral injury. However, primitive reflexes such as the palmar–mental reflex (tested by repeatedly scratching the base of the individual's thumb, with a positive response being slight downward movement of the lower lip and jaw) that occurs in 60% of normal elderly people, and the snout reflex, seen in a third of elderly individuals, are not diagnostically reliable for dementia.

Ocular findings such as nystagmus (as in brain stem lesions), ophthalmoplegia (Wernicke–Korsakoff syndrome), anisocoria, papilledema (hypertensive encephalopathy), cortical blindness (Anton's syndrome), visual field losses (CVA hemianopia), Kayser–Fleischer rings (Wilson's disease), and Argyll Robertson pupils (syphilis, diabetic neuropathy) can offer valuable clues to the etiology of the cognitive deficit.

Movement disorders including tremors (Parkinson's disease, drug intoxication, cerebellar dysfunction, Wilson's disease), chorea (Huntington's disease, other basal ganglia lesions), myoclonus (subacute sclerosing panencephalitis, Creutzfeldt–Jakob disease, Alzheimer's disease, anoxia), and asterixis (hepatic disease, uremia, hypoxia, carbon dioxide retention) should be noted.

Gait disturbances, principally apraxia (normal-pressure hydrocephalus, inhalant abuse, cerebellar dysfunction) and peripheral neuropathy (Korsakoff's syndrome, neurosyphilis, heavy metal intoxication, solvent abuse, isoniazid or phenytoin toxicity, vitamin deficiencies, and HIV spectrum illnesses), are also common in dementia. Extrapyramidal symptoms in the absence of antipsychotics may indicate substance abuse, especially phencyclidine abuse, or basal ganglia disease. Although the many and varied physical findings of dementia are too numerous to mention here in any detail, it should be obvious that the physical examination is an invaluable tool in the assessment of dementia (Table 11-6).

The prevalence of dementias is not precisely known. Estimates vary depending on the age range of the population studied and whether the individuals sampled were in the general community, acute care facilities, or long-term nursing institutions. A review of 47 surveys of dementia conducted between 1934 and 1985 indicated that the prevalence of dementia increased exponentially by age, doubling every 5 years up to age 95 years, and that this condition was equally

Table 11-6	Physical Signs Associated with Dementia or Delirium
Physical Sign	**Condition**
Myoclonus	Creutzfeldt–Jakob disease
	Subacute sclerosing panencephalitis
	Postanoxia
	Alzheimer's disease (10%)
	AIDS dementia
	Uremia
	Penicillin intoxication
	Meperidine toxicity
Asterixis	Hepatic encephalopathy
	Uremia
	Hypoxia
Chorea	Huntington's disease
	Wilson's disease
	Hypocalcemia
	Hypothyroidism
	Hepatic encephalopathy
	Oral contraceptives
	Systemic lupus erythematosus
	Carbon monoxide poisoning
	Toxoplasmosis
	Pertussis, diphtheria
Peripheral neuropathy	Wernicke–Korsakoff syndrome
	Neurosyphilis
	Heavy metal intoxication
	Organic solvent exposure
	Vitamin B_{12} deficiency
	Medications: isoniazid, phenytoin

distributed among men and women, with Alzheimer's dementia (AD) much more common in women. The National Institute of Mental Health Multisite Epidemiological Catchment Area study revealed a 6-month prevalence rate for mild dementia of 11.5% to 18.4% for persons older than 65 years living in the community. The rate for severe dementia was higher for the institutionalized elderly: 15% of the elderly in retirement communities, 30% of nursing home residents, and 54% of the elderly in state hospitals.

Studies suggest that the fastest growing segment of the US population consists of persons older than the age of 85 years, 15% of whom are demented. Half of the US population currently lives to the age of 75 years and one quarter lives to the age of 85. A study of 2000 consecutive admissions to a general medical hospital revealed that 9% were demented and, among those, 41% were also delirious on admission.

Course

The course of a particular dementia is influenced by its etiology. Although historically the dementias have been considered progressive and irreversible, there is, in fact, significant variation in the course of individual dementias. The disorder can be progressive, static, or remitting. In addition to the etiology, factors that influence the course of the dementia include (1) the time span between the onset and the initiation of prescribed treatment, (2) the degree of reversibility of the particular dementia, (3) the presence of comorbid mental disorders, and (4) the level of psychosocial support. The previous distinction between treatable and untreatable dementias has been replaced by the concepts of reversible, irreversible, and arrestable dementias. Most reversible cases of dementia are associated with shorter duration of symptoms, mild cognitive impairment, and superimposed delirium. Specifically, the dementias caused by drugs, depression, and metabolic disorders are most likely to be reversible. Other conditions such as normal-pressure hydrocephalus, subdural hematomas, and tertiary syphilis are more commonly arrestable.

Although potentially reversible dementias should be aggressively investigated, in reality, only 8% of dementias are partially reversible and about 3% are fully reversible. There is some evidence to suggest that early treatment of demented individuals, particularly those with Alzheimer's type, with such agents as donepe-

zil (Aricept), which acts as an inhibitor of acetylcholinesterase, and galanthamine (Reminyl) may slow down the rate of progression of the dementia.

Differential Diagnosis

Memory impairment occurs in a variety of conditions including delirium, amnestic disorders, and depression. In delirium, the onset of altered memory is acute and the pattern typically fluctuates (waxing and waning) with increased proclivity for confusion during the night. Delirium is more likely to feature autonomic hyperactivity and alterations in level of consciousness. In some cases, a dementia can have a superimposed delirium (Figure 11-2).

Individuals with major depressive disorder often complain of lapses in memory and judgment, poor concentration, and seemingly diminished intellectual capacity. Often, these symptoms are mistakenly diagnosed as dementia, especially in elderly individuals. A thorough medical history and mental status examination focusing on such symptoms as hopelessness, crying

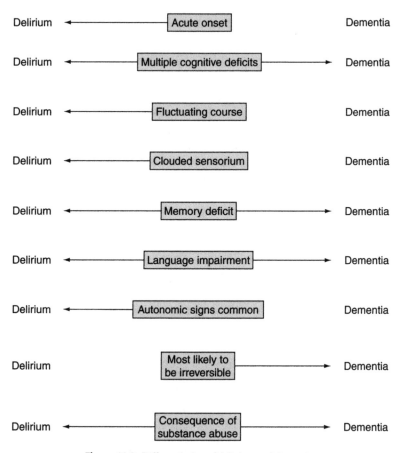

Figure 11-2 *Differentiation of delirium and dementia.*

episodes, and unrealistic guilt, in conjunction with a family history of depression, can be diagnostically beneficial. The term *pseudodementia* has been used to denote cognitive impairment secondary to a functional mental disorder, most commonly depression. In comparison with demented individuals, those with depressive pseudodementia exhibit better insight regarding their cognitive dysfunction, are more likely to give "I don't know" answers, and may exhibit neurovegetative signs of depression. Pharmacological treatment of the depression should improve the cognitive dysfunction as well. Because of the rapid onset of their antidepressant action, the use of psychostimulants (e.g., methylphenidate, dextroamphetamine) to differentiate between dementia and pseudodementia has been advocated by some authors. Some authors have proposed abandonment of the term pseudodementia, suggesting that most individuals so diagnosed have both genuine dementia and a superimposed affective disorder (Figure 11-3).

Amnestic disorder also presents with a significant memory deficit, but without the other associated features such as aphasia, agnosia, and apraxia. If cognitive impairment occurs only in the context of drug use, substance intoxication or substance withdrawal is the appropriate diagnosis. Although mental retardation implies below-average intellect and subsequent impairment in other areas of function, the onset is before 18 years of age and abnormalities of memory do not always occur. Mental retardation must be considered in the differential diagnosis of dementias of childhood and adolescence along with such disorders as Wilson's disease (hepatolenticular degeneration), lead intoxication, subacute sclerosing panencephalitis, HIV spectrum disorders, and substance abuse, particularly abuse of inhalants. If an individual develops dementia before age 18 years and has an IQ in the mentally retarded range (i.e., below 70), an additional diagnosis of mental retardation may be justified.

Individuals with schizophrenia may also exhibit a variety of cognitive abnormalities, but this condition also has an early onset, a distinctive constellation of other symptoms (e.g., delusions, hallucinations, disorganized speech), and does not result from a medical condition or the persisting effects of a substance. Factitious disorder and malingering must be distinguished from dementia. The individual with factitious disorder and psychological symptoms may have some apparent cognitive deficits reminiscent of a dementia.

Dementia must also be distinguished from age-related cognitive decline (also known as benign senescence). Only when such changes exceed the level of altered function to be expected for the individual's age is the diagnosis of dementia warranted.

Dementia of the Alzheimer Type

DIAGNOSIS

The course and clinical features of Dementia of the Alzheimer Type (DAT) (see diagnostic criteria for Dementia of Alzheimer Type, page 98) parallel those discussed for dementia in general. Typically, the early course of DAT is difficult to ascertain because the individual is usually an unreliable informant, and the early signs may be so subtle as to go unnoticed even by the individual's closest associates. These early features include impaired memory, difficulty with problem solving, preoccupation with long past events, decreased spontaneity, and an inability to respond to the environment with the individual's usual speed and accuracy. Individuals with DAT may forget names, misplace household items, or forget what they were about to do. Often the individuals have insight into these memory deficits and occasionally convey their concerns to family members. Such responses as "You're just getting older," and "I do that sometimes myself" are common from these family members and as a result the individual becomes depressed, which can further affect cognitive functioning. Anomia, or difficulty with word finding, is common in this middle stage of Alzheimer's disease. Eventually the individual develops schemes, word associations, and excuses ("I never was very good in math") to assist in retention and cover up deficits. The individual may also employ family members as a surrogate memory.

Because memory loss is usually most obvious for newly acquired material, the individual with DAT tries to avoid unfamiliar activities. Typically, the individual is seen by the clinician when confusion, aggression, wandering, or some other socially undesirable behavior ensues. At that time, disorders of perception and language may appear. The individual often turns to a spouse to answer questions posed during the history taking. By this time, the affected individual has lost insight into his or her dementia and abandons attempts to compensate for memory loss. Finally, in the late stage of Alzheimer's disease, physical and cognitive effects are marked. Disorders of gait, extremity paresis and paralysis, seizures, peripheral neuropathy, extrapyramidal signs, and urinary incontinence are seen, and the individual is often no longer ambulatory. The aimless wandering of the middle stage has been replaced by a mute, bedridden state and decorticate posture. Myoclonus occasionally occurs. Significantly, affective disturbances remain a distinct possibility throughout the course of the illness. Alzheimer's disease progresses at a slow pace for 8 to 10 years to a state of complete helplessness.

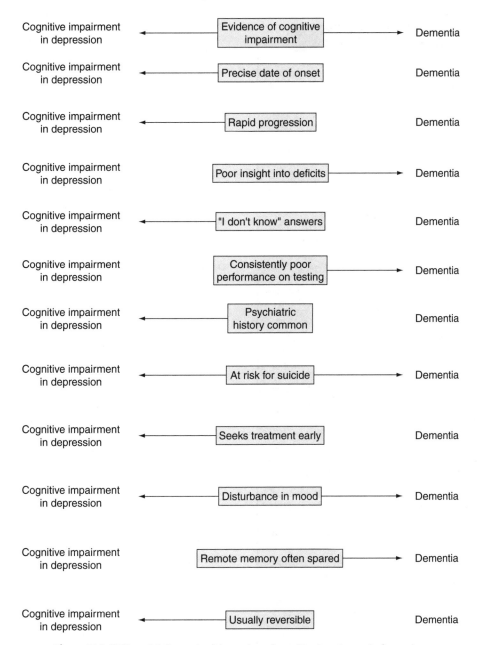

Figure 11-3 *Differential diagnosis of dementia and cognitive impairment in depression.*

The role of laboratory determinations in the evaluation for AD is to exclude other causes of dementia, especially those that may prove reversible or arrestable. Before death, AD is largely a diagnosis of exclusion. Throughout the course of this disorder, laboratory values are essentially normal. Some nonspecific changes may occur, but electroencephalography and lumbar puncture are not diagnostic. As the disease progresses, computed tomography (CT) and magnetic resonance imaging (MRI) may show atrophy in the cerebral cor-

tex and hydrocephalus *ex vacuo*. MRI may show nonspecific alteration of white matter (leukoariosis), and eventually EEG shows diffuse-background slowing. Pneumoencephalography has demonstrated enlarged ventricles and widening of cortical sulci in Alzheimer's disease, and positron emission tomography in the later stages shows decreased cerebral oxygen and glucose metabolism in the frontal lobes. At present, in the workup of an individual with a slowly progressive dementia, a good family history, physical examination,

294.1x DEMENTIA OF THE ALZHEIMER TYPE

A. The development of multiple cognitive deficits manifested by both

   (1) memory impairment (impaired ability to learn new information or to recall previously learned information)

   (2) one (or more) of the following cognitive disturbances:

      (a) aphasia (language disturbance)

      (b) apraxia (impaired ability to carry out motor activities despite intact motor function)

      (c) agnosia (failure to recognize or identify objects despite intact sensory function)

      (d) disturbance in executive functioning (i.e., planning, organizing, sequencing, abstracting)

B. The cognitive deficits in criteria A1 and A2 each cause significant impairment in social or occupational functioning and represent a significant decline from a previous level of functioning.

C. The course is characterized by gradual onset and continuing cognitive decline.

D. The cognitive deficits in criteria A1 and A2 are not due to any of the following:

   (1) other central nervous system conditions that cause progressive deficits in memory and cognition (e.g., cerebrovascular disease, Parkinson's disease, Huntington's disease, subdural hematoma, normal-pressure hydrocephalus, brain tumor)

   (2) systemic conditions that are known to cause dementia (e.g., hypothyroidism, vitamin B_{12} or folic acid deficiency, niacin deficiency, hypercalcemia, neurosyphilis, HIV infection)

   (3) substance-induced conditions

E. The deficits do not occur exclusively during the course of a delirium.

F. The disturbance is not better accounted for by another Axis I disorder (e.g., major depressive disorder, schizophrenia).

Code based on presence or absence of a clinically significant behavioral disturbance:

294.10 Without Behavioral Disturbance: if the cognitive disturbance is not accompanied by any clinically significant behavioral disturbance.

294.11 With Behavioral Disturbance: if the cognitive disturbance is accompanied by a clinically significant behavioral disturbance (e.g., wandering, agitation).

Specify subtype:

With Early Onset: if onset is at age 65 years or below

With Late Onset: if onset is after age 65 years

Coding note: Also code 331.0 Alzheimer's disease on Axis III. Indicate other prominent clinical features related to the Alzheimer's disease on Axis I (e.g., 293.83 Mood Disorder Due to Alzheimer's Disease, With Depressive Features, and 310.1 Personality Change Due to Alzheimer's Disease, Aggressive Type. Code based on type of onset and predominant features.

and laboratory and radiographic tests to rule out other causes of dementia are the most effective tools in the diagnosis of Alzheimer's disease.

Alzheimer's disease is the most common cause of dementia, accounting for 55–65% of all cases. There were fewer than 3 million cases diagnosed in the United States in 1980, but the Census Bureau predicts that there will be more than 10 million American citizens with Alzheimer's disease by the year 2050. Prevalence of the disease doubles with every 5 years between the ages of 65 and 85 years.

Alzheimer's disease affects women three times as often as men, for unknown reasons. Furthermore, at least one study suggests that dementia, including Alzheimer's, is more common in black than in white American women. Comparison of population studies in diverse countries shows strikingly similar prevalence rates.

TREATMENT

The two principles of management in AD are to treat what is treatable without aggravating existing symptoms and to support caregivers who are also victims of this disease. Given the significant decrease in ACh seen in AD, cholinesterase inhibitors which work by increasing the central nervous system concentrations of ACh have shown some promise in improving cognitive impairments early in the course of AD. Four acetylcholinesterase inhibitors (donepezil, tacrine, rivastigmine, galantamine) have been approved for use in the United States for the treatment of mild to moderate dementia. Side effects, particularly hepatic and cholinergic, are potentially problematic. Furthermore, improvement in cognitive functioning is often modest at best and ultimately temporary as the illness inevitably progresses.

The *N*-methyl-D-aspartate (NMDA) receptor, a glutamate receptor subtype, has important effects in learning and memory. Stimulation by the excitatory amino acid glutamate results in long-term potentiation of neuronal activity basic to memory formation. There appears to be a decrease in cerebral cortcial and hippocampal NMDA receptors in Alzheimer's disease. Memantine is a moderate affinity noncompetitive NMDA receptor antagonist approved in the US in 2003 for the treatment of moderate to severe dementia. A postmarketing surveillance study conducted among German physicians who treated dementia patients with memantine in combination with an anticholinesterase inhibior (mainly Aricept) suggests that this combination is safe and well tolerated.

Depression is often associated with AD. If antidepressant medication is to be used, low doses (about one-third to one-half of the usual initial dose) are advised and only agents with minimal anticholinergic activity should be employed. Appropriate choices would be the selective serotonin reuptake inhibitors such as paroxetine, fluoxetine, sertraline, citalopram, and escitalopram. Although sertraline, citalopram and escitalopram are least likely to cause drug–drug interactions, even these agents have the potential to increase confusion in Alzheimer's individuals. Agents such as trazodone and mirtazapine have occasionally been employed because of their sedating properties. If tricyclic antidepressants are used, the secondary amines (e.g., desipramine, nortriptyline) are recommended over the tertiary ones (e.g., amitriptyline, doxepin). Careful attention to the possible side effects of these agents, particularly orthostatic hypotension, lowering of the seizure threshold, excessive fatigue, urinary retention, constipation, confusion, and accelerated memory impairment, is suggested. Most clinicians now feel that tricyclic antidepressants are inappropriate for this population.

Anxiety and psychosis, particularly paranoid delusions, are common in AD. Benzodiazepines can be disinhibiting in such individuals and may exacerbate confusion and should be avoided if possible. If minor tranquilizers are required, agents with a shorter duration of action (e.g., lorazepam, oxazepam) are preferred. Antipsychotic medications with high anticholinergic potential (e.g., thioridazine, chlorpromazine) may also affect memory adversely. While these agents have been favored in the past because of their tendency to produce sedation, newer agents such as olanzapine (Zyprexa), risperidone (Risperdal), quetiapine (Seroquel) ziprasidone (Geodon) and aripipevazole (Abilify) have been reported to have lower incidences of neuroleptic-related side effects. However, a reported increase in cerebrovascular events (e.g., stroke, TIA) in elderly patients taking these newer agents raises questions about their safety, especially in patients with risk factors for vascular disease. Haloperidol has less anticholinergic activity but has a greater tendency toward extrapyramidal effects.

The appropriate management of AD entails more than psychopharmacological intervention. Other elements of the treatment plan should include environmental manipulation and support for the family. In the attempt to maintain individuals with Alzheimer's disease in their homes for as long as possible, some adjustments of their environment are important. Written daily reminders can be helpful in the performance of daily activities. Prominent clocks, calendars, and windows are important. An effort should be made to minimize changes in the individual's daily activities and environment. Repeated demonstrations of how to lock doors and windows and operate appliances are helpful and arranging for rapid dialing of essential telephone numbers can be useful. Maintaining adequate hydration, nutrition, exercise, and cleanliness is essential.

The family of the individual with Alzheimer's disease is also a victim of the disease. Family members must watch the gradual deterioration of the individual and accept that a significant part of their own lives must be devoted to the care of the individual. Difficult decisions about institutionalization and termination of life support are distinct possibilities, and individuals with AD often turn their anger and paranoia toward the caregiver. Education is a valuable treatment tool for families. Information about the disease and peer support are available through Alzheimer's associations, and many such agencies provide family members with a companion for the individual with AD to allow the family some time away. For these reasons, family members are at risk for depression, anxiety disorders, insomnia, and a variety of other psychological manifestations. Should these occur, they should be promptly treated.

Vascular Dementia

DIAGNOSIS

Vascular dementia usually results from multiple CVAs or one significant CVA. It is generally considered the second most common cause of dementia after Alzheimer's disease, accounting for about 10% of all cases. Men are twice as likely as women to be diagnosed with this condition. Vascular dementia is characterized by a stepwise progression of cognitive deterioration with accompanying lateralizing signs. (See DSM-IV-TR diagnostic criteria, page 100) It is always associated with evidence of systemic hypertension and usually involves renal and cardiac abnormalities. Risk factors for the development of a vascular dementia include those generally associated with obstructive coronary artery disease, including obesity, hypercholesterolemia, smoking, hypertension, stress, and lack of exercise. The actual incidence of vascular dementia has decreased somewhat with better standards of care, improved diagnostic techniques, and lifestyle changes.

Vascular dementia is characterized by the early appearance of localizing neurological signs. Spasticity, hemiparesis, ataxia, and pseudobulbar palsy are common. Pseudobulbar palsy is associated with injury to the frontal lobes and results in impairment of the corticobulbar tracts. It is characterized by extreme emotional lability, abnormal speech cadence, dysphagia, hyperactive jaw jerk, hyperactive deep tendon reflexes, and Babinski's reflex.

DSM-IV-TR Diagnostic Criteria

290.4x VASCULAR DEMENTIA

A. The development of multiple cognitive deficits manifested by both
(1) memory impairment (impaired ability to learn new information or to recall previously learned information)
(2) one (or more) of the following cognitive disturbances:

   (a) aphasia (language disturbance)
   (b) apraxia (impaired ability to carry out motor activities despite intact motor function)
   (c) agnosia (failure to recognize or identify objects despite intact sensory function)
   (d) disturbance in executive functioning (i.e., planning, organizing, sequencing, abstracting)

B. The cognitive deficits in criteria A1 and A2 each cause significant impairment in social or occupational functioning and represent a significant decline from a previous level of functioning.
C. Focal neurological signs and symptoms (e.g., exaggeration of deep tendon reflexes, extensor plantar response, pseudobulbar palsy, gait abnormalities, weakness of an extremity) or laboratory evidence indicative of cerebrovascular disease (e.g., multiple infarctions involving cortex and underlying white matter) that are judged to be etiologically related to the disturbance.
D. The deficits do not occur exclusively during the course of a delirium.

Code based on predominant features:

290.41 With Delirium: if delirium is superimposed on the dementia

290.42 With Delusions: if delusions are the predominant feature

390.43 With Depressed Mood: if depressed mood (including presentations that meet full symptom criteria for a major depressive episode) is the predominant feature. A separate diagnosis of mood disorder due to a general medical condition is not given.

209.40 Uncomplicated: if none of the above predominates in the current clinical presentation

Specify if:

With behavioral disturbance

Coding note: Also code cerebrovascular condition on Axis III.

Reprinted with permission from the *Diagnostic and Statistical Manual of Mental Disorders*, 4th ed., Text Rev. Copyright 2000 American Psychiatric Association.

CT, MRI, and gross specimens show cerebral atrophy and infarctions, with the radiological procedures showing multiple lucencies and the gross specimens revealing distinct white-matter lesions. The EEG is abnormal but nonspecific, and positron emission tomography reveals hypometabolic areas. Vascular dementia is differentiated from AD on the basis of its mode of progression, early appearance of neurological signs, and radiographical evidence of cerebral ischemia.

TREATMENT

Primary prevention and secondary prevention are important in the treatment of cerebrovascular disorders. Lifestyle changes are effective in arresting the progress of the disease; however, no known pharmacological treatment can reverse the effects of a completed stroke. Such interventions as anticoagulants for frequent transient ischemic attacks after a hemorrhagic lesion has been investigated but excluded; aspirin for decreasing platelet aggregation, and surgical removal of obstructing plaques probably do not reverse the mental state.

Depression occurs in 50–60% of individuals with CVAs and responds to traditional antidepressants. Tricyclic antidepressants, such as amitriptyline, in less than antidepressant doses, improve both CVA depression and pseudobulbar palsy. Physical rehabilitation is essential and often results in an improvement in mood and outlook.

Dementia Due to HIV Disease

DIAGNOSIS

Acquired Immunodeficiency Syndrome (AIDS) was first described in the United States in 1979. In the developed countries, the death rate from AIDS has been on the decline since the advent of new medication regimens utilizing traditional antiretrovirals and the newer protease inhibitors. These medication cocktails have also decreased the incidence of AIDS–dementia complex, so that physicians are now more likely to see AIDS-related delirium secondary to infection, metabolic disarray, and medication rather than traditional AIDS dementia. In the truest sense, AIDS is not a disease but an increased susceptibility to a variety of diseases caused by loss of immunocompetence due to HIV infection.

AIDS is now best considered as part of the spectrum of HIV infection. There are four stages of infection.

- *Stage 1: Acute Infection.* Most infected persons remember no signs or symptoms at the time of the initial infection. The acute syndrome follows infection by 4 to 6 weeks and is characterized by fevers, rigors, muscle aches, maculopapular rash, diarrhea, and abdominal cramps. These symptoms, often mistaken for those of influenza, resolve spontaneously after 2 to 3 weeks.
- *Stage 2: Asymptomatic carrier.* This stage follows the acute infection. The infected individual is without symptoms for a variable amount of time. The mean symptom-free period has increased significantly since the disease was first identified and is

now about 10 years. Most of the estimated 2 million infected Americans are at this stage. Even though these individuals are asymptomatic, they are carriers of the disease and can infect others.

- *Stage 3: Generalized adenopathy.* In older terminology, this stage was referred to as the AIDS-related complex. It is characterized by palpable lymph nodes that persist for longer than 3 months. These nodes must be outside the inguinal area and due to no other condition except HIV.
- *Stage 4: Other diseases.*

  – Constitutional symptoms such as lingering fever, wasting syndromes, and intractable diarrhea.
  – Secondary infections including *P. carinii* pneumonia, cytomegalovirus retinitis, parasitic colitis, and oral esophageal thrush.
  – Secondary neoplasms such as Kaposi's sarcoma and B-cell lymphomas.
  – Neurological diseases (AIDS dementia complex).

Thus, the diagnosis of AIDS is made when an infected individual develops either a $CD4^+$ cell count of less than 200 or a certain condition listed in the stages.

Initially, the behavioral abnormalities observed in HIV-positive individuals were attributed to the emotional reaction to the disease. Subsequent investigations demonstrated that neurological complications occur in 40–45% of individuals with AIDS, and in about 10% of cases, neurological signs are the first feature of the disease. The neurological signs present in AIDS are believed to be related to both the direct effects of the virus on cells (such as macrophages) that enter the central nervous system and the neurological conditions that opportunistically affect these individuals.

Individuals with AIDS dementia present with impairments of cognitive, behavioral, and motor systems. The cognitive symptoms include memory impairment, confusion, and poor concentration. Behavioral features include apathy, reclusivity, anhedonia, depression, delusions, and hallucinations. Motor symptoms include incoordination, lower extremity paresis, unsteadiness, and difficulty with fine motor movements like handwriting and buttoning clothes. As the disease progresses, parkinsonism and myoclonus develop. Localizing signs such as tremors, focal seizures, abnormal reflexes, and hemiparesis can result. The protozoan *Toxoplasma gondii* commonly infects the central nervous system and can be diagnosed by CT or by increased toxoplasmosis antibody titers. Discrete cerebral lesions are also produced by fungi such as *Candida* and *Aspergillus, Mycobacterium tuberculosis*, and viruses such as cytomegalovirus and papovavirus. Papovavirus causes progressive

multifocal leukoencephalopathy. Tertiary syphilis has increased significantly since the advent of AIDS, and neoplasms such as lymphomas, metastatic Kaposi's sarcoma, and gliomas are also causes of AIDS dementia.

Many confounding factors can increase cognitive dysfunction in AIDS, including a high incidence of drug and alcohol abuse; medications such as histamine H_2 receptor antagonists (cimetidine), corticosteroids, narcotics, and antiviral drugs (e.g., zidovudine [formerly azidothymidine, AZT]) that increase confusion; and coexistent depression (Table 11-7).

The CT scan shows cerebral atrophy and MRI reveals nonspecific white-matter abnormalities. Neoplasms and lesions such as toxoplasmosis are also

Table 11-7	Neuropsychiatric Effects of AIDS-related Drugs	
Drug	**Use**	**Effect**
Ketoconazole (Nizoral)	Antifungal	Severe depression
		Suicidality (rare)
Foscarnet	Cytomegalovirus retinitis	Depression
	Herpes	Confusion
Ganciclovir	Cytomegalovirus retinitis	Anxiety
		Psychosis
Bactrim	*Pneumocystis* pneumonia	Hallucinations
		Depression
		Apathy
Pentamidine	*Pneumocystis* pneumonia	Delirium
		Hallucinations
Interferon alpha	Cancer	Depression
Rifampin	Tuberculosis	Delirium
		Behavioral changes
Isoniazid	Tuberculosis	Memory disturbance
		Psychosis
Dronabinol (Marinol)	Appetite stimulant	Wasting syndrome
		Nausea
		Depression
		Anxiety
		Psychosis
		Euphoria
Zalcitabine (DDC)	Antiviral	Psychosis
		Amnesia
		Confusion
		Depersonalization
		Depression
		Mania
		Suicidality
		Mood swings
Didanosine	Antiviral	Anxiety
Zidovudine (AZT)	Antiviral	Confusion, mania
		Depression, anxiety

visible. Lumbar puncture reveals a pleocytosis and elevated protein levels, and autopsy demonstrates an atrophic brain with demyelination, multinuclear giant cells, and gliosis of the cerebral cortex.

TREATMENT

The treatment of neuropsychiatric disorders in AIDS involves utilizing agents that are least likely to interfere with other medications prescribed, or to exacerbate the symptoms of the disease. AIDS-related depression has responded well to the selective serotonin reuptake inhibitors (SSRIs) and to psychostimulants. Some HIV drugs can have interactions with SSRIs, and SSRIs can interact with other agents the individual with HIV may have been prescribed, such as antiarrhythmics, benzodiazepines, and anticonvulsants, by inhibiting the cytochrome P-450 enzyme system. Some individuals have suggested that citalopram and escitalopram are less likely to inhibit this enzyme system. Careful attention to drug–drug interactions, using lower starting doses of certain psychiatric drugs, and monitoring of blood levels of affected medications are recommended. Among the psychostimulants, methylphenidate is preferred to dextroamphetamine because of the latter's tendency to produce dyskinesias. Use of stimulants for treating individuals with a history of substance abuse is not recommended. Anticholineric agents have a number of side effects such as mydriasis, decreased gastrointestinal motility, and postural hypotension. However, low-dose tricyclic antidepressants are often used for their sedative, analgesic, and appetite stimulant properties. Most antidepressants and some mood stabilizers and antipsychotics can cause bone marrow suppression, so they should be used with care, and hematologic parameters should be routinely monitored. Lithium carbonate, which produces a leukocytosis, may be of benefit in recurrent unipolar and treatment-resistant depression, but may potentiate AIDS-related diarrhea. Many of the drugs used to treat AIDS-related conditions may produce untoward psychiatric effects. Depression has been well documented as a side effect of indinavir (Crixivan), and nelfinavir (Viracept) has been associated with anxiety, depression, mood lability, and even suicidality. St. John's Wort may decrease the concentration of many of the protease inhibitors and is therefore contraindicated in individuals taking these agents.

In summary, AIDS dementia is best treated by identifying the associated medical condition, instituting appropriate therapy, and managing behavior in the interim.

Dementia Due to Other General Medical Conditions

Dementia Due to Pick's Disease

Pick's disease is a rare form of progressive dementia clinically indistinguishable from Alzheimer's disease. It is about one-fifth as common as AD. Pick's disease occurs in the sixth and seventh decades of life and has a duration that varies from 2 to 15 years. ACh levels are reduced. The pathology of Pick's disease involves prominent changes (e.g., sclerosis, atrophy) in the frontal and temporal lobes with sparing of the parietal and occipital lobes.

The clinical features of Pick's disease are quite similar to those of Alzheimer's disease, and since neither condition is curable, an elaborate differential diagnosis is unnecessary. Because of parietal sparing, features such as apraxia and agnosia are less common in Pick's disease, and visual–spatial ability, often impaired in Alzheimer's disease, is preserved. Given the prominent changes in the frontal lobe, disinhibited behavior, loss of social constraints, and lack of concern about appearance and matters of personal hygiene occur relatively early in Pick's disease. Such speech disorders as echolalia and logorrhea are common, and individuals with Pick's disease are more likely to develop Klüver–Bucy syndrome (orality, hyperphagia, hypersexuality, placidity) indicative of damage to the temporal lobes. Significant memory impairment may occur relatively late in the course, and eventually the individual becomes listless, mute, and ultimately decerebrate and comatose. Like Alzheimer's disease, the treatment of Pick's disease is symptomatic.

Dementia Due to Parkinson's Disease

Although dementia rarely occurs as an initial symptom of Parkinson's disease, it is found in nearly 40% of such individuals older than 70 years of age. The prevalence in persons over 60 is 1%. The disease results from loss of dopamine production in the basal ganglia, and can be idiopathic or postencephalitic. Usually, the individual is 50 years of age or older, and unlike Alzheimer's and Pick's dementias, this disease occurs slightly more often in men. Dementia most commonly occurs in cases of Parkinson's disease in which the decline has been rapid and response to anticholinergics has been poor.

The clinical features of Parkinson's disease are well described, with the cardinal triad being tremor, rigidity, and bradykinesia. Associated features include postural instability, a festinating gait, micrographia, seborrhea, urinary changes, constipation, hypophonia, and an expressionless facial countenance. The tremor in Parkinson's disease has a regular rate and is most prominent when the individual is sitting with arms supported; and has been described as an intention tremor. Paranoid delusions and visual hallucinations may occur, but auditory hallucinations are rare. Antipsychotics with low incidence of extrapyramidal symptoms such as quetiapine, olanzapine, and ziprasidone are recommended. The pharmacological treatment of Parkinson's disease involves the use of a number of types of medication. These include selegiline (Eldepryl), a selective monoamine oxidase inhibitor, levodopa, other dopamine agonists (pramipexole [Mirapex], bromocriptine, pergolide mesylate [Permax], amantadine), and various anticholinergic agents (e.g., benztropine). Selegiline should not be given to individuals on antidepressant medication as there is a risk that dopaminergic agents may activate psychosis or mania. When discontinuing levodopa after a long course of treatment, the drug should be tapered so as to prevent a discontinuation syndrome similar in nature to the neuroleptic malignant syndrome. Some medications (metoclopramide, droperidol, several antipsychotics) may produce parkinsonian features such as masked facies, sparsity of speech, and tremor, and in those cases, the appropriate course of treatment is to discontinue the offending medication.

Dementia Due to Huntington's Disease

Dementia is also a characteristic of Huntington's disease, an autosomal, dominant, inheritable condition localized to chromosome 4. Unfortunately, this condition does not become apparent until age 35 to 45 years, usually after childbearing has occurred. Fifty percent of offspring are affected. There is also a juvenile form of the disease. Huntington's disease affects about 4 in 100,000 people, making it a significant cause of dementia in middle-aged adults.

The most noticeable clinical feature of Huntington's disease is the movement disorder, which involves both choreiform movements (frequent movements that cause a jerking motion of the body) and athetosis (slow writhing movements). In the juvenile form of Huntington's disease, which represents about 3% of all cases, the chorea is replaced by dystonia, akinesia, and rigidity, and the course of the disease is more rapid than in the adult form. In the early stages of the disease, the chorea is not as noticeable and may be disguised by the individual by making the movements seem purposeful.

The dementia typically begins 1 year before or 1 year after the chorea and, unlike individuals with other dementias, individuals with Huntington's disease are often well aware of their deteriorating mentation. This may be a factor in the high rates of suicide and alcoholism associated with this condition. Although attempts have been made to increase ACh and GABA concentrations in these individuals, such pharmacological interventions have been unsuccessful, and the dementia is untreatable. Genetic counseling is indicated.

Subacute Sclerosing Panencephalitis

Subacute sclerosing panencephalitis is an infectious cause of dementia that usually appears in childhood. The average age at onset is 10 years, and most individuals are male and live in rural areas. It is diagnosed on the basis of periodic complexes on the EEG and an elevated measles titer in the cerebrospinal fluid (CSF). The CT scan shows cerebral atrophy and dilated ventricles. Myoclonus and dementia are prominent features. It has been postulated that a mutant measles virus is the infectious agent, on the basis of the high CSF measles antibody titer and the fact that the disease is virtually nonexistent in children who have been vaccinated for measles. Affected individuals show an insidious onset of impairment of cognition usually preceded by behavioral problems.

Creutzfeldt–Jakob Disease

The primary features of Creutzfeldt–Jakob disease are dementia, basal ganglia and cerebellar dysfunction, myoclonus, upper motor neuron lesions, and rapid progression to stupor, coma, and death in a matter of months. The disease generally affects people 65 years of age or older, with a duration of 1 month to 6 years and an average life span of 15 months after the onset of the disease.

The clinical and pathological features of Creutzfeldt–Jakob have been produced experimentally by injecting animals with brain tissue from affected adults. The agent of transmission is believed to be a prion-containing protein (not DNA or RNA). These prions have been detected in the cerebral cortex of autopsy specimens of both individuals with Creutzfeldt–Jakob disease and victims of kuru, a fatal disease transmitted by cannibalism. Slow viruses have also been implicated as infectious agents in kuru. Creutzfeldt–Jakob has been accidentally transferred to humans by corneal and pituitary gland transplantation, electroencephalogram electrodes and ingesting meat infected with the disease (mad cow disease).

The memory loss in Creutzfeldt–Jakob disease involves all phases of memory, with recent (secondary) memory being the most impaired. Personality changes, immature behavior, and paranoia are early signs, and virtually every aspect of brain functioning can be involved. Motor disorders including rigidity, incoordination, paresis, and ataxia usually follow. As with subacute sclerosing panencephalitis, the EEG in Creutzfeldt–Jakob disease shows periodic complexes and biopsy specimens that reveal a characteristic spongiform encephalopathy and occasional amyloid plaques.

Neurosyphilis

During the late 19th century, neurosyphilis was responsible for a significant number of admissions to psychiatric hospitals. The condition decreased in incidence after the causative agent (*Treponema pallidum*) was identified and penicillin treatment became readily available. The rise of AIDS in the 1980s and 1990s has led to an increase in the number of diagnosed cases of neurosyphilis.

Dementia, secondary to neurosyphilis, produces various physical findings in advanced cases. These may include dysarthria, Babinski's reflex, tremor, Argyll Robertson pupils, myelitis, and optic atrophy. Although notorious, delusions of grandeur in neurosyphilis are rare. A reactive CSF VDRL result or a positive serum fluorescent treponemal antibody result in an individual with neurological symptoms who cannot document treatment should be treated with appropriate therapy. Penicillin often improves cognitive deficits and corrects CSF abnormalities, but complete recovery is rare.

Dementia Due to Head Trauma

Head trauma is the leading cause of brain injury for children and young adults. Traumatic head injuries result in concussions, contusions, or open head injuries, and the physical examination often reveals such features as blood behind the tympanic membranes (Battle's sign), infraorbital ecchymosis, and pupillary abnormalities. The psychiatric manifestations of an acute brain injury are generally classified as a delirium or an amnestic disorder; however, head trauma-induced delirious states often merge into a chronic dementia. Episodes of repeated head trauma, as in *dementia pugilistica* (punchdrunk syndrome), can lead to permanent changes in cognition and thus are appropriately classified as demented states. The punchdrunk syndrome is seen in aging boxers and includes dysarthric speech, emotional lability, slowed thought, and impulsivity. A single head injury may result in a postconcussional syndrome with resultant memory impairment, alterations in mood and personality, hyperacusis, headaches, easy fatigability, anxiety, belligerent behavior,

and dizziness. Alcohol abuse, postural hypotension, and gait disturbances are often associated with head injuries that result in dementia.

Normal-Pressure Hydrocephalus

Normal-pressure hydrocephalus is generally considered the fifth leading cause of dementia after Alzheimer's, vascular, alcohol-related, and AIDS dementias. Long considered reversible but often merely arrestable, normal-pressure hydrocephalus is a syndrome consisting of dementia, urinary incontinence, and gait apraxia. It results from subarachnoid hemorrhage, meningitis, or trauma that impedes CSF absorption.

Unlike other dementias, the dementia caused by normal-pressure hydrocephalus has physical effects that often overshadow the mental effects. Psychomotor retardation, marked gait disturbances, and, in severe cases, complete incontinence of urine occur. A cisternogram is often helpful in the diagnosis, and CT and MRI show ventricular dilatation without cerebral atrophy. CSF analysis reveals a normal opening pressure, and glucose and protein determinations are within the normal range. The hydrocephalus can be relieved by insertion of a shunt into the lateral ventricle to drain CSF into the chest or the abdominal cavity, where it is absorbed. Clinical improvement with shunting approaches 50% with a neurosurgical complication rate of 13–25%.

Wilson's Disease

Hepatolenticular degeneration (Wilson's disease) is an inherited autosomal recessive condition associated with dementia, hepatic dysfunction, and a movement disorder. Localized to chromosome 13, this disorder features copper deposits in the liver, brain, and cornea. Symptoms begin in adolescence to the early twenties and cases are often seen in younger children. Wilson's disease should be considered along with Huntington's disease, AIDS dementia, substance abuse dementia, head trauma, and subacute sclerosing panencephalitis in the differential diagnosis of dementia that presents in adolescence and early adulthood. Personality, mood, and thought disorders are common, and physical findings include a wing-beating tremor, rigidity, akinesia, dystonia, and the pathognomonic Kayser–Fleischer ring around the cornea. Wilson's disease can mimic other conditions, including Huntington's disease, Parkinson's disease, atypical psychosis, and neuroleptic-induced dystonia. Slit-lamp ocular examination, abnormal liver function tests, and markedly decreased serum ceruloplasmin levels are diagnostic. Chelating agents such as penicillamine, if administered early, can reverse central nervous system and nonneurological findings in about 50% of cases.

Other Medical Conditions

In addition to the conditions mentioned previously, other medical illnesses can be associated with dementia. These include endocrine disorders (hypothyroidism, hypoparathyroidism), chronic metabolic conditions (hypocalcemia, hypoglycemia), nutritional deficiencies (thiamine, niacin, vitamin B_{12}), structural lesions (brain tumors, subdural hematomas), and multiple sclerosis.

Substance-Induced Persisting Dementia

DIAGNOSIS

In instances in which the features of dementia result from central nervous system effects of a medication, toxin, or drug of abuse (including alcohol), the diagnosis of dementia due to the persisting effects of a substance should be made. The most common dementias in this category are those associated with alcohol abuse, accounting for about 10% of all dementias. The diagnosis of alcohol persisting dementia requires that the cognitive changes persist after the cessation of alcohol use and are not the result of changes in mentation associated amnestic episodes (blackouts), or Wernicke–Korsakoff syndrome. In addition to various nutritional deficiencies and the toxic effects of alcohol itself, alcohol abusers are more prone to develop dementia as a result of head trauma and chronic hepatic encephalopathy.

Severe alcohol dependence is the third leading cause of dementia. Alcohol-induced dementia is a relatively late occurrence, generally following 15 to 20 years of heavy drinking. Dementia is more common in individuals with alcoholism who are malnourished. The CT scan shows cortical atrophy and ventricular dilatation after about 10 years with neuronal loss, pigmentary degeneration, and glial proliferation. The frontal lobes are the most affected, followed by parietal and temporal areas. The amount of deterioration is related to age, number of episodes of heavy drinking, and total amount of alcohol consumed over time.

Alcohol-induced dementia, secondary to the toxic effects of alcohol, develops insidiously and often presents initially with changes in personality. Increasing memory loss, worsening cognitive processing, and concrete thinking follow. The dementia may be affected by periodic superimposed delirious states including those

Table 11-8	Central Nervous System Sequelae of Alcohol Abuse

Blackouts
Dementia
Marchiafava–Bignami disease
Wernicke–Korsakoff syndrome
Hepatic encephalopathy
Delirium tremens
Withdrawal seizures
Episodic dyscontrol (pathological intoxication)
Alcoholic hallucinosis
Head injury

caused by recurrent use of alcohol and cross-sensitive drugs, respiratory disease related to smoking, central nervous system hemorrhage secondary to trauma, chronic hypoxia related to recurrent seizure activity, folic acid deficiency, and higher rates of some neoplasms among those with alcoholism (Table 11-8).

Many other agents can produce dementia as a result of their persisting effects. Exposure to such heavy metals as mercury and bromide, chronic contact with various insecticides, and use of various classes of drugs of abuse may produce dementia. In particular, the abuse of organic solvents (inhalants) has been associated with neurological changes (see Chapter 20). The inhalants are generally classified as anesthetics (halothane, chloroform, ether, nitrous oxide), solvents (gasoline, paint thinner, antifreeze, kerosene, carbon tetrachloride), aerosols (insecticides, deodorants, hair sprays), and nitrites (amyl nitrite). The solvent category is particularly toxic to the brain. In addition, acute anoxia may result from the common practice of inhaling a substance with a plastic bag around the head. Such neurological findings as peripheral neuropathy, paresis, paresthesias, areflexia, seizures, signs of cerebellar damage, and Babinski's sign are common. Although the cerebellum is often involved, any area of the cerebral cortex may be affected (Table 11-9).

TREATMENT

The presence of dementia makes the treatment of alcoholism or other drug dependence more difficult. Most treatment programs depend on education about substance abuse, working the 12 steps, some degree of sociability, and such relatively abstract concepts as secondary gratification and a higher power. Such treatment programs are often reluctant to engage in the painstaking repetition that individuals with substance-induced persisting dementia often require. These individuals may become frustrated in peer support groups such as Alcoholics Anonymous. Despite these obstacles, individuals with alcoholism who complete a treatment

Table 11-9	Neurological Effects of Selected Inhalants	
Agent	**Use**	**Effect**
n-Hexane	Organic solvent	Peripheral neuropathy
Methyl butyl ketone	Paint thinner	Polyneuropathy
Toluene	Paint thinner	Cognitive dysfunction
		Cerebellar ataxia
		Optic neuropathy
		Sensorineural hearing loss
		Dementia
Trichloroethylene	Metal degreasing	Trigeminal neuropathy
	Extracting oils	
Methylene chloride	Paint stripping	Carbon monoxide poisoning
	Aerosol propellant	
		Hypoxic encephalopathy
1,1,1-trichloroethane	Solvent	Cerebral hypoxia
	Industrial degreasing	

program and remain sober do have some improvement in their mental state. There is an initial improvement that peaks at 3 to 4 weeks, followed by a slow but steady improvement detected at 6 to 8 months. In general, the presence of a cognitive deficit (dementia) dictates an alcohol treatment program that is behavior-based, concrete, structured, supportive, and repetitive.

Dementia Due to Multiple Etiologies

Dementia may have more than one cause in a particular individual. Certain types of dementia tend to occur together, including alcohol persisting dementia and dementia caused by head trauma, vascular dementia and dementia of the Alzheimer type, and alcohol persisting dementia and a nutritional dementia. For the purpose of DSM-IV-TR diagnosis, all conditions contributing to the dementia should be diagnosed by coding the various types of dementia on Axis I, for example alcohol persisting dementia and dementia due to head trauma.

Amnestic Disorders

DIAGNOSIS

The amnestic disorders are characterized by a disturbance in memory related to the direct effects of a general medical condition or the persisting effects of a substance. The impairment should interfere with social and occupational functioning and represent a significant decline from the previous level of functioning. The

DSM-IV-TR Diagnostic Criteria

DSM-IV-TR DIAGNOSTIC CRITERIA FOR AMNESTIC DISORDER

A. The development of memory impairment as manifested by impairment in the ability to learn new information or the inability to recall previously learned information.
B. The memory disturbance causes significant impairment in social or occupational functioning and represents a significant decline from a previous level of functioning.
C. The memory disturbance does not occur exclusively during the course of a delirium or a dementia.

Note: Further criteria are based on etiology—see specific disorders for discussion.

Reprinted with permission from *DSM-IV-TR Guidebook*. Copyright 2004, Michael B First, Allen Frances, and Harold Alan Pincus.

amnestic disorders are differentiated on the basis of the etiology of the memory loss. These disorders should not be diagnosed if the memory deficit is a feature of a dissociative disorder, is associated with dementia, or occurs in the presence of clouded sensorium, as individuals with amnestic disorder have impaired ability to learn new information (anterograde amnesia) or cannot remember material previously learned (retrograde amnesia). Memory for the event that produced the deficit (e.g., a head injury in a motor vehicle accident) may also be impaired. Remote recall (tertiary memory) is generally good, so individuals may be able to accurately relate incidents that occurred during childhood but not remember what they had for breakfast. As illustrated by such conditions as thiamine amnestic syndrome, immediate memory is often preserved. In some instances, disorientation to time and place may occur, but disorientation to person is unusual.

The onset of the amnesia is determined by the precipitant and may be acute as in head injury or insidious as in poor nutritional states. DSM-IV-TR characterizes short-duration amnestic disorder as lasting less than 1 month and long-duration disorder lasting 1 month or longer. Often, individuals lack insight into the memory deficit and vehemently insist that their inaccurate responses on a Mental Status Examination are correct.

The exact prevalence and incidence of the amnestic disorders are unknown. Memory disturbances related to specific conditions such as alcohol dependence and head trauma have been studied and these appear to be the two most common causes of amnestic disorders.

Differential Diagnosis

Amnestic disorders must be differentiated from the less disruptive changes in memory that occur in normal aging, the memory impairment that is accompanied by other cognitive deficits in dementia, the amnesia that might occur with clouded consciousness in delirium, the stress-induced impairment in recall seen in dissociative disorders, and the inconsistent amnestic deficits seen in factitious disorder and malingering.

The specific causes of amnestic disorders include (1) systemic medical conditions such as thiamine deficiency; (2) brain conditions, including seizures, cerebral neoplasms, head injury, hypoxia, carbon monoxide poisoning, surgical ablation of temporal lobes, electroconvulsive therapy, and multiple sclerosis; (3) altered blood flow in the vertebral vascular system, as in transient global amnesia; and (4) effects of a substance (drug or alcohol use and exposure to toxins). Conditions that affect the temporal lobes such as herpes infection and Klüver–Bucy syndrome can produce amnesia. Among drugs that can cause amnestic disorders, triazolam (Halcion) has received the most attention, but all benzodiazepines can produce memory impairment, with the dose utilized being the determining factor (Table 11-10).

Selected Amnestic Disorders

Blackouts. Blackouts are periods of amnesia for events that occur during heavy drinking. Typically, a person awakens the morning after consumption and does not remember what happened the night before. Unlike delirium tremens, which is related to chronicity of alcohol abuse, blackouts are more a measure of the amount of alcohol consumed at any one time. Thus, blackouts are common in binge pattern drinkers and may occur the first time a person ingests a large amount of alcohol. Blackouts are generally transient phenomena,

but some individuals may continue to have blackouts for weeks even after they have stopped using alcohol. These memory lapses are similar to blackouts experienced while using alcohol. With continued sobriety, the blackouts should end, but information forgotten during past blackouts is never remembered. Blackouts may also be produced by agents with cross-sensitivity to alcohol, such as benzodiazepines. Blackouts should not be confused with alcohol-induced dementia, which presents with cortical atrophy on CT scans, associated features of dementia, and a usually irreversible course.

Korsakoff's Syndrome. Korsakoff's syndrome is an amnestic disorder caused by thiamine deficiency. Although generally associated with alcohol abuse, it can occur in other malnourished states such as marasmus, gastric carcinoma, and HIV spectrum disease. This syndrome is usually associated with Wernicke's encephalopathy, which involves ophthalmoplegia, ataxia, and confusion. Korsakoff's syndrome is often associated with a neuropathy and occurs in about 85% of untreated individuals with Wernicke's disease. Complete recovery from Korsakoff's syndrome is rare.

Head Injury. Head injuries can produce a wide variety of neurological and mental disorders even in the absence of radiological evidence of structural damage. Delirium, dementia, mood disturbances, behavioral disinhibition, alterations of personality, and amnestic disorders may result. Amnesia in head injury is for events preceding the incident and the incident itself, leading some clinicians to mistakenly consider these individuals as having factitious disorders or being malingerers. The eventual duration of the amnesia is related to the degree of memory recovery that occurs in the first few days after the injury.

TREATMENT

As in delirium and dementia, the primary goal in the amnestic disorders is to discover and treat the underlying cause. Because some of these causes of amnestic disorder are associated with dangerous self-damaging behavior (e.g., suicide attempts by hanging, carbon monoxide poisoning, deliberate motor vehicle accidents, self-inflicted gunshot wounds to the head, and chronic alcohol abuse), some form of psychiatric management is often necessary. In the hospital, continuous reorientation by means of verbal redirection, clocks, and calendars can allay the individual's fears. Supportive individual psychotherapy and family counseling are beneficial.

Table 11-10	Causes of Amnestic Disorders
Types simplex encephalopathy	
Substance-induced (alcohol) blackouts	
Wernicke–Korsakoff syndrome	
Multiple sclerosis	
Klüver–Bucy syndrome	
Electroconvulsive therapy	
Seizures	
Head trauma	
Carbon monoxide poisoning	
Metabolic	
Hypoxia	
Hypoglycemia	
Medications	
Triazolam	
Barbiturates (thiopental sodium)	
Diltiazem (Cardizem)	
Zalcitabine (DDC)	
Cerebrovascular disorders	

Comparison of DSM-IV-TR and ICD-10 Diagnostic Criteria

The overall construct of delirium is similar in DSM-IV-TR and ICD-10 (i.e., a disturbance in consciousness and cognition with an acute onset and fluctuating course). The ICD-10 Diagnostic Criteria for Research include some additional items: impairment in short-term memory with intact long-term memory, disorientation, psychomotor disturbances, and problems with sleep. ICD-10 does not include the DSM-IV-TR category delirium due to multiple etiologies.

Similarly, the overall construct of dementia is similar in DSM-IV-TR and ICD-10 (i.e., memory impairment plus a decline in other cognitive abilities). The ICD-10 Diagnostic Criteria for Research are more narrowly defined in several ways: the minimum duration of the disturbance is 6 months as compared with DSM-IV-TR, which does not specify any minimum duration. Required cognitive deficits, in addition to memory loss, are restricted to a deterioration in judgment and thinking (as opposed to DSM-IV-TR, which requires any one of aphasia, apraxia, agnosia, or disturbance in executive functioning); and there must also be a "decline in emotional control or motivation or a change in social behavior."

Like DSM-IV-TR, ICD-10 includes two subtypes of dementia of the Alzheimer's type: early-onset and late-onset. However, in contrast to DSM-IV-TR, the ICD-10 Diagnostic Criteria for Research for these subtypes also specify characteristic course features and types of deficits: early-onset cases must have a "relatively rapid onset and progression" and a characteristic type of cognitive impairment (e.g., aphasia), whereas late-onset cases have a very slow and gradual onset with a predominance of memory impairment over other intellectual deficits. In ICD-10, this disorder is referred to as *Dementia in Alzheimer's Disease*.

For vascular dementia, the ICD-10 Diagnostic Criteria for Research are more narrowly defined than the DSM-IV-TR criteria in that ICD-10 specifies that the deficits in higher cognitive functions are unevenly distributed and that there be both clinical *and* laboratory evidence of focal brain damage. Furthermore, ICD-10 subspecifies vascular dementia based on acute onset and multi-infarct, subcortical, and mixed cortical and subcortical types.

For amnestic disorder, the ICD-10 Diagnostic Criteria for Research are more narrowly defined than the criteria in DSM-IV-TR by virtue of requiring both an impaired ability to learn new information *and* a reduced ability to recall past experiences, as well as a requirement that immediate recall be preserved. In ICD-10, this disorder is referred to as *Organic Amnestic Syndrome*.

12 Mental Disorders Due to a General Medical Condition

This chapter describes disorders characterized by mental symptoms, which occur due to direct physiological effect of a general medical condition. In evaluating individuals with mental symptoms of any sort, one of the first questions to ask is whether those symptoms are occurring as part of a primary mental disorder or are caused by a general medical condition, and Figure 12-1 presents a decision tree designed to help in making this decision. The first step is to review the history, physical examination, and laboratory tests to see if there is evidence for the presence of a general medical condition that could plausibly cause the mental symptoms in question. In making this determination, one looks not only for a temporal correlation (e.g., the onset of a psychosis shortly after starting or increasing the dose of a medication), but also keeps in mind well-documented associations between certain mental symptoms (e.g., depression) and certain general medical conditions (e.g., Cushing's syndrome). If it appears, at this point, that the mental symptoms could indeed be occurring secondary to a general medical condition, the next step involves determining whether these symptoms could be better accounted for by a primary mental disorder. For example, consider the case of a 45-year-old man with a history of recurrent major depressive disorder, currently euthymic, who begins a course of steroids for asthma and then, within a week, becomes depressed. The steroids are stopped but the depression continues. In this case, if the depression had cleared shortly after stopping the steroids, one might make the case that the depression occurred secondary to the steroid treatment; the persistence of the symptoms, however, argues strongly that this depression represents rather a recurrence of the major depressive disorder.

Once it appears that the mental symptoms in question could directly result from a general medical condition and could not be better accounted for by a primary mental disorder, then it remains to classify these symptoms into one of the specific types noted in Figure 12-1. There is also, at the end of the decision tree, a residual category for "unspecified" mental symptoms.

In caring for individuals with mental disorders due to a general medical condition, the question arises as to whether symptomatic treatment for these mental symptoms should be offered. Figure 12-2 provides a general treatment algorithm designed to help answer this question. First, one must determine whether the mental symptoms demand *emergent* treatment. Consider, for example, a postictal psychosis characterized by delusions of persecution, which prompt the individual to become assaultive: here, even though the condition itself will eventually resolve spontaneously, symptomatic treatment of the psychosis is required to protect the individual or others. In cases in which the mental symptoms do not present an emergency, one looks to whether the underlying general medical condition is treatable or not. For example, in the case of psychosis due to Huntington's disease, as the underlying condition is not treatable, one generally proceeds directly to symptomatic treatment. In cases in which the underlying condition is treatable, one must make a judgment as to whether, with treatment of the underlying general medical condition, the mental symptoms will resolve at a clinically acceptable rate. Consider, for example, an individual with anxiety due to hyperthyroidism who has just begun treatment with an antithyroid drug. In such a case, the decision as to whether to offer a benzodiazepine as symptomatic treatment for the anxiety depends not only on the severity and tolerability of the anxiety but also on the expected time required for the antithyroid drug to resolve the hyperthyroidism: here, clearly, considerable clinical judgment is required.

Clinical Guide to the Diagnosis and Treatment of Mental Disorders. M. B. First and A. Tasman
© 2006 John Wiley & Sons, Ltd.   ISBN 0 470 019158

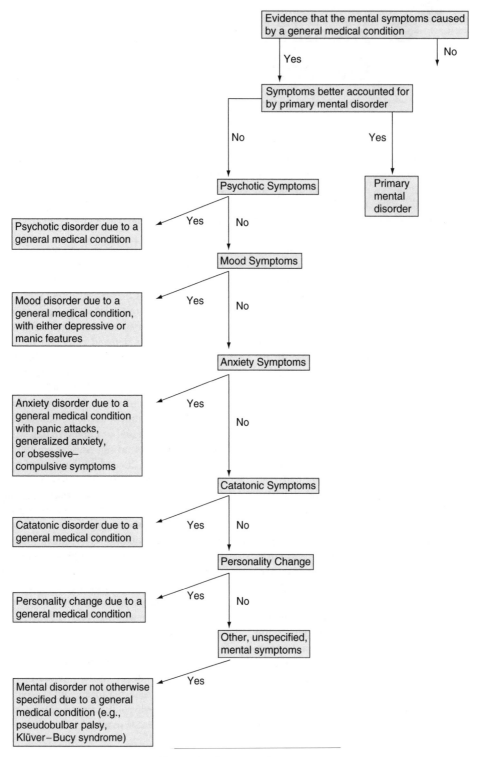

Figure 12-1 *Diagnostic decision tree.*

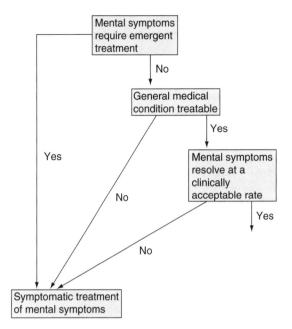

Figure 12-2 *General treatment algorithm.*

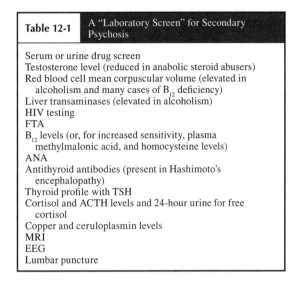

Table 12-1	A "Laboratory Screen" for Secondary Psychosis

Serum or urine drug screen
Testosterone level (reduced in anabolic steroid abusers)
Red blood cell mean corpuscular volume (elevated in
　alcoholism and many cases of B_{12} deficiency)
Liver transaminases (elevated in alcoholism)
HIV testing
FTA
B_{12} levels (or, for increased sensitivity, plasma
　methylmalonic acid, and homocysteine levels)
ANA
Antithyroid antibodies (present in Hashimoto's
　encephalopathy)
Thyroid profile with TSH
Cortisol and ACTH levels and 24-hour urine for free
　cortisol
Copper and ceruloplasmin levels
MRI
EEG
Lumbar puncture

Psychotic Disorder Due to a General Medical Condition

DIAGNOSIS

A psychotic disorder due to a general medical condition is characterized clinically by hallucinations or delusions occurring in a clear sensorium, without any associated decrement in intellectual abilities. Furthermore, one must be able to demonstrate, by history, physical examination, or laboratory findings, that the psychosis is occurring on the basis of a general medical condition.

Psychotic disorder due to a general medical condition is a disorder that by definition occurs in a clear sensorium, without any associated decrement in intellectual abilities; both delirium and dementia are commonly accompanied by hallucinations and delusions, but these conditions are clearly distinguished from psychotic disorder due to a general medical condition by the presence of confusion or significant intellectual deficits. When these features are present, one should proceed to the differential for delirium and dementia described in the preceding chapter of this book.

In most cases, a thorough history and physical examination will disclose evidence of the underlying cause of the psychosis in question. In those cases, however, in which the individual's symptomatology is atypical for one of the primary causes of psychosis (e.g., schizophrenia), yet the history and physical examination fail

to disclose clear evidence for another cause, a "laboratory screen," as listed in Table 12-1, may be appropriate. Clearly, one does not order all these tests at once, but begins with those most likely, given the overall clinical picture, to be the most informative.

Table 12-2 lists the various secondary causes of psychosis, dividing them into those occurring *secondary to precipitants* (e.g., medications), those occurring *secondary to diseases with distinctive features* (e.g., the chorea of Huntington's disease), and finally a group occurring *secondary to miscellaneous causes* (e.g., cerebral tumors).

Psychosis occurring *secondary to precipitants* is perhaps the most common form of secondary psychosis. Among the various possible precipitants, substances are perhaps the most common, but these are covered in the various chapters on specific substances known to cause psychotic symptoms, like stimulants, hallucinogens, phencyclidine, cannabis, and alcohol. After drugs of abuse, various medications are the next most common precipitants, and of the medications listed in Table 12-1, the most problematic are the neuroleptics themselves. It appears that in a very small minority of individuals treated chronically with neuroleptics, a "supersensitivity psychosis" (or, as it has also been called, on analogy with tardive dyskinesia, "tardive psychosis") may occur. Making such a diagnosis in the case of individuals with schizophrenia may be difficult, as one may well say that any increase in psychotic symptoms, rather than evidence for a supersensitivity psychosis, may merely represent an exacerbation of the schizophrenia; in the case of individuals treated with antipsychotics for other conditions (e.g., Tourette's

Table 12-2	Causes of Psychosis due to a General Medical Condition

Secondary to Precipitants
Medications
  Neuroleptics (supersensitivity psychosis)
  Dopaminergic drugs
  Disulfiram
  Sympathomimetics
  Bupropion
  Fluoxetine
  Baclofen (upon discontinuation)
Other precipitants
  Postencephalitic psychosis
  Posthead trauma

Secondary to Diseases with Distinctive Features
Associated with epilepsy
  Ictal psychosis
  Postictal psychosis
  Psychosis of forced normalization
  Chronic interictal psychosis
Encephalitic onset
  Herpes simplex encephalitis
  Encephalitis lethargica
  Infectious mononucleosis
With other specific features:
  Huntington's disease (chorea)
  Sydenham's chorea
  Chorea gravidarum
  Manganism (parkinsonism)
  Creutzfeldt–Jakob disease (myoclonus)
  Hashimoto's encephalopathy (myoclonus)
  Wilson's disease (various abnormal involuntary movements)
  AIDS (thrush, *Pneumocystis* pneumonia)
  Systemic lupus erythematosus (arthralgia, rash, pericarditis, pleurisy)
  Hyperthyroidism (tremor, tachycardia)
  Hypothyroidism (cold intolerance, voice change, constipation, hair loss, myxedema)
  Cushing's syndrome ("Cushingoid" habitus, e.g., "moon" facies)
  Adrenocortical insufficiency (abdominal complaints and dizziness)
  Hepatic porphyria (abdominal pain)
  Autosomal dominant cerebellar ataxia
  Dentatorubropallidoluysian atrophy (ataxia)
  Prader–Willi syndrome (massive obesity)

Secondary to Miscellaneous Causes
Cerebral tumors
Cerebral infarction
Multiple sclerosis
Neurosyphilis
Vitamin B$_{12}$ deficiency
Metachromatic leukodystrophy
Subacute sclerosing panencephalitis
Fahr's syndrome
Thalamic degeneration
Velo-cardio-facial syndrome

ing dopamine agonists as bromocriptine and lergotrile. The other medications noted in Table 12-1 very rarely cause a psychosis.

Of the psychoses *secondary to diseases with distinctive features*, the psychoses of epilepsy are by far the most important, and these may be ictal, postictal, or interictal. Ictal psychoses represent complex partial seizures and are immediately suggested by their exquisitely paroxysmal onset. Postictal psychoses are typically preceded by a "flurry" of grand mal or complex partial seizures and, importantly, are separated from the last of this "flurry" of seizures by a "lucid" interval lasting from hours to days. Interictal psychoses appear in one of two forms, namely, the psychosis of forced normalization and the chronic interictal psychosis. The psychosis of forced normalization appears when anticonvulsants have not only stopped seizures but also have essentially "normalized" the EEG; a disappearance of the psychosis with the resumption of seizure activity secures the diagnosis. The chronic interictal psychosis, often characterized by delusions of persecution and of reference and auditory hallucinations, appears subacutely, over weeks or months, in individuals with long-standing, uncontrolled grand mal or complex partial seizures.

Encephalitic psychoses are suggested by typical "encephalitic" features such as headache, lethargy, and fever. Prompt diagnosis is critical, especially in the case of herpes simplex encephalitis, given its treatability.

Of the *miscellaneous causes* capable of causing psychosis, cerebral tumors are perhaps the most important, with psychosis being noted with tumors of the frontal lobe, *corpus callosum*, and temporal lobe. Suggestive clinical evidence for such a cause includes prominent headache, seizures, or certain focal signs, such as aphasia. Cerebral infarction is likewise an important cause, and is suggested not only by accompanying focal signs but also by its acute onset; infarction of the frontal lobe, temporoparietal area, and thalamus have all been implicated. Neurosyphilis should never be forgotten as a differential possibility in cases of psychosis of obscure origin, and a Fluorescent Treponemal Antibody (FTA) is appropriate in such cases. Vitamin B$_{12}$ deficiency, likewise, should be borne in mind, especially as this may present with psychosis without any evidence of spinal cord or hematologic involvement. The remaining disorders listed in Table 12-2 are extremely rare causes of psychosis, and represent the "zebras" of this differential listing. Among these "zebras," however, one is of particular interest, namely, velo-cardio-facial syndrome. This genetic disorder, characterized by cleft palate, cardiovascular malformations, and dysmorphic

syndrome), however, the appearance of a psychosis is far more suggestive, as it could not be accounted for on the basis of the disease for which the neuroleptic was prescribed. Dopaminergic drugs capable of causing a psychosis include levodopa itself and such direct-act-

facies (micrognathia and prominent nose), and, often, mental retardation, also appears, in a substantial minority of cases, to cause a psychosis phenotypically very similar to that caused by schizophrenia.

TREATMENT

Treatment, if possible, is directed at the underlying cause. In those cases in which such treatment is unavailable or ineffective, or in which control of the psychosis is emergently required, neuroleptics are indicated. Although conventional neuroleptics, such as haloperidol, have long been used successfully, newer atypical agents, such as olanzapine or risperidone, may be better tolerated. In general, it is best to start with a low dose (e.g., 2.5 mg of haloperidol, 5 mg olanzapine or 1 mg of risperidone) with gradual incremental increases, if necessary.

Mood Disorder Due to a General Medical Condition with Depressive Features

DIAGNOSIS

A mood disorder secondary to a general medical condition with depressive features is characterized by a prominent and persistent depressed mood or loss of interest, and by the presence of evidence, from the history, physical examination or laboratory tests, of a general medical condition capable of causing such a disturbance. Although other depressive symptoms (e.g., lack of energy, sleep disturbance, appetite change, or psychomotor change) may be present, they are not necessary for the diagnosis.

The various secondary causes of depression are listed in Table 12-3. In utilizing Table 12-3, the first question to ask is whether the depression could be *secondary to precipitants*. Of the various possible precipitants, substances of abuse (e.g., as seen in alcoholism or during stimulant withdrawal) are very common causes, and these are discussed in their respective chapters. Medications are particularly important; however, it must be borne in mind that most individuals are able to take the medications listed in Table 12-3 without untoward effect. Consequently, before ascribing a depression to any medication, it is critical to demonstrate that the depression did not begin before the medication was begun, and, ideally, to demonstrate that the depression resolved after the medication was discontinued. Anticholinergic withdrawal may occur within days after abrupt discontinuation of highly anticholinergic medications, such

Table 12-3	Causes of Depression due to a General Medical Condition

Secondary to Precipitants
Medications
  Propranolol
  Interferon
  ACTH
  Prednisone
  Reserpine
  Alpha-methyldopa
  Nifedipine
  Ranitidine
  Bismuth subsalicylate
  Pimozide
  Subdermal estrogen/progestin
Anticholinergic withdrawal ("cholinergic rebound")
Poststroke depression
Head trauma
Whiplash

Secondary to Diseases with Distinctive Features
Hypothyroidism (hair loss, dry skin, voice change)
Hyperthyroidism (weight loss with *increased* appetite, tachycardia, and, in the elderly, atrial fibrillation or congestive heart failure)
Cushing's syndrome (moon facies, hirsutism, acne, "buffalo hump", and abdominal striae)
Chronic adrenocortical insufficiency (nausea, vomiting, abdominal pain, and postural dizziness)
Obstructive sleep apnea (severe snoring)
Multiple sclerosis (various focal findings)
Down syndrome
Epilepsy
  Ictal depression
  Chronic interictal depression

Occurring as Part of Certain Neurodegenerative or Dementing Disorders
Alzheimer's disease
Multi-infarct dementia
Diffuse Lewy body disease
Parkinson's disease
Fahr's syndrome
Tertiary neurosyphilis
Limbic encephalitis

Miscellaneous or Rare Causes
Cerebral tumors
Hydrocephalus
Pancreatic cancer
New-variant Creutzfeldt–Jakob disease
Hyperparathyroidism
Systemic lupus erythematosus
Pernicious anemia
Pellagra
Lead encephalopathy
Hyperaldosteronism

as benzotropine or certain tricyclic antidepressants, and is characterized by depressed mood, malaise, insomnia and gastrointestinal symptoms such as nausea, vomiting, abdominal cramping, and diarrhea. Poststroke depression is not uncommon, and may be more likely when the anterior portion of the left frontal lobe is involved; although spontaneous remission within a year is the rule, depressive symptoms, in the meantime, may be quite severe. Both head trauma and whiplash injuries may be followed by depressive symptoms in close to half of all the cases.

Depression may occur *secondary to diseases with distinctive features*, and keeping such features in mind whenever evaluating depressed individuals will lead to a gratifying number of diagnostic "pick-ups." These features are noted in Table 12-3, and are for the most part self-explanatory; depression associated with epilepsy, however, may merit some further discussion. Ictal depressions are, in fact, simple partial seizures whose symptomatology is for the most part restricted to affective changes. The diagnosis of ictal depression is suggested by the paroxysmal onset of depression (literally over seconds); although such simple partial seizures may last only minutes, longer durations, up to months, have also been reported. Interictal depressions, rather than occurring secondary to paroxysmal electrical activity within the brain, occur as a result of long-lasting changes in neuronal activity, perhaps related to "kindling" within the limbic system, in individuals with chronically recurrent seizures, either grand mal or, more especially, complex partial. Such interictal depressions are of gradual onset and are chronic.

Depression *occurring as part of certain neurodegenerative or dementing disorders* is immediately suggested by the presence of other symptoms of these disorders, such as dementia or distinctive physical findings, for example, parkinsonism.

The *miscellaneous or rare causes* represent, for the most part, the "zebras" in the differential for depression, and should be considered when, despite a thorough investigation, the diagnosis of a particular case of depression remains unclear.

Course

Most medication-induced depressions begin to clear within days of discontinuation of the offending medication; depression as part of withdrawal from stimulants or anabolic steroids clears within days or weeks, and from anticholinergics, within days. Poststroke depression, as noted above, typically remits within a year. The course of depression secondary to head trauma or whiplash is generally prolonged, though quite variable. Most of the other conditions or disorders in the list are chronic, and depression occurring secondary to them likewise tends to be chronic; exceptions include depression in multiple sclerosis, which may have a relapsing and remitting course, corresponding to the appearance and disappearance of appropriately situated plaques.

TREATMENT

Treatment efforts should be directed at relieving, if possible, the underlying cause. When this is not possible, antidepressants should be considered. Controlled studies have demonstrated the effectiveness of both nortriptyline and citalopram for poststroke depression, and nortriptyline for depression seen in Parkinson's disease. For other secondary depressions, citalopram (or escitalopram) is probably a good choice, given its benign side-effect profile and notable lack of drug–drug interactions; nortriptyline should be used with caution in individuals with cardiac conduction defects (as it may prolong conduction time) and in those at risk for seizures as in head trauma as this agent may also lower the seizure threshold.

Mood Disorder Due to a General Medical Condition with Manic Features

DIAGNOSIS

Mood disorder due to a general medical condition with manic features is characterized by a prominent and persistently elevated, expansive, or irritable mood which, on the basis of the history, physical, or laboratory examinations, can be attributed to an underlying general medical condition. Other manic symptoms, such as increased energy, decreased need for sleep, hyperactivity, distractibility, pressured speech, and flight of ideas, may or may not be present.

As a rule, it is very rare for mania to constitute the initial presentation of any of the diseases or disorders listed in Table 12-4; thus, other evidence of their presence will become evident during the routine history and physical examination. Exceptions to the rule include neurosyphilis, vitamin B_{12} deficiency, and Creutzfeldt–Jakob disease; however, in all these cases continued observation will eventually disclose the appearance of other evidence suggestive of the correct diagnosis.

Table 12-4 lists secondary causes of elevated or irritable mood, with these causes divided into categories designed to facilitate the task of differential diagnosis. In utilizing Table 12-4, the first step is to determine whether the mania could be *secondary to precipitants*. Substance-induced mood disorder related to drugs of abuse is covered in the relevant substance-related disorders chapters in this textbook. Of the precipitating factors listed in Table 12-4, medications are the most common offenders. However, before attributing the mania to one of these medications,

Table 12-4	Causes of Mania due to a General Medical Condition

Secondary to Precipitants
Medications
  Corticosteroids or adrenocorticoptrophic hormone
  Levodopa
  Zidovudine
  Oral contraceptives
  Isoniazid
  Buspirone
  Procyclidine
  Procarbazine
  Propafenone
  Baclofen, upon discontinuation after long-term use
  Reserpine, upon discontinuation after long-term use
  Methyldopa, upon discontinuation after long-term use
Closed head injury
Hemodialysis
Encephalitis
Aspartame
Metrizamide

Secondary to Diseases with Distinctive Features
Hyperthyroidism (proptosis, tremor, tachycardia)
Cushing's syndrome (moon facies, hirsutism, acne, "buffalo hump", abdominal striae)
Multiple sclerosis (various focal findings)
Cerebral infarction (sudden onset with associated localizing signs)
Sydenham's chorea
Chorea gravidarum
Hepatic encephalopathy (asterixis, delirium)
Uremia (asterixis, delirium)
Epilepsy
  Ictal mania
  Postictal mania

Occurring as part of Certain Neurodegenerative or Dementing Diseases
Alzheimer's disease
Neurosyphilis
Huntington's disease
Creutzfeldt–Jakob disease

Miscellaneous or Rare Causes
Cerebral tumors
Systemic lupus erythematosus
Vitamin B_{12} deficiency
Metachromatic leukodystrophy
Adrenoleukodystrophy
Tuberous sclerosis

nia, and such a syndrome occurring in "bulked up" individuals should prompt a search for other clinical evidence of abuse, such as gynecomastia and testicular atrophy. Closed head injury may be followed by mania either directly upon emergence from postcoma delirium, or after an interval of months. Hemodialysis may cause mania, and in one case, mania occurred as the presenting sign of an eventual dialysis dementia. Encephalitis may cause mania, as, for example, in postinfectious encephalomyelitis, with the correct diagnosis eventually being suggested by more typical signs such as delirium or seizures. Encephalitis lethargica (Von Economo's disease; European sleeping sickness) may also be at fault, with the diagnosis suggested by classic signs such as sleep reversal or oculomotor paralyses. Aspartame taken in very high dose caused mania and a seizure in one individual, and metrizamide myelography prompted mania in another. Mania occurring *secondary to disease with distinctive features* is immediately suggested by these features, as listed in Table 12-4. Some elaboration may be in order regarding mania secondary to cerebral infarction. This cause, of course, is suggested by the sudden onset of the clinical disturbance, with the mania being accompanied by various other more or less localizing signs; what is most remarkable here is the variety of structures that, if infarcted, may be followed by mania. Thus, mania has been noted with infarction of the midbrain, thalamus (either on the right side or bilaterally), anterior limb of the internal capsule and adjacent caudate on the right, and subcortical white matter or cortical infarction on the right in the frontoparietal, or temporal areas. Mania associated with epilepsy may also deserve additional comment. Ictal mania is characterized by its paroxysmal onset, over seconds, and the diagnosis of postictal mania is suggested when mania occurs shortly after a "flurry" of grand mal or complex partial seizures.

Mania *occurring as part of certain neurodegenerative or dementing diseases* is suggested, in general, by a concurrent dementia, and in most cases the mania plays only a minor role in the overall clinical pictures. Neurosyphilis, however, is an exception to this rule, for in individuals with general paresis of the insane (dementia paralytica) mania may dominate the picture.

Of the *miscellaneous or rare causes* of mania, cerebral tumors are the most important to keep in mind, with mania being noted with tumors of the midbrain, tumors compressing the hypothalamus (e.g., a craniopharyngioma), or a pituitary adenoma, and tumors of the right thalamus, right cingulate gyrus, or one or both frontal lobes.

it is critical to demonstrate that the mania occurred only after initiation of that medication; ideally, one would also want to show that the mania spontaneously resolved subsequent to the medication's discontinuation. Of the medications listed, corticosteroids, such as prednisone, are most likely to cause mania, with the likelihood increasing in direct proportion to dose: in one study, 80 mg of prednisone produced mania within five days in 75% of subjects. Levodopa is the next most likely cause, and in the case of levodopa the induced mania may be so pleasurable that some individuals have ended up abusing the drug. Anabolic steroid abuse may cause an irritable ma-

Course

Most cases of medication-induced mania begin to clear in a matter of days; for other causes, the course of the mania generally reflects the course of the underlying disease.

TREATMENT

Treatment, if possible, is directed at the underlying cause. In cases where such etiologic treatment is not possible, or not rapidly effective enough, pharmacologic measures are in order. Mood stabilizers, such as lithium or divalproex used in a fashion similar to that for the treatment of mania occurring in bipolar disorder, are commonly used: both lithium and divalproex are effective in the prophylaxis of mania occurring secondary to prednisone; case reports also support the use of lithium for mania secondary to zidovudine and divalproex for mania secondary to closed head injury. In choosing between lithium and divalproex, in cases where there is a risk for seizures (e.g., head injury, encephalitis, stroke, or tumors), divalproex clearly is preferable.

In cases where emergent treatment is required, before lithium or divalproex could have a chance to become effective, oral or intramuscular lorazepam or haloperidol (in doses of 2 mg and 5 mg, respectively) may be utilized, again much as in the treatment of mania in bipolar disorder.

Anxiety Disorder Due to a General Medical Condition with Panic Attacks or with Generalized Anxiety

DIAGNOSIS

Pathologic anxiety secondary to a general medical condition may occur in the form of well-circumscribed and transient panic attacks or in a generalized, more chronic form. As the differential diagnoses for these two forms of anxiety are quite different, it is critical to clearly distinguish among them.

Panic attacks have an acute or paroxysmal onset, and are characterized by typically intense anxiety or fear which is accompanied by various "autonomic" signs and symptoms, such as tremor, diaphoresis, and palpitations. Symptoms rapidly crescendo over seconds or minutes and in most cases the attack will clear anywhere from within minutes up to a half-hour. Although attacks tend to be similar to one another in the same individual, there is substantial inter-individual variability in the symptoms seen.

Table 12-5	Causes of Panic Attacks due to a General Medical Condition

Partial seizures
Paroxysmal atrial tachycardia
Hypoglycemia
Angina or acute myocardial infarction
Pulmonary embolus
Acute asthmatic attack
Pheochromocytoma
Parkinson's disease

Generalized anxiety tends to be of subacute or gradual onset, and may last for long periods of time, anywhere from days to months, depending on the underlying cause. Here, some individuals, rather than complaining of feeling anxious *per se*, may complain of being worried, tense, or ill at ease. Autonomic symptoms tend not to be as severe or prominent as those seen in panic attacks: shakiness, palpitations (or tachycardia), and diaphoresis are perhaps most common.

The causes of secondary panic attacks are listed in Table 12-5. Substance-induced anxiety disorder related to drugs of abuse (e.g., cannabis, LSD) is covered in the relevant substance-related disorders chapters in this textbook. Partial seizures and paraoxysmal atrial tachycardia are both characterized by their exquisitely paroxysmal onset, over a second or two; in addition, paroxysmal atrial tachycardia is distinguished by the prominence of the tachycardia and by an ability, in many cases, to terminate the attack with a Valsalva maneuver. Hypoglycemia is often suspected as a cause of anxiety, but before the diagnosis is accepted, one must demonstrate the presence of "Whipple's triad": hypoglycemia (blood glucose ≤ 45 mg/dL), typical symptoms, and the relief of those symptoms with glucose. Angina or acute myocardial infarction can present with a panic attack, with the diagnosis being suggested by the clinical setting, for example, multiple cardiac risk factors. A pulmonary embolus, at the moment of its lodgment in a pulmonary artery, may also present with a panic attack, and again here the correct diagnosis is suggested by the clinical setting, for example, situations, such as prolonged immobilization, which favor deep venous thrombosis. Acute asthmatic attacks are suggested by wheezing, and pheochromocytoma by associated hypertension. Individuals with Parkinson's disease treated with levodopa may experience panic attacks during "off" periods.

The secondary causes of generalized anxiety are listed in Table 12-6. Sympathomimetics and theophylline, as used in asthma and chronic obstructive pulmonary disease (COPD) are frequent causes, as are many of the antidepressants. Hyperthyroidism is suggested by heat intolerance and proptosis, and Cushing's

Table 12-6	Causes of Generalized Anxiety due to a General Medical Condition

Sympathomimetics
Theophylline
Various antidepressants (tricyclics, SSRIs, etc.)
Hyperthyroidism
Cushing's syndrome
Hypocalcemia
Chronic obstructive pulmonary disease
Congestive heart failure
Poststroke
Post-head trauma

Table 12-7	Causes of Obsessions and Compulsions due to a General Medical Condition

Postencephalitic
Postanoxic
Post-closed head injury
Clozapine
Sydenham's chorea
Huntington's disease
Simple partial seizures
Infarction of the basal ganglia or right parietal lobe
Fahr's syndrome

syndrome by the typical Cushingoid habitus (i.e., moon facies, hirsutism, acne, "buffalo hump," and abdominal striae). Hypocalcemia may be suggested by a history of seizures or tetany. Both COPD and congestive heart failure are suggested by marked dyspnea. Stroke and severe head trauma may be followed by chronic anxiety, but this is seen in only a minority of these individuals.

TREATMENT

Treatment is directed at the underlying cause, and this is sufficient for all cases of secondary panic attacks and most cases of secondary generalized anxiety; exceptions include poststroke and post-head trauma anxiety, and in these cases benzodiazepines have been used with success.

Anxiety Disorder Due to a General Medical Condition with Obsessive–Compulsive Symptoms

DIAGNOSIS

Obsessions consist of unwanted, and generally anxiety-provoking, thoughts, images or ideas, which repeatedly come to mind despite attempts to stop them. Allied to this are compulsions that consist of anxious urges to do or undo things, urges which, if resisted, are followed by rapidly increasing anxiety that can often only be relieved by giving into the compulsion to act. The acts themselves that the individuals feel compelled to perform are often linked to an apprehension on the individuals' part that they have done something that they ought not to have done or have left undone something that they ought to have done. Thus, one may feel compelled to repeatedly subject the hands to washing to be sure that all germs have been removed, or to repeatedly go back and check on the gas to be sure that it has been turned off.

Secondary obsessions and compulsions are relatively rare.

In the vast majority of cases, obsessions and compulsions occur as part of certain primary mental disorders, including obsessive–compulsive disorder, depression, schizophrenia, and Tourette's syndrome. Those rare instances where obsessions and compulsions are secondary to a general medical condition or medication are listed in Table 12-7.

In most cases, these causes of secondary obsessions or compulsions are readily discerned, as for example, a history of encephalitis, anoxia, closed head injury, or treatment with clozapine. Sydenham's chorea is immediately suggested by the appearance of chorea; however, it must be borne in mind that obsessions and compulsions may constitute the presentation of Sydenham's chorea, with the appearance of chorea being delayed for days. Ictal obsessions or compulsions, constituting the sole clinical manifestation of a simple partial seizure, may, in themselves, be indistinguishable from the obsessions and compulsions seen in obsessive–compulsive disorder, but are suggested by a history of other seizure types, for example, complex partial or grand mal seizures. Infarction of the basal ganglia or parietal lobe is suggested by the subacute onset of obsessions or compulsions accompanied by "neighborhood" symptoms such as abnormal movements or unilateral sensory changes. Fahr's syndrome, unlike the foregoing, may be an elusive diagnosis, only suggested perhaps when CT imaging incidentally reveals calcification of the basal ganglia.

Course

Although the course of obsessions and compulsions due to fixed lesions, such as those seen with head trauma or cerebral infarction, tends to be chronic, some spontaneous recovery may be anticipated over the following months to a year.

TREATMENT

When treatment of the underlying cause is not possible, a trial of an SSRI, as used for obsessive–compulsive disorder, might be appropriate.

Catatonic Disorder Due to a General Medical Condition

DIAGNOSIS

Catatonia can develop as a result of the direct effects of a general medical condition on the central nervous system. Catatonia exists in two subtypes, namely, stuporous catatonia (also known as the akinetic or "retarded" subtype) and excited catatonia, and each will be described in turn.

Stuporous catatonia is characterized by varying combinations of mutism, immobility, and waxy flexibility; associated features include posturing, negativism, automatic obedience, and "echo" phenomena. Mutism ranges from complete to partial: some individuals may mumble or perhaps utter brief, often incomprehensible, phrases. Immobility, likewise, ranges in severity: some individuals may lie in bed for long periods, neither moving, blinking or even swallowing; others may make brief movements, perhaps to pull at a piece of clothing or to assume a different posture. Waxy flexibility, also known by its Latin name *cerea flexibilitas*, is characterized by a more or less severe "lead pipe" rigidity combined with a remarkable tendency for the limbs to stay in whatever position they are placed, regardless of whether the individual is asked to maintain that position or not. Posturing is said to occur when individuals spontaneously assume more or less bizarre postures, which are then maintained: one individual crouched low with his arm wrapped over his head, another stood with one arm raised high and the other stuffed inside his belt. Negativism entails a mulish, intractable, and automatic resistance to whatever is expected, and may be either "passive" or "active." Passively negativistic individuals simply fail to do what is asked or expected: if clothes are laid out they will not dress; if asked to eat or take pills, their lips remain frozen shut. Active negativism manifests in doing the opposite of what is expected: if asked to come into the office, the individual may back into the hallway or if asked to open the eyes wide to allow for easier examination, they may cramp the eyes closed. Automatic obedience, as may be suspected, represents the opposite of negativism, with affected individuals doing exactly what they are told, even if this places them in danger. Echo phenomena represent a kind of automatic obedience: in echolalia individuals simply repeat what they hear and in echopraxia they mimic the gestures and activity of the examiner. It should be noted that in negativism, automatic obedience, and echo phenomena there is nothing natural or fluid about the individual's behavior. To the contrary, movements are often awkward, wooden, and tinged with the bizarre.

Excited catatonia manifests with varying degrees of bizarre, frenzied, and purposeless behavior. Such individuals typically keep to themselves: one marched in place, all the while chanting and gesticulating; another tore at his hair and clothing, broke plates in a corner then crawled under the bed where he muttered and thrashed his arms.

Stuporous catatonia occurring in association with epilepsy is often suggested by a history of grand mal or complex partial seizures. Ictal catatonia is further suggested by its exquisitely paroxysmal onset, and postictal catatonia by an immediately preceding "flurry" of grand mal or complex partial seizures. Psychosis of forced normalization is an interictal condition distinguished by the appearance of symptoms subsequent to effective control of seizures. The chronic interictal psychosis is also, as suggested by the name, an interictal condition, which however, appears not after seizures are controlled but rather in the setting of ongoing, chronic uncontrolled epilepsy. Of medications capable of causing catatonia, neuroleptics are by far the most common. Viral encephalitis is suggested by concurrent fever and headache: herpes simplex encephalitis should always be considered in such cases, given its treatability; further, it must be kept in mind that although encephalitis lethargica no longer occurs in epidemics, sporadic cases still do occur. Focal lesions capable of causing catatonia are typically found in the medial or inferior portions of the frontal lobes. The miscellaneous conditions listed are all quite rare causes of catatonia.

DSM-IV-TR Diagnostic Criteria

293.89 CATATONIC DISORDER DUE TO ... [INDICATE THE GENERAL MEDICAL CONDITION]

A. The presence of catatonia as manifested by motoric immobility, excessive motor activity (that is apparently purposeless and not influenced by external stimuli), extreme negativism or mutism, peculiarities of voluntary movement, or echolalia or echopraxia.
B. There is evidence from the history, physical examination, or laboratory findings that the disturbance is the direct physiological consequence of a general medical condition.
C. The disturbance is not better accounted for by another mental disorder (e.g., a Manic Episode).
D. The disturbance does not occur exclusively during the course of a delirium.

Coding note: Include the name of the general medical condition on Axis I. e.g., 293.89 Catatonic Disorder Due to Hepatic Encephalopathy: also code the general medical condition on Axis III (see Appendix G for codes).

Reprinted with permission from the *Diagnostic and Statistical Manual of Mental Disorders*, 4th ed., Text Rev. Copyright 2000 American Psychiatric Association.

Excited catatonia, in the vast majority of cases, is caused by either schizophrenia or bipolar disorder (during a manic episode); only rarely is it seen because of a general medical condition, as for example, a viral encephalitis.

Differential Diagnosis

Stuporous catatonia must be distinguished from akinetic mutism and from stupor of other causes. Akinetic mutes appear quite similar to immobile and mute catatonics; they, however, lack such signs as waxy flexibility, posturing, and negativism, all of which are typically seen in catatonia. Stupor of other causes is readily distinguished from catatonic stupor by the salient fact that catatonics remain alert, in stark contrast with the somnolence or decreased level of consciousness seen in all other forms of stupor.

Excited catatonia must be distinguished from mania. Mania is typified by hyperactivity, which at times may be quite frenzied: the difference with catatonia is that individuals with mania want to be involved, whereas those with catatonia keep to themselves.

Stuporous catatonia, in the majority of cases, occurs as part of such primary mental disorders as schizophrenia or a depressive episode of either major depressive or bipolar disorder. The causes of catatonia due to a general medical condition or medications are listed in Table 12-8.

Table 12-8	Causes of Catatonia Due to a General Medical Condition

Stuporous Catatonia
Associated with epilepsy
  Ictal catatonia
  Postictal catatonia
  Psychosis of forced normalization
  Chronic interictal psychosis
Medication
  Neuroleptics
  Disulfiram
  Benzodiazepine withdrawal
Viral encephalitis
  Herpes simplex encephalitis
  Encephalitis lethargica
Focal lesions, especially of the frontal lobes
Miscellaneous conditions
  Hepatic encephalopathy
  Limbic encephalitis
  Systemic lupus erythematosus
  Lyme disease, in stage III
  Subacute sclerosing panencephalitis, in stage I
  Tay–Sachs disease
  Thrombotic thrombocytopenic purpura

Excited Catatonia
Viral encephalitis

TREATMENT

In addition to treating, if possible, the underlying cause, catatonia may be symptomatically relieved by lorazepam given parenterally in a dose of 2 mg; in severe cases wherein lorazepam is not sufficiently effective and the individual is at immediate risk, consideration should be given to emergency ECT, which is typically dramatically effective, generally bringing relief after but a few treatments.

Personality Change Due to a General Medical Condition

DIAGNOSIS

The personality of an adult represents a coalescence of various personality traits present in childhood and adolescence, and is generally quite enduring and resistant to change. Thus, the appearance of a significant change in an adult's personality is an ominous clinical sign and indicates the presence of intracranial pathology. Individuals themselves may not be aware of the change. However, to others, who have known the individual over time, the change is often quite obvious. Such observers often note that the individual is "not himself" anymore.

In most cases, the change is nonspecific in nature: there may be either a gross exaggeration of hitherto minor aspects of the individual's personality or the appearance of a personality trait quite uncharacteristic for the individual. Traits commonly seen in a personality change, as noted in DSM-IV-TR, include lability, disinhibition, aggressiveness, apathy, or suspiciousness (see DSM-IV-TR diagnostic criteria, page 120).

In addition to these nonspecific changes, there are two specific syndromes which, though not listed in DSM-IV-TR, are well described in the literature, namely, the *frontal lobe syndrome* and the *interictal personality syndrome* (also known as the "Geschwind syndrome").

The *frontal lobe syndrome* is characterized by a variable mixture of disinhibition, affective changes, perseveration, and abulia. Disinhibition manifests with an overall coarsening of behavior. Attention to manners and social nuances is lost: individuals may eat with gluttony, make coarse and crude jokes, and may engage in unwelcome and inappropriate sexual behavior, perhaps by propositioning much younger individuals or masturbating in public. Affective changes tend toward a silly, noninfectious euphoria; depression, however, may also be seen. Perseveration presents with a tendency to persist in whatever task is currently at hand,

DSM-IV-TR Diagnostic Criteria

310.1 PERSONALITY CHANGE DUE TO ... [INDICATE THE GENERAL MEDICAL CONDITION]

A. A persistent personality disturbance that represents a change from the individual's previous characteristic personality pattern. (In children, the disturbance involves a marked deviation from normal development or a significant change in the child's usual behavior patterns lasting at least 1 year).
B. There is evidence from the history, physical examination, or laboratory findings that the disturbance is the direct physiological consequence of a general medical condition.
C. The disturbance is not better accounted for by another mental disorder (including other Mental Disorders Due to a General Medical Condition).
D. The disturbance does not occur exclusively during the course of a delirium.
E. The disturbance causes clinically significant distress or impairment in social, occupational, or other important areas of functioning.

Specify type:

Labile Type: if the predominant feature is affective lability
Disinhibited Type: if the predominant feature is poor impulse control as evidenced by sexual indiscretions, etc.
Aggressive Type: if the predominant feature is aggressive behavior
Apathetic Type: if the predominant feature is marked apathy and indifference
Paranoid Type: if the predominant feature is suspiciousness or paranoid ideation
Other Type: if the predominant feature is not one of the above, e.g., personality change associated with a seizure disorder
Combined Type: if more than one feature predominates in the clinical picture

Unspecified Type
Coding note: Include the name of the general medical condition on Axis I, e.g., 310.1 Personality Change Due to Temporal Lobe Epilepsy: also code the general medical condition on Axis III (see Appendix G for codes).

Reprinted with permission from the *Diagnostic and Statistical Manual of Mental Disorders*, 4th ed., Text Rev. Copyright 2000 American Psychiatric Association.

and individuals may repeatedly button and unbutton clothing, open and close a drawer or ask the same question again and again. Abulia is characterized by an absence of desires, urges, or interests, and such individuals, being undisturbed by such phenomena, may be content to sit placidly for indefinite periods of time. Importantly, such abulic individuals are not depressed, nor are they incapable of activity. Indeed, with active supervision they may be able to complete tasks; however, once supervision stops, so too do the individuals, as they lapse back into quietude.

The *interictal personality syndrome*, a controversial entity, is said to occur as a complication of long-standing uncontrolled epilepsy, with repeated grand mal or complex partial seizures. The cardinal characteristic of this syndrome is what is known as "viscosity," or, somewhat more colloquially, "stickiness." Here, individuals seem unable to let go or diverge from the current emotion or train of thought: existing effects persist long after the situation that occasioned them, and a given train of thought tends to extend itself indefinitely into a long-winded and verbose circumstantiality or tangentiality. This viscosity of thought may also appear in written expression as individuals display "hypergraphia," producing long and rambling letters or diaries. The inability to "let go" may even extend to such simple acts as shaking hands, such that others may literally have to extract their hand to end the handshake. The content of the individual's viscous speech and writing generally also changes, and tends toward mystical or abstruse philosophical speculations. Finally, there is also a tendency to hyposexuality, with an overall decrease in libido.

Personality change is common, and is especially frequent after closed head injury and as a prodrome to the dementia occurring with such neurodegenerative disorders as Pick's disease, fronto-temporal dementia, and Alzheimer's disease.

Personality change of the nonspecific or of the frontal lobe type, as noted in Table 12-9, may occur *secondary to precipitants* (e.g., closed head injury), *secondary to cerebral tumors* (especially those of the frontal or temporal lobes) or *as part of certain neurodegenerative or dementing disorders*. Finally, there is a group of *miscellaneous causes*. In Table 12-9, those disorders or diseases that are particularly prone to cause a personality change of the frontal lobe type are indicated by an asterisk. The interictal personality syndrome occurs only in the setting of chronic repeated grand mal or complex partial seizures, and may represent microanatomic changes in the limbic system which have been "kindled" by the repeated seizures.

In the case of personality change occurring *secondary to precipitants*, the etiology is fairly obvious; an exception might be cerebral infarction, but here the acute onset and the presence of "neighborhood" symptoms are suggestive. In addition to infarction of the frontal lobe, personality change has also been noted with infarction of the caudate nucleus.

Personality change occurring s*econdary to cerebral tumors* may not be accompanied by any distinctive features, and indeed a personality change may be the only clinical evidence of a tumor for a prolonged period of time.

Personality change *occurring as part of certain neurodegenerative or dementing disorders*

Table 12-9	Causes of Personality Change of the Nonspecific or Frontal Lobe Type

Secondary to Precipitants
Closed head injury
Head trauma with subdural hematoma
Postviral encephalitis
Gunshot wounds
Cerebral infarction

Secondary to Cerebral Tumors
Frontal lobe*
Corpus callosum* (in its anterior part)
Temporal lobe

Occurring as Part of Certain Neurodegenerative or Dementing Disorders
Pick's disease*
Fronto-temporal dementia*
Alzheimer's disease*
Amyotrophic lateral sclerosis*
Progressive supranuclear palsy*
Cortico-basal ganglionic degeneration*
Multiple system atrophy*
Huntington's disease
Wilson's disease
Lacunar syndrome*
Normal pressure hydrocephalus
AIDS
Neurosyphilis
Creutzfeldt–Jakob disease

Miscellaneous Causes
Granulomatous angiitis
Vitamin B_{12} deficiency
Limbic encephalitis
Metachromatic leukodystrophy
Adrenoleukodystrophy
Mercury intoxication
Manganism

*Particularly likely to cause a frontal lobe syndrome.

deserves special mention, for in many instances the underlying disorder may present with a personality change—this is particularly the case with Pick's disease, fronto-temporal dementia, and Alzheimer's disease. The inclusion of amyotrophic lateral sclerosis here may be surprising to some, but it is very clear that, albeit in a small minority, cerebral symptoms may not only dominate the early course of amyotrophic lateral sclerosis (ALS) but may also constitute the presentation of the disease. In the case of the other neurodegenerative disorders (i.e., progressive supranuclear palsy, cortico-basal ganglionic degeneration, multiple system atrophy, Huntington's disease, and Wilson's disease), a personality change, if present, is typically accompanied by abnormal involuntary movements of one sort or other, such as parkinsonism, ataxia, or chorea. The lacunar syndrome, occurring secondary to multiple lacunar infarctions affecting the thalamus, internal capsule, or basal ganglia, deserves special mention as it very commonly causes a personality change of the frontal lobe type by interrupting the connections be-

tween the thalamus or basal ganglia and the frontal lobe. Normal-pressure hydrocephalus is an important diagnosis to keep in mind, as the condition is treatable. Other suggestive symptoms include a broad-based shuffling gait and urinary urgency or incontinence. AIDS should be suspected whenever a personality change is accompanied by clinical phenomena suggestive of immunodeficiency, such as thrush. Neurosyphilis may present with a personality change characterized by slovenliness and disinhibition. Creutzfeldt–Jakob disease may also present with a personality change, and this appears particularly likely with the "new variant" type (i.e., associated with Mad Cow disease); the eventual appearance of myoclonus suggests the correct diagnosis.

The *miscellaneous causes* represent the diagnostic "zebras" in the differential for personality change. Of them two deserve comment, given their treatability: granulomatous angiitis is suggested by prominent headache, and vitamin B_{12} deficiency by the presence of macrocytosis or a sensory polyneuropathy.

Course

This is determined by the underlying cause; in the case of the interictal personality syndrome, it appears that symptoms persist even if seizure control is obtained.

Differential Diagnosis

Personality change must be clearly distinguished from a personality disorder. The personality disorders (e.g., antisocial personality disorder, borderline personality disorder), all in Chapter 42, do not represent a change in the individual's personality but rather have been present in a lifelong fashion. In gathering a history of an individual with a personality change, one finds a more or less distinct time when the "change" occurred; by contrast, in evaluating an individual with a personality disorder, one can trace the personality traits in question in a more or less seamless fashion back into adolescence, or earlier.

The frontal lobe syndrome, at times, may present further diagnostic questions, raising the possibility of either mania, when euphoria is prominent, or depression, when abulia is at the forefront. Mania is distinguished by the quality of the euphoria, which tends to be full and infectious in contrast with the silly, shallow, and noninfectious euphoria of the frontal lobe syndrome. Depression may be distinguished by the quality of the individuals' experience: depressed individuals definitely feel something, whether it be a depressed mood or simply a weighty sense of oppression. By contrast, the individual with abulia generally feels nothing: the "mental horizon" is clear and undisturbed by any dysphoria or unpleasantness. MRI scanning is diagnostic in most cases, and where this is uninformative, further testing is dictated by one's clinical suspicions (e.g., HIV testing).

The interictal personality syndrome must be distinguished from a personality change occurring secondary to a slowly growing tumor of the temporal lobe. In some cases, very small tumors, which may escape detection by routine MRI scanning, may cause epilepsy, and then, with continued growth, also cause a personality change. Thus, in the case of an individual with epilepsy who develops a personality change, the diagnosis of the interictal personality syndrome should not be made until a tumor has been ruled out by repeat MRI scanning.

TREATMENT

Treatment, if possible, is directed at the underlying cause. Mood stabilizers (i.e., lithium, carbamazepine, or divalproex) may be helpful for lability, impulsivity, and irritability; propranolol, in high dose, may also have some effect on irritability. Neuroleptics (e.g., olanzapine, risperidone, and haloperidol) may be helpful when suspiciousness or disinhibition are prominent. Antidepressants (e.g., an SSRI) may relieve depressive symptoms. Regardless of which agent is chosen, it is prudent, given the general medical condition of many of these individuals, to "start low and go slow." In many cases, some degree of supervision will be required.

COMPARISON OF DSM-IV-TR AND ICD-10 DIAGNOSTIC CRITERIA

The DSM-IV-TR category Psychotic Disorder Due to a General Medical Condition is referred to in ICD-10 as "organic hallucinosis" or "organic delusional disorder" depending on the type of presenting symptom.

In contrast to DSM-IV-TR, which requires clinically significant mood symptoms of any type, the ICD-10 Diagnostic Criteria for Research for Mood Disorder due to a General Medical Condition require that the full symptomatic and duration criteria be met for a hypomanic, manic, or major depressive episode. This disorder is referred in ICD-10 as "organic mood disorder." Also in contrast to DSM-IV-TR, which requires anxiety symptoms of any type, the ICD-10 Diagnostic Criteria for Research for Anxiety Disorder Due to a General Medical Condition require that the clinical picture meet full symptomatic and duration criteria for panic disorder or generalized anxiety disorder.

For catatonic disorder due to a general medical condition, the ICD-10 Diagnostic Criteria for Research are more narrowly defined than the criteria in DSM-IV-TR by virtue of requiring both catatonic stupor/negativism and excitement and that there be a rapid alternation of stupor and excitement. In ICD-10, this disorder is referred to as "organic catatonic disorder."

The DSM-IV-TR category of Personality Change Due to a General Medical Condition corresponds to two ICD-10 categories: "organic personality disorder" and "organic emotionally labile disorder." The ICD-10 Diagnostic Criteria for Research for Organic Personality Disorder are probably more narrowly defined in that "at least three" features characteristic of a personality change are required.

Substance-Related Disorders: General Approaches to Substance and Polysubstance Use Disorders/Other Substance Use Disorders

This chapter provides an overview of the substance-use disorders (SUDs) (those disorders that represent maladaptive pattern of substance use, i.e., substance abuse and dependence), and the substance-induced disorders (those disorders that represent psychiatric symptoms that result from the direct effects of a substance on the central nervous system, i.e., substance intoxication, substance withdrawal, and the other specific substance-induced mental disorders). Many of the general principles outlined in this chapter are elaborated on in later chapters with regard to specific abused substances. Note that the DSM-IV-TR diagnostic criteria sets included in this chapter are *generic* in that they potentially apply across all of the classes of substances included in DSM-IV-TR. In fact, only some of the generic criteria sets apply to each of the classes of substance (e.g., there is no Nicotine Abuse and no Opioid-Induced Mood Disorders). Please refer to Table 13-1 for a cross-listing of which substance-related diagnoses apply to each class of substance. Polysubstance dependence and some substances that do not clearly meet standards for abuse and dependence (e.g., steroids) are covered in this chapter.

DIAGNOSIS

Substance Dependence

The severity of dependence can be indicated by the number of criteria met (from a minimum of 3 to a maximum of 7) and by whether or not physiological dependence occurs (i.e., whether there is tolerance or withdrawal), because physiological dependence is associated with a higher risk for immediate general medical problems and a higher relapse rate (see DSM-IV-TR diagnostic criteria, page 125). The five criteria indicating compulsive use alone may define substance dependence if at least three occur at any time in the same 12-month period. Physiological dependence is much more likely with some drugs, such as opioids and alcohol, and is infrequent with other classes of drugs, such as hallucinogens.

Treatment-seeking opioid users are likely to meet most of the dependence syndrome criteria and therefore their pattern of use is at the high end of severity. Cannabis users, in contrast, are likely to meet relatively few dependence syndrome criteria and therefore their pattern of use is of a lesser degree of severity. Individuals with alcohol or cocaine dependence tend to demonstrate a much wider variability in the number of dependence criteria met, with the proportion of individuals having relatively low levels of dependence approximately equal to those having extremely high levels of dependence. Thus, the severity of substance dependence is variable depending on the type of drug abused. Some substances such as steroids are of research interest but have not been clearly identified as producing the acute reinforcement or dependence and withdrawal symptoms that characterize the abuse of other substances. The heavy use of anabolic steroids

Clinical Guide to the Diagnosis and Treatment of Mental Disorders. M. B. First and A. Tasman
© 2006 John Wiley & Sons, Ltd.   ISBN 0 470 019158

Table 13-1   DSM-IV-TR Substance Diagnoses Associated with Class of Substance

	Dependence	Abuse	Intoxication	Withdrawal	Intoxication Delirium	Withdrawal Delirium	Dementia	Amnestic Disorder	Psychotic Disorders	Mood Disorders	Anxiety Disorders	Sexual Dysfunctions	Sleep Disorders
Alcohol	X	X	X	X	I	W	P	P	I/W	I/W	I/W	I	I/W
Amphetamines	X	X	X	X	I				I	I/W	I	I	I/W
Caffeine			X								I		I
Cannabis	X	X	X		I				I		I		
Cocaine	X	X	X	X	I				I	I/W	I/W	I	I/W
Hallucinogens	X	X	X		I				I*	I	I		
Inhalants	X	X	X		I		P		I	I	I		
Nicotine	X			X									
Opioids	X	X	X	X	I				I	I		I	I/W
Phencyclidine	X	X	X		I				I	I	I		
Sedatives, hypnotics, or anxiolytics	X	X	X	X	I	W	P	P	I/W	I/W	W	I	I/W
Polysubstance	X												
Other	X	X	X	X	I	W	P	P	I/W	I/W	I/W	I	I/W

*Also Hallucinogen Persisting Perception Disorder (Flashbacks).

Note: X, I, W, I/W, or P indicates that the category is recognized in DSM-IV-TR. In addition, I indicates that the specifier With Onset During Intoxication may be noted for the category (except for Intoxication Delirium); W indicates that the specifier With Onset During Withdrawal may be noted for the category (except for Withdrawal Delirium); and I/W indicates that either With Onset During Intoxication or With Onset During Withdrawal may be noted for the category. P indicates that the disorder is persisting.

DSM-IV-TR Diagnostic Criteria

SUBSTANCE DEPENDENCE

A maladaptive pattern of substance use, leading to clinically significant impairment or distress, as manifested by three (or more) of the following, occurring at any time in the same 12-month period:

(1) tolerance, as defined by either of the following:

    (a) a need for markedly increased amounts of the substance to achieve intoxication or desired effect

    (b) markedly diminished effect with continued use of the same amount of the substance

(2) withdrawal, as manifested by either of the following:

    (a) the characteristic withdrawal syndrome for the substance (refer to criteria A and B of the criteria sets for withdrawal from the specific substances)

    (b) the same (or a closely related) substance is taken to relieve or avoid withdrawal symptoms

(3) the substance is often taken in larger amounts or over a longer period than was intended

(4) there is a persistent desire or unsuccessful effort to cut down or control substance use

(5) a great deal of time is spent in activities necessary to obtain the substance (e.g., visiting multiple doctors or driving long distances), use the substance (e.g., chain-smoking), or recover from its effects

(6) important social, occupational, or recreational activities are given up or reduced because of substance use

(7) the substance use is continued despite knowledge of having a persistent or recurrent physical or psychological problem that is likely to have been caused or exacerbated by the substance (e.g., current cocaine use despite recognition of cocaine-induced depression, or continued drinking despite recognition that an ulcer was made worse by alcohol consumption)

Specify if:

With physiological dependence: evidence of tolerance or withdrawal (i.e., either item 1 or 2 is present)

Without physiological dependence: no evidence of tolerance or withdrawal (i.e., neither item 1 nor 2 is present)

Course specifiers (see text for definitions):

Early full remission

Early partial remission

Sustained full remission

Sustained partial remission

On agonist therapy

In a controlled environment

Reprinted with permission from the *Diagnostic and Statistical Manual of Mental Disorders*, 4th ed., Text Rev. Copyright 2000 American Psychiatric Association.

DSM-IV-TR Diagnostic Criteria

SUBSTANCE ABUSE

A. A maladaptive pattern of substance use leading to clinically significant impairment or distress, as manifested by one (or more) of the following, occurring within a 12-month period:

    (1) recurrent substance use resulting in a failure to fulfill major role obligations at work, school, or home (e.g., repeated absences or poor work performance related to substance use; substance-related absences, suspensions, or expulsions from school; neglect of children or household)

    (2) recurrent substance use in situations in which it is physically hazardous (e.g., driving an automobile or operating a machine when impaired by substance use)

    (3) recurrent substance-related legal problems (e.g., arrests for substance-related disorderly conduct)

    (4) continued substance use despite having persistent or recurrent social or interpersonal problems caused or exacerbated by the effects of the substance (e.g., arguments with spouse about consequences of intoxication, physical fights)

B. The symptoms have never met the criteria for substance dependence for this class of substance.

Reprinted with permission from the *Diagnostic and Statistical Manual of Mental Disorders*, 4th ed., Text Rev. Copyright 2000 American Psychiatric Association.

Substance Abuse

Substance abuse is a maladaptive pattern of substance use leading to significant adverse consequences manifested by psychosocial, medical, or legal problems or use in situations in which it is physically hazardous occurring within a 12-month period. Since a diagnosis of substance dependence preempts a diagnosis of abuse, tolerance, withdrawal, and compulsive use are generally not present in individuals with a diagnosis of substance abuse.

Substance Intoxication

Substance intoxication is a reversible substance-specific syndrome with maladaptive behavioral or psychological changes developing during or shortly after using the substance (see DSM-IV-TR diagnostic criteria, page 126). It does not apply to nicotine. Recent use can be documented by history or toxicological screening of body fluids (urine or blood). Different substances may produce similar or identical syndromes and, in polydrug users, intoxication may involve a complex mixture of disturbed perceptions, judgment, and behavior that can vary in severity and duration

by body builders, with the associated possible medical complications, has raised important public health issues, however.

DSM-IV-TR Diagnostic Criteria

SUBSTANCE INTOXICATION

A. The development of a reversible substance-specific syndrome due to recent ingestion of (or exposure to) a substance. Note: Different substances may produce similar or identical syndromes.
B. Clinically significant maladaptive behavioral or psychological changes that are due to the effect of the substance on the central nervous system (e.g., belligerence, mood lability, cognitive impairment, impaired judgment, impaired social or occupational functioning) and develop during or shortly after use of the substance.
C. The symptoms are not due to a general medical condition and are not better accounted for by another mental disorder.

Reprinted with permission from the *Diagnostic and Statistical Manual of Mental Disorders*, 4th ed., Text Rev. Copyright 2000 American Psychiatric Association.

---

according to the setting in which the substances were taken. Physiological intoxication is not in and of itself necessarily maladaptive and would not justify a diagnosis of the DSM-IV-TR category substance intoxication. For example, caffeine-induced tachycardia with no maladaptive behavior does not meet the criteria for substance intoxication.

Substance Withdrawal

Substance withdrawal is a syndrome due to cessation of, or reduction in, heavy and prolonged substance use. It causes clinically significant impairment or distress and is usually associated with substance dependence. Most often, the symptoms of withdrawal are the opposite of intoxication with that

---

DSM-IV-TR Diagnostic Criteria

SUBSTANCE WITHDRAWAL

A. The development of a substance-specific syndrome due to the cessation of (or reduction in) substance use that has been heavy and prolonged.
B. The substance-specific syndrome causes clinically significant distress or impairment in social, occupational, or other important areas of functioning.
C. The symptoms are not due to a general medical condition and are not better accounted for by another mental disorder.

Reprinted with permission from the *Diagnostic and Statistical Manual of Mental Disorders*, 4th ed., Text Rev. Copyright 2000 American Psychiatric Association.

---

substance. The withdrawal syndrome usually lasts several days to 2 weeks.

Other Substance-Induced Disorders

Not infrequently, substance intoxication and substance withdrawal are characterized by psychopathology that mimics the other disorders contained in the rest of DSM-IV-TR. When this occurs, if the symptoms are in excess of those usually associated with the intoxication or withdrawal syndrome, and if they are sufficiently severe to warrant independ-

---

DSM-IV-TR Diagnostic Criteria

SUBSTANCE INDUCED DISORDER

A. Presence of the particular psychiatric symptom.
B. There is evidence from the history, physical examination, or laboratory findings of either (1) or (2)

 (1) the symptoms in Criterion A developed during, or within a month of, Substance Intoxication or Withdrawal
 (2) medication use is etiologically related to the disturbance

C. The disturbance is not better accounted for by a mental disorder that is not substance-induced. Evidence that the symptoms are better accounted for by a mental disorder that is not substance-induced might include the following: the symptoms precede the onset of the substance use (or medication use); the symptoms persist for a substantial period of time (e.g., about a month) after the cessation of acute withdrawal or severe intoxication, or are substantially in excess of what would be expected given the type or amount of the substance used or the duration of use; or there is other evidence that suggests the existence of an independent non-substance-induced mental disorder (e.g., a history of recurrent non-substance-related episodes).

Note: This diagnosis should be made instead of a diagnosis of Substance Intoxication or Substance Withdrawal only when the symptoms are in excess of those usually associated with the intoxication or withdrawal syndrome and when the symptoms are sufficiently severe to warrant independent clinical attention.

Specify if:

With Onset During Intoxication: if the criteria are met for Intoxication with the substance and the symptoms develop during the intoxication syndrome

With Onset During Withdrawal: if criteria are met for Withdrawal from the substance and the symptoms develop during, or shortly after, a withdrawal syndrome

Note: This is a summary of six criteria sets.

Reprinted with permission from *DSM-IV-TR Guidebook*. Copyright 2004, Michael B First, Allen Frances, and Harold Alan Pincus.

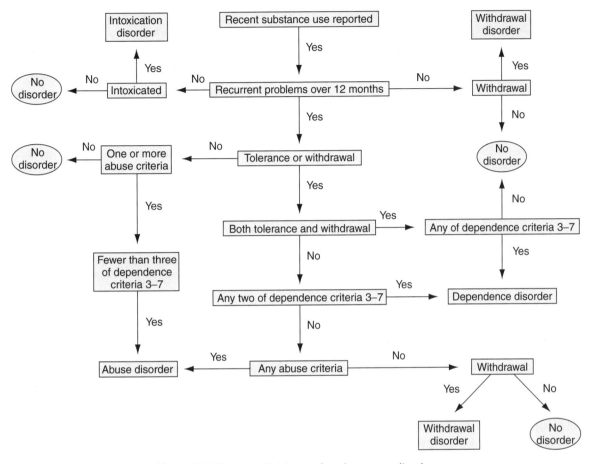

Figure 13-1 *Diagnostic decision tree for substance-use disorders.*

ent clinical attention, a specific substance-induced mental disorder should be diagnosed. For example, since dysphoric mood is commonly seen as a result of cocaine withdrawal, the mere presence of depression after stopping cocaine would not ordinarily warrant a diagnosis of Cocaine-Induced Mood Disorder; typically a diagnosis of Cocaine Withdrawal would suffice. However, if the depressed mood is especially severe and prolonged and is associated with suicidal ideation, then a diagnosis of Cocaine-Induced Mood Disorder would make clinical sense.

DSM-IV-TR includes nine substance-induced disorders (see summary of DSM-IV-TR diagnostic criteria for Substance-Induced Disorders, page 126). Seven of these (Substance Intoxication Delirium, Substance Withdrawal Delirium, Substance-Induced Psychotic Disorder, Substance-Induced Mood Disorder, Substance-Induced Anxiety Disorder, Substance-Induced Sexual Dysfunction,

and Substance-Induced Sleep Disorder) represent disorders that begin during acute intoxication or withdrawal and subside within 4 weeks of stopping the substance. A specifier is available to indicate whether the substance-induced disorder had its onset during intoxication or withdrawal (see Table 13-1 to determine which classes of substances lead to psychopathology during intoxication versus withdrawal). To facilitate differential diagnosis, these disorders have been placed in the DSM-IV-TR within the diagnostic groupings with which they share phenomenology (e.g., Substance-Induced Anxiety Disorder is included within the Anxiety Disorder section of DSM-IV-TR). Two of them (Substance-Induced Persisting Dementia and Substance-Induced Persisting Amnestic Disorder) represent psychopathology resulting from more or less permanent damage to the central nervous system, a consequence of prolonged periods of heavy substance use.

The diagnosis of substance abuse and dependence is made by eliciting an appropriate history, performing laboratory tests to confirm drug use, and observing the physiological manifestations of tolerance and withdrawal (see Figure 13-1 for a diagnostic decision tree for SUDs).

The phenomenology and variations in presentation among abused substances are related to the wide range of substance-induced states as well as the conditions under which the individual using substances is brought to treatment. Many individuals who use illicit *street* drugs may not know precisely what drugs they have ingested and certainly will not have a good idea of the precise amount. In addition, individuals who are dependent on substances producing significant withdrawal syndromes, such as opioids and alcohol, may have a mixed picture of early intoxication and overdose followed by an evolving withdrawal syndrome; alcohol and sedative withdrawal may produce psychiatric complications (e.g., hallucinations) as well as medical complications (e.g., seizures).

The severity of withdrawal symptoms may, in part, be determined by the setting. For example, studies of opioid-dependent individuals have shown that the expression of withdrawal symptoms may be substantially less when no medication treatment is available for symptom relief. As a further example of this phenomenon, individuals with opioid addiction who have been in prison without access to opioids for several years may experience precipitous opiate withdrawal when they return to the neighborhoods where they previously used heroin. This conditioned withdrawal phenomenon further supports the importance of setting in the presentation of withdrawal symptoms.

Finally, the issues of motivation for seeking treatment and a tendency to deny substance abuse can have important influence on the individual's presentation. The individual who presents for treatment because of dysphoric feelings in the context of drug dependence is likely to articulate the severity of his or her problem adequately and even exaggerate some aspects of present discomfort. In contrast, the automobile driver forced to come to a treatment program because of a driving-while-intoxicated offense is likely to minimize her or his alcohol use or any associated complications.

Two special issues in the psychiatric examination of substance dependence are (1) the source of information when obtaining the history of the substance abuse and (2) the management of aberrant behaviors. Information about an individual's substance-abuse history can be provided not only by the individual but also by employers, family members, and school officials.

When individuals self-report the amount of substance abused, there is a tendency to underreport the severity and duration of abuse, particularly if the person is being referred to treatment by an outside source such as the family, the employer, or the legal system. In general, significant others' estimates of the amount of drug use by the individual can be a good source of data.

Aberrant behaviors potentially requiring management include intoxication, violence, suicide, impaired cognitive functioning, and uncontrolled affective displays. The evaluation of an intoxicated substance abuser can address only a limited number of issues. These issues are primarily related to the safety of the substance abuser and other individuals who may be affected by his or her actions. Thus, a medical evaluation for signs of overdose or major cognitive impairment is critical, with consideration of detaining the individual for several hours or even days, if severe complications are evident.

Temporary suicidal behavior may be encountered in a variety of substance addictions, particularly those with alcohol and stimulants. Suicidal ideation may be intense but may clear within hours. During the evaluation session, it is important to elicit the precipitants that led the individual to seek treatment at this time and to keep the evaluation focused on specific data needed for the evaluation of substance dependence, its medical complications, and any comorbid mental disorders. Many individuals spend a great deal of time detailing their drug-abusing careers, but, in general, these stories do not provide useful material for the evaluation or for future psychotherapeutic interventions. Similarly, the evaluation should not become focused on the affective aspects of a individual's recent life because affect is frequently used as a defense to avoid discussing issues of more immediate relevance such as precipitants or to act as a pretext for obtaining benzodiazepines or other antianxiety agents from the physician. Abused substances have generally been a way of managing affect and these individuals need to develop alternative coping strategies.

Physical examination is critical for the assessment of substance addiction, particularly before pharmacotherapy is initiated. Many signs of drug withdrawal require a physical examination and cannot rely entirely on history. Because the general medical complications of substance addiction are also substantial, the most clearly ill individuals must have a formal general medical evaluation. Vital signs (blood pressure, pulse, and so on) are an essential beginning but a full examination of heart, lungs, and nervous system is minimally necessary. Transmissible infectious diseases such as AIDS, tuberculosis, and venereal diseases are common among illicit drug users and require screening for adequate detection. This screening for HIV infection also protects health care personnel as well as individuals undergoing treatment. A wide variety of other infectious diseases, including hepatitis and endocarditis, are also associated with intravenous drug use and require appropriate blood studies. With alcohol dependence, a wide range of gastrointestinal complications have been described, particularly liver dysfunction.

Urine toxicological screens can be sensitive for detecting drug use within 3 days of use of opiates and cocaine. Urine screens for other abused drugs such as cannabis can remain positive for as long as a month in heavy users. A breathalyzer can be used for detecting alcohol use within an 8- to 12-hour period after use. Specific biological tests can also aid in the diagnosis of dependence, for example, a naloxone challenge test assesses opioid dependence by precipitating withdrawal symptoms. Associated medical findings on physical examination include *track marks* in intravenous drug users, nasal damage in intranasal drug users, and pulmonary damage in drug smokers.

Cultural differences in the presentation of drug addiction can be striking. For example, the use of hallucinogens by Native Americans in religious ceremonies shows none of the abusive characteristics of adolescent hallucinogen addiction in middle-class America. Alcohol abuse can also show widely varying presentations based on the amount of alcohol that is considered culturally acceptable in various geographical settings.

Wide cultural variations in attitudes toward substance consumption have led to widely varying patterns of substance misuse and prevalence of substance-related disorders. Relatively high prevalence rates for the use of virtually every substance occur between the ages of 18 and 24 years, with intoxication being the initial substance-related disorder, usually beginning in the teens. Tolerance and withdrawal require a sustained period of use and these manifestations of physical dependence for most drugs of abuse typically begin in the twenties and early thirties. Although most substance-related disorders are more common in men than in women, sex ratios can vary considerably with different drugs of abuse.

In both the Epidemiological Catchment Area study and the National Comorbidity Survey, substance abuse and dependence were the most common comorbid disorders, usually appearing in combination with affective and anxiety disorders. In the National Comorbidity Survey, the lifetime rate of substance abuse was 27% and the rate of comorbid depression among these substance abusers was 19%. Furthermore, 80% of these depressed substance-abusing subjects had more than one mental disorder; only 20% had only one mental disorder. In the Epidemiological Catchment Area study, 75% of daily substance users had a comorbid mental disorder. In studies of treatment-seeking substance abusers, the rates of other mental disorders are almost uniformly higher than those in community samples, but the rates of excess comorbidity in these abusers varies with the specific abused drug. For example, in the Epidemiological Catchment Area study, the lifetime rate of major depression in the community was 7%, whereas the major depression rates for substance users seeking treatment were 54% for opioids, 38% for alcohol, and 32% for cocaine. Rates for other disorders are compared in Table 13-2.

Table 13-2	Lifetime diagnoses in SUD and Community Sample			
	Patients with Opioid Dependence ($N = 533$)	**Patients with Alcoholism** ($N = 321$)	**Cocaine Users** ($N = 149$)	**New Haven Community** ($N = 3058$)
Major depression	53.9	38	31.5	6.7
Bipolar disorder I (mania)	0.6	2	3.4	1.1
Schizophrenia	0.8	2	0.7	1.9
Phobia	9.6	27	11.4	7.8
Antisocial personality	25.5	41	34.9	2.1
Alcoholism	34.5	100	63.8	11.5
Drug abuse	100	43	100	5.8

COURSE SPECIFIERS AVAILABLE FOR SUBSTANCE DEPENDENCE

The following remission specifiers can be applied only after no criteria for dependence or abuse have been met for at least 1 month. Note that these specifiers do not apply if the individual is on agonist therapy or in a controlled environment (see below).

- Early Full Remission. This specifier is used if, for at least 1 month, but for less than 12 months, no criteria for dependence or abuse have been met.
- Early Partial Remission. This specifier is used if, for at least 1 month, but less than 12 months, one or more criteria for dependence or abuse have been met (but the full criteria for dependence have not been met).
- Sustained Full Remission. This specifier is used if none of the criteria for dependence or abuse have been met at any time during a period of 12 months or longer.
- Sustained Partial Remission. This specifier is used if full criteria for dependence have not been met for a period of 12 months or longer; however, one or more criteria for dependence or abuse have been met.

The following specifiers apply if the individual is on agonist therapy or in a controlled environment:

- On Agonist Therapy. This specifier is used if the individual is on a prescribed agonist medication such as methadone and no criteria for dependence or abuse have been met for that class of medication for at least the past month (except tolerance to, or withdrawal from, the agonist). This category also applies to those being treated for dependence using a partial agonist or an agonist/antagonist.
- In a Controlled Environment. This specifier is used if the individual is in an environment in which access to alcohol and controlled substances is restricted, and no criteria for dependence or abuse have been met for at least the past month. Examples of these environments are closely supervised and substance-free jails, therapeutic communities, or locked hospital units

Reprinted with permission from the *Diagnostic and Statistical Manual of Mental Disorders*, 4th ed., Text Rev. Copyright 2000 American Psychiatric Association.

Course

The natural history of substance dependence characteristically follows the course of a chronic relapsing disorder, although a large number of individuals who experiment with potentially abusable drugs in adolescence do not go on to acquire dependence.

The course of substance dependence is variable and may involve full or partial remission with six course specifiers available in the DSM-IV-TR.

Population surveys, such as the high school senior surveys and National Institute on Drug Abuse household survey, have provided repeated cross-sectional data on changing trends in substance use and its associated problems. These surveys have increasingly recognized cultural differences in the course of drug use. Thus, the natural history of substance abuse and dependence is determined by the type of substance used and, for polysubstance dependence, can be complicated by changing secular trends and epidemics lasting from months to decades.

Differential Diagnosis

The differential diagnosis of substance-induced intoxication and withdrawal can involve a wide range of mental disorders. Distinguishing substance abuse from these disorders is usually facilitated by a structured interview to elicit a wide range of psychiatric symptoms appropriately timed after the most recent substance use. During acute intoxication in polydrug users, the differential diagnosis might include an acute psychotic disorder, mania, delirium, dementia, or several specific anxiety disorders. Among these anxiety disorders are generalized anxiety disorder, panic disorder, and obsessive–compulsive disorder. Distinguishing these disorders from acute intoxication or withdrawal with a mixture of drugs most frequently requires that the clinician wait 24 to 72 hours to determine whether the symptoms persist and, therefore, whether they are independent of the drug use. A previous history of schizophrenia, bipolar disorder, or other major psychiatric disorder that is consistent with the presenting symptoms may also be helpful in arriving at an accurate diagnosis. When individuals present with psychotic or manic behavior during drug intoxication, it may be necessary to use symptomatic treatment such as a benzodiazepine or neuroleptic agent to conduct an examination.

Antisocial and borderline personality disorders are commonly considered in the differential diagnosis of substance-dependent individuals. Many of the behaviors that characterize these personality disorders are also common to the use of illegal and illicit drugs. In establishing these personality disorders, particularly antisocial personality, it is important to ascertain whether the behaviors are independent of the activities needed to obtain drugs. The symptoms of drug withdrawal frequently overlap with those of depressive disorders, and this differential diagnosis can be particularly difficult. Furthermore, the syndrome of protracted withdrawal can include sleep and appetite disturbance as well as dysphoria that mimics dysthymic disorder and other affective disorders. Thus, conservatively, the clinician should wait 4 to 6 weeks after acute detoxification to determine a diagnosis of affective disorder in these substance-dependent individuals. However, waiting this long is often impractical in the clinical setting in which the maintenance of sustained abstinence may depend on relief of depressive symptoms using either medications or psychotherapy.

TREATMENT

The most important goal of any treatment is abstinence from the abused drug. Issues of *controlled use* are debated by some mental health professionals, but this is usually not a realistic goal for dependent individuals. A critical, first treatment goal with substance addiction is often acute treatment of overdose. A clinician must be aware of specific therapies such as naloxone for opioid overdose and flumazenil for benzodiazepine or other sedative overdose. The polydrug user often has combined toxicity from drug interactions such as alcohol with barbiturates or phencyclidine with cocaine. For dependence on a drug with a significant withdrawal syndrome, such as opioids or alcohol, the initial treatment involves either agonist stabilization, such as methadone maintenance, or medical detoxification when necessary. After detoxification or stabilization, prevention of relapse may occur through a variety of behavioral or other psychotherapeutic approaches. Reduction in drug use without total abstinence using agonist maintenance (e.g., methadone) may be an early priority, together with the provision of essential social services for legal problems, housing, and food. After this stabilization, vocational rehabilitation and various psychotherapeutic issues may be addressed, including the management of affect such as depression. For individuals with psychosis, inpatient treatment or interventions with medication may be required before detoxification can occur.

Other treatment goals in longer-term management include total abstinence and family involvement. A common treatment goal in the longer-term management of individuals who abuse substances is abstinence from all drugs, although the individual often advocates for controlled use of some substances. For example, alcohol use by the individual receiving methadone maintenance or the continued smoking of marijuana or even tobacco by individuals formerly suffering from alcoholism can lead to a serious conflict in treatment goals. Another goal is to change the role of family members from *enablers* or codependents with

the substance user to treatment allies. These family members need to be engaged in treatment to work as active collaborators in the therapeutic plan for the individual. Although family treatment is commonly applied to many mental disorders, it can have a particularly powerful impact with adolescent substance users to eliminate family behaviors that reinforce the drug taking.

Psychiatric assessment is critical because of the high rates of depression and risk of suicide in this population. A full medical assessment generally is essential because of the high rates of infectious and gastrointestinal diseases directly related to substance abuse and dependence. Medical assessment is also essential to determine whether active medical detoxification is necessary. Finally, a psychotherapeutic issue early in treatment may be distinguishing between *slips* and a full relapse. Slips are common in substance users, and individuals must be prepared for them and not consider them failures that will inevitably lead to full relapse and dependence.

Somatic Treatments

Pharmacotherapy can have several roles in substance dependence treatment, including treatment of overdose and acute intoxication (naloxone, flumazenil), detoxification or withdrawal symptom relief (benzodiazepines, clonidine), blockage of drug reinforcement (naltrexone), development of responses to the abused substance (disulfiram), treatment of psychiatric comorbidity (antidepressants), and substitution agents to produce cross-tolerance and reduce drug craving (methadone). A key element in the treatment of many dependence-producing drugs is the need for detoxification, which may last from 3 days to as long as 2 weeks. Detoxification is essential if antagonist pharmacotherapies, such as naltrexone for opioid dependence, or aversive agents, such as disulfiram for alcoholism, are to be employed. Conversely, agonist maintenance treatment, such as methadone or buprenorphine for heroin dependence, does not require detoxification before beginning treatment. Using these agonists usually requires regular clinic attendance by the substance user and relatively prolonged treatment of 1 to 2 years, with some individuals continuing agonist therapy for up to 20 years.

Figure 13-2 outlines potential roles for pharmacotherapy and psychotherapy. The general treatment approaches, along with their indications and side effects, are seen in Table 13-3.

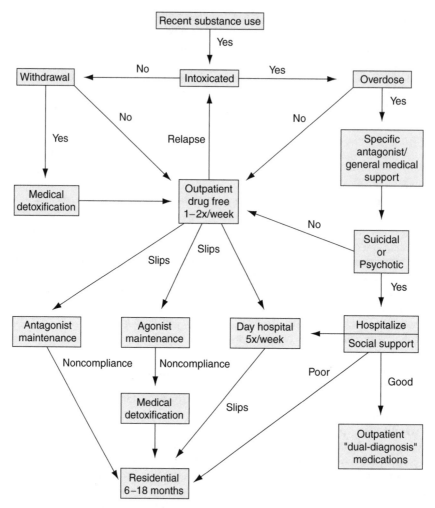

Figure 13-2 *Treatment decision tree for substance use disorders.*

Table 13-3	General Treatment Approaches: Indications and Side Effects	
Treatment	**Indication**	**Side Effects**
Pharmacotherapy Detoxifications	Dependence on Alcohol Opioids Sedatives	Overmedication, if not carefully monitored
		Undermedication, leading to seizures
Antagonists	Drug-free therapy failed	Precipitated withdrawal
Aversive agents		
Agonists		Illness from use of abused drugs
Continued dependence		
Psychotherapy	Lower level intervention failed	
Self-help		
Outpatient		
Day hospital		
Residential		
Inpatient	Medical detoxification	Social cost
	Psychotic behavior	
	Suicidal behavior	
Urine monitoring	Outpatient treatment	None
Breath alcohol		

Psychosocial Treatments

A wide range of psychosocial treatments are available in SUDs, ranging from long-term residential treatments (6 to 8 months) to relatively low-intervention outpatient medication-free treatments with once-weekly hour-long therapy. In these outpatient treatments, professional interventions may be unavailable, and counseling is provided by nonprofessionals using group therapy. These groups may be based on extensions of self-help groups, such as Alcoholics Anonymous or Narcotics Anonymous, and use a 12-step program and the associated traditions of these fellowships.

Behavioral treatments that have frequently been used include relapse prevention therapy and contingency contracting, in which various aversive contingencies are put in place for periods of up to 6 months to prevent a relapse to substance abuse and potential dependence.

Special Treatment Factors

Comorbid mental disorders, particularly depressive and anxiety disorders, are extremely common in substance abuse, with lifetime rates approaching 50% in individuals addicted to opioids. Although the rate of major psychotic disorders among SUDs is relatively low, the rate of substance abuse in individuals with schizophrenia or bipolar disorder may be as high as 50%.

Splitting treatment between a mental health clinic and substance-abuse clinic can be a significant problem for the coordinated management of the dual-diagnosis individual. A prominent problem in the management of SUDs with comorbid mental disorders is medication management within a substance-abuse treatment setting, because of limited psychiatric resources. In mental health settings, the need for monitoring, using urine toxicological screens for illicit drugs, and breath testing for alcohol can pose difficult logistic and boundary problems. Integrated dual-diagnosis treatments have been developed using social skills training combined with relapse prevention behavioral therapies as well as pharmacological adjuncts to either typical or atypical neuroleptics for individuals with schizophrenia.

Treatment of a comorbid medical condition is essential in SUDs because many substance users do not seek medical care and may be seen only by a mental health professional. The most important current comorbid disorder in SUDs is AIDS that is spread primarily by intravenous drug use but, increasingly, is also spread through sexual activity among drug users.

Other areas of medical comorbidity include vitamin deficiencies, infectious diseases, and gastrointestinal disorders such as cirrhosis, gastrointestinal bleeding, and peptic and duodenal ulcers. Stimulant users may experience cerebrovascular accidents. Also, dementing disorders need particular consideration in conjunction with alcoholism, inhalant abuse, and sedative dependence.

Two clinical questions often arise: is use of addictive medication flatly contraindicated in individuals with any kind of substance-abuse history, or is such medication prohibited only in instances of use of drugs of the same class (e.g., alcohol and benzodiazepines, and methylphenidate and cocaine)? In general, a physician should never rule out the use of any addictive drug if there are good symptom-based reasons for prescribing it. Nor should the physician assume that an addicting drug of one class (e.g., opiates) will be safe for an individual who abused another class such as stimulants. However, in any situation in which a potentially addicting drug is considered for use in a remitted substance abuser, considerable caution and limit setting is warranted. Finally, inpatient management may become necessary for the evaluation and use of these risky treatment interventions.

Treatment-Refractory Individuals

A variety of escalating treatment interventions can be applied to individuals with substance abuse or dependence who are refractory to treatment. If initial detoxification with outpatient follow-up care is ineffective, several levels of intensified interventions can be applied, such as agonist maintenance with methadone for individuals addicted to opioids, disulfiram treatment for individuals with alcoholism, and perhaps antidepressants for stimulant use disorders. Further interventions can include residential placement for up to 2 years to enable full psychosocial rehabilitation of refractory individuals.

Polysubstance Dependence

Two typical patterns of drug use fall under the category of polysubstance dependence. In one such pattern, the individual indiscriminantly uses a number of different drugs, so that he or she does not really care what drug is being used, so long as a *high* results. The second pattern is analogous to the old concept of *mixed personality disorder* in which an individual would have features from a number of different personality disorders but not one would predominate the picture. In this case, one or two dependence criteria are met for each of several different classes of drug but full criteria for dependence are only met when the drug classes are grouped together as a whole. For example, a diagnosis of polysubstance dependence applies to an individual who, during the same 12-month period, missed work because of his heavy use of alcohol, continued to use marijuana despite the fact that it led to asthma attacks, and was repeatedly unable to stay within his self-imposed limits regarding his use of cocaine. In this instance, although his problems associated with the use of any one drug were not severe enough to justify a diagnosis of dependence on that drug, his overall use of substances significantly impaired his functioning and thus warrants a diagnosis of polysubstance dependence, that is, on the group of substances taken as a whole.

Other Substance-Use Disorders: Anabolic Steroids and Nitrites

This group of substance-induced conditions most notably includes anabolic steroids and nitrite inhalants. Both have psychoactive effects and can have consequences for the individual and broad public health.

The clinical effects of anabolic steroids are related to a typical *cycle* of 4 to 18 weeks on steroids and 1 month to 1 year off. While taking the steroids, the primary effects sought by abusers are increasing muscle mass and strength, and not euphoria. In the context of an adequate diet and significant physical activity, these individuals appear quite healthy and they are unlikely to appear for treatment of their anabolic steroid abuse. However, some of the adverse cardiovascular, hepatic, and musculoskeletal effects of steroids as well as virilization in women may bring these users to medical attention. Severe cases of acne can also bring some adolescents to medical attention. Abuse of other psychoactive drugs may occur in up to a third of these steroid users, but is generally relatively low compared to other substance abusers.

Heavy use can increase aggression, change libido and sexual functions, and induce mood changes with occasional psychotic features. Androgenic steroids' tendency to provoke aggression and irritability has raised concerns about violence toward family members by abusers. Mood disturbances may be present in over 50% of body builders using anabolic steroids, as well as cognitive impairment including distractibility, forgetfulness, and confusion.

Dependence symptoms have included a withdrawal syndrome, with common symptoms being fatigue, depressed mood, and desire to take more steroids. Other common dependence symptoms are as follows: using the substance more than intended, continuing to use steroids despite problems worsened by its use, and the excessive spending of time relating to obtaining steroids. Because few clinical laboratories are equipped to conduct steroid tests and because these tests are quite expensive, these signs of dependence and some common laboratory abnormalities are usually used to make the diagnosis.

Anabolic steroid abuse leads to hypertrophied muscles, acne, oily skin, needle punctures over large muscles, hirsutism in females, and gynecomastia in males. Heavy users can also develop edema and jaundice. Common laboratory abnormalities include elevated hemoglobin and hematocrit, elevated low-density lipoprotein cholesterol, elevated liver function tests, and reduced luteinizing hormone levels.

Mental health professionals may have these individuals come to their attention because of the excessive aggression, loss of sexual ability, or mood disturbances. Treatment approaches are generally symptomatically oriented toward controlling the depressed mood and the psychotic features, but longer-term interventions such as peer counseling by former body builders and group support may be of value for these users.

Nitrite inhalants are sometimes considered within the category of inhalant abuse and produce an intoxication with mild euphoria, muscle relaxation, and a change in time perception. Concern has been raised about their impairing immune functioning, a decrease in oxygen-carrying capacity of the blood, and toxicity with severe headache, vomiting, and hypotension. No physical dependence or withdrawal syndrome has been described with these drugs.

COMPARISON OF DSM-IV-TR AND ICD-10 DIAGNOSTIC CRITERIA

The ICD-10 Diagnostic Criteria for Research for Substance Dependence are close, but not identical, to the DSM-IV-TR criteria. ICD-10 has included all seven of the DSM-IV-TR items but condenses these into five criteria and adds a sixth item tapping drug-craving behavior. Furthermore, the method for establishing clinical significance differs in the two systems. DSM-IV-TR specifies that there be a maladaptive pattern of substance use leading to clinically significant impairment or distress, whereas the ICD-10 Diagnostic Criteria for Research indicate either a one-month duration or repeated occurrences within a 12-month period.

The ICD-10 Diagnostic Criteria for Research corresponding to Substance Abuse are less specific than the criteria in DSM-IV-TR, requiring that there be "clear evidence that substance use was responsible for (or substantially contributed to) physical or psychological harm, including impaired judgment or dysfunctional behavior, which may lead to disability or have adverse consequences for interpersonal relationships." In ICD-10, this disorder is referred to as *Harmful Use*.

The ICD-10 Diagnostic Criteria for Research for Intoxication are nearly equivalent to the DSM-IV-TR criteria. However, in contrast to the DSM-IV-TR definition of Withdrawal, which specifies that the withdrawal symptoms cause clinically significant distress or impairment, the ICD-10 Diagnostic Criteria for Research for Withdrawal indicates only the presence of characteristic signs and symptoms.

14 Substance-Related Disorders: Alcohol

DIAGNOSIS

Alcohol consumption occurs along a continuum, with considerable variability in drinking patterns among individuals. There is no sharp demarcation between "social" or "moderate" drinking and "problem" or "harmful" drinking. It is clear, however, that as average alcohol consumption and frequency of intoxication increase, so does the incidence of medical and psychosocial problems.

The most visible group of people affected by alcohol problems are those who have developed a syndrome of alcohol dependence and who are commonly referred to as alcoholics. In this chapter, the term *alcoholic* is applied specifically to those individuals with alcohol dependence. A less prominent group consists of those persons who experience problems with their drinking but who are not dependent on alcohol. These individuals are variously termed alcohol abusers, problem drinkers, and harmful drinkers. These two "worlds" of alcohol problems may require different approaches to diagnosis and clinical management.

Alcohol Dependence and Abuse

The DSM-IV-TR diagnosis of *alcohol dependence* is given when three or more of the seven criteria are present (see generic DSM-IV-TR criteria for Substance Dependence, Chapter 13, page 125). Because physiological dependence is associated with greater potential for acute medical problems (particularly, acute alcohol withdrawal), the first criteria to be considered are tolerance and withdrawal. The remaining criteria reflect the behavioral and cognitive dimensions of alcohol dependence: (1) impaired control (i.e., alcohol is consumed in larger amounts or over a longer period of time than was intended; there is a persistent desire or unsuccessful efforts to cut down or control drinking; the individual continues to drink despite knowledge of a persistent or recurrent physical or psychological problem), and

(2) increased salience of alcohol (i.e., a great deal of time spent drinking or recovering from its effects; important social, occupational, or recreational activities are given up or reduced because of drinking).

Alcohol abuse is considered to be present only if the individual's drinking pattern has never met criteria for alcohol dependence and he or she demonstrates a pattern of drinking that leads to clinically significant impairment or distress, as evidenced by one or more of the four criteria in DSM-IV-TR for alcohol abuse (see generic DSM-IV-TR criteria for Substance Abuse, Chapter 13, page 125).

Alcohol Intoxication

A DSM-IV-TR diagnosis of alcohol intoxication is given when, shortly after alcohol consumption, there are maladaptive behaviors such as aggression or inappropriate sexual behavior, or there are psychological changes such as labile mood and impaired judgment (see DSM-IV-TR diagnostic criteria, page 137). Clinical signs indicative of alcohol intoxication include slurred speech, lack of coordination, unsteady gait, nystagmus, impairment of attention and memory, and in the most severe cases, stupor and coma. Alcohol intoxication may also present with severe disturbances in consciousness and cognition (alcohol intoxication delirium), especially when large amounts of alcohol have been ingested or after alcoholic intoxication has been sustained for extended periods. Usually, this condition subsides shortly after alcohol intoxication ends. Physical and mental status examinations accompanied by analysis of blood and urine allow the clinician to rule out general medical conditions or mental disorders mimicking this condition. In this regard, urine toxicology is a valuable tool in ruling out intoxication with benzodiazepines, barbiturates, or other sedatives that can present with a similar clinical picture. Collateral information from relatives or friends confirming

Clinical Guide to the Diagnosis and Treatment of Mental Disorders. M. B. First and A. Tasman
© 2006 John Wiley & Sons, Ltd. ISBN 0 470 019158

DSM-IV-TR Diagnostic Criteria

303.00 ALCOHOL INTOXICATION

A. Recent ingestion of alcohol.
B. Clinically significant maladaptive behavioral or psychological changes (e.g., inappropriate sexual or aggressive behavior, mood lability, impaired judgment, impaired social or occupational functioning) that developed during, or shortly after, alcohol ingestion.
C. One (or more) of the following signs, developing during, or shortly after, alcohol use:

(1) slurred speech
(2) incoordination
(3) unsteady gait
(4) nystagmus
(5) impairment in attention or memory
(6) stupor or coma

D. The symptoms are not due to a general medical condition and are not better accounted for by another mental disorder

Reprinted with permission from the *Diagnostic and Statistical Manual of Mental Disorders*, 4th ed., Text Rev. Copyright 2000 American Psychiatric Association.

DSM-IV-TR Diagnostic Criteria

291.81 ALCOHOL WITHDRAWAL

A. Cessation of (or reduction in) alcohol use that has been heavy and prolonged.
B. Two (or more) of the following, developing within several hours to a few days after Criterion A:

(1) autonomic hyperactivity (e.g., sweating or pulse rate greater than 100)
(2) increased hand tremor
(3) insomnia
(4) nausea or vomiting
(5) transient visual, tactile, or auditory hallucinations or illusions
(6) psychomotor agitation
(7) anxiety
(8) grand mal seizures

C. The symptoms in Criterion B cause clinically significant distress or impairment in social, occupational, or other important areas of functioning.
D. The symptoms are not due to a general medical condition and are not better accounted for by another mental disorder.

Specify if:

With Perceptual Disturbances.

Reprinted with permission from the *Diagnostic and Statistical Manual of Mental Disorders*, 4th ed., Text Rev. Copyright 2000 American Psychiatric Association.

the ingestion of alcohol is also useful and should be actively pursued by the clinician.

The blood alcohol level (BAL) is frequently used as a measure of alcohol intoxication, although this measure is less reliable in persons with a high degree of tolerance to alcohol. Euphoria, anxiolysis, and mild deficits in coordination, attention, and cognition can be observed at levels between 0.01 and 0.10%. Marked deficits in coordination and psychomotor skills, decreased attention, ataxia, impaired judgment, slurred speech, and mood lability can be observed at a greater BAL. Severe intoxication, characterized by lack of coordination, incoherent thoughts, confusion, nausea, and vomiting can be observed at BALs between 0.20 and 0.30. However, at these levels, some heavy-drinking individuals who have developed tolerance to the effects of alcohol may not appear intoxicated and may perform well on psychomotor or cognitive tasks. Stupor and loss of consciousness often occur when the BAL is between 0.30 and 0.40. Beyond this level, coma, respiratory depression, and death are possible outcomes. It should also be noted that alcohol intoxication is often associated with toxicity and overdose with other drugs, particularly those with depressant effects on the CNS.

Alcohol Withdrawal

Alcohol withdrawal is a condition that follows a reduction in alcohol consumption or an abrupt cessation of drinking in alcohol-dependent individuals. In addition to significant distress, alcohol withdrawal is also associated with impairment of social, occupational, and other areas of functioning. Uncomplicated cases

of alcohol withdrawal are characterized by signs and symptoms of autonomic hyperactivity, and may include increased heart rate, increased blood pressure, hyperthermia, diaphoresis, tremor, nausea, vomiting, insomnia, and anxiety. Onset of symptoms of uncomplicated alcohol withdrawal usually occurs between 4 and 12 hours following the last drink. Symptom severity tends to peak around the second day, usually subsiding by the fourth or fifth day of abstinence. After this period, less severe anxiety, insomnia, and autonomic symptoms may persist for a few weeks, with some individuals experiencing a protracted alcohol-withdrawal syndrome up to 5 or 6 months after cessation of drinking. A small but significant number of alcohol-dependent individuals (10%) can experience complicated alcohol-withdrawal episodes. Alcohol-withdrawal delirium (also known as delirium tremens) can occur in 5% of the cases, usually between 36 and 72 hours following alcohol cessation. In addition to signs of autonomic hyperactivity, this condition is characterized by illusions, auditory, visual, or tactile hallucinations, psychomotor agitation, fluctuating cloudiness of consciousness, and disorientation. Grand mal seizures associated with alcohol withdrawal occur in 3–5% of the cases, typically within the first 48 hours following reduction or cessation of drinking. In both instances of complicated alcohol withdrawal, lack or delay in instituting proper treatment is associated with an increased mortality rate. Prior history of delirium tremens and/or alcohol-withdrawal seizures, older age, poor nutritional status, comorbid medical conditions, and history of high tolerance to alcohol are predictors of increased severity of alcohol withdrawal.

Alcohol-Induced Persisting Dementia

Continuous heavy drinking is also associated with progressive and gradual development of multiple cognitive deficits characterized by memory impairment, apraxia, agnosia, or disturbances in executive functioning. These deficits cause serious impairment in social and occupational functioning and persist beyond the duration of alcohol intoxication and alcohol withdrawal. History, physical examination, and laboratory tests should be utilized to determine whether these deficits are etiologically related to the toxic effects of alcohol use. Other factors associated with this condition are poor nutritional status and vitamin deficiencies as well as history of head trauma. It is believed that this condition is associated with the repeated occurrence of Wernicke's encephalopathy. Atrophy of frontal lobes and increased ventricular size have been described in this condition. Continuous alcohol consumption exacerbates the dementia, whereas drinking cessation is associated with improvement and even recovery of cognitive deficits.

Alcohol-Induced Persisting Amnestic Disorder

Continuous heavy alcohol consumption can lead to several neurological deficits caused by thiamine deficiency. Among them, alcohol-induced persisting amnestic disorder (AIPAD, also known as a Korsakoff's psychosis due to the fantastic confabulatory stories described by individuals suffering this condition) is prominent. Profound deficits in anterograde memory and some deficits in retrograde memory characterize this condition. Individuals cannot retain or learn new information and experience profound disorientation to time and place. The severity of anterograde memory deficits typically leads individuals suffering from Korsakoff's psychosis, who are unaware of their deficit, to reconstruct forgotten events by confabulating. Korsakoff's amnestic disorder is usually preceded by several episodes of Wernicke's encephalopathy, characterized by confusion, ataxia, nystagmus, and gaze palsies. When this condition subsides, the characteristic memory deficits of Korsakoff's psychosis become prominent.

Cessation of drinking can lead to an improvement in memory, with approximately 20% of the cases demonstrating complete recovery. However, in most cases, memory deficits remain unchanged, and in some instances, long-term care is needed despite sobriety.

Alcohol-Induced Psychotic Disorder

This disorder is characterized by prominent hallucinations or delusions that are judged by the clinician to be due to the effects of alcohol. The psychotic symptoms usually occur within a month of an alcohol intoxication or withdrawal episode, and the individual is characteristically fully alert and oriented, lacking insight that these symptoms are alcohol-induced. Although onset of psychotic symptoms can occur during or shortly after alcohol intoxication, delirium or alcohol-withdrawal delirium, alcohol-induced hallucinations, and/or delusions do not occur exclusively during the course of these conditions. Evidence that hallucinations and delusions are not part of a primary psychotic disorder include: atypical or late age of onset of psychotic symptoms, onset of alcohol drinking preceding the onset of psychiatric symptoms, and remission of psychotic episodes during extended periods of abstinence. Usually, alcohol-induced psychotic symptoms tend to subside within a few weeks of abstinence, although in a subset of individuals, psychotic symptoms can become chronic, requiring long-term treatment with antipsychotic medication. In these cases, clinicians are obligated to consider schizophrenia or delusional disorder as part of the differential diagnosis.

Alcohol-Induced Mood Disorder

Alcohol-induced mood disorder (AIMD), characterized by depressed mood and anhedonia, as well as elevated, expansive, or irritable mood, frequently develops as a consequence of heavy drinking. Although mood disturbances are common among alcoholic individuals entering treatment (occurring in up to 80% of individuals), alcohol-induced mood symptoms tend to subside within 2 to 4 weeks following alcohol cessation. Evidence that the mood disturbances are not better explained by a primary mood disorder should be sought by the clinician. Evidence suggesting a primary mood disorder includes onset of mood symptoms preceding onset of alcohol abuse and persistence of mood symptoms after alcohol cessation or during extended periods of abstinence. Regardless of the primary or secondary nature of mood symptoms, given the high prevalence of suicide among alcoholics, clinicians should closely monitor the individual for emerging suicidal thoughts, implementing more intensive treatment (discussed later) if necessary.

Alcohol-Induced Anxiety Disorder

Although alcohol has anxiolytic properties at low doses, heavy alcohol consumption can induce prominent anxiety symptoms. Alcohol-induced anxiety (AIA) symptoms more commonly include generalized anxiety symptoms, panic attacks, and phobias. An onset of drinking preceding the anxiety syndrome, and improvement or remission of anxiety during periods of abstinence, suggest alcohol-induced anxiety disorder (AIAD). Monitoring the course of these symptoms for several weeks after alcohol cessation can be useful in determining their nature. Usually, a substantial improvement of anxiety will be observed during this period, suggesting a direct relationship of anxiety to alcohol. In some cases, a full remission of symptoms is not observed until after 3 to 4 weeks of abstinence.

Alcohol-Induced Sleep Disorder

Heavy alcohol consumption can be associated with a prominent disturbance of sleep. At intoxicating BALs, especially when BALs are declining, sedation and sleepiness can be observed. Alcohol intoxication induces an increase in nonrapid eye movement (NREM) sleep, whereas rapid eye movement (REM) sleep density decreases. Subsequently, there is an increase in wakefulness, restless sleep, and vivid dreams or nightmares related to a reduction in NREM sleep and a rebound in REM sleep density. During alcohol withdrawal, sleep is fragmented and discontinuous with an increase in REM sleep. After withdrawal, individuals frequently complain of sleep difficulties and may experience superficial and fragmented sleep for months or years.

Alcohol-Induced Sexual Dysfunction

Although small doses of alcohol in healthy individuals appear to enhance sexual receptivity in women and facilitate arousal to erotic stimuli in men, continuous and/or heavy drinking may cause significant sexual impairment. Alcohol-induced sexual dysfunction is characterized by impaired desire, impaired arousal, and impaired orgasm, or sexual pain Use of other substances, particularly those prescribed for the treatment of alcohol withdrawal such as benzodiazepines or barbiturates, should be ruled out as a cause of the sexual dysfunction.

Comprehensive assessment provides the basis for an individualized plan of treatment. Depending upon the severity of alcohol dependence, the nature of comorbid medical and psychiatric pathology, the presence of social supports, and evidence of previous response to treatment, decisions can be made concerning the most appropriate intensity, setting, and modality of treatment.

Although denial of alcohol-related problems is legendary among alcoholics, there is substantial evidence that a valid alcohol history can be obtained, given adequate assessment procedures and the right conditions. A complete alcohol history should include specific questions concerning average alcohol consumption, maximal consumption per drinking occasion, frequency of heavy-drinking occasions, and drinking-related social problems (e.g., objections raised by family members, friends, or people at work), legal problems (including arrests or near-arrests for driving while intoxicated (DWI)), psychiatric symptoms (e.g., precipitation or exacerbation of mood or anxiety symptoms), and alcohol-related medical problems (e.g., alcoholic gastritis or pancreatitis).

Systematic clinical assessment often begins with routine screening to identify active cases, as well as persons at risk. Perhaps the most widely used alcohol-screening test is the CAGE, which contains only four questions: (1) Have you ever felt you ought to *cut* (the "C" in CAGE) down on your drinking? (2) Have people *annoyed* (A) you by criticizing your drinking? (3) Have you ever felt bad or *guilty* (G) about your drinking? (4) Have you ever had a drink first thing in the morning to steady your nerves or get rid of a hangover, that is, an *eye* opener (E)? Reliability and validity studies of this test have been conducted in diverse samples (e.g., psychiatric inpatients, ambulatory medical patients, prenatal clinics), with generally acceptable levels of sensitivity.

The Alcohol Use Disorders Identification Test (AUDIT), a 10-item screening instrument, may be used as the first step in a comprehensive and sequential alcohol use history. The AUDIT (Table 14-1) covers the domains of alcohol consumption, symptoms of alcohol dependence, and alcohol-related consequences.

Medical illness is a common consequence of heavy drinking and may be present in the absence of physical dependence. Early in the course, individuals with alcoholism may show no physical or laboratory abnormalities. But as it progresses, it is widely manifested throughout most organ systems. A thorough physical examination is indicated if, in the history, there is evidence of medical problems. The physical examination provides essential information about the presence and extent of end-organ damage, and should be focused on the systems most vulnerable to developing alcohol-related pathology: the cardiovascular system, the gastrointestinal system, and the central and peripheral nervous systems. The physician should also be alert

Table 14-1	Alcohol Use Disorders Identification Test

1. How often do you have a drink containing alcohol?
   - (0) Never
   - (1) Monthly or less
   - (2) Two to four times a month
   - (3) Two or three times a week
   - (4) Four or more times a week

2. *How many drinks containing alcohol do you have on a typical day when you are drinking? (Code number of standard drinks)
   - (0) 1 or 2
   - (1) 3 or 4
   - (2) 5 or 6
   - (3) 7 or 8
   - (4) 10 or more

3. How often do you have 6 or more drinks on one occasion?
   - (0) Never
   - (1) Less than monthly
   - (2) Monthly
   - (3) Weekly
   - (4) Daily or almost daily

4. How often during the last year have you found that you were not able to stop drinking once you had started?
   - (0) Never
   - (1) Less than monthly
   - (2) Monthly
   - (3) Weekly
   - (4) Daily or almost daily

5. How often during the last year have you failed to do what was normally expected from you because of drinking?
   - (0) Never
   - (1) Less than monthly
   - (2) Monthly
   - (3) Weekly
   - (4) Daily or almost daily

6. How often during the last year have you needed a first drink in the morning to get yourself going after a heavy-drinking session?
   - (0) Never
   - (1) Less than monthly
   - (2) Monthly
   - (3) Weekly
   - (4) Daily or almost daily

7. How often during the last year have you had a feeling of guilt or remorse after drinking?
   - (0) Never
   - (1) Less than monthly
   - (2) Monthly
   - (3) Weekly
   - (4) Daily or almost daily

8. How often during the last year have you been unable to remember what happened the night before because you had been drinking?
   - (0) Never
   - (1) Less than monthly
   - (2) Monthly
   - (3) Weekly
   - (4) Daily or almost daily

9. Have you or someone else been injured as a result of your drinking?
   - (0) No
   - (2) Yes, but not in the last year
   - (4) Yes, during the last year

10. Has a relative or friend or a physician or other health care worker been concerned about your drinking or suggested you cut down?
   - (0) No
   - (2) Yes, but not in the last year
   - (4) Yes, during the last year

Record sum of individual item scores here _____ .

*In determining the response categories, it has been assumed that one "drink" contains 10 g of alcohol.

to other acute alcohol-related signs, including alcohol withdrawal or delirium, intoxication or withdrawal from other drugs, and the acute presentation of psychiatric symptomatology. Other systemic or nonspecific health problems associated with alcoholism include malnutrition, muscle wasting, neuritis, specific vitamin deficiencies, infectious diseases (such as tuberculosis, dermatitis, pediculosis, and hepatitis), and trauma secondary to fights and accidents (Table 14-2).

Several laboratory tests, particularly those related to hepatic function (e.g., serum transaminases, bilirubin, prothrombin time, and partial thromboplastin time) have been commonly used by clinicians. Other laboratory tests (e.g., gamma-glutamyl transpeptidase

Table 14-2	Health Problems Commonly Associated with Alcoholism

Malnutrition, muscle wasting, neuritis, vitamin deficiencies
Infectious diseases (e.g., tuberculosis)
Hepatitis, pancreatitis, gastritis
Trauma secondary to fights, accidents
Cardiovascular disease (e.g., myocardial infarction)

[GGTP], mean corpuscular volume [MCV]) of erythrocytes can be used as objective indicators of heavy drinking. Elevation in GGTP occurs in approximately three-fourths of alcoholics before there is clinical evidence of liver disease. It is often considered to be the earliest indication of heavy alcohol consumption and is widely available clinically. GGTP levels usually return to normal limits after 4 to 5 weeks of abstinence.

CDT is more sensitive than most routine laboratory tests for the identification of heavy alcohol consumption. In one study, CDT was found to have a sensitivity of 91% and a specificity of 100% in distinguishing alcoholics from light drinkers/abstainers. In contrast to GGTP, CDT elevations are associated with few conditions other than heavy drinking. CDT and GGTP appear to identify two different subsets of alcoholic individuals. Elevations in GGTP values detect alcoholics with hepatic damage secondary to heavy drinking, whereas CDT appears to be more directly related to heavy drinking. Whenever possible, CDT and GGTP should be used together by classifying as a case the individuals who have elevated scores in either test.

This approach increases the likelihood of identifying individuals experiencing alcohol use disorders. CDT appears to detect relapse to heavy drinking among individuals in alcohol treatment more accurately than other laboratory tests.

In a clinical setting where laboratory results are generally not immediately available, the alcohol breath test, which measures the amount of alcohol in expired air (providing an estimate of venous ethanol concentration), is valuable. Although its accuracy depends on the individual's cooperation (which in an intoxicated individual is often problematic), the alcohol breath test can be a reliable and inexpensive method for assessing recent alcohol consumption. Venous blood levels should be obtained if dangerously high levels of intoxication are suspected, when an individual is comatose, or for medical–legal purposes. A BAL greater than 150 mg/dL in an individual showing no signs of intoxication (i.e., no dysarthria, motor incoordination, gait ataxia, nystagmus, or impaired attention) can be interpreted to reflect physiological tolerance. In nontolerant individuals, a BAL in excess of 400 mg/dL can result in death, and 300 mg/dL indicates a need for emergency care.

Another laboratory evaluation that is indicated in alcoholics is a urine toxicology screen. To identify drug use that the individual may not recognize or which he or she denies is a problem, the screen should include opiates, cocaine, cannabis, and benzodiazepines. Routine urinalysis, blood chemistries, hepatitis profile, complete blood count, and serologic test for syphilis and (for women) serum testing for pregnancy should also be obtained.

Course

A typical sequence of the symptoms of alcohol dependence appears as follows: heavy drinking during the late twenties; interference with functioning in multiple life areas during their early thirties; loss of control, followed by an intensification of social- and work-related problems, and onset of medical consequences in the mid- to late thirties; and severe long-term consequences by the late thirties and early forties. Women appear to experience many of these milestones at a later age than men.

There are few effects of onset age, family history of alcoholism, or comorbid psychiatric diagnoses on the order of symptom appearance. However, other features defining the course of alcoholism, particularly the response to treatment, vary as a function of variables related to the individual, including age of onset, severity of alcohol dependence, and comorbid mental disorders. There is consistent evidence that early age of onset is a predictor of greater severity of alcoholism

and a poorer response to treatment. Greater severity of alcohol dependence has also been shown to predict poorer treatment outcome.

While considered to be important in the development of alcoholism, comorbid mental disorders also have prognostic significance. Among males, the presence of a comorbid lifetime diagnosis of ASPD, major depressive disorder, or drug abuse/dependence was associated with poorer drinking outcomes. Among females, the presence of major depressive disorder predicted a better outcome on drinking-related measures, while those individuals with ASPD or drug abuse/dependence had a poorer prognosis. Three-year posttreatment outcomes in this group of alcoholics also showed comorbid ASPD, major depressive disorder, and drug abuse/dependence to be associated with poorer outcomes, irrespective of gender. Alcoholics with comorbid depression have greater psychiatric severity at follow-up than primary alcoholics. Variable findings have also been reported concerning the prognostic significance of ASPD and drug abuse among alcoholics.

TREATMENT

When a determination has been made that an individual is drinking excessively, the nature, setting, and intensity of the intervention must be determined in order to address the specific treatment needs of the individual. Among heavy drinkers without evidence of alcohol dependence, a brief intervention aimed at the reduction of drinking may suffice. In contrast, among alcoholics, there are typically a variety of associated disabilities, so it is necessary to address both the excessive drinking *and* problems related to it. Consequently, alcoholism treatment is best conceived of as multimodal. Table 14-3 provides an overview of the goals of

Table 14-3	Goals of Alcoholism Treatment

Promote complete abstinence from alcohol.
Stabilize acute medical (including alcohol withdrawal) and psychiatric conditions, as needed.
Increase motivation for recovery.
Initiate treatment for chronic medical and psychiatric conditions, as needed.
Assist the patient in locating suitable housing (e.g., moving from a setting where drinking is widespread), as needed.
Enlist social support for recovery (e.g., introduce to 12-step programs and, when possible, help the patient to repair damaged marital and other family relationships).
Enhance coping and relapse prevention skills (including social skills, identification and avoidance of high-risk situations).
Improve occupational functioning.
Promote maintenance of recovery through ongoing participation in structured treatment or self-help groups.

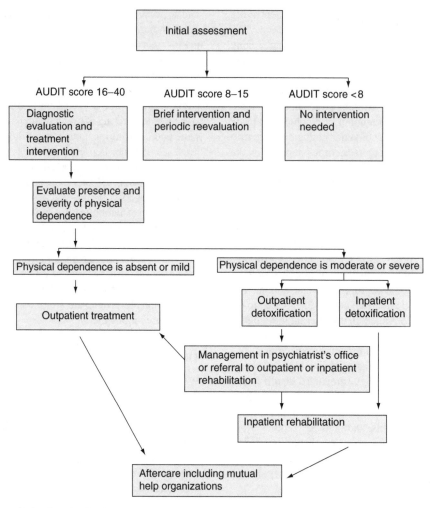

Figure 14-1 *Algorithm for the identification and management of patients with alcohol abuse and dependence.*

alcoholism treatment. It should be noted that while total abstinence is a primary goal of treatment for persons with alcohol dependence, moderate drinking can be considered as a goal for persons with alcohol abuse.

Figure 14-1 describes a process for the management of individuals with alcohol abuse and dependence. The algorithm is written from the perspective of a community-based or consultation/liaison clinician who does not necessarily have specialized training in addiction medicine. Following the initial assessment, using a screening test such as the CAGE or AUDIT, the individual is referred to either a diagnostic evaluation with a likely treatment recommendation or a brief intervention with further monitoring. Brief interventions are characterized by their low intensity and short duration. They are intended to provide early intervention, before or soon after the onset of alcohol-related problems. Brief interventions seek to motivate high-risk drinkers

to moderate their alcohol consumption, rather than promote total abstinence with specialized treatment techniques. They are simple enough to be delivered by primary care practitioners and are especially appropriate for individuals whose at-risk drinking meets criteria for alcohol abuse rather than dependence. The cumulative evidence shows that clinically significant effects on drinking behavior and related problems, though not on alcohol dependence, can follow from brief interventions.

If the individual's screening results and diagnostic evaluation provide evidence of alcohol dependence, the next step is to differentiate between mild and more severe levels of physical dependence to determine the need for detoxification. If withdrawal risk is low, the individual may be referred directly to outpatient therapy. If the withdrawal risk is moderate or high, outpatient or inpatient detoxification is indicated.

There are a number of potentially life-threatening conditions for which alcoholics are at increased risk. The presence of any of the following requires immediate attention: acute alcohol withdrawal (with the potential for seizures and delirium tremens), serious medical or surgical disease (e.g., acute pancreatitis, bleeding esophageal varices), and serious psychiatric illness (e.g., psychosis, suicidal intent). In the presence of any of these emergent conditions, acute stabilization should be the first priority of treatment.

The presence of complicating medical conditions or mental disorders is an important determinant of whether detoxification and rehabilitation are initiated in an inpatient or an outpatient setting. Other considerations are the alcoholic's current living circumstances and social support network. Women with children are sometimes unwilling to enter residential treatment unless their family needs are taken care of. Homeless people may be eager to enter residential treatment even when their medical or psychiatric condition does not warrant it.

In the alcoholic individual whose condition is stabilized or in the individual without these complicating features, the major focus should be on the establishment of a therapeutic alliance, which provides the context within which rehabilitation can occur. The presence of a trusting relationship facilitates the individual's acknowledgement of alcohol-related problems and encourages open consideration of different treatment options. In addition to participation in structured rehabilitation treatment, the individual should be made aware of the widespread availability of Alcoholics Anonymous (AA) and the wide diversity of its membership.

Despite treatment, some alcoholics relapse repeatedly. For many emergency department personnel, the multiple recidivist alcoholic has come to personify the disorder. For clinicians involved in the delivery of alcoholism rehabilitation services, these individuals' apparent unresponsiveness to treatment may contribute to frustration and a sense of futility. Presently, long-term residential treatment appears to be the only option for alcoholics who do not respond to more limited efforts at rehabilitation. Unfortunately, the availability of such care in many states is limited as a consequence of the effort to deinstitutionalize psychiatric patients.

Management of Alcohol Withdrawal

An important initial intervention for a substantial number of alcohol-dependent individuals is the management of alcohol withdrawal through detoxification. The objectives in treating alcohol withdrawal are the relief of discomfort, prevention or treatment of complications, and preparation for rehabilitation. Successful management of the alcohol-withdrawal syndrome provides a basis for subsequent efforts at rehabilitation.

Careful screening for concurrent medical problems is an important element in detoxification. Administration of thiamine (50–100 mg by mouth or IM) and multivitamins is a low-cost, low-risk intervention for the prophylaxis and treatment of alcohol-related neurological disturbances. Good supportive care and treatment of concurrent illness, including fluid and electrolyte repletion, are essential.

Social detoxification, which involves the nonpharmacological treatment of alcohol withdrawal, has been shown to be effective. It consists of frequent reassurance, reality orientation, monitoring of vital signs, personal attention, and general nursing care. Social detoxification is most appropriate for individuals in mild-to-moderate withdrawal. The medical problems commonly associated with alcoholism may substantially complicate therapy, so care must be taken to refer those individuals whose condition requires medical management.

Increasingly, detoxification is being done on an ambulatory basis, which is much less costly than inpatient detoxification. Inpatient detoxification is indicated for serious medical or surgical illness, and for those individuals with a past history of adverse withdrawal reactions or with current evidence of more serious withdrawal (e.g., delirium tremens.)

Owing to their favorable side effect profile, the benzodiazepines have largely supplanted all other medications for the treatment of alcohol withdrawal. Although any benzodiazepine will suppress alcohol-withdrawal symptoms, diazepam and chlordiazepoxide are often used, since they are metabolized to long-acting compounds, which in effect are self-tapering. Because metabolism of these drugs is hepatic, impaired liver function may complicate their use. Oxazepam and lorazepam are not oxidized to long-acting metabolites and thus carry less risk of accumulation.

Although carbamazepine appears useful as a primary treatment of withdrawal, the liver dysfunction that is common in alcoholics may affect its metabolism, which makes careful blood level monitoring necessary. Antipsychotics are not indicated for the treatment of withdrawal except in those instances where hallucinations or severe agitation are present, in which case they should be added to a benzodiazepine. In addition to their potential to produce extrapyramidal side effects, antipsychotics lower seizure threshold, which may be particularly problematic during alcohol withdrawal.

Psychosocial Treatments

A variety of treatment components are delivered within the context of rehabilitation services. In many programs, a combination of therapeutic interventions is provided to all individuals, based on the assumption that multiple components have a greater chance of meeting at least some of each individual's needs. Therapeutic approaches most often employed in both residential and outpatient programs include behavior therapy, group therapy, family treatment, and pharmacotherapy. Regarding specific treatment modalities, the weight of evidence suggests that behavioral treatments are likely to be more effective than insight-oriented or family therapies.

Behavioral elements most frequently employed in treatment programs are relapse prevention, social skills and assertiveness training, contingency management, deep muscle relaxation, self-control training, and cognitive restructuring.

Behavior therapists stress the importance of teaching new, adaptive skills designed to alter the conditions that precipitate and reinforce drinking, as well as developing alternative ways of coping with persons, events, and feelings that serve to maintain drinking. A model of treatment, characterized as "relapse prevention" because of its focus on identifying and coping with situations that represent high risk for heavy drinking, has been used increasingly. Individuals who received skills training attend aftercare more regularly and have less severe (though no less frequent) relapses than individuals in control groups.

The deleterious effects of alcoholism on marriages and families have been a source of concern to both clinicians and researchers. Alcoholism creates major stress on the family system by threatening health, interpersonal relations, and the economic functioning of family members.

In addition to specific treatment for alcoholic couples or families, self-help groups for family members of alcoholics have grown substantially. Al-Anon, although not formally affiliated with AA, shares the structure and many of the tenets of the 12 steps of AA. Al-Anon and AA meetings are often held jointly. Alateen groups, sponsored by Al-Anon for children of alcoholics, are available as well.

Somatic Treatments

In the following sections, we discuss two types of pharmacotherapy for alcoholics: alcohol-sensitizing drugs and medications to directly reduce drinking.

Alcohol-Sensitizing Drugs. Medications such as disulfiram or calcium carbimide cause an unpleasant reaction when combined with alcohol. The efficacy of such drugs in the prevention or limitation of relapse in alcoholics has not been demonstrated. However, these drugs may be of utility in selected samples of alcoholics with whom special efforts are made to ensure compliance.

Disulfiram (Antabuse) is the most commonly used alcohol-sensitizing medication and the only one approved for use in the United States. When given in a single daily dose of 125–500 mg, disulfiram binds irreversibly to ALDH, permanently inactivating this enzyme. When alcohol is consumed, it is metabolized to acetaldehyde, which accumulates because of inhibition of the enzyme that metabolizes it. Elevated levels of acetaldehyde are responsible for the aversive effects associated with the disulfiram–ethanol reaction (DER).

Although disulfiram has been used in the treatment of alcoholism for more than 50 years, the few placebo-controlled studies that have been conducted have not shown the drug to have substantial efficacy. Given the limited efficacy of disulfiram for the prevention of relapse, it should not be used as a first-line treatment for alcohol dependence. However, if an individual has not responded to other pharmacological treatments and is motivated to take disulfiram, it may be beneficial. Whenever disulfiram is prescribed, individuals should be warned about its hazards, including the need to avoid over-the-counter (OTC) preparations with alcohol and drugs that interact adversely with disulfiram, as well as the potential for a DER to result from alcohol used in food preparations.

Drugs that May Directly Reduce Alcohol Consumption. Efforts to use medications to treat excessive drinking have increasingly focused on agents that have selective effects on specific neurotransmitter systems.

An extensive literature supports the role of opioidergic neurotransmission in the pathophysiology of alcohol consumption and related phenomena. In contrast, opioid antagonists, such as naltrexone, decrease ethanol consumption and self-administration.

Naltrexone appears to produce a modest effect on drinking behavior among alcoholics. However, given the comparatively small overall effect of the medication, a variety of other factors, including medication compliance, the severity and chronicity of alcohol dependence, and the choice of concomitant psychotherapy, may determine whether an effect of the medication is observed.

Acamprosate was approved by the FDA in 2004 for the maintenance of abstinence from alcohol in individuals with alcohol dependence who are abstinent at treatment initiation. Acamprosate, an amino acid derivative, affects both gamma-aminobutyric acid (GABA) and excitatory amino acid (i.e., glutamate) neurotransmission (the latter effect most likely being the one that is important for its therapeutic effects in alcoholism). Together, studies involving more than 4000 individuals provide consistent evidence of the efficacy of acamprosate in alcoholism rehabilitation. On the basis of these findings, and the benign side effect profile of the medication, it appears to hold considerable value for the treatment of alcohol dependence.

Other drugs, including SSRIs such as fluoxetine and citalopram, and ondansetron have been used with variable success in reducing alcohol intake.

Considerable additional research is required before medications are likely to play a meaningful role in the postwithdrawal treatment of alcohol dependence. One currently useful strategy is the identification of comorbid psychopathology in alcoholics, with pharmacotherapy directed toward reducing both psychiatric symptoms and alcohol consumption. In addition, the opioid antagonist naltrexone, which is capable of yielding a modest effect overall in reducing drinking behavior, appears to be of considerable value in some individuals. Further research is required with naltrexone to determine the optimal dosage, duration of treatment, and psychosocial treatment strategies with which to use the medication. The question of whether the medication is most efficacious for alcoholics with high levels of craving for alcohol remains an important one. The SSRIs fluoxetine, citalopram, and sertraline may be of value in subgroups of heavy drinkers, particularly those with a later onset of problem drinking. In contrast, ondansetron may be useful in alcoholics with an early onset of problem drinking. Prospective replication of this serotonergic matching strategy is required, however, before it can be recommended for general clinical use.

Alcoholics Anonymous (AA) and Mutual Help Organizations

Although mutual help societies composed of recovering alcoholics are not considered a formal treatment, they are often used as a substitute, an alternative, and an adjunct to treatment. Mutual help groups based on the Twelve Steps of AA have proliferated throughout the world. To the extent that AA and other mutual help groups are more numerous than outpatient treatment, they may constitute a significant resource for problem drinkers who are attempting to reduce or stop drinking.

With an estimated 87,000 groups in 150 countries, AA is by far the most widely utilized source of help for

Table 14-4	The 12 Steps of Alcoholics Anonymous

1. We admitted we were powerless over alcohol—that our lives had become unmanageable.
2. Came to believe that a Power greater than ourselves could restore us to sanity.
3. Made a decision to turn our will and our lives over to the care of God *as we understood Him.*
4. Made a searching and fearless moral inventory of ourselves.
5. Admitted to God, to ourselves, and to another human being the exact nature of our wrongs.
6. Were entirely ready to have God remove all these defects of character.
7. Humbly asked Him to remove our shortcomings.
8. Made a list of all persons we had harmed, and became willing to make amends to them all.
9. Made direct amends to such people wherever possible, except when to do so would injure them or others.
10. Continued to take personal inventory and when we were wrong, promptly admitted it.
11. Sought through prayer and meditation to improve our conscious contact with God *as we understood Him,* praying only for knowledge of His will for us and the power to carry that out.
12. Having had a spiritual awakening as the result of these steps, we tried to carry this message to alcoholics, and to practice these principles in all our affairs.

Source: The 12 Steps are reprinted with permission of Alcoholics Anonymous World Services, Inc. Permission to reprint this material does not mean that AA has reviewed or approved the contents of this publication, nor that AA agrees with the views expressed herein. AA is a program of recovery from alcoholism. Use of the 12 Steps in connection with programs and activities that are patterned after AA but address other problems does not imply otherwise.

drinking problems in the United States and throughout the world. In addition, a number of self-help organizations have modeled themselves after AA, basing recovery from drug abuse, overeating, and other behavioral disorders on the 12 Steps of AA (see Table 14-4). Unfortunately, clinicians often refer individuals to self-help groups such as AA without consideration of the individual's needs and without adequate monitoring of the individual's response. Not all people are willing to endorse the AA emphasis on spirituality and its disease concept of alcoholism, which requires lifelong abstinence as the only means to recovery. Greater familiarity with AA may help clinicians to identify those individuals who might benefit from this approach.

Although it is regarded as one of the most useful resources for recovering alcoholics, the research literature supporting the efficacy of AA is limited. Attendance at AA tends to be correlated with longterm abstinence, but this may reflect motivation for recovery. The type of motivated alcoholic that persists with AA might do just as well with other forms of supportive therapy. In fact, the few random assignment studies that have been conducted do not indicate that AA (or similar programs) is more effective than other types of treatment. Personality variables do not appear to differentiate between alcoholics who affiliate with AA and those who do not, although there is some evidence that AA is less successful among persons with major psychiatric disorders and those of low socioeconomic status.

Treatment of Psychiatric Comorbidity

Comorbid mental disorders may contribute to the development or maintenance of heavy drinking. Efforts to treat the comorbidity may have beneficial effects on drinking outcomes. Following detoxification, many alcoholics complain of persistent anxiety, insomnia, and general distress. These symptoms may last for weeks or months and may be difficult to differentiate from the emergence of diagnosable mental disorders. Irrespective of their etiology, negative emotional states, including frustration, anger, anxiety, depression, and boredom, have been shown to contribute to relapse in a substantial proportion of alcoholics.

A variety of medications have been employed to treat comorbid psychiatric symptoms and disorders in alcoholics. Indications for the use of these medications in alcoholics are similar to those for nonalcoholic populations, but there is added potential for adverse effects due to comorbid medical disorders and the pharmacokinetic effects of acute and chronic alcohol consumption. The use of these medications in alcoholics therefore entails additional considerations that can only be arrived at through careful psychiatric diagnosis.

Treatment of Depressive Symptoms/Disorders. Depressive symptoms are common early in alcohol withdrawal, but they often remit spontaneously with time. For depression that persists beyond the period of acute withdrawal, an antidepressant is probably warranted.

Although it has been argued that most instances of postwithdrawal depression will spontaneously remit within a few days to several weeks, there are still a substantial number of individuals whose severe and persistent depression requires treatment. Given the superior safety profile of SSRIs, particularly in relation to risk of suicide by medication overdose, use of these drugs is preferable to the use of TCAs.

Treatment of Anxiety Symptoms/Disorders. While a number of studies have shown chlordiazepoxide to be effective in the maintenance of alcoholics in long-term outpatient treatment, the potential for additive CNS depression produced by the concurrent use of alcohol and benzodiazepines is well recognized. Furthermore, the use of benzodiazepines may itself result in tolerance and dependence and may increase depressive symptoms.

Buspirone is a non-benzodiazepine anxiolytic that is less sedating than diazepam or clorazepate, does not interact with alcohol to impair psychomotor skills, and has a low potential for abuse. When combined with appropriate psychosocial treatment, buspirone appears useful in the treatment of alcoholics with persistent anxiety.

Currently, antipsychotics are indicated only in alcoholics with a coexistent psychotic disorder or for the treatment of alcoholic hallucinosis. Several placebo-controlled studies have found no advantage in the use of phenothiazines for treatment of anxiety, tension, and depression following detoxification. Because of their capacity to lower seizure threshold, antipsychotics should be used with caution in this population.

COMPARISON OF DSM-IV-TR AND ICD-10 DIAGNOSTIC CRITERIA

The ICD-10 and DSM-IV-TR criteria sets are nearly identical except for the following: the ICD-10 Diagnostic Criteria for Research for Alcohol Intoxication also lists flushed face and conjunctival injection as symptoms but does not include the DSM-IV-TR item for impairment in attention; the ICD-10 Diagnostic Criteria for Research for Alcohol Withdrawal require three symptoms from a list of ten, which includes headache and splits tachycardia and sweating into two separate items.

Substance-Related Disorders: Amphetamine

Consistent with the schema put forward by the DSM-IV-TR, this chapter defines the amphetamine-like substances to include the Phenylisopropylamines Amphetamine (AMPH), methamphetamine (METH), and phenylpropanolamine (PPA), the natural substances ephedrine and pseudoephedrine, and phenylethylamines including methylphenidate. While METH and AMPH cause the vast majority of abuse and dependence, use of any of these substances has been associated with abuse and dependence, so as a class these will be referred to as amphetamine-type stimulants, or ATS, in this chapter.

By far, the most widely abused ATS is METH, which is commonly known as meth, speed, crank, CR, wire, and jib, and in its recrystallized smoked form, ice, crystal, or glass. Legitimate forms of METH prescribed for attention-deficit/hyperactivity disorder (ADHD) and weight control (Methedrine, Desoxyn, and Adipex) undoubtedly represent a miniscule source of the total amount abused each year. AMPH, most prevalent in Western Europe, is commonly known as amp, bennies, dex, or black beauties, and is prescribed as Adderall, Dexedrine, and Dextrostat in the treatment of ADHD, narcolepsy, weight control, and depression. Other agents that have been designated as Schedule II controlled substances by the Drug Enforcement Administration are methylphenidate (Ritalin, Concerta) and phenmetrazine (Preludin). On the street, Ritalin is known as Rits or Vitamin R. A large number of Schedule III and IV phenylethylamines (benzphetamine, diethylproprion, mazindol, phendimetrazine, phenmetrazine, and phentermine) are used for weight control. There is no specific evidence that these substances represent a significant source of illicit diversion, and they are not further discussed in this chapter. ATS agents are also widely available in over-the-counter (OTC) preparations. PPA has been removed from the market, but ephedrine and pseudoephedrine are still very widely used as decongestants, and less so, phenylephrine and propylhexidrine.

However, it is uncommon that those who go on to amphetamine dependence continue to supply their habit through licit sources. Further, medically appropriate use of synthetic stimulants does not appear to pose a significant risk for the induction of substance-use disorders. This has been most closely examined for the widely prescribed methylphenidate (Ritalin) for ADHD; in this case, treatment may actually reduce the risk of developing substance abuse by controlling ADHD, which is itself a risk factor for substance abuse. Further, methylphenidate poses a low risk for medical complications. It has been postulated that the persistence of peripheral autonomic effects, as well as much longer half-life in the striatum, accounts for its low abuse potential relative to cocaine.

DIAGNOSIS

Consistent with the DSM-IV-TR perspective functionally equating amphetamines with cocaine, those diagnostic categories that are included are identical to those for Cocaine-Related Disorders, with the sole exception of omitting the specifier "With Onset During Withdrawal" from the diagnostic category Amphetamine-Induced Anxiety Disorder. For the substance use disorders, amphetamine (ATS) abuse and dependence will be discussed below. Of the substance-induced disorders, the critical diagnoses of ATS intoxication and withdrawal are described. The specific complications of delirium, psychotic disorders, mood disorders, anxiety disorders, sexual dysfunctions, and sleep disorders all are described under intoxication. Amphetamine-induced mood and sleep disorders also allow for specifiers of onset during withdrawal.

Amphetamine Dependence

ATS dependence is diagnosed when a maladaptive pattern of use leads to clinically significant impairment or distress, as defined by three or more of the following that occur during the same 12-month period: (1) evidence of tolerance, (2) occurrence of withdrawal, or the reuse of the substance to alleviate withdrawal, and (3) compulsive use of amphetamines as defined by three or more of the following: using more than intended, (4) desire or efforts to reduce use, (5) occupying significant time in drug-related activities, (6) loss of social, occupational, or recreational pursuits, or (7) continued use despite known adverse, physical, or psychological consequences (see DSM-IV-TR diagnostic criteria for Substance Dependence in Chapter 13, page 125).

Amphetamine Abuse

The diagnosis of ATS abuse requires a maladaptive pattern of use that does not meet the criteria for dependence, and that results in clinically significant impairment or distress. In the preceding 12 months, recurrent substance use must result in one or more of the following: failure to meet major role obligations, placement of the user in physical danger, legal entanglements, or social/interpersonal problems (see DSM-IV-TR diagnostic criteria for Substance Abuse in Chapter 13, page 125).

Amphetamine Intoxication

Specific diagnostic criteria are provided for ATS intoxication. These include recent use of an ATS (criterion A), clinically significant maladaptive behavioral or psychological changes occurring after the use of the ATS (criterion B), two or more specified physiological changes after the use of the ATS (criterion C), and the requirement that the condition is not accounted for by another mental or medical condition (criterion D). A specifier "with perceptual disturbances" is included.

The specifics of criteria B and C provide a useful clinical consensus of the syndrome of ATS intoxication (see Table 15-1 for a list of the maladaptive behaviors of Criterion B, with comments in parentheses). Importantly, psychosis and paranoia are experienced by approximately one-third of ATS-dependent subjects and occur at a significantly greater rate than for cocaine or Ecstasy. With chronic use, the incidence of psychosis increases. Furthermore, the occurrence of psychotic symptoms correlates with heavier use, co-use of benzodiazepines, and preexisting mental illness. Cognitive disturbances include visual, tactile, and auditory hallucinations. Visual hallucinations often suggest an underlying "organic" cause to psychosis, and formication, the feeling of "bugs crawling under the skin" is highly suggestive of ATS or cocaine intoxication. Psychosis in the presence of an intact sensorium, where the subject is aware that the hallucinations are not real, may differentiate ATS-

induced psychosis from psychotic states such as schizophrenia. Nonetheless, ATS-induced psychosis shares many features with other acute psychotic states. Of concern, ATS-induced psychosis can sometimes persist for

DSM-IV-TR Diagnostic Criteria

292.89 AMPHETAMINE INTOXICATION AND 292.89 COCAINE INTOXICATION

A. Recent use of amphetamine or a related substance (e.g.,methylphenidate)/cocaine.
B. Clinically significant maladaptive behavioral or psychological changes (e.g., euphoria or affective blunting; changes in sociability; hypervigilance; interpersonal sensitivity; anxiety, tension, or anger, stereotyped behaviors; impaired judgment; or impaired social or occupational functioning) that developed during, or shortly after, use of amphetamine or a related substance/cocaine.
C. Two (or more) of the following, developing during, or shortly after, use of amphetamine or a related substance/cocaine:

(1) tachycardia or bradycardia
(2) pupillary dilation
(3) elevated or lowered blood pressure
(4) perspiration or chills
(5) nausea or vomiting
(6) evidence of weight loss
(7) psychomotor agitation or retardation
(8) muscular weakness, respiratory depression, chest pain, or cardiac arrhythmias
(9) confusion, seizures, dyskinesias, dystonias, or coma

D. The symptoms are not due to a general medical condition and are not better accounted for by another mental disorder.

Specify if:

With Perceptual Disturbances

Note: This is a summary of two criteria sets.

Reprinted with permission from *DSM-IV-TR Guidebook.* Copyright 2004, Michael B First, Allen Frances, and Harold Alan Pincus.

Table 15-1	Maladaptive Behaviors Listed in Criterion B of Amphetamine Intoxication, with Comments and Explications in Parentheses

Euphoria or affective blunting (felt to occur in longer-term users)
Changes in sociability (e.g., being hypertalkative, more interactive or more withdrawn, increased libido)
Hypervigilance (with ideas of reference that can proceed to frank paranoia)
Interpersonal sensitivity
Anxiety, tension, or anger (agitated behavior and altercations are common)
Stereotyped behavior (picking at skin, grooming, pacing, disassembly/reassembly of objects)
Impaired judgment (often seen as sexual promiscuity)
Impaired social or occupational functioning

Table 15-2	Physiological Disturbances Listed in Criterion C of Amphetamine Intoxication, with Comments and Explications in Parentheses

Tachycardia or reflex bradycardia
Papillary dilatation
Elevated or lowered blood pressure
Perspiration or chills
Nausea or vomiting
Evidence of weight loss
Psychomotor agitation or retardation (an excited delirium is described as for cocaine, along with tremor)
Muscle weakness, respiratory depression, chest pain, or cardiac arrhythmia
Confusion, seizures, dyskinesias, dystonias or coma (Headaches and tinnitus are additional neurological symptoms that have also been described as occurring)

months following cessation of drug use. The physiological disturbances in criterion C are listed in Table 15-2, again with comments in parentheses.

Amphetamine Withdrawal

While the intoxicated state is characterized as euphoric, expansive, and activated, and often presents with agitation, violence, and/or psychosis, ATS withdrawal is characterized by decreased energy and mood. The clinician often evaluates such individuals who become suicidal during the "crash." The period of most intense withdrawal may last days, though a protracted state of depression and low energy often persists for weeks. Resurgence of craving when exposed to drug-associated environmental cues probably persists for years, as is the case with other substance-dependence disorders. The occurrence of ATS withdrawal usually occurs in those who have progressed from the diagnosis of abuse to dependence.

The ATS withdrawal diagnosis requires cessation or reduction of ATS use that has been heavy or prolonged (criterion A), dysphoric mood, and at least two physiologic changes that occur from a few hours to days after cessation of use (i.e., fatigue; vivid, unpleasant dreams; insomnia and hypersomnia; increased appetite; psychomotor retardation or agitation) which cause clinically significant distress or impairment in social, occupational, or other important areas of functioning (criteria B and C); and the requirement that the condition is not accounted for by another mental or medical condition (criterion D).

Both the longer half-lives of ATS relative to other psychostimulants, as well as the broader-spectrum effects on nerve terminal catecholamine levels, result in prolonged withdrawal and abstinence states. ATS withdrawal states occur in some 87% of users. The acute phase appears to last up to 5 days, with some symptoms persisting for weeks, possibly months, following the acute phase.

DSM-IV-TR Diagnostic Criteria

292.0 AMPHETAMINE WITHDRAWAL AND 292.0 COCAINE WITHDRAWAL

A. Cessation of (or reduction in) amphetamine (or related substance)/cocaine use that has been heavy and prolonged.
B. Dysphoric mood and two (or more) of the following physiological changes, developing within a few hours to several days after Criterion A:

   (1) fatigue
   (2) vivid, unpleasant dreams
   (3) insomnia or hypersomnia
   (4) increased appetite
   (5) psychomotor retardation or agitation

C. The symptoms in Criterion B cause clinically significant distress or impairment in social, occupational, or other important areas of functioning.
D. The symptoms are not due to a general medical condition and are not better accounted for by another mental disorder.

Note: This is a summary of two criteria sets.

Reprinted with permission from *DSM-IV-TR Guidebook*. Copyright 2004, Michael B First, Allen Frances, and Harold Alan Pincus.

Since neurocognitive impairment occurs early in withdrawal, clinicians should be cognizant that instructions to individuals in withdrawal be kept simple and written out. Decision making, as has been known anecdotally for years, appears affected. Over months, these cognitive deficits may partially remit to a greater extent than in opiate abusers. Severe craving marks the early withdrawal phase, leading to high recidivism. Sleep disturbance is accompanied by increase in REM sleep.

Medical Complications

For heavy users, a number of general consequences of ATS dependence will be obvious; malnutrition and cachexia from sleep deprivation, exposure to the elements and so on. Skin disorders, including infections and lesions from "picking" are common. More serious are ATS-related deaths due to cardiac arrhythmias, stroke, and rhabdomyolysis that have been documented since the 1950s. These problems were similar to those reported for the more widely abused cocaine. A number of factors place ATS users at high risk for contraction of HIV, and likely Hepatitis B and C, infection.

Some of the medical complications result from exposure to contaminants during ATS use. The production methods for ATS determine what contaminants are present in illicit manufacture. Contaminants are both toxic, as well as stimulants in their own right.

Many of the cardiovascular complications for ATS result from peripheral catecholamine toxicity. This explains why the principal drug interactions of concern involve the psychotropics that are meant to augment catecholamine function. Of most concern are the monoamine oxidase inhibitors, whose action can potentiate ATS toxicity for 2 to 3 weeks following cessation of use. Similarly, tricyclic antidepressants can potentiate effects of ATS, as well as increase absorption and slow hepatic metabolism

HIV and Immunomodulatory Effects. Intravenous drug use is the fastest growing route for transmission of HIV infection. In addition, ATS use is associated with unsafe sexual behaviors, including participation in unprotected sex and involvement with multiple sexual partners. Once HIV has been contracted, ATS abuse leads to accelerated CNS and cardiovascular toxicity. METH and AMPH are immunomodulators, and in fact, may be immunotoxic to peripheral T cells, mitogen-stimulated lymphocytes, and spleen cells.

Pulmonary. In a large autopsy series of individuals who died from ATS use, pulmonary edema was present in 70% of cases, as well as pneumonia (8.2%), and emphysema (5.1%). Birefringent crystals at bifurcation of pulmonary vessels is associated with intravenous abuse of crushed pills that contain insoluble fillers such as talc, microcrystalline cellulose, corn starch, or cotton fibers. With sufficient deposition, small vessel thrombosis and granuloma formation ensues. The changes ultimately reduce pulmonary perfusion, and increase pulmonary vascular resistance.

Gastrointestinal. In METH-related deaths, the sum of liver-related complications is second highest among organ systems. Fatty liver (16.2%), cirrhosis (9.0%), portal triaditis (6.1%), and hepatitis (4.1%) have been detected. This may relate to the high comorbidity with alcohol dependence, though the exact contribution is unknown.

Cardiovascular. Both cocaine and ATS cause similar vascular toxicity, largely related to catecholamine excess. Hearts of stimulant abusers develop areas of fibrosis and contraction band necrosis, and usually are increased in weight. As well, coronary artery disease is accelerated. Aortic dissection is a less well known but catastrophic complication of METH use. Cardiotoxic effects are only partly reversible. Of note, heart failure in children treated with Ritalin is so rare as to be at the case report level.

Central Nervous System. As opposed to the medical complications described above, which often are discerned at autopsy, CNS effects including psychosis and stroke are common presenting symptoms in emergency departments.

Seizures are one of the most common presentations of ATS intoxication to emergency rooms. In association with an uncontrollable delirium, they can quickly lead to death if not controlled. Following decreases in ATS blood levels, individuals who abuse ATS are not left at increased risk for reoccurrence of seizures unless CNS lesions from prior stroke have developed.

Hyperthermia is related to a number of causes in those presenting with METH intoxication. Increased motor activity, with reduced heat dissipation from peripheral vasoconstriction, is the proximate cause. It is also likely that direct affects on hypothalamic thermal regulation exist.

Renal. Rhabdomyolysis is clearly the major concern for renal impairment; there does not appear to be independent toxicity to the kidney. METH, however, is an increasingly common cause of rhabdomyolysis, and is often associated with hyperthermia. Myoglobin and myoglobin breakdown products cause tubular obstruction. Renal damage results from hypotension and renal ischemia secondary to metabolic derangements secondary to rhabdomyolysis, including phosphorus and potassium imbalance, and tubular obstruction due to catabolic product accumulation.

Effects on the Fetus. Fetal loss, developmental delay, and subsequent learning disabilities are potential complications of ATS use during pregnancy. Most recent evidence suggests a small effect of newborn birthweight, and a low incidence (4%) of overt ATS withdrawal in newborns of METH-dependent mothers.

TREATMENT

There are few studies that specifically address the treatment of ATS use disorders. This reflects the traditional focus on cocaine use disorders. Even for cocaine, effective pharmacotherapies are lacking compared to treatment of alcohol- and opiate-dependent individuals. Behavioral treatment approaches remain the mainstay of treatment of psychostimulant use disorders, and those whose efficacy is supported in the cocaine use disorders are assumed will be effective for ATS use disorders. Outcomes in psychosocial treatment cohorts do appear to be similar.

Several unique aspects of ATS addiction must be addressed for treatment to be effective. Because ATS users begin to experience adverse consequences of their use later than comparable cocaine addicts, they appear to be more ambivalent to enter treatment, probably because they reason that since they have gotten along fairly well up to that point, why should they begin the difficult process of treatment? Thus, treatment entry and retention rates are lower than those for individuals with cocaine dependence, and necessitates outreach programs to enhance treatment engagement. A number of co-occurring problems, such as high HIV and hepatitis infection rates, homelessness, and child-rearing difficulties, must be integrated into the treatment approach. Further, the continued neurocognitive deficits in METH-dependent individuals increase the need to apply outreach attempts to noncompliant individuals. Association with difficult-to-alter behaviors (sexual/social and weight loss) means those "rewards" must be coopted by substitution of other options, such as referral to self-help groups for weight loss. As for any addiction, the need to separate reinforcing social contacts from the addict's lifestyle is a difficult process. Abuse by those seeking performance enhancement may be targeted through education programs and drug screening programs, such as those that have been so successful in the military.

Treatment of ATS Intoxication

Management of acute intoxication is guided by the presenting medical and psychiatric symptoms. In ATS intoxication, there are no direct receptor targets to achieve blockade; though dopamine receptor blockade theoretically should be useful in blocking acute and or chronic affects of ATS, this has not proven to be the case. Anxiety and agitation are first treated by an environment that reduces stimulation and provides orientation, with staff providing reassurance and talk downs. Physical restraints should be avoided, as these may worsen rhabdomyolysis or hyperthermia. When nonpharmacological means are insufficient, benzodiazepines, typically lorazepam or diazepam, are first-line treatments since they protect against imminent seizures. Antipsychotics for agitation should be avoided because of the risk of worsening hyperthermia or rhabdomyolysis if neuroleptic malignant syndrome were to occur, and their ability to lower seizure threshold. However, since benzodiazepines run the risk of disinhibiting some individuals, typical antipsychotics are often the preferred choice.

For psychosis and paranoia, high potency antipsychotics, typically haloperidol, are used. This avoids the

anticholinergic effects that may worsen delirium and hyperthermia. If oral use of the ATS is suspected or confirmed, charcoal gastric lavage is indicated. Acidification of the urine with ammonium chloride solution or cranberry juice may be used to enhance ATS excretion, though should be avoided if rhabdomyolysis is a concern, since this would worsen dissociation and precipitation of myoglobin or where renal or hepatic dysfunction are an issue. Basic life support and initial management are needed for critical conditions such as myocardial ischemia or arrythmia, stroke or seizures, hyperthermia, and rhabdomyolysis. Hypertension and tachycardia, if not responsive to benzodiazepine sedation, may require treatment with an alpha-adrenergic blocker, typically phentolamine. Agents with beta blockade activity, such as propanolol and labetolol, must be avoided as alpha-adrenergic tone can increase, leading to a worsening of the clinical condition.

Treatment of ATS Withdrawal

Emergency considerations in the withdrawal phase of ATS intoxication are principally psychiatric. The week following cocaine withdrawal is associated with increased risk of silent myocardial ischemia. Because this is hypothesized to result from coronary vasospasm, this may not generalize to ATS withdrawal. Otherwise, medical complications of ATS withdrawal, such as myalgias, involuntary motor movements, and so on can be treated symptomatically and should spontaneously remit.

The use of antidepressants for 3 to 4 weeks following cessation of ATS use is suggested, because depression is a hallmark of ATS withdrawal. Often, allowing the individual increased time to sleep and reestablishment of normal nutrition is quite helpful. Where needed, the use of trazodone for sleep or short-term benzodiazepines for anxiety is needed along with antidepressant therapy.

Psychosocial Treatments for ATS Dependence

Cognitive behavioral therapy forms the basis of many treatments for psychostimulant dependence. Contingency incentives, skills training, and family member participation are helpful for maintaining ATS abstinence. An extension of such a combined approach, termed the community-reinforcement-plus-vouchers approach, combines couples counseling, vocational training and skills training, and contingency management through rewards for negative urine testing. This combined approach, developed for the treatment of cocaine dependence, is shown to improve treatment retention and decrease drug use and is likely to be similarly useful for other ATS dependencies.

Several other psychosocial treatments might be applied to individuals with ATS use disorders. Relapse prevention, easily combined with widely used drug counseling, systematically teaches individuals the skills needed to avoid drug use through training in assertiveness and refusal skills, how to cope with craving, how to deal with relapses, and how to recognize patterns of behavior or thinking that lead to relapse. Network therapy, meant to engage family and community in supporting drug-free functioning, appears well suited to ATS abuse and dependence, where acquisition appears more linked to community networks than stressful street "buys."

Residential treatment for pregnant women and the homeless is likely to be of benefit for stabilization of ATS-dependent subjects, though there is no specific indication for stimulants. The prolonged nature of ATS-induced withdrawal, and the association with aggressivity and violence, will often make inpatient psychiatric stabilization necessary. It is unknown whether transition to therapeutic communities or half-way houses will be of greater benefit to ATS-dependent subjects that those with other substance use disorders, or be superior in outcome to outpatient-based programs.

Pharmacotherapy for ATS Dependence

As is the case with cocaine use disorders, effective pharmacotherapies for amphetamine use disorders are not available. The main role of pharmacotherapy is acute symptomatic relief, and treatment of comorbid conditions. Behavioral treatments and self-help groups remain the mainstay of treatment for the many individuals suffering from ATS dependence.

COMPARISON OF DSM-IV-TR AND ICD-10 DIAGNOSTIC CRITERIA

The ICD-10 criteria sets for other stimulant intoxication and withdrawal are almost the same as the DSM-IV-TR criteria sets for amphetamine intoxication and withdrawal except that the ICD-10 Diagnostic Criteria for Research include drug craving as an additional item. ICD-10 combines amphetamines and caffeine into a single substance class, referred to as "other stimulants, including caffeine."

16   Substance-Related Disorders: Caffeine

Caffeine is the most widely consumed psychoactive substance in the world. In North America, it is estimated that more than 80% of adults and children consume caffeine regularly. This cultural integration of caffeine use can make the recognition of mental disorders associated with caffeine use particularly difficult. It is important, however, for the clinician to recognize the role of caffeine as a psychoactive substance capable of producing a variety of psychiatric syndromes, despite the pervasive and well-accepted use of caffeine

Caffeine Intoxication

DIAGNOSIS

DSM-IV-TR defines caffeine intoxication as a set of symptoms that develop during or shortly after caffeine use. There may be two kinds of presentation associated with caffeine intoxication. The first presentation is associated with the *acute* ingestion of a large amount of caffeine and represents an acute drug overdose condition. The second presentation is associated with the *chronic* consumption of large amounts of caffeine and results in a more complicated presentation. Caffeine intoxication has long been recognized as a syndrome produced by the ingestion of an excessive amount of caffeine.

The primary features of caffeine intoxication can be found in the diagnostic criteria from DSM-IV-TR. The diagnostic decision tree for caffeine intoxication, caffeine-induced anxiety disorder, and caffeine-induced sleep disorder is shown in Figure 16-1. One study that utilized a random-digit-dial telephone interview survey of 162 users of caffeine examined the types of symptoms reported by persons who had experienced some features of caffeine intoxication. Results from that study showed that two-thirds of participants had experienced at least one of the DSM-IV-TR symptoms related to caffeine intoxication in the previous year. The most common symptoms reported in decreasing

---

DSM-IV-TR Diagnostic Criteria

305.90 CAFFEINE INTOXICATION

A. Recent consumption of caffeine, usually in excess of 250 mg (e.g., more than 2–3 cups of brewed coffee).
B. Five (or more) of the following signs, developing during, or shortly after, caffeine use:

    (1) restlessness
    (2) nervousness
    (3) excitement
    (4) insomnia
    (5) flushed face
    (6) diuresis
    (7) gastrointestinal disturbance
    (8) muscle twitching
    (9) rambling flow of thought and speech
    (10) tachycardia or cardiac arrhythmia
    (11) periods of inexhaustibility
    (12) psychomotor agitation

C. The symptoms in Criterion B cause clinically significant distress or impairment in social, occupational, or other important areas of functioning.
D. The symptoms are not due to a general medical condition and are not better accounted for by another mental disorder (e.g., an anxiety disorder).

Reprinted with permission from the *Diagnostic and Statistical Manual of Mental Disorders*, 4th ed., Text Rev. Copyright 2000 American Psychiatric Association.

---

order of frequency were frequent urination, restlessness, insomnia, nervousness, and excitement (all which were at rates greater than 20%). In addition, 24% reported heart pounding in response to high caffeine use (although this is not one of the DSM-IV-TR criteria).

In a study of 124 general hospital patients, the most common somatic symptoms that individuals reported as associated with caffeine intake (i.e., symptoms not specified as associated with either caffeine intoxication or caffeine withdrawal) were in descending order of frequency: diuresis, insomnia, withdrawal headaches, diarrhea, anxiety, tachycardia, and tremulousness.

In addition to the characteristics of caffeine intoxication noted in DSM-IV-TR, there have been reports of

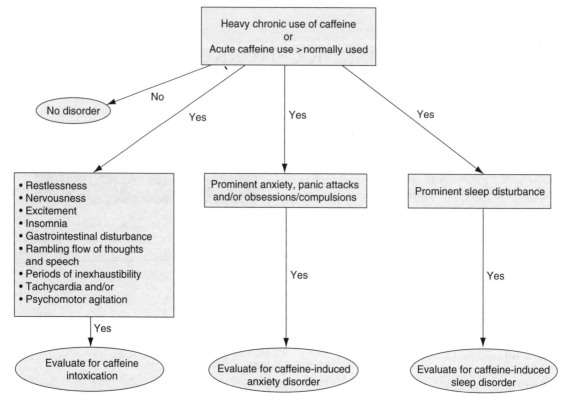

Figure 16-1 *Diagnostic decision tree for caffeine intoxication disorder, caffeine-induced anxiety disorder, and caffeine-induced sleep disorder.*

fever, irritability, tremors, sensory disturbances, tachypnea and headaches associated with cases of caffeine intoxication. Although a wide variety of symptoms of caffeine intoxication have been reported, the most common signs and symptoms appear to be anxiety and nervousness, diuresis, insomnia, gastrointestinal disturbances, tremors, tachycardia, and psychomotor agitation.

Course

In an individual who is not tolerant to caffeine, acute caffeine ingestion producing caffeine intoxication is a time-limited condition that will rapidly resolve with cessation of caffeine use, consistent with the relatively short half-life of caffeine (3–6 hours). In an individual who has caffeine intoxication superimposed on chronic caffeine use, abrupt termination of all caffeine use may lead to caffeine-withdrawal symptoms (described in detail in the section on caffeine withdrawal). Because symptoms of caffeine withdrawal can partially overlap with symptoms of caffeine intoxication (e.g., nervousness and anxiety), the time course of symptom resolution can be expected to be protracted, lasting several days to a week or more.

While many people may experience some of the symptoms of caffeine intoxication at some point in their lives, caffeine users do not generally seek out the experience of caffeine intoxication (unlike many other drugs of abuse). The symptoms of caffeine intoxication tend to be perceived as unpleasant, and caffeine users tend to titrate their dose of caffeine to avoid intoxication.

Although caffeine intoxication is clearly related to caffeine ingestion, it is not simply the result of a person consuming a high dose of caffeine. Rather, caffeine intoxication represents the relationship between the dose of caffeine consumed, the degree of acquired tolerance to caffeine in that person, and the individual's sensitivity to caffeine.

Tolerance represents an acquired change in responsiveness by an individual as a result of exposure to a drug, such that an increased amount of the drug is required to produce the same effect, or a lesser effect is produced by the same dose of the drug. In a person who regularly consumes caffeine, tolerance may occur to the acute effects of caffeine. Thus, a sensitive person with no tolerance to caffeine might have signs and symptoms of caffeine intoxication in response to a rela-

Table 16-1	Typical Caffeine Content of Foods and Medications
Substance	**Caffeine content**
Brewed coffee	100 mg/6 oz
Instant coffee	70 mg/6 oz
Espresso	40 mg/1 oz
Decaffeinated coffee	4 mg/6 oz
Brewed tea	40 mg/6 oz
Instant tea	30 mg/6 oz
Canned or bottled tea	20 mg/12 oz
Caffeinated soda	40 mg/12 oz
Cocoa beverage	7 mg/6 oz
Chocolate milk	4 mg/6 oz
Dark chocolate	20 mg/1 oz
Milk chocolate	6 mg/1 oz
Caffeinated water	100 mg/16.9 oz
Coffee ice cream or yogurt	50 mg/8 oz
Caffeinated gum	50 mg/stick
Caffeine-containing analgesics	32–65 mg/tablet
Stimulants	100–200 mg/tablet
Weight-loss aids	40–100 mg/tablet
Sports nutrition	100 mg/tablet

Source: Griffiths RR, Juliano LM, and Chausmer AL (2003) Caffeine pharmacology and clinical effects. In *Principles of Addiction Medicine*, Graham AN, Schultz TK, Mayo-Smith M, et al. (eds). ASAM, Chevy Chase, Maryland.

Table 16-2	Differential Diagnosis of Caffeine Intoxication
Manic episode	Panic disorder
Amphetamine/ cocaine intoxication	Generalized anxiety disorder
Sedative, hypnotic or anxiolytic withdrawal	Medication-induced side effects (e.g., akathisia)
Nicotine withdrawal	Sleep disorders

tively low dose of caffeine (such as 100 mg, the amount found in a typical cup of brewed coffee) (Table 16-1), whereas another person with a high daily consumption of caffeine would show no evidence of intoxication with a similar dose.

Although caffeine intoxication can occur in the context of habitual chronic consumption of high doses, probably most often it occurs after inadvertent overdosing. Examples include overdosing of intravenous caffeine to children in medical settings (e.g., for respiratory stimulating effects), excessive caffeine consumption in tablet form by students who fail to appreciate the dose being ingested (e.g., to study through the night), and the person who unknowingly consumes a highly concentrated form of caffeine (e.g., caffeinated coffee brewed with caffeine-containing water to create an especially high dose of caffeine in the coffee).

Differential Diagnosis

The diagnosis of caffeine intoxication is based on the history and clinical presentation of the individual. Ideally, the extent of caffeine exposure can also be assessed by a serum or saliva assay of the caffeine level. In the past, caffeine use has often been overlooked in individuals presenting with symptoms consistent with a caffeine use disorder. However, it may be that there is presently a greater awareness of the deleterious effects of caffeine, making clinicians more sensitive to

the inclusion of caffeine in a differential diagnosis, and individuals who ingest caffeine more aware of the possible role of excessive caffeine in somatic and psychological symptoms.

Several conditions should be included in the differential diagnosis of caffeine intoxication (Table 16-2). These include other substance-abuse-related disorders (amphetamine or cocaine intoxication; withdrawal from sedatives, hypnotics, anxiolytics, or nicotine), other psychiatric disorders (panic disorder, generalized anxiety disorder, mania, and sleep disorders), medication-induced side effects (e.g., akathisia), and somatic disorders (e.g., pheochromocytoma, hyperthyroidism, gastroesophageal reflux, and arrhythmia).

TREATMENT

The first step in evaluating an individual with a possible diagnosis of caffeine intoxication is to obtain a careful history about all recent caffeine consumption. The possible use of beverages and medications—both prescription and over-the-counter (OTC) diet aids and energy pills—should be reviewed. Some beverages (e.g., caffeine-containing soft drinks) and medications (e.g., energy pills, aids to combat sleep, or diet pills) may not be recognized by the individual as containing caffeine. The amount of caffeine acutely consumed should help clarify the diagnosis of caffeine intoxication, although it is important to determine whether the individual has been chronically consuming high doses of caffeine. If this is the case, the individual may be tolerant and therefore less likely to be experiencing caffeine intoxication. However, some clinicians have reported that caffeine intoxication can occur even in the context of chronic caffeine use.

If the individual is unable to provide an accurate history of recent caffeine consumption (e.g., because of delirium after a caffeine overdose), the individual should be evaluated on an emergency basis and medically monitored.

The primary approach to the treatment of caffeine intoxication is to teach the individual about the effects of excessive caffeine consumption. In individuals who are resistant to accepting the role of caffeine in their presenting symptoms, it may be useful to suggest a trial-off caffeine as both a diagnostic and a potentially therapeutic probe.

Caffeine Withdrawal

DIAGNOSIS

Like caffeine intoxication, there is a long history of recognition that some people also can experience symptoms of caffeine withdrawal. The observation of headaches associated with the cessation of caffeine use has been repeatedly observed and is now a well-established characteristic of caffeine withdrawal. Other symptoms, in roughly decreasing order of frequency, are fatigue, sleepiness/drowsiness, dysphoric mood (e.g., miserable, decreased well-being/contentedness), difficulty concentrating, work difficulty, depression, anxiety, irritability, and influenza-like symptoms (e.g., nausea/vomiting, muscle aches/stiffness, hot and cold spells, heavy feelings in arms or legs) (Table 16-3). In addition to these symptoms, caffeine withdrawal may produce impairment in psychomotor, vigilance, and cognitive performances, increases in cerebral blood flow, and changes in quantitative electroencephalography (EEG) activity.

The proposed criteria for a DSM-IV-TR research diagnosis of caffeine withdrawal require the presence of headache and one or more of the following: marked fatigue or drowsiness, marked anxiety or depression, and nausea or vomiting. Problems with this approach are that it does not reflect the independence of headache and nonheadache withdrawal symptoms and it excludes several withdrawal symptoms that have been repeatedly documented: difficulty concentrating, work difficulty or feeling unmotivated, and irritable or dysphoric mood.

On the basis of expanded literature, it is proposed that the diagnosis of caffeine withdrawal requires the

presence of three or more of the following five symptom clusters: (1) headache, (2) fatigue or drowsiness, (3) dysphoric mood (including irritability, depression, or anxiety), (4) difficulty concentrating or work difficulty, and (5) nausea or vomiting.

The key steps in establishing a diagnosis of caffeine withdrawal are to determine the history of the person's caffeine consumption from all dietary sources, and then establish whether there has been a significant decrease in caffeine intake. The diagnostic decision tree for caffeine dependence and caffeine withdrawal is shown in Figure 16-2. Caffeine withdrawal is probably more common than is generally recognized, and it seems there is a tendency for people to attribute the symptoms of caffeine withdrawal to other etiologies besides caffeine (e.g., having the flu, or a bad day). Caffeine withdrawal may be particularly common in medical settings where individuals are required to abstain from food and fluids, such as before surgical procedures and certain diagnostic tests. In addition, caffeine withdrawal may occur in settings where the use of caffeine-containing products is restricted or banned, such as inpatient psychiatric wards. The most common feature of caffeine withdrawal is headache (Table 16-4). Caffeine-withdrawal headache is typically described as gradual in development, diffuse, throbbing, and sometimes accompanied by nausea and vomiting. Caffeine-withdrawal headache usually resolves within 2 to 4 days, although some subjects continue to report sporadic headaches for as long as 11 days after cessation of caffeine use.

When symptoms of caffeine withdrawal occur, the severity can vary from mild to extreme. At its worst, caffeine withdrawal has been repeatedly documented to produce clinically significant distress or impairment in daily functioning and, on rare occasions, to be totally incapacitating.

Individuals with high daily caffeine consumption or individuals with a history of frequent headaches may be at increased risk for developing caffeine withdrawal or caffeine-withdrawal headaches.

Caffeine abstinence has been shown to contribute to the incidence and severity of postoperative headache after general anesthesia. In individuals with a history of caffeine consumption who received caffeine on the day of a surgical procedure, the rate of postoperative headaches was lower than in those who received placebo.

Table 16-3	Signs and Symptoms Associated with Caffeine Withdrawal

Headache
Fatigue, lethargy, sluggishness
Sleepiness, drowsiness
Dysphoric mood
Difficulty concentrating
Work difficulty, unmotivated
Depression
Anxiety
Irritability
Nausea or vomiting
Muscle aches or stiffness

Table 16-4	Features of Caffeine-Withdrawal—Headache

Gradual onset between 12 and 40 hours
Worse with exercise, Valsalva maneuver
Can be accompanied by flu-like symptoms (including nausea, vomiting)
Diffuse, throbbing, severe

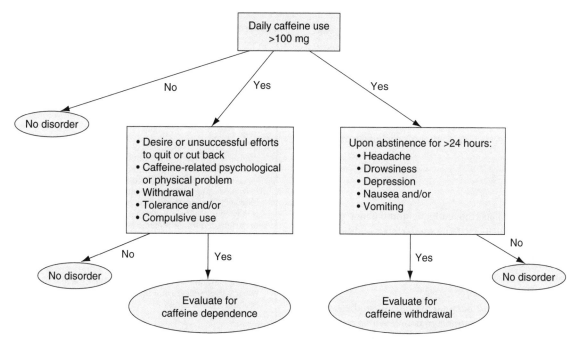

Figure 16-2 *Diagnostic decision tree for caffeine-dependence disorder and caffeine-withdrawal disorder.*

Differential Diagnosis

Caffeine withdrawal should be considered when evaluating individuals presenting with headaches, fatigue, sleepiness, mood disturbances, or impaired concentration. The differential diagnosis of caffeine withdrawal includes: viral illnesses; sinus conditions; other types of headaches such as migraine, tension, postanesthetic; other drug withdrawal states such as amphetamine or cocaine withdrawal; and idiopathic drug reactions.

TREATMENT

There have been few studies attempting to address the treatment of caffeine withdrawal, although it has frequently been observed that the symptoms of caffeine withdrawal can be alleviated with the consumption of caffeine If the medical recommendation is made to eliminate or substantially reduce caffeine consumption, then it may be useful to recommend a tapering dose schedule rather than abrupt discontinuation.

Caffeine Dependence

DIAGNOSIS

Caffeine dependence, a diagnosis not officially included in DSM-IV-TR, may be an unrecognized condition with a higher prevalence than is generally appreciated.

Clinicians do not typically think to inquire about caffeine use and about problematic use consistent with a diagnosis of caffeine dependence. However, probing for evidence of caffeine dependence may be useful, and it would be reasonable to focus upon the DSM-IV-TR criteria for dependence that are more appropriate for a substance that is widely available and generally culturally accepted. Thus, the clinician should probe for evidence of tolerance, withdrawal, and continued use despite a doctor's recommendation that the person cut down or stop using caffeine, use despite other problems associated with caffeine, often using larger amounts or over a longer period than intended, or persistent desires and/or difficulties in decreasing or discontinuing use.

Differential Diagnosis

The diagnosis of caffeine dependence includes symptoms that can also contribute to a diagnosis of caffeine intoxication and caffeine withdrawal, and both of these conditions should be included in the differential diagnosis of an individual with possible caffeine dependence. Since intoxication and withdrawal symptoms can contribute to the diagnosis of dependence, conditions that overlap with these caffeine-related disorders should also be considered (and are reviewed above in their respective sections). When considering an individual for a possible diagnosis of caffeine dependence, the clinician should also consider other substance-dependence syndromes—especially those related to stimulants—in the differential diagnosis. Finally, the possible presence of other psychiatric conditions, such as depressive and anxiety disorders, should be assessed. These disorders may be more commonly found among individuals with caffeine dependence, and some of their presenting features (e.g., low mood, anxiety, and disturbed sleep) can overlap with the symptoms of caffeine intoxication and withdrawal, which commonly occur in caffeine dependence.

TREATMENT

Medical specialists frequently recommend that patients reduce or eliminate caffeine for certain conditions, including anxiety, insomnia, arrhythmias, palpitations and tachycardia, esophagitis/hiatal hernia, and fibrocystic disease Stopping caffeine use, however, can be difficult for some people.

While there have been no systematic studies which have examined the treatment of people with a clearly established diagnosis of caffeine dependence, a structured caffeine reduction treatment program (i.e., caffeine fading) can be valuable in achieving substantial reductions in caffeine consumption. These reports have generally noted success with a combination of gradual tapering of caffeine, self-monitoring of daily caffeine use, and reinforcement for decreased use. When attempting to reduce or eliminate caffeine use, several steps may be useful (Table 16-5). Since many individuals are not knowledgeable about sources of caffeine in their diets, education and history taking are likely to be important components of treatment. During caffeine tapering it may be useful for the individual to consume extra non-caffeinated fluids, to avoid herbal preparations which contain caffeine or other psychoactive drugs, to avoid the use of anxiolytics, and to maintain a diary throughout the time they are progressively decreasing their caffeine use in order to monitor their progress. Abrupt cessation of caffeine should be avoided in order to minimize withdrawal symptoms and increase the likelihood of long-term compliance with the dietary change.

Caffeine-Induced Anxiety Disorder

DIAGNOSIS

In addition to the symptom of anxiety that can be a component of caffeine intoxication and caffeine withdrawal, caffeine can also produce an anxiety disorder, caffeine-induced anxiety disorder.

The diagnosis of caffeine-induced anxiety disorder is based on evidence of an anxiety disorder etiologically

Table 16-5	A Method for Eliminating or Reducing Caffeine Use

Step 1: Use a daily diary to have the person identify all sources of caffeine in their diet, including different forms (i.e., brewed vs. instant coffee) and doses, for 1 week.

Step 2: Educate the patient about sources of caffeine. For example, some individuals might not be aware that caffeine is present in noncola soft drinks or analgesics. Calculate the total milligrams of caffeine consumed on a daily basis.

Step 3: With the collaboration of the patient, generate a graded dose reduction (i.e., fading schedule) of caffeine use. Reasonable decreases would be 10% of the initial dose every few days. Allow for individualization of the caffeine fading. Rather than attempting to progressively eliminate consumption of the preferred caffeine beverage, it may be useful to suggest that the patient substitute decaffeinated for caffeinated beverages. In the case of coffee or tea, caffeine fading can be accomplished by mixing caffeinated and decaffeinated beverages together and progressively increasing the proportion of decaffeinated beverage. It may be useful to have the patient maintain a diary throughout the time they are progressively decreasing their caffeine use, in order to monitor their progress.

Step 4: Discuss the possibility of relapse with the patient. Discuss triggers (i.e., antecedent conditions) for caffeine use and offer coping suggestions for high-risk relapse situations. Suggest that the patient continue to self-monitor caffeine consumption.

related to caffeine (see Figure 16-1 for caffeine intoxication, caffeine-induced anxiety disorder, and caffeine-induced sleep disorder). Other diagnostic considerations besides caffeine-induced anxiety disorder include caffeine intoxication and caffeine withdrawal, a primary anxiety disorder, and an anxiety disorder due to a general medical condition. Caffeine-induced anxiety disorder can occur in the context of caffeine intoxication or caffeine withdrawal, but the anxiety symptoms associated with the caffeine-induced anxiety disorder should be excessive relative to the anxiety seen in caffeine intoxication or caffeine withdrawal. In addition to these conditions, substance-induced anxiety disorder can be produced by a variety of other psychoactive substances (e.g., cocaine).

TREATMENT

Although there are no studies on the treatment of caffeine-induced anxiety disorder, guidelines for treatment should generally follow those recommended for the treatment of caffeine dependence (see Caffeine Dependence). Thus, an initial, careful assessment of caffeine consumption should be conducted, and a program of gradual decreasing caffeine use should be instituted (see Table 16-5). Abrupt cessation of caffeine use should be avoided to minimize withdrawal symptoms and to increase the likelihood of long-term compliance with the dietary change. Given the etiological role of caffeine in caffeine-induced anxiety disorder, the prudent course of treatment would avoid the use of pharmacological agents such as benzodiazepines for the treatment of the anxiety disorder until caffeine use has been eliminated. A temporary caffeine-free trial may be useful in persuading skeptical individuals about the role of caffeine in their anxiety symptoms.

Caffeine-Induced Sleep Disorder

DIAGNOSIS

Psychoactive substances can produce sleep disorders distinct from the sleep disturbances associated with intoxication or withdrawal produced by that substance. It has long been recognized that caffeine-containing products can produce sleep disturbances, primarily in the form of insomnia

The primary feature of a substance-induced sleep disorder is a sleep disturbance directly related to a psychoactive substance. The form of the disorder can be insomnia, hypersomnia, parasomnia, or mixed, although caffeine typically produces insomnia. In general, sleep disturbance can often be a feature of substance intoxication or withdrawal (although sleep disturbance does not typically occur with caffeine withdrawal), and caffeine-induced sleep disorder should be diagnosed in individuals who are having caffeine intoxication only if the symptoms of the sleep disturbance are excessive relative to what would typically be expected.

In addition to caffeine-induced sleep disorder, it is worth noting that complaints of poor sleep that are not severe enough to qualify as a "disorder" may also be related to caffeine use. The diagnosis of a caffeine-induced sleep disorder is based on evidence of a sleep disorder etiologically related to caffeine (see Figure 16-1 for caffeine intoxication, caffeine-induced anxiety disorder, and caffeine-induced sleep disorder). Other diagnostic considerations include caffeine intoxication and caffeine withdrawal, a primary sleep disorder, insomnia or hypersomnia related to another

mental disorder, and a sleep disorder due to a general medical condition. A caffeine-induced sleep disorder can occur in the context of caffeine intoxication or caffeine withdrawal, but the sleep symptoms associated with the caffeine-induced sleep disorder should be excessive relative to the sleep disturbance seen in caffeine intoxication or caffeine withdrawal.

As with caffeine-induced anxiety disorder, a trial of caffeine abstinence may be useful in confirming the diagnosis and helping to convince a skeptical individual about the etiological significance of caffeine in their sleep disorder.

TREATMENT

There are no studies on the treatment of caffeine-induced sleep disorder. As for other conditions associated with caffeine use, such as caffeine dependence, caffeine intoxication, and caffeine-induced anxiety disorder, general guidelines for caffeine reduction can be recommended. These include an initial assessment of total caffeine consumption followed by a program of gradually decreasing caffeine use (see Table 16-5). Abrupt cessation of caffeine use should be avoided to minimize withdrawal symptoms and to increase the likelihood of long-term compliance with the dietary change. Given the etiological role of caffeine in caffeine-induced sleep disorder, the use of pharmacological agents or other interventions to improve sleep should be avoided until an adequate trial-off caffeine establishes the presence of a noncaffeine-related sleep disorder.

COMPARISON OF DSM-IV-TR AND ICD-10 DIAGNOSTIC CRITERIA

ICD-10 includes caffeine-related disorders in its "Other Stimulant" class which also includes amphetamines. This results in the ICD-10 Diagnostic Criteria for Research for Caffeine Intoxication being the same as those for amphetamine intoxication.

CHAPTER

17 Substance-Related Disorders: Cannabis

Cannabis preparations, derived from the female *Cannabis sativa* plant, have been widely used for their psychotropic effects since the beginning of history. The drug is prepared in different ways in different parts of the world. The flowering tops and resin secreted by the female plant contain the highest concentrations of Δ-9-tetrahydrocannabinol (Δ-9-THC), the primary psychoactive component. Marijuana, the most common preparation, is made by drying and shredding the upper leaves, tops, stems, flowers, and seeds of the plant. Hashish is a more potent preparation made by extracting and drying the resin and sometimes also the compressed flowers. Hashish oil, which is even more potent, is distilled from hashish. Marijuana and hashish can be smoked either in the form of cigarettes or by using a pipe. Hashish, hashish oil, and less commonly marijuana, can be mixed with tea or food and taken orally. For the remainder of this chapter, we will refer to these preparations collectively as *cannabis*.

Intoxication occurs within minutes after smoking cannabis and typically persists for several hours. After eating foods containing cannabis, intoxication occurs after approximately an hour and can persist for 8 to 24 hours. The onset of intoxication after drinking cannabis steeped in tea is shorter, but not as rapid as after smoking, and has an intermediate duration of intoxication. Smoking is the predominant method of taking cannabis in most parts of the world including the United States.

As with other substances of abuse, DSM-IV-TR distinguishes a number of different cannabis-related diagnoses. These fall into two basic groups. The first group is defined by adverse effects resulting from cannabis use; these include cannabis abuse and cannabis dependence. The category of cannabis dependence includes a number of specifiers that indicate the presence or absence of physiological dependence, type of remission, and whether or not the individual has been in a controlled environment. The second set of cannabis-related disorders in DSM-IV-TR includes psychiatric syndromes presumed to be induced by cannabis. This group includes the following: cannabis intoxication, which is almost certainly induced by cannabis and consists of the common signs and symptoms that normally follow cannabis use; cannabis intoxication delirium, a degree of disturbance beyond that normally expected with ordinary intoxication; cannabis-induced psychotic disorder, which is subdivided into categories of psychosis with delusions and psychosis with hallucinations; and cannabis-induced anxiety disorder, which is also subdivided into several types as shown in Table 17-1.

To diagnose any of the cannabis-related disorders, it is important to obtain a detailed history of the individual's pattern of substance abuse (including abuse not only of cannabis but also of other substances) and to attempt to substantiate this report with toxicology screening for

Table 17-1	Cannabis-Related Disorders
Cannabis-Use Disorders	
304.3	Cannabis dependence
	With physiological dependence
	Without physiological dependence
	Early full remission
	Early partial remission
	Sustained full remission
	Sustained total remission
	In a controlled environment
305.20	Cannabis abuse
Cannabis-Induced Disorders	
292.89	Cannabis intoxication
	With perceptual disturbances
292.81	Cannabis intoxication delirium
292.11	Cannabis-induced psychotic disorder, with delusions
	With onset during intoxication
292.12	Cannabis-induced psychotic disorder, with hallucinations
	With onset during intoxication
292.89	Cannabis-induced anxiety disorder
	With onset during intoxication
	With generalized anxiety
	With panic attacks
	With obsessive–compulsive symptoms
	With phobic symptoms
292.9	Cannabis-related disorder not otherwise specified

Clinical Guide to the Diagnosis and Treatment of Mental Disorders. M. B. First and A. Tasman
© 2006 John Wiley & Sons, Ltd.   ISBN 0 470 019158

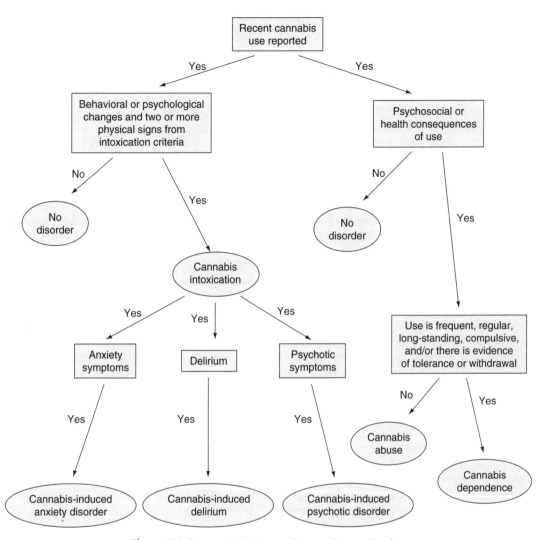

Figure 17-1 *Diagnostic decision tree for cannabis-use disorders.*

drugs of abuse. Individuals who smoke cannabis regularly can have substantial accumulations of THC in their fat stores. Thus, for weeks after cessation of smoking, detectable levels of cannabinoids may be found in the urine. However, a positive response on toxicology screening for cannabinoids cannot establish any of the cannabis-related diagnoses; it is useful only as an indicator that these diagnoses should be considered. A diagnostic decision tree for cannabis-related disorders is presented in Figure 17-1.

Cannabis-Use Disorders

DIAGNOSIS

Cannabis Dependence

It is uncommon to see individuals who exhibit cannabis dependence as their only diagnosis because such individuals rarely seek treatment, as they generally do not acknowledge that they have a problem and are unaware that treatment is available. Some individuals with this disorder will respond to offers for treatment because they realize that they are unable to stop use on their own and because they notice the deleterious effect of compulsive use. Therefore, the diagnosis of cannabis dependence will most often be made in individuals who present with other psychiatric problems, such as mood and anxiety disorders, and other substance-use disorders (see generic DSM-IV-TR diagnostic criteria for Substance Dependence, Chapter 13, page 125). Another manner in which individuals with cannabis dependence may come to the attention of clinicians is when they are arrested for possession of the substance or some crime related to cannabis abuse, such as driving under the influence of the drug. Nevertheless, cannabis dependence is probably underdiagnosed in both psychiatric and general medical populations because it is not considered.

The diagnosis of cannabis dependence cannot be made without obtaining a history indicating that the cannabis use is impairing the individual's ability to function either physically or psychologically. Areas to inquire about include the individual's performance at work, ability to carry out social and family obligations, and physical health. It is also important to find out how much of the individual's time is spent on cannabis-related activities and whether the individual has tried unsuccessfully to stop or cut down on use in the past. Although it has been our experience that people who have used cannabis daily over a period of years almost invariably report tolerance to many of the effects of cannabis and experience an unpleasant withdrawal state if use is discontinued, neither tolerance nor withdrawal is necessary for the diagnosis of cannabis dependence. When this diagnosis is made, it can be described further by the following specifiers: with or without physiological dependence, early full or partial remission, sustained full or partial remission, or in a controlled environment. These diagnostic distinctions must be based on the pattern of use reported by the individual.

Cannabis Abuse

Most individuals who are diagnosed with cannabis abuse have only recently started using cannabis (see DSM-IV-TR diagnostic criteria for Substance Abuse in Chapter 13 page 125). As with cannabis dependence, cannabis abuse is unlikely to be diagnosed unless some additional condition or circumstance brings the individual to medical attention. Teenagers often fall into this category because they spend time in supervised environments like school and home where responsible adults may intervene. Also, teenagers are more likely to have motor vehicle accidents while intoxicated because they are inexperienced drivers, and are more likely to be arrested for possession because they have a greater tendency to participate in risky behaviors of all types.

Although virtually all individuals with cannabis dependence meet the inclusion criteria for cannabis abuse, they cannot be given this diagnosis because the presence of cannabis dependence is an exclusion criterion. Undoubtedly, the vast majority of people with cannabis dependence would have been given the diagnosis of cannabis abuse until they developed dependence.

The difference between people with cannabis abuse and those with cannabis dependence is that the people with dependence have been using more regularly (one or more times per day) and for a longer duration (one or more years), and the acute problems associated with abuse have turned into the chronic problems associated with dependence.

Course

About a third of those adolescents who try cannabis will use it regularly for some period of time, whereas only about 10% will go on to develop long-term dependence lasting into adulthood. Even among these persistent users, the majority will stop use by age 30 years. Thus, it is possible to extrapolate from these figures that less than 2% of adults will exhibit cannabis dependence during their 20s and that probably less than 1% of adults will continue use into their 30s, suggesting a good prognosis for the majority of cannabis-dependent individuals under age 30 years. For the small minority who continue to suffer from cannabis dependence into their 30s, most follow a chronic or relapsing course similar to those who suffer from dependence on other substances

Cannabis abuse and dependence appear to pursue a benign course in many individuals; many studies have suggested that individuals suffering from these disorders do not differ in ability to function in society from matched control subjects who are not users. A few studies, have, however, described an "amotivational syndrome" associated with chronic cannabis use, characterized by subjective reports of lack of direction, motivation, and ambition. This "amotivational syndrome" appears to result from the effects of continuous intoxication and likely resolves when cannabis is discontinued.

TREATMENT

Up until the last few years, the prevailing opinion was that cannabis use did not produce addiction and dependence and that cannabis users could discontinue use without the help of treatment programs. Although it is undeniably true that the majority of cannabis users are able to stop without assistance, it is also becoming apparent that many cannabis-dependent individuals cannot stop without help.

With the recognition that cannabis use produces dependence and withdrawal, and that cannabis-dependent individuals may benefit from treatment, many substance abuse programs have started offering treatment to people whose primary drug of abuse or dependence is marijuana. Unfortunately, these programs are not generally designed specifically for cannabis dependence and they have not achieved high success rates. Similarly, many nonprofessional organizations that offer support groups, such as Alcoholics Anonymous (AA), Narcotics Anonymous (NA), and Self-Management and Recovery Training (SMART), have also begun to welcome people whose primary drug is cannabis. In addition, there is now a nonprofessional support organization, Marijuana Anonymous (MA), started by and run for cannabis-dependent individuals.

The strongest predictor of successful outcome is longer retention in treatment programs. Predictors of dropping out of an outpatient treatment program and presumably continuing use are young age, financial difficulties, and psychological stress.

To help an individual tolerate the 7- to 10-day withdrawal period, practitioners should provide psychological support (e.g., reassurance that the symptoms will resolve in a little over a week) and in some cases, provide pharmacological support.

Decisions regarding pharmacotherapy must be influenced by the fact that there is no strong evidence for positive benefits. Thus, brief courses of symptom-focused treatment are most appropriate, if needed at all.

The foundation of maintenance treatment, as with other types of substance-use disorders, is regular attendance at groups that provide education and support. Since cannabis dependence, like other types of substance abuse, is characterized by a chronic, relapsing course, these groups provide an important function by addressing issues around relapse prevention and provide support for dealing with relapses when they do occur.

Several approaches that are more important to the treatment of cannabis dependence should be employed in addition to the basic, general substance abuse program. For example, recent studies have found that both adolescent and adult cannabis users frequently report that they use cannabis to relax, or as a stress reduction or coping mechanism. This observation suggests that treatment programs should teach healthier and more effective coping mechanisms and cognitive behavioral strategies for relaxation and stress reduction.

The most salient feature of cannabis abuse or dependence is that it is often comorbid with other Axis I disorders as discussed earlier. Toxicology screening for other drugs of abuse is imperative because the most common comorbid Axis I disorders are other types of substance abuse. Even in the absence of an obvious Axis I diagnosis, psychological reasons for cannabis use should be investigated.

It is a reasonable assumption that at least some individuals with Axis I disorders are adversely affected by cannabis use even if they use the drug only occasionally. In such cases, the role of cannabis as an exacerbating factor must be assessed and discussed with the individual. These patients may or may not be suitable for support groups directed primarily at substance abuse because cannabis may represent a relatively minor portion of the individual's overall clinical picture.

Refractory Individuals

Like alcohol, the most common problem in managing cannabis-use disorders is the high rate of relapse due to the wide availability of the drug and the large number of people who are users. Users are therefore tempted to resume use soon after a period of treatment when they find themselves in situations where they are surrounded by people using the substance. It is often useful for families and other people important in the individual's life to get involved in the treatment to understand the role that they play in the individual's substance abuse. Some treaters advocate periodic random urine testing, which is an inexpensive and reliable method of monitoring abstinence, because THC remains present for a long time and can be detected with infrequent testing.

Cannabis-Induced Disorders

DIAGNOSIS

Cannabis Intoxication

There are four criteria necessary to make this diagnosis. The first is that recent use of cannabis must be established. This cannot be done with toxicology screening because the result may be negative after a single episode

---

DSM-IV-TR Diagnostic Criteria

292.89 CANNABIS INTOXICATION

A. Recent use of cannabis.
B. Clinically significant maladaptive behavioral or psychological changes (e.g., impaired motor coordination, euphoria, anxiety, sensation of slowed time, impaired judgment, social withdrawal) that developed during or shortly after cannabis use.
C. Two (or more) of the following signs, developing with 2 hours of cannabis use:

    (1) conjunctival injection
    (2) increased appetite
    (3) dry mouth
    (4) tachycardia

D. The symptoms are not due to a general medical condition and are not better accounted for by another mental disorder.

of smoking or, alternatively, may be positive even if the individual has not used the drug for a time much longer than the period of intoxication. In addition, the symptoms resulting from cannabis use must produce "clinically significant maladaptive behavioral or psychological changes." Third, the individual must exhibit some physical signs of cannabis use. DSM-IV-TR requires the individual to have at least two of four signs—conjunctival injection, increased appetite, dry mouth, and tachycardia—within 2 hours of cannabis use. Fourth, symptoms cannot be accounted for by a general medical condition or another mental disorder. There is a specifier, "with perceptual disturbances," that can be used if the individual is experiencing illusions or hallucinations while not delirious and while maintaining intact reality testing.

There has been extensive research on the effects of acute cannabis intoxication. In addition to the symptoms and signs required for a DSM-IV-TR diagnosis, many psychological and physiological effects have been reported. Awareness of these may enhance the clinician's ability to recognize cannabis intoxication. Physiological effects are listed in Table 17-2, and are divided into commonly observed effects and rare effects that have been described only after the use of very high doses of cannabis. Cannabis has low toxicity and no deaths from cannabis overdose have been reported. Similarly, psychological effects are listed in Table 17-3, divided into commonly observed effects and uncommon effects. Most people find the commonly

Table 17-2	Physiological Effects of Cannabis Intoxication

Common and Transient
Tachycardia
Hypertension
Thirst
Increased appetite
Constipation
Decreased intraocular pressure
Mydriasis
Mild bronchoconstriction followed by bronchodilation
Increased reaction time
Impaired coordination
Distorted time perception
Decreased libido
Mild analgesia
Mild anti-emetic effects

Uncommon and Transient
Ataxia
Ptosis
Miosis
Drowsiness
Bradycardia
Hypotension
Peripheral vasoconstriction
Hypothermia

Table 17-3	Psychological Effects of Cannabis Intoxication

Common and Transient
Euphoria
Distortions in perception, including time perception
Enhancement of sensations

Uncommon and Transient
Dysphoria
Anxiety, and less commonly panic reactions
Restlessness
Depersonalization
Derealization
Paranoid ideation

experienced psychological effects enjoyable. However, some individuals, especially women and inexperienced users in an unfamiliar environment, find them frightening and experience anxiety and even have panic reactions. Although all of these effects typically persist only for the period of acute intoxication, some reports have described individuals who report "flashbacks" of cannabis intoxication long after use, and depersonalization persisting long after acute intoxication. At this time, there is insufficient evidence to ascertain whether these reports are attributable to cannabis itself, to confounding factors such as the concomitant use of other drugs, or the presence of other Axis I disorders.

In addition, cannabis use produces deficits in a number of neuropsychological functions, both during acute intoxication and after up to a week or more of abstinence in chronic, long-term users. These tasks include short-term memory, sustained or divided attention, and complex decision making. A study of chronic, long-term users found that these deficits were generally reversible after 28 days of abstinence.

Cannabis Intoxication Delirium

We have not located any original reports of this entity, although it is mentioned in various reviews and is included in DSM-IV-TR. Thus, if cannabis intoxication delirium does occur in neurologically intact individuals, it is probably a rare complication. If the delirium does not resolve within 24 to 48 hours, it is almost certainly a result of an underlying neurological or medical condition. Therefore, in an individual with delirium, even if recent cannabis use has been reported, a full diagnostic workup should be performed to rule out a concomitant, treatable neurological condition.

Cannabis-induced psychotic disorder or cannabis-induced anxiety disorder are not generally diagnosed unless the symptoms are in excess of those usually associated with the intoxication or withdrawal state and are sufficiently severe to warrant independent clinical attention.

Cannabis-Induced Psychotic Disorder

There are two subtypes of cannabis-induced psychotic disorder: one featuring delusions, the other hallucinations. The diagnosis of this disorder is readily made in individuals who have psychotic symptoms that appear immediately after ingestion of cannabis. However, a careful history is required to establish whether the individual has a preexisting psychotic disorder (as is often the case in such situations) or whether the symptoms arose *de novo* after cannabis consumption. There is little evidence that cannabis-induced psychotic disorders can arise in previously asymptomatic individuals.

Cannabis-Induced Anxiety Disorder

This disorder may be further described by the following specifiers: with generalized anxiety, with panic attacks, with obsessive–compulsive symptoms, and with phobic symptoms. People who experience anxiety after using cannabis are typically inexperienced users who react to the novel experiences of perceptual distortions and intensified sensations with anxiety and even panic reactions, rather than enjoyment. Women are more likely than men to experience cannabis-induced anxiety. If symptoms of severe anxiety or panic persist for 24 to 48 hours after the period of acute intoxication, they are likely due to an underlying mental disorder that must be diagnosed and treated.

Course

Cannabis intoxication is a self-limiting state that remits as cannabis is metabolized and eliminated from the body. If symptoms suggestive of cannabis intoxication persist, other diagnoses should be considered. Similarly, although there are few data regarding the course of the other cannabis-induced disorders, it appears that cannabis-induced psychotic and anxiety disorders as well as cannabis intoxication delirium rarely persist beyond the period of acute intoxication with the drug.

TREATMENT

Uncomplicated cannabis intoxication rarely comes to clinical attention, and if it does, it does not require treatment other than reassurance, as it is a self-limiting condition. Similarly, as suggested in the previous sections, symptoms of delirium, psychosis, or anxiety associated with cannabis use typically resolve promptly after the period of acute intoxication is past. Again, no treatment is necessary other than keeping the individual safe and providing reassurance that symptoms caused by the drug will stop, as these are also self-limiting conditions. If the symptoms continue after more than 24 to 48 hours of abstinence from the drug, the possibility of another Axis I diagnosis must be considered. In such cases, treatment should then be directed at the primary Axis I disorder.

COMPARISON OF DSM-IV-TR AND ICD-10 DIAGNOSTIC CRITERIA

The ICD-10 and DSM-IV-TR criteria sets for cannabis intoxication are virtually identical. While DSM-IV-TR does not include a category for cannabis withdrawal, ICD-10 does include such a category (called "Cannabinoid Withdrawal State") without the inclusion of "definitive diagnostic criteria."

Substance-Related Disorders: Cocaine

Cocaine, a central nervous system stimulant produced by the coca plant, is consumed in several preparations. Cocaine hydrochloride powder is usually snorted through the nostrils, or it may be mixed in water and injected intravenously. Cocaine hydrochloride powder is also commonly heated ("cooked up") with ammonia or baking soda and water to remove the hydrochloride, thus forming a gel-like substance that can be smoked ("freebasing"). "Crack" cocaine is a precooked form of cocaine alkaloid that is sold on the street as small "rocks."

DIAGNOSIS

The state of intense euphoria produced by cocaine intoxication is a powerful reinforcer and can lead to the development of cocaine-use disorders in many individuals, although only 10–16% of those who try the drug go on to develop these disorders. The route of administration is strongly correlated with the development of cocaine-use disorders, in that the intravenous and smoked routes of administration allow rapid transport of the drug to the brain, producing intense effects that are short-lived. Rapid tolerance to euphoria occurs and plasma concentrations are not correlated with peak euphoria, producing a need for frequent dosing to regain euphoric effects (binge use) that can place the cocaine abuser at a risk for medical and psychiatric complications of cocaine abuse.

While the question of whether cocaine is physiologically addictive is not completely clear, the psychological addiction alone is powerful and can completely dominate the life of the cocaine abuser. Binge use of cocaine may be followed by what has been described as a mild withdrawal syndrome characterized by dysphoria and anhedonia. Cocaine withdrawal may resemble a depressive disorder, in some cases requiring emergent treatment. Some combinations of these consequences of cocaine abuse are usually responsible for the identification and diagnosis of individuals with cocaine-use disorders and referral to substance-abuse treatment.

When evaluating an individual regarding the possible presence of a cocaine-related disorder, the initial evaluation period should include the collection of a complete history of all substance abuse, which is essential to accurate diagnosis and appropriate treatment. Figure 18-1 shows a diagnostic decision tree for cocaine-related disorders. The history includes the circumstances under which each drug was used, the psychoactive effects sought and obtained, the route of administration, and the frequency and amount of each drug used. Cocaine abusers frequently abuse other drugs and alcohol to enhance euphoria or to alleviate dysphoric effects associated with cocaine abuse (agitation, paranoia). A thorough history with diagnosis of other substance-use disorders is important to treatment planning. Individuals may need detoxification from other substances prior to initiation of cocaine abuse treatment. It is also important to monitor clinically for relapses to any substance abuse during treatment for cocaine-use disorders because the use of other drugs and alcohol often leads to resumption of cocaine abuse. In addition, a thorough history of current and previous substance abuse is important so that treatment can be individualized and individuals can be helped in developing coping skills that will assist them in specific situations that they identify as placing them at high risk for relapse.

A careful psychiatric history with particular attention to onset of psychiatric symptoms in relation to drug use is essential. The determination of a premorbid psychiatric illness is critical to providing appropriate treatment. For persons in whom substance abuse is an attempt to self-medicate an underlying mental illness, the introduction of psychotropic medication in conjunction with ongoing treatment for the substance abuse will improve both the mental disorder as well as the substance-use disorder(s). Conversely, the evaluation of temporal onset of psychiatric symptoms may preclude erroneous use of psychotropic medication in cases in which the psychiatric symptoms are in fact

Clinical Guide to the Diagnosis and Treatment of Mental Disorders. M. B. First and A. Tasman
© 2006 John Wiley & Sons, Ltd.   ISBN 0 470 019158

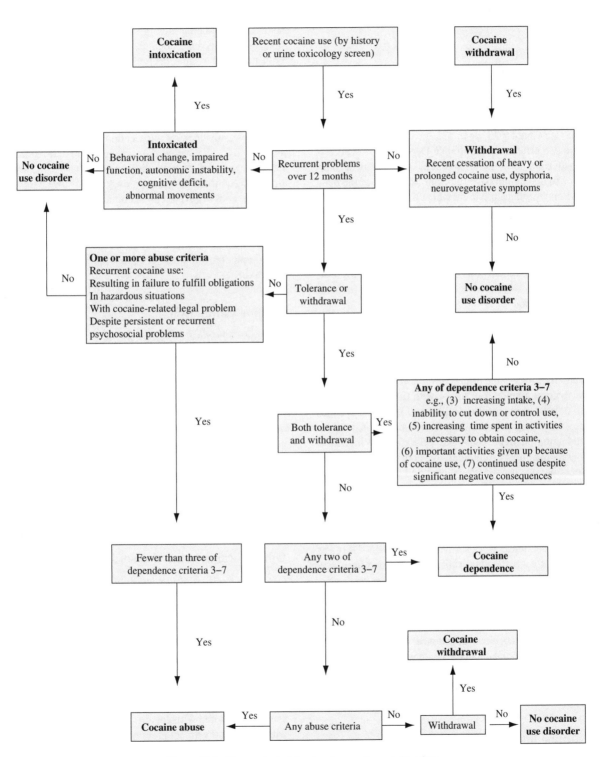

Figure 18-1 *Diagnostic decision tree for cocaine-use disorders.*

cocaine-induced and spare the individual exposure to the potential side effects of these medications.

Cocaine Dependence

The DSM-IV-TR defines the essential features of substance dependence as a cluster of cognitive, behavioral, and physiological symptoms indicating continued use of the substance despite significant consequences of use (see Chapter 13, page 125 for the DSM-IV-TR diagnostic criteria for Substance Dependence). There is a pattern of administration that usually results in tolerance to and compulsive self-administration of the drug and may produce a withdrawal syndrome on cessation of drug use. Cocaine dependence can develop quickly after initiation of use because of the potent euphoria produced by the drug. The route of administration is related to the development of cocaine dependence; smoked and intravenous routes are more highly correlated with dependence than the intranasal route of administration.

Cocaine has a short half-life requiring frequent dosing to maintain the "high" (binge use). Binges may be separated by several days while the individual recovers or attempts to obtain more money for drug purchase. Tolerance to cocaine effects develops quickly, resulting in larger amounts of drug use with time. This is often associated with mental or physical complications of use, including paranoia, aggressive behavior, anxiety and agitation, depression, and weight loss. Withdrawal symptoms, most prominently dysphoric mood, may be seen, but are usually short-lived and clear within several days of abstinence.

Cocaine Abuse

Substance abuse is described by DSM-IV-TR as a maladaptive pattern of substance use demonstrated by recurrent and significant adverse consequences related to repeated use (see Chapter 13, page 125 for the DSM-IV-TR diagnostic criteria for Substance Abuse). The intensity and frequency of use are less in cocaine abuse than in cocaine dependence. Episodes of abuse may occur around paydays or special occasions and may be characterized by brief periods (hours to days) of high-dose binge use followed by longer periods of abstinence or nonproblem use.

Cocaine Intoxication

The clinical effects of cocaine intoxication are characterized initially by euphoria (referred to as "high") and also include agitation, anxiety, irritability or affective

lability, grandiosity, impaired judgment, increased psychomotor activity, hypervigilance or paranoia, and sometimes hallucinations (visual, auditory, or tactile) may occur. Because cocaine and amphetamines are both part of the same drug class, i.e., stimulants, the criteria set for cocaine intoxication and withdrawal are identical to the criteria sets for amphetamine intoxication and withdrawal (see DSM-IV-TR diagnostic criteria, Chapter 15, page 148–149). Physical symptoms that can accompany cocaine intoxication include hypertension, tachycardia, hyperthermia, pupillary dilation, nausea, vomiting, tremor, diaphoresis, chest pain, arrhythmia, confusion, seizures, dyskinetic movements, dystonia, and, in severe cases, coma. These effects are more frequently seen in high-dose binge users of cocaine. Cardiovascular effects are probably a result of sympathomimetic properties of cocaine (i.e., release of norepinephrine and blockade of norepinephrine reuptake).

Cocaine Withdrawal

Cocaine withdrawal develops within a few hours to a few days after stopping or reducing cocaine use that has been heavy and prolonged (see DSM-IV-TR diagnostic criteria, Chapter 15, page 149). The syndrome is characterized by dysphoria and two or more physiological changes including fatigue, vivid and unpleasant dreams, insomnia or hypersomnia, increased appetite, and psychomotor agitation or retardation. Anhedonia and craving for cocaine can be part of the withdrawal syndrome. Depression and suicidal ideation are the most serious complications and require individualized assessment and treatment. The syndrome may last up to several days but generally resolves without treatment.

Other Cocaine-Induced Disorders

DSM-IV-TR also specifies additional cocaine-induced disorders described in other diagnostic groupings with which they share phenomenology (Table 18-1). These include cocaine intoxication delirium, cocaine-induced psychotic disorder, cocaine-induced mood disorder, cocaine-induced anxiety disorder, cocaine-induced sleep disorder, and cocaine-induced sexual dysfunction. These disorders are diagnosed instead of intoxication or withdrawal only if symptoms are in excess of those usually associated with cocaine intoxication or cocaine withdrawal and warrant independent clinical attention. In addition, the clinician should pay careful attention to the temporal relationship of the psychiatric symptoms and cocaine abuse. Symptoms that are severe enough to warrant consideration of one of these diagnoses should

Table 18-1	Other DSM-IV-TR Cocaine-Induced Disorders
292.89	Cocaine intoxication
	Specify if: with perceptual disturbances
292.0	Cocaine withdrawal
292.81	Cocaine intoxication delirium
292.11	Cocaine-induced psychotic disorder, with delusions
	Specify if: with onset during intoxication
292.12	Cocaine-induced psychotic disorder, with hallucinations
	Specify if: with onset during intoxication
292.84	Cocaine-induced mood disorder
	Specify if: with onset during intoxication/ with onset during withdrawal
292.89	Cocaine-induced anxiety disorder
	Specify if: with onset during intoxication/ with onset during withdrawal
292.89	Cocaine-induced sexual dysfunction
	Specify if: with onset during intoxication
292.89	Cocaine-induced sleep disorder
	Specify if: with onset during intoxication/ with onset during withdrawal
292.9	Cocaine-related disorder not otherwise specified

Source: Data Reprinted with permission from the *Diagnostic and Statistical Manual of Mental Disorders*, 4th ed., Text Rev. Copyright 2000 American Psychiatric Association.

also dissipate with continued abstinence from cocaine. Symptoms that worsen after cessation of cocaine use in a period of 1 to 4 weeks should be reevaluated and other Axis I or Axis III disorders considered, with modification of the treatment plan as clinically indicated.

Course

Cocaine produces a sense of intensified pleasure in most activities and a heightened sense of alertness and well-being. Anxiety and social inhibition are decreased. Energy, self-esteem, and self-perception of ability are increased. There is enhancement of emotion and sexual feeling. Pleasurable experiences, although heightened, are not distorted and hallucinations are usually absent. The person engaging in low-dose cocaine use often receives positive feedback from others responding to the user's increased energy and enthusiasm. This, in combination with the euphoria experienced by the user, can be reinforcing, and cocaine use is perceived as free of any adverse consequences. The duration of cocaine's euphoric effects depends on the route of administration. The faster the drug is absorbed and occupies receptors of the "brain rewarding region," the more intense the euphoric effects.

Cocaine users quickly learn that higher doses are associated with intensified and prolonged euphoria, resulting in increasing use of the drug and progression to cocaine dependence. The abuser is focused on the cocaine-induced euphoria and begins to compulsively pursue this effect. These behaviors become pivotal in the lives of cocaine abusers, who continue drug abuse despite the presence of increasing personal and social consequences.

The psychoactive effects of cocaine are similar to those of amphetamine; the main difference in terms of abuse liability is in cocaine's much shorter duration of action. Whereas the plasma elimination half-life for cocaine is approximately 90 minutes, this drug produces pharmacodynamic tachyphylaxis, resulting in rapidly diminishing psychoactive effects in the presence of continued cocaine in the plasma. This phenomenon explains the "half-life" of cocaine-induced euphoria, (which is approximately 45 minutes after intranasal use and 5 minutes after intravenous and smoking administration), as well as characteristic binge use in which cocaine is repetitively administered over short intervals. During binge use, the drug may be administered as frequently as every 10 minutes, resulting in rapid mood changes. Cocaine binges reportedly can last as long as 7 days, although the average length is 12 hours.

Uncontrolled use of cocaine often begins with either increased access and resultant escalating dosages and frequency of administration or a change from intranasal use to a route of administration with more rapid onset of effects (i.e., intravenous or smoked). These characteristics are integral to the development of high-dose binging with cocaine. Such binges produce extreme euphoria and vivid memories. These memories are later contrasted with current dysphoria to produce intense craving, which perpetuates the binge-use pattern. Addicts report that during binge use, thoughts are focused exclusively on the cocaine-induced effects. Normal daily needs, including sleep and nourishment, are neglected. Responsibilities to family and employer and social obligations are given up. This continues until the supply of cocaine is exhausted.

Binges are often separated by several days of abstinence; cocaine-dependent individuals average one to three binges per week. This is in contrast to use patterns for opiate and alcohol dependence, which often produce physiological dependence necessitating daily consumption to prevent withdrawal symptoms. This differentiation is crucial to an understanding of the syndrome of cocaine dependence. Although the prediction of development of cocaine-use disorders is not possible on an individual basis, it is clear that those who progress to binge use of the drug will be significantly affected and constitute the treatment-seeking population. The cocaine abuser is likely to be ambivalent about the need for treatment, and the treatment dropout rate is high (ranging from 38% to 73%). Dropout usually occurs early in treatment (during the initial evaluation process).

Newly abstinent cocaine abusers may experience a triphasic abstinence pattern, although this varies by individual, that includes a period of acute abstinence, sometimes referred to as the "crash," lasting several hours to several days consisting of dysphoria, fatigue, insomnia or hypersomnia, increased appetite, and either psychomotor agitation or retardation, subsequent to the more intensive "crash" phase. A more chronic withdrawal period sometimes occurs characterized by minor depressive symptoms and cocaine craving lasting 2 to 10 weeks. This may then be followed by an extinction phase characterized by intermittent drug craving that becomes increasingly manageable with continued abstinence.

Like other drug- and alcohol-use disorders, cocaine-use disorders are chronic relapsing illnesses that present substantial challenges in the treatment process. Cocaine abusers are at high risk for relapse, particularly in the first few months of treatment related to acute craving often in the context of ongoing psychosocial stressors that result from or have been exacerbated by cocaine abuse. Newly abstinent cocaine abusers often lack adequate coping skills necessary to avoid cocaine use, which take time to acquire in the treatment process. Although the ability to cope with cocaine craving improves with continued abstinence, relapse to cocaine abuse or other drug and alcohol abuse will continue to be a risk for those with a history of a cocaine-use disorder who relapse to cocaine abuse. Repeated treatments may be required for those with cocaine-use disorders. Treatment modalities include inpatient hospitalization for medical or psychiatric complications of cocaine abuse, partial hospital programs, self-help groups, psychotherapy (usually group or family therapy for individuals with primary cocaine-use disorders), or some combination of these treatments according to the clinical presentation of the individual (see later in the chapter).

Comorbidity with Other Mental Disorders

Comorbid conditions related to cocaine abuse are abuse of other substances and comorbid mental disorder. Several studies have documented the high rate of comorbid mental disorders in cocaine abusers entering treatment. These disorders include mood disorders (major depressive disorder, bipolar disorders), schizophrenia, posttraumatic stress disorder, attention-deficit/hyperactivity disorder, anxiety disorders, and antisocial personality disorder.

It is important to note that comorbid psychiatric illnesses are common among cocaine users. Furthermore, the diagnosis of a comorbid primary mental disorder can be challenging to make in cocaine abusers because psychiatric symptoms may be the result of cocaine abuse or acute abstinence. When mental disorders co-occur with cocaine-use disorders, it is important to provide treatment for both disorders. Cocaine-use disorders will not generally resolve with treatment of the mental disorder alone, nor will substance-abuse treatment resolve a comorbid mental disorder.

Medical Complications of Cocaine Abuse

Cardiac toxicity is one of the leading causes of morbidity and mortality associated with cocaine use. The risk of myocardial infarct is well established in cocaine use and is not related to dose, route, or frequency of administration. The risk of acute myocardial infarction is increased 24-fold in 1 hour immediately following cocaine use in persons who are otherwise at a relatively low risk for such events.

Cocaine use also is associated with a wide range of cardiac dysrhythmias, including sinus tachycardia, sinus bradycardia, supraventricular and ventricular tachycardia, ventricular premature contractions, ventricular tachycardia and fibrillation, torsades des pointes, and asystole. Life-threatening dysrhythmia caused by cocaine in the absence of myocardial ischemia is rare.

Intranasal abuse of cocaine has been associated with a number of medical complications including chronic sinusitis, septal perforation, subperiosteal abscess, pneumomediastinum, pneumothorax, and pulmonary edema. The presence of pulmonary edema in a young, otherwise healthy individual, without predisposing risk factors, should alert the physician to the possibility of cocaine abuse.

Cerebrovascular accidents related to cocaine use have been well documented in the medical literature. Cerebral infarct, subarachnoid hemorrhage, intraparenchymal hemorrhage, and intraventricular hemorrhage have been observed as acute complications of cocaine use. Seizures were one of the earliest known complications of cocaine abuse. Cocaine produces hyperpyrexia, which in combination with its effects on neurotransmitters may contribute to the development of seizures. Seizures may occur as a primary effect of cocaine owing to its ability to lower the seizure threshold or may be secondary to other central nervous system or cardiac events precipitated by cocaine use.

Recently, acute renal failure as a result of rhabdomyolysis has been recognized as an important complication of cocaine abuse. Pregnancy may increase the risk of rhabdomyolysis and renal failure. Renal failure may progress rapidly in the context of cocaine-induced

Table 18-2	Major Medical Complications Associated with Cocaine Abuse

Cardiovascular
Myocardial infarct
Arrhythmias
Aortic dissection
Cardiomyopathy

Respiratory
Pneumonitis (associated with smoked cocaine)
Pulmonary edema
Nasal septal perforation, chronic sinusitis (associated with intranasal inhalation)

Central Nervous System
Hyperpyrexia
Seizure
Cerebral infarct
Subarachnoid hemorrhage
Intraparenchymal hemorrhage
Intraventricular hemorrhage

Renal
Renal failure secondary to rhabdomyolysis
Obstetrical
Premature labor
Placental abruption

Complications of Intravenous Use
Infectious diseases (HIV, hepatitis)
Endocarditis
Cellulitis Abscesses

Psychiatric
Depression
Suicidality
Psychosis

rhabdomyolysis and dialysis may be necessary for some individuals.

The major medical complications of cocaine abuse are summarized in Table 18-2.

TREATMENT

Treatments for cocaine-use disorders continue to evolve and have been shown to be effective. In a large-outcome study, a comparison of short-term inpatient treatment programs, outpatient drug-free programs, and long-term residential programs specifically for those with cocaine-use disorders was undertaken. Of those who received any treatment, 24% relapsed to weekly cocaine use, a large decrease over the 73% relapse rate in the year prior to treatment. Some required an additional treatment program (18%) in the year following treatment, which is not an uncommon scenario for this chronic, relapsing disorder. Those with high levels of psychosocial, medical, or psychiatric problems at intake or less than 90 days of treatment had higher cocaine use in the follow-up period. Treatment periods of 90 days or more were associated with better substance-abuse outcomes.

The two primary goals of cocaine treatment are (1) the initiation of abstinence through disruption of binge cycles and (2) the prevention of relapse. Treatment planning to achieve these goals must be considered in the context of the individual clinical presentation of the patient. Initial assessment to determine immediate needs is necessary to determine the most appropriate level of care (inpatient or outpatient treatment) as well as other psychiatric and medical considerations important to the development of the treatment plan.

The majority of those with cocaine-use disorders are most appropriately treated in an outpatient setting. Outpatient treatment may vary with provider but generally includes multiple weekly contacts for the initial months of treatment because less frequent contact is not effective in the initiation or maintenance of abstinence. These sessions consist of some combination of individual drug counseling, peer support groups, family or couples therapy, urine toxicology monitoring, education sessions, psychotherapy, and psychiatric treatment that may include pharmacotherapy for cocaine addiction or comorbid mental disorders. Inpatient treatment is reserved for those who have been refractory to outpatient treatment, whose compulsive use of cocaine represents an imminent danger (e.g., suicidality associated with cocaine toxicity or acute abstinence), who have other comorbid mental disorders or general medical conditions, or who are dependent on more than one substance and require monitored detoxification.

The treatment of cocaine-use disorders should be undertaken in the context of a thorough understanding of the disease (Table 18-3). One of the greatest challenges in the early stages of cocaine treatment is to prevent an early dropout. It has been estimated that up to 80% of individuals drop out of treatment programs. Frequent clinical contacts especially in the early weeks of treatment can help establish a therapeutic alliance that will assist in engaging the cocaine user in the treatment process. Many programs offer 3 to 6 days per week of substance-abuse treatment sessions within outpatient partial hospital programs or intensive outpatient chemical dependency programs. Assessments by the program physician and counseling staff can identify other areas requiring specific interventions (comorbid general medical condition or mental disorders) and can expedite the initiation of appropriate pharmacotherapies. These interventions will increase treatment retention.

Initial treatment should include the encouragement of abstinence from all drug and alcohol use. Individuals who abuse alcohol and marijuana often do not perceive these drugs as problems. Education regarding the

Table 18-3	Cocaine-use Disorders: Recovery and Treatment		
Parameter	**Acute Abstinence**	**Withdrawal Phase**	**Extinction Phase**
Duration	Several hours to four days	2 to 10 weeks	3 to 12 months
Treatment	Symptomatic May need hospitalization for medical or psychiatric care and assessment	Initiate psychotherapy Individual/group therapy Self-help groups, other therapies, e.g., family, marital, individual, as needed	Continue psychotherapy, decrease intensity with continued abstinence; self-help groups and additional interventions developed for patients as needed
Pharmacotherapy	Benzodiazepines for anxiety, agitation, paranoia Antipsychotics (sparingly) for severe psychosis or agitation	None approved specific for cocaine-use disorders Consider disulfiram for cocaine–alcohol abuse previously refractory to treatment; psychotropics for comorbid psychiatric disorders or cocaine-related disorders; pharmacotherapies for other substance use disorders	Unusual to initiate in this phase Taper and discontinue pharmacotherapy for cocaine abuse and monitor clinically

use of such drugs as conditioned stimuli to the use of cocaine should be emphasized. The "disease model" of chemical dependency may be used to assist in the initiation of abstinence. Emphasis is placed on the individuals recognizing chemical dependency as a disease needing treatment to control, but one for which there is no cure. Comprehensive drug education should also be provided in the initial treatment phase. Frequent contact with a drug counselor is an important part of treatment. Individual, group, and (where clinically indicated) family or marital therapy should be available. Attendance at 12-step or other self-help groups is often a useful adjunct to treatment and can be particularly helpful during the early stages of treatment when support for sobriety is essential.

The early recovery phase of treatment varies in duration from 3 to 12 months and is characterized by multiple weekly contacts and participation in therapeutic modalities with the goal of initiation and maintenance of abstinence. The focus during early recovery should be on relapse prevention and development of new and adaptive coping skills, healthy relationships, and lifestyle changes that will facilitate abstinence.

Relapses are common during early recovery. Individuals often feel pleased about their progress in treatment, become overly confident about their ability to control use, and test themselves by deliberately encountering what they know to be a high-risk situation for their drug use. Individuals should be informed about the potential for relapse from the start of the treatment process. Relapse should, however, also trigger a review of the treatment plan and consideration of the need for additional interventions or whether a higher level of care is needed to assist the individual in the recovery process.

Success with initiating and maintaining abstinence over several months is followed by a reduced frequency of contact (e.g., a decrease to weekly group or individual therapy sessions). The focus should be on maintaining a commitment to abstinence, addressing renewed denial, and continued improvement of interpersonal skills. Participation in self-help groups should continue to be encouraged. Self-help groups based on 12-step principles encourage individuals to continue to view themselves as addicts in recovery—a cognitive structuring that many recovering drug abusers find helpful in maintaining sobriety.

Psychosocial Treatments

A variety of psychotherapeutic strategies for the treatment of cocaine-use disorders have been described (Table 18-4). In contrast to opiate addiction, for which psychotherapies alone are insufficient, there appear to be at least some subpopulations of cocaine abusers for whom psychotherapy alone may be adequate. Behavioral therapies, in particular cognitive–behavioral therapy and contingency management approaches, have been demonstrated to be effective treatments for some cocaine-dependent individuals.

Table 18-4	Psychotherapies: the Mainstay of Treatment for Cocaine-use Disorders

Interpersonal therapy
Supportive expressive therapy
Cognitive–behavioral therapy/Relapse-prevention therapy
Voucher-based treatment
Individual and group drug counseling
Systematic cue exposure
Self-help groups (e.g., Cocaine Anonymous)

Although the name implies focus on the prevention of relapse, in fact this method employs several strategies intended to facilitate abstinence. Specific techniques in cocaine-addiction treatment include exploring the positive and negative consequences of continued use, self-monitoring to recognize drug cravings early on and to identify high-risk situations for use, and developing strategies for coping with and avoiding high-risk situations and the desire to use. Research indicates that the skills individuals learn through relapse-prevention therapy remain after the completion of treatment. In two long-term outcome studies, most people receiving this cognitive–behavioral approach maintained the gains they made in treatment throughout the year following treatment and a proportion of study participants continued to make gains following the termination of the 12-week CBT treatment period.

Psychotherapeutic approaches are often delivered in the context of multimodal treatment programs and nearly all substance-abuse clinicians emphasize the importance of self-help groups such as Cocaine Anonymous.

Individual and group drug counseling focuses directly on reducing or stopping the use of drugs. It also addresses related areas of impaired social and occupational function as well as the content and structure of the patient's individualized recovery program. Through its emphasis on short-term behavioral goals, drug counseling helps the patient develop coping strategies and tools for abstaining from drug use and then maintaining abstinence.

Somatic Therapies

The development of pharmacological treatments for cocaine abuse has been based on the premise that an altered neurochemical substrate underlies the chronic, high-intensity (binge) use and acute abstinence/withdrawal that follows binge use. This neuroadaptation model has also served as a basis for a number of studies that have evaluated the clinical utility of psychotropic agents that, based on their pharmacological profile, might possess anticraving properties, block euphoria, or decrease cocaine abstinence symptoms. To date, no medication has emerged as an accepted effective pharmacotherapy.

Treatment Refractoriness

The term "treatment refractoriness" sometimes implies a lack of response to a therapeutic trial of a pharmacotherapy. In the case of cocaine dependence, however, there is no effective pharmacotherapy with which to treat the disorder; therefore, the term relates to a different set of occurrences in the treatment setting. Recidivism to cocaine use, treatment dropout, and multiple treatment experiences are common. Such problems are a reflection of the severity of illness and parameters of relative treatment refractoriness. Comorbid substance use and mental disorders contribute to treatment refractoriness. Lack of accurate diagnosis and treatment contributes to relapse potential in the form of continued exposure to high-risk situations and lifestyle instability that are associated with ongoing substance abuse. Continued psychiatric symptoms that individuals attempt to relieve through cocaine use contribute to poor treatment outcome.

The psychological addiction associated with cocaine abuse can be disabling. Because physiological dependence, if it does occur, generally does not require pharmacotherapy, treatment referrals for individuals with primary cocaine dependence but no other acute mental disorder or general condition, are generally to an outpatient drug abuse treatment clinic. Those unable to initiate and maintain sobriety in an outpatient drug treatment program should be evaluated for more intensive forms of treatment. Management of these individuals should include consideration of a variety of options including pharmacotherapy (see the earlier section on somatic therapies for cocaine abuse) and programs that offer a graded increase in structure. Such individuals may need initial detoxification from another drug or alcohol that could require several days of inpatient treatment. Those who are determined to need intensive outpatient treatment often attend these programs 5 days a week initially, and sessions last an average of about 4 hours. There is a gradual reduction in the number of sessions per week as the period of sobriety lengthens. Such programs are of flexible duration, but a full program usually requires at least 12 weeks. This program can be followed with resumption of the outpatient treatment clinic level of care, which takes place fewer days per week and with shorter sessions. Those with comorbid psychiatric disorders should be referred to dual diagnosis specialty treatment programs when available. Dual diagnosis speciality programs differ from traditional substance-abuse treatment programs in that they have a dual diagnosis treatment orientation, with an increased use of psychotropic medication, longer lengths of stay, and greater tolerance for relapse and medication nonadherence.

Individuals who have failed other forms of treatment may be referred to residential programs, although the number of these programs is shrinking, given the constraints on treatment that have occurred as a result of managed care and erosion of benefits provided by health insurers for treating substance-use disorders. Residential programs vary in length and must be tailored to the needs of the patient. Such programs can be important to the initiation of abstinence. These programs allow sufficient time in a drug-free and supportive environment so that the recovery process can begin, as well as provide adequate time for reduc-

tion of drug craving and acquisition of effective relapse-prevention skills.

COMPARISON OF DSM-IV-TR AND ICD-10 DIAGNOSTIC CRITERIA

The ICD-10 and DSM-IV-TR criteria sets for cocaine intoxication and withdrawal are almost the same except that the ICD-10 criteria set for withdrawal includes drug craving as an additional item.

Substance-Related Disorders: Hallucinogens and MDMA

Human ingestion of hallucinogens can be traced back thousands of years. In the Americas, Europe, and Africa, hallucinogens were used for consecration during religious ceremonies, for divination, and as tools for rites of passage and shamanic healing. The majority of these botanicals grow in the Americas. In South and North America, cacti containing the hallucinogen mescaline are still widely used by a number of Native American tribes. In South America, boiled potions are made from *Trichocereus* species, a cactus containing about 1% mescaline. A much more potent mescaline-containing cactus, peyote (*Lophophora williamsii*), grows naturally in northern Mexico and along a long strip of the Texas–Mexico border. The Huichol of Mexico have used peyote as a religious sacrament continuously for 3000 years, as have the Native American Church (NAC) of the United States and Canada. In the NAC, peyote is treasured as the holy sacrament from God to be ingested in all-night prayer vigils.

Hallucinogenic mushrooms containing psilocybin (4-phosphoryloxy-*N*,*N*-dimethyltryptamine) and psilocin (4-hydroxy-*N*,*N*-dimethyltryptamine), especially from the genus *Psilocybe*, are found throughout the Americas, Europe, and Asia. *Psilocybe cubensis* typically contains 1.6 mg psilocybin per gram of dried mushroom; a dose of 40 μg/kg induces a 3- to 4-hour intoxication. Easily grown and indigenous to many parts of the United States, *Psilocybe* mushrooms are commonly trafficked as hallucinogens in the illicit market. Dimethyltryptamine (DMT), a short-acting hallucinogen, is also present in a wide variety of botanicals. Many tribes of the Amazon and elsewhere ingest potent DMT snuffs prepared from seeds of *Anadenanthera peregrina*, *Anadenanthera columbrina*, and other botanicals.

The dawn of modernity for hallucinogenic drugs can be placed to the moment in 1943 when Albert Hofmann, a Swiss chemist, discovered the potent psychological effects of LSD. Within a decade the drug was being tested as an agent of chemical warfare in the United States and Europe. Within two decades it assumed cult status among the ministry, academics, and students, culminating in an epidemic of abuse in its third decade starting in the late 1960s. Congressional reaction came in the form of the Drug Abuse Control Amendments of 1965 and 1968, which choked off drug supplies to researchers, and criminalized drug sale and use. The scientific impact of these laws was to retard the advance of knowledge in this field for a generation.

The development and chemical identification of additional agents causing LSD-like mental symptoms, however, proceeded apace. This work has both clarified aspects of their mechanisms of action, and created a challenge to defining hallucinogens. Two classes of drugs appear to have more in common with LSD than not. These include other substituted indolealkylamines (psilocybin, psilocin, ibogaine, dimethyltryptamine, and bufotenine, *inter alia*) and phenethylamines (mescaline, MDMA, MDA, 2CB [4-bromo-2,5-dimethoxyphenethylamine], and DOM [2,5-dimethoxy-4-methylamphetamine] *inter alia*). Nearly 200 compounds, largely of the phenethylamine class, for hallucinogenic properties, have been synthesized.

The definition of a hallucinogenic drug has been a matter of controversy. More than 90 species of hallucinogenic plants afford an anthropological definition. Hundreds of substituted phenylethylamines and tryptamines lend themselves to chemical characterization. Because few have been systematically studied in humans, hallucinogens have been defined by their botanical or chemical rubrics rather than their psychophysiological affects. To address the problem of classification, one may define as hallucinogenic any agent which has alterations in perception, cognition, or mood as its primary psychobiological actions in the presence of an otherwise clear sensorium. Most commonly this includes indolealkylamines and phenethylamines, and excludes, *inter alia*, the anticholinergics, the arylcyclohexylamine dissociative anesthetics such as phencyclidine, stimulants such as amphetamine and cocaine, bromism, and heavy metal intoxication (either because changes in perception, mood, or cognition are not the primary effect or because they cloud the sensorium).

Hallucinogen Intoxication

DIAGNOSIS

The DSM-IV-TR criteria for the diagnosis of acute hallucinogen intoxication are shown below.

The acute effects of "tripping" on LSD-like (i.e., with similar psychic effects, e.g., psilocybin or mescaline) hallucinogens are variable and profound. Subjects given LSD without their knowledge suffer more anxiety, hypomotility, and speech disruption than those who take it knowingly. LSD is active within 30 minutes of the ingestion of a dose of 50 to 100 μg. Physically the drug stimulates the autonomic nervous system rapidly, resulting in tachycardia, hypertension, and dilated pupils, the last being present for much of the trip. The flood of rapidly changing perceptual, affective, and cognitive effects are by alternate turns exhilarating, nerve wracking, and incapacitating. Table 19-1 illustrates a typical time course for the psychiatric effects of LSD.

Table 19-1	Time Course for the Psychiatric Effects of LSD-like Hallucinogens
Time	**Psychiatric Effects**
0–30 minutes	Dizziness, nausea, weakness, anxiety
30–60 minutes	Blurred vision, visual pseudohallucinations and hallucinations, afterimagery, geometric and imagistic imagery with eyes closed, decreased concentration, dissociation, depersonalization, out of body sensations, reduced coordination
60–240 minutes	Intensified afterimagery, false perceptions of movement (walls appearing to breathe or melt), loss of rectilinearity of perceptions, a rapid flood of emotions including anxiety, euphoria, and oceanic unity, loss of the sense of time
4–12 hours	Gradual return to previous mental state, but with continued arousal, headache, fatigue, contemplative frame of reference, sense of profundity

Source: Modified from Hollister L (1984) Effects of hallucinogens in humans. In *Hallucinogens: Neurochemical, Behavioral, and Clinical Perspectives*, Jacobs B (ed). Raven Press, New York.

DSM-IV-TR Diagnostic Criteria

292.89 HALLUCINOGEN INTOXICATION

A. Recent use of a hallucinogen.
B. Clinically significant maladaptive behavioral or psychological changes (e.g., marked anxiety or depression, ideas of reference, fear of losing one's mind, paranoid ideation, impaired judgment, or impaired social or occupational function) that developed during, or shortly after, hallucinogen use.
C. Perceptual changes occurring in a state of full wakefulness and alertness (e.g., subjective intensification of perceptions, depersonalization, derealization, illusions, hallucinations, synesthesias) that developed during, or shortly after, hallucinogen use.
D. Two (or more) of the following signs, developing during, or shortly after, hallucinogen use:

   (1) pupillary dilation
   (2) tachycardia
   (3) sweating
   (4) palpitations
   (5) blurring of vision
   (6) tremors
   (7) incoordination

E. The symptoms are not due to a general medical condition and are not better accounted for by another mental disorder.

Because chemical identification of hallucinogens in emergency specimens with methods such as gas chromatography–mass spectrometry remain costly and time consuming, clinicians in emergency settings must rely on a careful drug history, the information from the less drug-affected friends of the individual, the mental status examination, and signs apparent from the physical examination. Routes of administration other than by ingestion are rare.

Motor function is reduced, so that such individuals are not likely to act out aggressively. Emergency presentations of the proverbial "bad trip" have apparently declined in recent years despite continued use by a significant percentage of American youth. "Bad trips" are drug-induced panic attacks in the context of a hallucinogenic experience, associated with prepossessing feelings of unreality, confusion, and the flooding of the senses with unbidden imagery.

Differential Diagnosis

The differential diagnosis of an acute hallucinogenic intoxication includes intoxication by other agents (such as phencyclidine [PCP], cocaine, amphetamines, anticholinergics, and inhalants, among others). It also includes acute schizophrenia or affective disorder, panic disorder, head injury, sedative, hypnotic, anxiolytic, or alcohol withdrawal (including gamma-hydroxybutyrate [GHB]), metabolic disorders such as hypoglycemia and hyperthyroidism, epilepsy, acute vascular events, release hallucinations of ophthalmologic disease, and the complications of central nervous system (CNS) tumors. Age, along with prior clinical history, the history of the current event, physical examination, and toxicology screen for suspected nonhallucinogenic agents usually reveal the diagnosis.

An individual presenting with a history of taking LSD is only correct approximately 50% of the time, judging from analysis of street samples analyzed by the Massachusetts Department of Public Health in the last decade. The street practice of adulteration or mislabeling of the drug is common. Psychosis following a smoked agent suggests phencyclidine. Differentiating between PCP and LSD is clinically important, since LSD-induced panic responds well to oral benzodiazepines, while PCP delirium requires high potency antipsychotic medications such as haloperidol.

TREATMENT

Treatment of hallucinogen intoxication with panic is easily managed with oral benzodiazepines (diazepam 20 mg or lorazepam 2 mg), which bring the terror, as well as the trip, to an end within 30 minutes. This knowledge, along with the availability of benzodiazepines in the environment, has reduced the need for psychiatric emergency interventions.

Hallucinogen-Induced Psychotic Disorders

Among the hallucinogens, LSD has been associated with the majority of, but not all, prolonged psychotic reactions following acute drug use. Psychoses are apparently rare with the abuse of botanical preparations, in all likelihood because such agents are of low potency, not widely abused, and often controlled by religious sanctions.

In addition to exhibiting positive signs of schizophrenia, individuals with post-LSD psychoses show affective lability and the novel addition of visual hallucinations less common in non-drug-related psychoses.

Differential Diagnosis

The differential diagnosis of posthallucinogen psychosis is the same as that for any acute psychotic disorder. This includes protracted psychoses following the use of the dissociative anesthetics phencyclidine and ketamine, amphetamines, and cocaine; schizophrenia and affective disorders, migraine, deliria from CNS infections, closed head injuries, tumors, vascular events, and the toxic effects of bromine, heavy metals, and

anticholinergic drugs. Central to diagnosis is a careful premorbid history, complemented by data from friends and family on the individual's recent medical history and behavior. Neurological examination, urine for toxicological screening, and computed tomography or magnetic resonance imaging of the brain are helpful in ruling out treatable non-LSD-related psychotic disorders.

TREATMENT

Treatment for post-LSD psychoses has been described in a number of case series. Neuroleptics, ECT, lithium, and 5-hydroxytryptophan have all been reported to be useful.

Hallucinogen Persisting Perception Disorder (HPPD)

DIAGNOSIS

The DSM-IV-TR diagnostic criteria for hallucinogen persisting perception disorder are shown below.

It is not uncommon for an individual suffering from HPPD to consult multiple clinicians before a diagnosis is made. Because the symptoms are primarily perceptual, an HPPD subject may consult an ophthalmologist, neurologist, or psychologist before seeing a mental health professional. Often individuals come for help having made their own diagnoses using the DSM-IV-TR or internet chat groups devoted to HPPD.

DSM-IV-TR Diagnostic Criteria

292.89 HALLUCINOGEN PERSISTING PERCEPTION DISORDER (FLASHBACKS)

A. The reexperiencing, following cessation of use of a hallucinogen, of one or more of the perceptual symptoms that were experienced while intoxicated with the hallucinogen (e.g., geometric hallucinations, false perception of movement in the peripheral visual fields, flashes of color, intensified colors, trails of images of moving objects, positive afterimages, halos around objects, macropsia, and micropsia).

B. The symptoms in Criterion A cause clinically significant distress or impairment in social, occupational, or other important areas of functioning.

C. The symptoms are not due to a general medical condition (e.g., anatomical lesions and infections of the brain, visual epilepsies) and are not better accounted for by another mental disorder (e.g., delirium, dementia, schizophrenia) or hypnopompic hallucinations.

Reprinted with permission from the *Diagnostic and Statistical Manual of Mental Disorders*, 4th ed., Text Rev. Copyright 2000 American Psychiatric Association.

Despite an individual's certainty about their diagnosis, the clinician is obligated to rule out other sources of chronic organic hallucinosis, including other drug toxicities, strokes, CNS tumors, infections, and head trauma. Magnetic resonance images of the brain are usually negative. Quantitative electroencephalography shows accelerated alpha and visual evoked potentials, especially in the posterior cerebrum.

TREATMENT

Treatment at the present time is palliative. Benzodiazepines, olanzapine, sertraline, naltrexone, and clonidine have anecdotally been reported to help in selected cases. Risperidone has been reported to exacerbate HPPD symptoms. Marijuana can chronically induce an exacerbation of HPPD. Because HPPD is also exacerbated by CNS arousal, affect, stress, and stimulants, these are to be reduced or avoided. HPPD is worse with one's eyes closed, or when entering a dark environment. Thus, sunglasses, which serve to reduce the difference between outdoor and indoor luminance, may reduce HPPD symptoms when the individual enters an interior space.

MDMA ("Ecstasy")-Related Disorders

3,4-Methylenedioxymethamphetamine (MDMA, commonly known as "ecstasy," and chemically N-methyl-1-[3,4-methylene-dioxyphenyl]-2-aminopropane) is a synthetic amphetamine analogue that is also similar to mescaline. It was originally synthesized by Dr E. Merck and patented in Germany as an appetite suppressant in 1914. It was never marketed and did not attract attention until the 1970s when it was studied as a hallucinogen analogue. During the "psychedelic" 1970s, recreational use of MDMA took root because of its psychological effects and the fact that it was available legally. Recreational use was partially fueled by reports of the use of MDMA as a psychotherapeutic adjunct. In 1985, guided by reports that a structurally related congener, 3,4-methylenedioxyamphetamine (MDA), damages serotonergic neurons in rodents, the Drug Enforcement Administration (DEA) placed MDMA on Schedule 1 of controlled substances. The actions of the DEA were validated when subsequent reports found that MDMA is toxic to the animal and the human brain. This is not surprising since MDA is the major metabolite of MDMA.

The publicity that followed the scheduling of MDMA only served to increase its popularity, particularly in college campuses. Recently, the use of MDMA has increased and its pattern of use has changed. These

factors have heightened public awareness of the drug and paradoxically led to an increase in use and adverse consequences. Emerging evidence supports the hypothesis that MDMA is a neurotoxin in humans with long-lived sequelae on cognition, memory, and emotions.

DIAGNOSIS

A typical MDMA user is a college student. MDMA users are more likely to use marijuana, smoke cigarettes, and engage in binge alcohol consumption. While other drug use appears more common in subjects using MDMA, it is of interest to note that in over a third, their first exposure to illicit drugs is in the setting of MDMA use.

Unlike many drugs of abuse that are frequently used alone, MDMA is almost always used in the company of others. Most MDMA users report positive mood and emotional effects as they relate to others. In a survey of 44 experienced MDMA users, subjects reported a greater capacity for empathy, communication, and understanding (Table 19-2). Subjects also reported increased self-esteem, high energy, relaxation, and dissociation.

Altered perceptions may be experienced by some MDMA users as a negative consequence of the drug. In a double-blind, placebo-controlled study of 13 MDMA-naïve subjects, most reported anxiety, a mild depersonalization or derealization, a moderate thought disorder, and poor coordination. Worsening or precipitation of panic attacks has been reported in different settings. At least 12 cases of acute psychosis associated with MDMA use have been reported. In most of these cases, there is use of concomitant substances. In at least one case with long-term follow-up, psychotic symptoms were evident 6 months later. A wide range of impulsive or irrational behaviors have been associated with MDMA use. Most of these reports were published because they resulted in a major medical problem or death. There is no *a priori* reason to expect that MDMA

Table 19-2	A Survey of 44 Experienced MDMA Users Regarding Reported Effects of Ecstasy Use
Reported Effect of MDMA in the	**% Reporting**
Range of 50 to 700 mg	80
Increase in communication and empathy	68
Changes in cognition or mental associations	68
Increase in euphoria or ecstasy	63
Changes in perception[*]	44

[*]Illusions or hallucinations are usually associated with higher doses.

Reprinted with permission from Cohen S (1960) Lysergic acid diethylamide: side effects and complications. *J Nerv Ment Disord* **130**, 20–40. Copyright, Lipincott, Williams & Wilkins.

use would produce impulsivity, but many "ecstasy" users have an increase in impulsive behaviors.

MDMA users generally limit the frequency of use of the drug. Most report limiting use of MDMA to twice per month or less. Fridays and Saturdays are the most common days of use because users say they need one day to recover after use. More frequent use is associated with a loss of the desired effect of the drug.

Physical Consequences of MDMA Use

Users exhibit complications that are related to both the sympathomimetic and serotonergic properties of MDMA. These include nausea, vomiting, anorexia, hypertension, palpitations, diaphoresis, headaches, difficulty walking, muscle aches and tension, hot and cold flashes, urinary urgency, nystagmus, blurred vision, insomnia, and dry mouth. The common complaints of trismus and bruxism may reflect MDMA enhancement of serotonin activation of the $5HT_{1B}$ receptors of the trigeminal motor nuclei.

Other frequently reported acute physical consequences of MDMA use are muscle tension, diaphoresis, blurred vision, ataxia, hyperreflexia, tachycardia, and hypertension.

The acute motoric abnormalities have been related to driving impairment.

MDMA has been associated with a wide range of somatic toxic events. These include thrombotic or hemorrhagic strokes, leukoencephalopathy, myocardial infarction, arrhythmias, and pneumothorax. The wide range of manifestations suggests that many of these cases are either idiosyncratic or related to impurities remaining from the synthetic process.

There have been cases of severe medical illness or death due to electrolyte and fluid abnormalities and cases of multiple organ system failure. These complications may be related to the specific environment in raves, where people are exposed to hot, crowded environments. In association with the increased body temperature caused by MDMA, dehydration and its consequences are likely. Crowding has been shown to increase amphetamine toxicity in animals, a phenomenon labeled *aggregation toxicity*. A similar phenomenon may occur in crowded raves in humans.

MDMA may also cause serotonergic hyperstimulation and produce a fatal serotonin–syndrome-like illness.

Clinical Manifestations of Long-Term MDMA Neurotoxicity

Former chronic "ecstasy" users (an average of 527 tablets) have higher self-reported depression as measured by the Beck's Depression Scale than non-drug-using controls. Heavy MDMA use has also been associated with higher rates of psychopathology, including obsessive and compulsive behaviors, anxiety, somatization, and loss of libido. The cause-and-effect relationship between MDMA use and these psychiatric syndromes is unclear, but since these syndromes involve serotonergic mechanisms, additional investigation into these potential long-term sequelae is warranted.

MDMA users have been noted to have problems with memory, attention, reasoning, impulse control, and sleep abnormalities in numerous studies.

All subjects exposed to MDMA, no matter how significant the history of use, may have decreased verbal fluency, decreased immediate prose recall, and decreased delayed prose recall, but no change in visual recall. Most investigators agree regarding the potential for neurotoxicity after even minimal use.

TREATMENT

There have been no studies examining the treatment of MDMA use. This may be due to the rarity of presentation of subjects seeking treatment for MDMA addiction. Nonetheless, MDMA has abuse potential. Although not well studied, serotonin reuptake inhibiting antidepressants may offer a possible treatment for individuals who present with an MDMA addiction.

COMPARISON OF DSM-IV-TR AND ICD-10 DIAGNOSTIC CRITERIA

The ICD-10 and DSM-IV-TR diagnostic criteria are nearly identical.

20 Substance-Related Disorders: Inhalants

The term *inhalant abuse* is used to describe a variety of drug-using behaviors that cannot be classified by their pharmacology or toxicology but are grouped on the basis of their primary mode of administration. Although other substances can be inhaled (e.g., tobacco, marijuana with or without phencyclidine, and even heroin or crack), this is not the primary route of administration; therefore, they do not fall into this classification. Several subcategories of inhalants can be established on the basis of chemical classes of products and primary abuse groups as follows: (1) industrial or household cleaning and paint-type solvents including paint thinners or solvents, degreasers or dry cleaning solvents, solvents in glues, art or office supply solvents such as correction fluids, and solvents in magic markers (gasoline is similar to these products); (2) propellant gases used in household or commercial products, such as butane in lighters, or fluorocarbons in electronic (personal computer, office equipment) cleaners or refrigerant gases; (3) household aerosol sprays such as paint, hair, and fabric protector sprays; (4) medical anesthetic gases such as ether, chloroform, halothane, and nitrous oxide; and (5) aliphatic nitrites. Most of the foregoing compounds affect the central nervous system (CNS) directly, whereas nitrites act on cardiovascular smooth muscle rather than as an anesthetic in the CNS. The nitrites are also used primarily as sexual enhancers rather than as mood alterants. Therefore, when discussing "inhalant abuse," we will be referring primarily to substances other than nitrites. One item worthy of note: the exclusion of anesthetics from the inhalant-related disorders section in the DSM-IV-TR is not medically correct, as almost all of the inhalants act physiologically as would any anesthetic and some, particularly the anesthetics nitrous oxide and trichloroethylene (TCE), are abused by the primary inhalant abuser discussed herein. Thus, the following discussion includes the abuse of selected anesthetics but does not discuss the problems of the anesthetic state.

Table 20-1 enumerates the solvents (frequently noted on the labels) contained in corresponding popular products currently used for recreational purposes. The term "glue sniffing" is still widely used today to describe the abuse of most of these substances. It is important to keep in mind that there are many different chemicals in these different products, all of which have different physiological effects and toxicities as well as different chemical properties. Sometimes the substances are listed on the product label; however, many times the container lacks sufficient detail to identify the potential toxin(s).

The disorders described in this chapter are classified under the inhalant-related disorders section in DSM-IV-TR and are subdivided into two groups: inhalant use disorders and inhalant-induced disorders.

DIAGNOSIS

The practice of "sniffing," "snorting," "huffing," "bagging," or inhaling to get high describes various methods of inhalation. These terms refer to the inhalation of volatile substances from (1) filled balloons, (2) bags, and (3) soaked rags and/or sprayed directly into oral orifices. Abusers can be identified by various telltale clues such as organic odors in the breath or clothes, stains on the clothes or around the mouth, empty spray paint or solvent containers, and other unusual paraphernalia. These clues may enable one to identify a serious problem of solvent abuse before it causes serious health problems or death.

The following Inhalant-Related Disorders are included in DSM-IV-TR:

- *Inhalant Dependence*. Dependence on inhalants is primarily psychological, with a less dramatic associated physical dependence occurring in some heavy

Clinical Guide to the Diagnosis and Treatment of Mental Disorders. M. B. First and A. Tasman
© 2006 John Wiley & Sons, Ltd.   ISBN 0 470 019158

Table 20-1	Chemicals Commonly Found in Inhalants
Inhalant	**Chemicals**
Adhesives	
Airplane glue	Toluene, ethyl acetate
Other glues	Hexane, toluene, methyl chloride, acetone, methyl ethyl ketone, methyl butyl ketone
Special cements	Trichloroethylene, tetrachloroethylene
Aerosols	
Paint sprays	Butane, propane, fluorocarbons, toluene, hydrocarbons
Hair sprays	Butane, propane
Deodorants, air fresheners	Butane, propane
Analgesic spray	Fluorocarbons
Asthma spray	Fluorocarbons
Fabric spray	Butane, trichloroethane
Personal computer cleaners	Dimethyl ether, hydrofluorocarbons
Anesthetics	
Gaseous	Nitrous oxide
Liquid	Halothane, enflurane
Local	Ethyl chloride
Cleaning Agents	
Dry cleaners	Tetrachloroethylene, trichloroethane
Spot removers	Xylene, petroleum distillates, chlorohydrocarbons
Degreasers	Tetrachloroethylene, trichloroethane, trichloroethylene
Solvents and Gases	
Nail polish remover	Acetone, ethyl acetate, toluene
Paint remover	Toluene, methylene chloride, methanol, acetone, ethyl acetate
Paint thinners	Petroleum distillates, esters, acetone
Correction fluids and thinners	Trichloroethylene, trichloroethane
Fuel gas	Butane, isopropane
Cigar or cigarette lighter fluid	Butane, isopropane
Fire extinguisher propellant	Bromochlorodifluoromethane
Food Products	
Whipped cream aerosols	Nitrous oxide
Whippets	Nitrous oxide
Room Odorizers	
Poppers, fluids (Rush, Locker Room)	Isoamyl, isobutyl, isopropyl, or butyl nitrite (now illegal) or cyclohexyl

users (see generic DSM-IV-TR diagnostic criteria, Chapter 13, page 125). Physical tolerance of some solvents has been documented by animal studies only under unusual conditions. The urgent need to continue use of inhalants has been reported among individuals with heavy use, although the nature of this phenomenon is unknown. There is at least a psychological dependence and often a weak physical dependence on these substances. A mild withdrawal syndrome occurs in 10 to 24 hours after cessation of use (only in those who have excessively abused inhalants) and lasts for several days. Symptoms include general disorientation, sleep disturbances, headaches, muscle spasms, irritability, nausea, and fleeting illusions. However, this is not an easily identified or a characteristic withdrawal syndrome that is useful for many practitioners in a clinical setting. The need to continue use is undeniably strong in many individuals; specific treatments for inhalant dependence, other than the drug therapy and/or psychotherapy used for other drug dependence, need to be developed.

• *Inhalant Abuse*. Abuse of inhalants may lead to harm to individuals (e.g., accidents involving automobiles, falling from buildings when in an impaired or intoxicated state (illusionary feelings), or self-inflicted harm such as attempted or successful suicide) (see generic DSM-IV-TR diagnostic criteria, Chapter 13, page 125). Frozen lips caused by rapidly expanding gases or serious burns may also occur. Chronic inhalant use is often associated with familial conflict and school problems.

• *Inhalant-Induced Disorders*. The primary disorder is inhalant intoxication, which is characterized by the presence of clinically significant maladaptive behavioral or psychological changes (e.g., belligerence, assaultiveness, apathy, impaired judgment, impaired social or occupational functioning) that develop during the intentional short-term, high-dose exposure to volatile inhalants (see DSM-IV-TR diagnostic criteria for inhalant intoxication, page 182). The maladaptive changes occurring after intentional and nonintentional exposure include disinhibition, excitedness, light-headedness, visual disturbances (blurred vision, nystagmus), incoordination, dysarthria, an unsteady gait, and euphoria. Higher doses of inhalants may lead to depressed reflexes, stupor, coma, and death, sometimes caused by cardiac arrhythmia. Lethargy, generalized muscle weakness, and headaches may occur some hours later depending on the dose.

There is little evidence that inhalant abuse either coexists with other mental disorders or leads to any such altered state. There have been few studies of comorbidity in psychiatric hospital populations and almost no studies in other populations.

On the other hand, there is clinical experience which strongly suggests that personality disorders of an antisocial type are common in solvent abusers.

DSM-IV-TR Diagnostic Criteria

292.89 INHALANT INTOXICATION

A. Recent intentional use or short-term, high-dose exposure to volatile inhalants (excluding anesthetic gases and short-acting vasodilators).

B. Clinically significant maladaptive behavioral or psychological changes (e.g., belligerence, assaultiveness, apathy, impaired judgment, impaired social or occupational functioning) that developed during, or shortly after, use of or exposure to volatile inhalants.

C. Two (or more) of the following signs developing during, or shortly after, inhalant use or exposure:

   (1) dizziness
   (2) nystagmus
   (3) incoordination
   (4) slurred speech
   (5) unsteady gait
   (6) lethargy
   (7) depressed reflexes
   (8) psychomotor retardation
   (9) tremor
   (10) generalized muscle weakness
   (11) blurred vision or diplopia
   (12) stupor or coma
   (13) euphoria

D. The symptoms are not due to a general medical condition and are not better accounted for by another mental disorder.

Reprinted with permission from the *Diagnostic and Statistical Manual of Mental Disorders*, 4th ed., Text Rev. Copyright 2000 American Psychiatric Association.

Table 20-2 | Symptoms Related to Solvent Abuse (Not All for Gases and Nitrites)

Moderate Intoxication
Dizziness
Headache
Lethargy
Disorientation, incoherence
Ataxia, gait (uncoordinated movement)
Odoriferous, foul breath (solvent vapors)

Strong Intoxication
Blurred vision
Belligerence
Nausea, vomiting
Irritability
Delirium
Slurred speech

Severe (Rare)
Seizures
Violent actions

Toxicology of Inhalant Abuse

The majority of inhalant abusers are never seen in a hospital or outpatient facility. Although many do not need medical attention for their inhalant habit, of those who do, many often die before reaching the hospital as a result of asphyxia, cardiac arrhythmia, or related overdose effects after inhaling fluorocarbons, low-molecular-weight hydrocarbon gases (butane, propane), nitrous oxide, or other solvents including toluene during either the first or a subsequent episode. Death may also occur after inhalation of toluene-containing substances as a result of metabolic acidosis or related kidney failure if left untreated. Although it is not common, anesthetics abused by medical personnel or others have also been a cause of death; death related to nitrous oxide use is often due to asphyxia. Some of the more common acute syndromes of the intoxicated state are listed in Table 20-2.

Neurotoxic Manifestations

Chronic high-level exposure to organic solvents occurs in the inhalant abuse setting at levels several thousand times higher than in the occupational setting and results in numerous irreversible disease states. Table 20-3 describes several well-characterized disorders and identifies the solvent when corroborated by animal studies. Some substances have been strongly correlated with the development of a disorder through numerous case studies.

Many organic solvents produce nonspecific effects (e.g., encephalopathy) after exposure to extremely high concentrations; a few produce relatively specific neurological syndromes with chronic administration. Two specific neurotoxic syndromes, a peripheral neuropathy and an ototoxicity, are well correlated with organic solvents. Most common, however, is a clinical syndrome consisting of cognitive impairment, cerebellar ataxia, and spasticity syndrome. In addition, a myopathy may occur alone or in combination with any of these clinical syndromes.

Most reports emphasize the cerebellar and cognitive dysfunction, with most cases showing combined impairment of cerebral and cerebellar functions as well as pyramidal changes. Neurological abnormalities vary from mild cognitive impairment to severe dementia, associated with elemental neurological signs such as cerebellar ataxia, corticospinal tract dysfunction, oculomotor abnormalities, tremor, deafness, and hyposmia. Cognitive dysfunction is the most disabling and frequent feature of chronic toluene toxicity and may be the earliest sign of permanent damage. Dementia, when present, is typically associated with cerebellar ataxia and other signs.

Ototoxicity. Sensorineural hearing loss is one of the more commonly occurring clinical neurotoxic syndromes related to inhalant abuse, along with a related

Table 20-3	Diseases Observed in Humans After Chronic Inhalant Abuse		
Condition	**Syndrome**	**Substance**	**Animal Studies**[*]
Slowly Reversible and/or Irreversible Syndromes			
Encephalopathy	Cognitive dysfunction	"Toluene,"[†] other solvents	—
Cerebellar syndrome	Limb dysmetria	"Toluene"	Rat
	Dysarthria		—
Sensorineural optic	High-frequency hearing loss	TCE, toluene	Rat, mouse
Sensorineural			
Optic nerve	Visual loss	"Toluene"	—
Oculomotor	Oculomotor disturbances (nystagmus)	Xylene, TCE	Rabbits
Myeloneuropathy	Sensory loss	Nitrous oxide	Rat, mouse
	Spasticity		
Axonal neuropathy	Distal sensory loss, limb weakness	Hexane, methyl butyl ketone	Rat, monkey
Cardiotoxicity	Arrhythmia	Chlorofluorocarbons, butanes, propanes	Mouse, rat, dog
Leukemia	Myelocytic	Benzene	Rat, mouse
Mostly Reversible Syndromes			
Trigeminal neuropathy	Numbness, paresthesia	TCE and/or dichloroacetylene	Rat
Renal acidosis	Metabolic acidosis	"Toluene"	Rat
	Hypokalemia		—
Carboxyhemoglobin	Hypoxia	Methylene chloride, tobacco	Human, rat
Methemoglobinemia	Syncope, blue	Nitrites, organic	Rat
Neonatal syndrome	Retarded growth, development	"Toluene"	Rat
Hepatotoxicity	Fatty vacuoles, plasma liver enzymes	Chlorohydrocarbons	Rat
Immunomodulatory	Loss of immune cell function	Nitrites, organic	Rat

[*]Symptoms observed in animal studies with these solvents.
[†]Quotation marks around substance indicates uncertainty about this solvent (alone) producing these symptoms.

equilibrium disorder. Neural conduction, most readily diagnosed by brain stem auditory evoked responses, is often abnormal. Brain stem auditory evoked responses may be a sensitive screening test for monitoring individuals at risk from toluene exposure and for early detection of CNS injury. However, although specific in revealing abnormalities characteristic of CNS involvement in chronic inhalant abuse, brain stem auditory evoked responses reveal abnormalities only in a small number of individuals of a chronic inhalant abuse population.

Other Cranial Nerve Involvement. A wide variety of neuropathic manifestations have been reported, and all of these neuropathies can be identified with specific cranial nerves (Table 20-4).

Anosmia is an often described syndrome of inhalant abuse. It would be expected that solvents would diminish the olfactory responses; however, it has seldom been studied.

Trigeminal Neuropathy. One neurological manifestation associated with TCE intoxication is a slowly reversible trigeminal neuropathy. Individuals developed paresthesia around the lips, which then spreads to involve the entire trigeminal distribution bilaterally. Motor weakness also occasionally occurred. Resolution of the trigeminal neuropathy occurs slowly, which is thought to indicate segmental or nuclear trigeminal involvement.

High levels of nitrous oxide exposure produce a myeloneuropathy with both central and peripheral components, even in the presence of adequate oxygen. The symptoms include numbness and weakness in the limbs, loss of dexterity, sensory loss, and loss of balance. The early neurological features indicate sensorimotor polyneuropathy; however, with persistent abuse, a myelopathy with severe spasticity may develop. There is also a combined degeneration of the posterior and lateral columns of the spinal cord resembling that in vitamin B_{12} deficiency, and other neuropathic symptoms resulting from spinal cord degeneration were produced after prolonged anesthesia in vitamin B_{12}-deficient individuals. Administration of vitamin B_{12} (or folinic acid) dramatically aids recovery of these surgical patients and may assist recovery in solvent abusers, especially once the myelopathy appears.

Table 20-4	Cranial Nerve Abnormalities Noted in Inhalant Abuse
Cranial Nerve	**Dysfunction**
I	Hyposmia, anosmia
II	Optic neuropathy
III, IV, VI	Oculomotor disorders: nystagmus, opsoclonus, ocular dysmetria
VIII	Sensorineural hearing loss

Peripheral Neuropathy. Cases of *n*-hexane polyneuropathy have been reported both after occupational exposure and after deliberate inhalation of vapors from products containing *n*-hexane such as glues gasoline, and naphtha.

Clinically and pathologically, the neuropathy occurring with *n*-hexane or MBK is that of a distal axonopathy. The clinical syndrome is an initially painless sensorimotor polyneuropathy, which begins after chronic exposure; weight loss may be an early symptom. Sensory and motor disturbances are noted initially in the hands and feet, and sensory loss involves primarily small fiber sensation (i.e., light touch, pin prick, temperature) with relative sparing of large fiber sensation (i.e., position and vibration).

Prognosis for recovery correlates directly with the intensity and duration of the toxic exposure and the severity of the neuropathy. Residual neuropathy is seen only in the most severely affected individuals with motor as well as sensory involvement, some of whom still continue to inhale despite warnings of further debilitation.

Nonnervous System Toxicity

Most of the known adverse clinical effects of inhalant abuse relate to its effects on the nervous system. There are, however, other significant adverse effects on other organ systems including the kidney, liver, lung, heart, and hemopoietic systems.

TREATMENT

Individuals need different treatments based on the severity of the dependence and any medical complications. Primary care physicians should address the medical issues identified earlier as well as other medical concerns before dealing with the dependence on solvents and other drugs. During this period, sedatives, neuroleptics, and other forms of pharmacotherapy are not useful in the treatment of inhalant abusers and should be avoided in most cases as they are likely to exacerbate the depressed state. Once it is determined that the individual is detoxified, that is, has low levels of solvent or other depressant drug, then therapy with other drugs, such as antianxiety drugs, may be useful. The determination of detoxification, even in the absence of drug (solvent) administration, is not well defined or systematic. It may take several days for the major "reversible" intoxication state to be reduced to a level at which coherent cognition can occur. The use of various psychological assessment tools can assist not only in evaluating the intoxication but also in following the progress of the treatment. Little can be done during this period other than to facilitate improvement of the basic health of these individuals, provide supportive care, and build the individual's self-esteem.

There is no accepted treatment approach for inhalant abuse. It should also be emphasized that there are various categories of solvent abusers, from those who may use only one substance (e.g., only nitrous oxide or butanes) to heavy users of a variety of solvents and gases. Many drug treatment facilities refuse treatment of the inhalant abuser because many feel that inhalant abusers are resistant to treatment or that there is no standard or accepted treatment. One facility that focuses solely on the comprehensive treatment of inhalant abusers, the International Institute on Inhalant Abuse based in Colorado (www.allaboutinhalants. com), uses a three-phase model that allows longer periods of treatment. Longer periods of treatment are needed to be able to address the complex psychosocial, economic, and biophysical issues of the inhalant abuser. When brain injury, primarily in the form of cognitive dysfunction, is present, the rate of progression in the treatment process is even slower and assumes a comprehensive neurological rehabilitation approach similar to that in individuals with traumatic brain injury. As few treatment approaches with solvent abusers have been evaluated, none on a broad scale, all treatments should consider several important parameters including the following:

- Culture
- Family structure
- Living environment
- Peer interactions
- Individual's ability to learn and adapt
- Establishment of self-image
- Individual attitudes and behavioral characteristics
- Building basic life skills
- Social bonding.

Some of these issues may be dealt with only through treating these individuals separately, especially in the early periods of treatment.

The inhalant abuser typically does not respond to usual drug rehabilitation treatment modalities. Several factors may be involved, particularly for the chronic abuser who may have significant psychosocial problems as well as irreversible brain injury. Treatment becomes slower and progressively more difficult when the severity of brain injury worsens as abuse progresses through transient social use (experimenting in groups) to chronic use in isolation. For these and other reasons, longer therapies are necessary than are utilized in most drug treatment facilities. Also, neurological impairment, the breadth of which still needs to be established, may be a major complication slowing the progress of rehabilitation. This is not as significant a problem with other forms of drug abuse.

Drug screening would be useful in monitoring inhalant abusers. Routine urine screening for hippuric acid (the major metabolite of toluene metabolism) performed two or three times weekly can detect the high level of exposure to toluene commonly seen in inhalant abusers. More frequently performed expired breath analysis for toluene or other abused compounds is also available. As alcohol is a common secondary drug of abuse among inhalant abusers, alcohol abuse should be monitored and considered in the approach to treatment.

COMPARISON OF DSM-IV-TR AND ICD-10 DIAGNOSTIC CRITERIA

The DSM and ICD-10 criteria are nearly identical.

Substance-Related Disorders: Nicotine

Nicotine dependence is the most common substance use disorder in the United States with about 25% of the population addicted to tobacco. Tobacco addiction has serious health consequences for the user, family members, and others who breathe second-hand environmental tobacco smoke or are exposed during pregnancy. Tobacco addiction increases morbidity and mortality. Many individuals with mental illness or other addictions are nicotine dependent, and about half of all the cigarettes consumed in the United States are by these individuals.

DIAGNOSIS

Nicotine Dependence

In the DSM-IV-TR, a specifier is used to designate the presence or absence of physiological dependence, depending on whether tolerance or withdrawal is present or whether both are absent (see generic DSM-IV-TR diagnostic criteria for Substance Dependence in Chapter 13, page 125). Further specifiers can be used to denote course (e.g., early full remission or sustained partial remission). Of note, the DSM distinguishes nicotine from other substances by not including a diagnosis of nicotine abuse because most individuals transit quickly and directly from use to dependence (meeting criteria of tolerance and withdrawal).

The DSM-IV-TR nicotine withdrawal syndrome describes a characteristic set of symptoms that develops after abrupt cessation or a reduction in the use of nicotine products after at least several weeks of daily use. Other symptoms that may be associated with nicotine withdrawal include craving for nicotine, a factor thought to be significant in relapse; a desire for sweets; and impaired performance on tasks requiring vigilance. To some extent, the degree of physiological dependence predicts severity of the withdrawal syndrome and difficulty stopping smoking. In addition to frank

> ### DSM-IV-TR Diagnostic Criteria
>
> **292.0 NICOTINE WITHDRAWAL**
>
> A. Daily use of nicotine for at least several weeks.
> B. Abrupt cessation of nicotine use, or reduction in the amount of nicotine used, followed within 24 hours by four (or more) of the following signs:
>
>   (1) dysphoric or depressed mood
>   (2) insomnia
>   (3) irritability, frustration, or anger
>   (4) anxiety
>   (5) difficulty concentrating
>   (6) restlessness
>   (7) decreased heart rate
>   (8) increased appetite or weight gain
>
> C. The symptoms in Criterion B cause clinically significant distress or impairment in social, occupational, or other important areas of functioning.
> D. The symptoms are not due to a general medical condition and are not better accounted for by another mental disorder.
>
> Reprinted with permission from the *Diagnostic and Statistical Manual of Mental Disorders*, 4th ed., Text Rev. Copyright 2000 American Psychiatric Association.

symptoms, other objective biological and physiological changes are associated with nicotine withdrawal, such as generalized slowing of electroencephalographic activity, decreases in catecholamine and cortisol levels, changes in rapid eye movement, impairment on neuropsychological testing, and decreased metabolic rate.

Nicotine dependence and smoking are two to three times more common in individuals with mental and other substance use disorders than in the general population. Smoking-related illnesses are the primary cause of death among those in recovery from other substances. It is estimated that 55–90% of individuals with mental disorders smoke versus 23% of the general population. The prevalence of smoking is especially high in individuals with schizophrenia (70–90%), affective disorders (42–70%), and alcohol

Clinical Guide to the Diagnosis and Treatment of Mental Disorders. M. B. First and A. Tasman
© 2006 John Wiley & Sons, Ltd.   ISBN 0 470 019158

dependence (60–90%) or other substance use disorders (70–95%). The odds ratio for "ever smoked" is 4.7 in persons suffering from alcohol dependence, 2.4 for individuals with major depressive disorder (MDD), 1.8 for persons with agoraphobia, 1.6 for individuals with dysthymia, and 1.6 for individuals with panic disorder (PD). Conversely, there is also evidence that affective, anxiety, and substance use disorders may be more common in individuals who smoke than in those who do not or in those who have never smoked. Finally, there is evidence to suggest that in one study up to 75% of smokers with a history of MDD developed depressed mood during the first week of withdrawal versus only 30% of those with no depressive history, and that the withdrawal syndrome may be more severe in smokers with a history of depression. The presence of depressive symptoms during withdrawal is also associated with failed cessation attempts. Self-reported depressive symptoms during adolescence also predict later frequency and duration of smoking. Several studies suggest a genetic predisposition to both nicotine dependence and co-occurring depression.

There is no simple reason why so many individuals with a mental disorder smoke. As with other addictive disorders, a combination of complex biological and psychosocial factors is likely. Potential biological factors in this group include a greater likelihood of susceptibility to nicotine dependence, with persons experiencing a greater sense of reward from nicotine. Other possibilities include using nicotine to reduce the side effects of psychiatric medications, both as a stimulant to counter sedation as well as a dopamine modulator that can diminish neuroleptic-induced parkinsonism. Subjectively, individuals report that using nicotine improves their cognitive functioning and reduces stress, although research data is mixed in this regard. In individuals with schizophrenia, an abnormality in P50 gating, which is believed to relate clinically to the ability to filter out distracting auditory stimuli, is reversed with nicotine. Social and behavioral factors are also important in understanding nicotine dependence, and psychiatric and addictive comorbidity. Smoking has been ignored and is a part of the pervasive culture in most mental health and substance abuse treatment centers and residential facilities. This is beginning to change. Historically, smoking was often used as a behavioral reward in psychiatric inpatient units and continues to serve as a social connector for many individuals with a mental disorder. Additionally, individuals coping with persistent psychiatric symptoms and reduced social and occupational functioning report smoking to fill the voids of boredom and disappointment.

Course

The National Health Interview Survey found that 70% of smokers interviewed reported they wanted to quit smoking at some point in their lifetime, and about 33% of smokers try to quit each year. Only about 3% of quit attempts without formal treatment are successful, and in recent years, about 30% of smokers who want to quit are seeking treatment. Outcomes for nicotine dependence treatment vary by the type of treatment and the intensity of treatment with specific reports ranging from about 15% to 45% 1-year abstinence rates following treatment. Cessation attempts result in high relapse rates, with the relapse curve for smoking cessation paralleling that for opiates. Most individuals relapse during the first 3 days of withdrawal and most others will relapse within the first 3 months. Withdrawal symptoms are most severe within the first 1 to 3 days of abstinence, often continue for 3 to 4 weeks, and in some persons last for up to 6 months or longer. Current depressive symptoms and a history of depression are predictors of relapse. Weight gain may also contribute to relapse, particularly in women. In contrast, several factors have been found to predict worse outcomes at smoking cessation (Table 21-1). Predictors include individual factors, manifestations of the addiction such as severity of withdrawal, and social and environmental circumstances.

Nicotine dependence, like other substance use disorders, can be thought of as a chronic relapsing illness with a course of intermittent episodes alternating with periods of remission for most smokers. About 65% of those who stop smoking relapse in 3 months and another 10% relapse in 3 to 6 months, and with treatment the overall relapse rate is still about 75–80% by 1 year. However, these reported lower outcome rates do not consider the additive effects over time related to multiple quit attempts, since about 40–50% of smokers in the United States have been able to quit smoking in their lifetime. Less than 25% of the individuals who have quit smoking are successful in their first attempt.

Table 21-1	Factors Predicting Worse Outcomes in Nicotine Dependence Treatment

Physical reactivity (pulse, blood pressure, etc.) to smoking-related cues
Family and friends who are current smokers
Lack of social support from spouses, partners, family members, friends
Deficits in social skills and assertiveness
Higher severity of withdrawal symptoms
Limited ability to cope with effects occurring in response to cues or triggers
Depressed mood

Repeated failures are common before successful abstinence, with the average smoker attempting to quit five
or six times before success. Recent prior attempts at
quitting do increase the odds that individuals will be
able to quit smoking on a future attempt. Relapse can
occur even after a long time of abstinence, with about
33% of former smokers who are abstinent for 1 year
eventually relapsing 5 to 10 years after cessation.

Treatment of nicotine dependence with resultant abstinence can result in highly beneficial health effects.
Educating individuals and families about these benefits
of abstinence from smoking can be helpful. Short-term
effects (within 1 month) include a significant reduction in respiratory symptoms and respiratory infections
such as influenza, pneumonia, and bronchitis. Excess
risk of death from coronary heart disease is reduced
after 1 year and continues to decline over time. In individuals with coronary heart disease, smoking cessation
decreases the risk of recurrent myocardial infarction
and cardiovascular death by 50%. By 10 to 15 years of
abstinence, the mortality rate from all causes returns
to that of a person who has never smoked. Pulmonary
function can also return to normal if chronic obstructive changes have not already occurred at the time of
cessation, and even with obstructive changes pulmonary function can improve with abstinence.

TREATMENT

Nicotine dependence treatment targets severity of the
problem, co-occurring disorders, and the different motivational levels to change. Treatment is provided in a
range of levels of intensity of care (self-help, brief treatment, and once or twice per week outpatient treatment)
and may include different modalities (self-help guides,
internet resources, medications, and individual or group
therapy). Formal treatment options have expanded rapidly in the past 25 years to include six FDA-approved
medications, and a range of effective psychosocial interventions including internet and phone-line services.
(Table 21-2). Unfortunately, most insurance plans do
not cover nicotine dependence treatment, and only
some prescription plans will cover the medications. Few

individuals receive combined medications and therapy
treatment. Most receiving treatment get medication
treatments, and only about 3% of the individuals receiving medication treatments will also receive psychosocial treatment despite the fact that this combination
improves outcomes by 50%. Primary care treatment
providers tend to offer brief counseling treatment services with follow-up visits. In addition, many individuals
receive minimal formal treatment and either purchase
over-the-counter nicotine replacement patch or gum, or
go to Nicotine Anonymous or other self-help groups in
attempting to quit on their own.

Before formal intervention is undertaken, it is beneficial and important to perform a comprehensive
evaluation to determine the biological, psychological,
and social factors that are most significant in the initiation and maintenance of nicotine use and dependence.
Comprehensive evaluation of the individual is outlined
in Table 21-3. The assessment often begins with an assessment of the patterns of tobacco usage (number of
cigarettes smoked per day, times during the day, location, and circumstances). In addition, the amount of
tobacco usage can be assessed through cotinine levels
or carbon monoxide (CO) levels. Cotinine levels can
be obtained from the urine, blood, or saliva to assess
the amount of nicotine ingested. The expired-air test
for a CO level is not costly and can be obtained within
a minute by any clinician with a CO meter. The CO
meter is useful at intake and to monitor for relapse.

A history of prior cessation attempts should include
the nature of prior treatments, length of abstinence,
timing of relapse, and factors specifically related to
relapse (e.g., environmental or interpersonal triggers).
Assessing prior treatments includes assessing medications and psychosocial treatments. The five Food and

Table 21-2	Effectiveness of Nicotine Dependence Treatment Interventions
No professional or formal intervention	5%
Physicians' advice	10%
Nicotine polacrilex	15–20%
Nicotine patch, gum, inhaler	20–25%
Bupropion	25%
Behavioral therapy	25–30%
Medication and behavioral therapy	40%

Table 21-3	Assessing Nicotine Use and Nicotine Dependence

Current and past patterns of tobacco use
(include multiple sources of nicotine)
Current motivation to quit
Objective measures: breath CO level or cotinine level
  (saliva, blood, urine)
Assess prior quit attempts (number and what happened in
  each attempt)
  Why quit? How long abstinent? Why relapsed?
  What treatment was used (how used and for how long)
Assess withdrawal symptoms and dependence criteria
Psychiatric and other substance use history
Medical conditions
Their common triggers (car, people, moods, home, phone
  calls, meals, etc.)
Perceived barriers against and supports for treatment
  success
Preference for treatment strategy

Drug Administration (FDA)-approved medications for nicotine dependence treatment are the four nicotine replacement therapies (NRT) of the patch, gum, spray, and inhaler, and the nonnicotine pill bupropion (Zyban). Sometimes, other medications have been prescribed for nicotine dependence treatment. Assessment about medications includes asking about what dose of medications and how long it was taken, any side effects that developed, and how the individual actually took the medication (especially relevant for NRT). For example, the individual may report taking off the NRT patch prior to a shower and then replacing the same patch, rendering it ineffective. Psychosocial treatments might include group or individual treatment, American Lung Association and other community support groups, hypnosis, acupuncture, or Nicotine Anonymous. A history of specific withdrawal symptoms and their severity and duration is critical, as is an assessment of the smoker's social and environmental contexts, for example, whether other household members smoke, and available family and social supports.

An assessment should be made of the person's reasons for quitting, his or her motivation and commitment and self-efficacy (perceived ability to quit). The individual's stage of readiness for stopping smoking is also important; that is, whether the person is not yet seriously considering stopping smoking (precontemplation), is considering attempting to quit but not for several months (contemplation), is seriously considering quitting in the next month and has begun to think about the necessary steps to stop smoking (preparation), or is actually attempting to stop smoking (action). It is also important to access the smoker's knowledge about smoking and nicotine dependence because deficits in knowledge and information can have a deleterious effect on smoking cessation attempts.

Assessment of the psychiatric history is also important. Numerous studies have shown the significance of current and past depression in relation to smoking, as well as the increased prevalence rates of cigarette smoking in individuals with a variety of mental disorders, such as MDD, schizophrenia, and alcohol and substance abuse. The presence of these comorbid disorders may also make successful smoking cessation less likely, especially if undiagnosed and untreated.

Assessing the individual for a history of current alcohol or other substance abuse is also important, as the prevalence of smoking in persons with alcohol dependence as well as in other substance abusers is much higher than in the general population. It may also be more difficult for individuals with current or prior substance abuse or dependence to stop smoking, as there is evidence that persons with alcohol dependence and other substance abusers start smoking earlier and are more physiologically dependent on nicotine. In addition, the use of alcohol or other substances may be intimately linked to smoking cigarettes and can serve as a strong trigger for craving and ultimate relapse.

A careful medical history should also be obtained. The presence of significant tobacco-related medical illness can sometimes serve as crucial leverage to help motivate the individual to attempt cessation. Current medications and medical conditions may also be important considerations in determining the approach to cessation, especially with regard to pharmacotherapy. For example, a history of seizures or an eating disorder is usually a contraindication to the use of bupropion/Zyban (nonnicotine pill medication). The individual should be assessed for pulmonary symptoms and signs (cough), and if there is a long history of significant nicotine use, pulmonary function tests should be considered. The presence of significant cardiovascular disease, especially a history of recent myocardial infarction, is especially relevant to planning psychopharmacological interventions. If the individual is already taking a psychiatric medication, consider it important to realize that quitting smoking may result in an increase in medication blood levels and side effects.

Phases of Treatment

The general approach to the treatment of nicotine dependence considers three phases of treatment (engagement, quitting, and relapse prevention) (Table 21-4). Each phase of treatment includes consideration of three primary biological, psychological, and social factors affecting nicotine dependence outcomes. The biological or physiological dependence parallels the characteristics of other physiologically addicting substances (dose-related effects, rapid tolerance leading to increased intake and the presence of a withdrawal syndrome, compulsive use). Psychological dependence involves the perceived benefits/reasons a person smokes, such as a perception that they are able to improve mood and sense of well-being, to satisfy craving, and to provide stimulation and relaxation. The social component involves environmental and social cues that become associated with the behavior of smoking cigarettes, such as the association with drinking coffee or alcohol, talking on the telephone, taking a work break, or smoking at parties or social functions. The direct beneficial effects of nicotine on mood and concentration become highly positive reinforcements, as do associated social context and behaviors linked with smoking, which then can act as powerful triggers for relapse during attempts at cessation.

Table 21-4	Three Phases of Nicotine Dependence Treatment

Engagement Phase
- Do a comprehensive evaluation of nicotine use and dependence
- Provide MET personalized feedback from the assessment
- Assess motivational level to quit and attempt to set a target quit date
- Explore previous quit attempts. What worked? What did not work? What triggered the return to tobacco use?
- Assess patient preference for treatment (medications, psychosocial treatments, group vs. individual, self-help, etc.) and provide education on treatment
- Create a treatment plan
- Strengthen and renew patient's motivation to quit smoking (MET orientation)
- Identify cues and triggers for usage
- Self-monitoring of smoking behavior (write down when use)
- Help patients gain understanding of their own tobacco use patterns
- Help increase knowledge about triggers and cues
- Help patients understand environmental influences on their smoking
- Begin education about nicotine, tobacco addiction, withdrawal symptoms, etc.
- Begin disconnecting smoking behavior and linked behaviors (no smoking while driving car, talking on phone, during meal time, etc.)
- Help them get medication evaluation and medications for the quitting phase

Quitting Phase
- Start medications on quit date (NRT) or before quit date (bupropion), sometimes begin NRT (gum, spray, inhaler, not patch) in small amounts and reduce tobacco usage in an equivalent or greater amount
- Teach specific coping techniques for handling withdrawal symptoms, cues/triggers, and how to enhance social support
- Help patient prepare emotionally, behaviorally, and physically for the quit date and the early abstinence period
- Help identify support systems, anticipate challenges, and address ways to handle people, places, things, and mood challenges
- Address nutrition and exercise components
- Address role of family/friends in supporting or sabotaging treatment
- Continue to strengthen client's resolve to quit
- Continue relapse prevention therapy approaches
- Assess triggers to craving and use and high-risk situations
- Coping with cravings, thoughts, and urges
- Problem solving
- Smoke refusal skills
- Planning for emergencies
- Seemingly irrelevant decisions
- Relapse analysis for slips

Relapse Prevention Phase
- Continue relapse prevention strategies for long-term abstinence
- Reinforce specific coping skills, including mood management and patient specific triggers
- Teach positive coping skills for dealing with frustration and anxiety
- Compliment success and provide encouragement
- Continue focus on maintaining motivation and commitment for abstinence
- Monitor progress
- Provide treatment within your discipline and make referrals when appropriate
- Encourage the use of peer support such as Nicotine Anonymous, help the client gain personal insight, and keep growing in their recovery
- Manage any relapses/slips to continue the course
- Continue medications as needed

The importance of each of the biopsychosocial factors in initiating and maintaining smoking can vary considerably in different individuals. As a result, smoking cessation interventions should be tailored to the individual and his or her particular circumstances. This may be one reason why "one size fits all" generic treatment interventions have had such a low success rate. It must also be kept in mind that nicotine dependence is as complex in its components and determinants as other addictions and that more comprehensive multicomponent treatments may be required.

When a smoker is ready for a cessation attempt, a "quit date" should be selected. After cessation, close monitoring should occur during the early period of abstinence. Before the quit date, the person should be encouraged to explore and organize social support for the self-attempt. Plans to minimize cues associated with smoking (e.g., avoiding circumstances likely to contribute to relapse) are important, as is considering alternative coping behaviors for situations with a higher potential for relapse. A telephone or face-to-face follow-up during the first few days after cessation is critical because this is the time that withdrawal symptoms are most severe, with 65% of individuals relapsing by 1 week. A follow-up face-to-face meeting within 1 to 2 weeks allows a discussion of problems that have occurred (e.g., difficulties managing craving) and serves as an opportunity to provide reinforcement for ongoing abstinence. Even after the early period of abstinence, periodic telephone or face-to-face contacts can provide continued encouragement to maintain abstinence, allow problems with maintaining abstinence to be addressed, and provide feedback regarding the health benefits of abstinence.

If an initial attempt at cessation using only information and brief advice from the physician has been unsuccessful, pharmacotherapy may be used unless contraindications are present or unless the person has had few or no significant withdrawal symptoms. The most common pharmacotherapy approaches are NRTs (patch, gum, spray, or inhaler) or bupropion (Zyban for nicotine dependence = Wellbutrin for depression). Combining different types of NRT and bupropion is becoming more common in clinical practice, including using these medications for at least several months and in some cases 1 year or longer. Maintenance medications are being considered in an effort of harm reduction in a more select group of individuals. If a detoxification/quit attempt with pharmacotherapy alone fails, psychosocial treatments and the use of higher NRT dosages/multiple medications are the next possible clinical steps. Psychosocial treatments are often available through organizations such as the American Cancer Society, the American Lung Association, the American Heart Association, or through local hospitals that provide health prevention and public education programs. If pharmacotherapy is unacceptable or contraindicated, behavioral therapy (BT) alone should be provided. Failure with pharmacotherapy or BT alone suggests the need for more detailed in-depth assessment and more intensive and multimodal interventions.

Self-Help

Many smokers have successfully quit smoking without participating in formal treatment. Although only about 3–4% are successful during the past year, this success rate improves with multiple attempts and probable self-learning through trial and error and learning from others. Eventually, about 50% of smokers are able to quit and more than 90% of successful quitters have been able to do so without the assistance of professionals or formal programs. These numbers reflect multiple factors, including the limitations on access to treatment (nonexistent health insurance coverage and limited number of providers with expertise to help), the cumulative process of multiple attempts, learning from others and from self-help materials, and the severity of the nicotine dependence. The primary unassisted method of detoxification from nicotine dependence is precipitous cessation (cold turkey), which is used by more than

80% of smokers. This is followed by spontaneous strategies to handle cravings and triggers. Some smokers attempt to limit intake, taper the number of cigarettes smoked, or switch to a reduced tar or nicotine brand.

Some geographical areas have Nicotine Anonymous groups that are structured similar to Alcoholics Anonymous or Narcotics Anonymous groups. These groups are based on the 12-Step approach to recovery from addictions. Nicotine Anonymous is a relatively new organization (founded in 1985) and does not have the extensive network that other 12-Step programs like Alcoholics Anonymous or Narcotics Anonymous have developed.

Brief or Minimal Medical Professional-Delivered Interventions/Advice

Even a brief face-to-face intervention by a physician or other medical staff can increase the likelihood of cessation two- to tenfold. The impact of physicians' brief advice to quit has received the most study relative to other disciplines such as nursing; however, clearly all disciplines have opportunity to make an impact. Physicians can inquire about an individual's smoking status, urge the individual to stop smoking, and spend a brief time counseling the individual about cessation strategies. Multiple follow-up interventions, even telephone contacts by other medical staff, can further improve the cessation rate. Resources are available to assist physicians in providing effective antismoking interventions, which can even be used by those not highly skilled in counseling. Physicians' advice appears to be most successful with individuals with a serious medical problem or specific medical reason for quitting (e.g., pregnancy or congestive heart disease). In addition, because an estimated 70% of smokers in the United States visit their physicians at least once a year, an important opportunity exists for providing this type of smoking cessation intervention.

Formal Treatment Options

There are now numerous effective psychosocial and pharmacological approaches that can be used in nicotine dependence treatment. Psychosocial intervention alone, pharmacotherapy alone, or combined approaches may be used. Given individuals' preferences and current concerns with cost-effectiveness, less costly single-modality interventions are often used initially, whereas more costly multimodal interventions are often reserved for persons for whom cessation attempts have failed. This may not be the wisest strategy, but it is the most common. Whether failure with unaided or minimal intervention attempts may have a negative effect on future cessation attempts is not known; however, some research suggests that with each repeated cessation attempt, the person gains additional knowledge and experience that may contribute to success in future cessation attempts.

Somatic Treatments

Pharmacological interventions have become an important component of treating nicotine dependence. Approaches used parallel other addictions in treating acute withdrawal (detoxification), protracted withdrawal, and even maintenance for harm reduction. The primary medications are NRT and bupropion. All six of these modalities are FDA approved and have demonstrated efficacy. Other medications may have some potential; however, they are not FDA approved and have limited empirical foundation to support their use (Table 21-5).

NRT is the most widely used medication option and is available over the counter (patch and gum) or by prescription (patch, gum, spray, and inhaler). The substituted nicotine initially prevents significant withdrawal symptoms that may lead to relapse during the early period of smoking cessation. The substituted nicotine is then gradually tapered and discontinued. Replacement produces a lower overall plasma level of nicotine than that experienced with smoking. Replacement not only avoids the strongly reinforcing peaks in plasma level but also prevents the emergence of withdrawal symptoms by maintaining the nicotine plasma level above a threshold.

Nicotine gum, approved in 1984, was the first NRT approved. It slowly releases nicotine. The NRT gum is available in doses of 2 and 4 mg, and the recommended dosing is in the range of 9 to 16 pieces per day. Nicotine gum is more effective when used in conjunction with some type of psychosocial intervention, particularly BT. Outcome is more positive when a definite schedule for gum use is prescribed—for example, one piece of gum per hour while awake—than when used on an as-needed basis. Some studies suggest that it is also more effective when used for longer than 3 months. Tapering may be necessary after 4 to 6 months of use, especially for individuals using higher total daily doses of gum. Nicotine gum requires a highly motivated individual and a good deal of time in instructing the individual in proper use of the gum. Many individuals find the gum difficult to learn to use properly. Side effects and adverse effects include local irritation in the mouth, tongue, and throat, mouth ulcers, hiccups, jaw ache, gastrointestinal symptoms (flatulence, indigestion, nausea), anorexia, and palpitations.

The *nicotine patch* transdermal delivery system provides continual sustained release of nicotine, which is absorbed through the skin. This form of nicotine replacement more than doubles the 1-year cessation rate. There is a dose–response relationship, with individuals receiving higher doses attaining higher cessation rates. The nicotine patch eliminates the conditioning of repeated nicotine use, which remains present with the use of other NRT products. Compliance rates are higher because it involves once-daily dosing and its administration is simple and discreet. The typical starting dose of NRT patch is 21 or 15 mg patch; however, in some cases multiple patches are used. Lower dose patches available at 7 and 14 mg are used to taper after smoking cessation. The nicotine patch is often used for a total of 6 to 12 weeks but can be used for much longer. The transdermal patch does not allow for self-titrated dosing, craving, and nicotine withdrawal symptoms like the other NRT routes (gum, spray, inhaler); however, the nicotine blood levels are significantly less than with smoking. The patch can be used more discreetly and can be used despite dental or temporomandibular joint problems.

Although the nicotine patch is well tolerated, about 25% of individuals have significant local skin irritation or erythema and 10% discontinue the patch because of intolerable side effects. Other side effects include sleep problems with the 24-hour patches. In a few cases, nicotine toxicity developed when smokers continued their usual heavy cigarette smoking while using the transdermal nicotine patch.

The *nicotine nasal spray* is rapidly absorbed and produces a higher nicotine blood level than does transdermal nicotine or gum. It has been suggested that the effective daily dose in nicotine dependent smokers is 15 to 20 sprays (8–10 mg) per day. Onset of action of the spray is the most rapid of all nicotine replacements. An initial concern about the nasal spray had been the potential for abuse because it has the most rapid absorption rate of the NRTs. It replicates repeated administration of nicotine in smoking, resulting in reinforcing

Table 21-5	Approaches to the Pharmacological Treatment of Nicotine Dependence

Nicotine replacement or substitution (agonist administration)—FDA-approved nicotine patch, gum, spray, lozenge, and inhaler
Nonnicotine pill—bupropion/Zyban—FDA approved
Combinations of nicotine replacement types and/or bupropion
Non-FDA-approved experimental options:
  Blockade therapy (antagonist administration)
  Nonspecific attenuation therapy
  Deterrent therapy

peaks in the plasma level of the drug. Side effects of the spray include local airway irritation (i.e., coughing, rhinorrhea, lacrimation, nasal irritation), but tolerance to these local effects appears to develop. Systemic effects include nausea, headache, dizziness, tachycardia, and sweating.

The *nicotine inhaler* provides nicotine through a cartridge that must be "puffed." It mimics the upper airway stimulation experienced with smoking; however, absorption is primarily through the oropharyngeal mucosa. Side effects of the inhaler and spray include local irritation, cough, headache, nausea, dyspepsia, the need for multiple dosing, and the impossibility of discreet use.

Bupropion, the nonnicotine pill FDA-approved medication option, is an atypical antidepressant. The effects in smoking cessation appear to be unrelated to its antidepressant properties. Smoking cessation rates appear to improve further when bupropion is combined with the nicotine patch. Adverse events have a low incidence and include dry mouth, insomnia, nausea, and skin rash. There have been no reports of seizures in any smoking cessation studies to date; however, this agent should not be used in individuals with a history of seizure disorders.

Other Antidepressants. Antidepressants have been used in an attempt to attenuate withdrawal symptoms, to treat or prevent emergent depressive symptoms or episodes in the early phase of cessation, and to prevent relapse of depressive episodes in individuals with a history of depression. Antidepressants may provide significant benefits in special populations of individuals with current or prior major depressive disorder (MDD), dysthymic disorder, or current depressive symptoms when these factors predict a poor outcome. Given that negative affect has been shown to be the most common antecedent of a smoking relapse, this approach appears promising. If antidepressants are used, pretreatment is necessary because the benefit of the medication may not be apparent for 1 to 3 weeks.

Combined NRTs/bupropion or serial pharmacotherapeutic approaches may also be beneficial, especially in more difficult to treat cases of nicotine dependence. The combination approach offers the advantage of multiple neurobiological mechanisms of actions. In addition, many researchers increasingly believe that periods of pharmacotherapy should be extended, although the issue of whether longer-term pharmacotherapy is beneficial in improving cessation rates remains unresolved. There may be some smokers who are unable to stop smoking without ongoing nicotine replacement, similar to individuals dependent on heroin who must be

maintained on methadone. Although long-term/maintenance use of NRT requires further study, successful maintenance in smokers who have chronic relapses would potentially reduce a number of the serious health risks associated with smoking, in spite of individuals still being exposed to the effects of nicotine. Ongoing maintenance antidepressant treatment may also be necessary for a time for some individuals with a history of serious depressive illness or for those who have had significant depressive symptoms emerge on cessation that do not improve with time.

Psychosocial Treatments

In contrast with the treatment of other substance use disorders, psychosocial treatment is underutilized and has not evolved to be the cornerstone of treatment. This limited utilization of psychosocial treatments does not match the very positive outcomes from either psychosocial treatments alone (25% 1-year abstinence with BT) or when combined with NRT or bupropion (50% improvement compared to NRT or bupropion alone); however, it does match the lack of health care coverage for this service. The underutilization of psychosocial treatment has become the cultural norm in nicotine dependence treatment. This may be due to several important considerations. These include the following: (1) primary care practitioners most frequently attempt to address nicotine dependence and do not traditionally integrate BTs; (2) nicotine dependence treatment is often not paid for by health care insurance companies; (3) few behavioral health specialists have been formally trained in nicotine dependence treatments; (4) mental health and addiction treatment programs have ignored addressing tobacco in those treatment settings, although this appears to be changing; and (5) individuals are unaware of this treatment modality and its success rates, and believe that medications or quitting cold turkey are all that is needed.

A great variety of psychosocial interventions have been developed to help in the treatment of nicotine dependence (Table 21-6). As in treating other substance

Table 21-6	Psychosocial Interventions for the Treatment of Nicotine Dependence

Self-help materials
Brief advice from the physician
Multiple component therapies
Motivational enhancement therapy
Cognitive–behavioral therapies/relapse prevention
Nicotine fading
Nicotine Anonymous
Others used, but with limited empirical support: hypnosis and acupuncture

use disorders, the core psychotherapy approaches are motivational enhancement therapy (MET), cognitive–behavioral therapy (CBT) (relapse prevention), and 12-Step facilitation. Psychosocial interventions, particularly BT, have been shown to increase abstinence rates significantly. However, only 7% of smokers attempting to quit smoking are willing to participate in BT. In addition, it is more expensive than pharmacotherapy and more labor-intensive.

Despite the fact that there has been little controlled research examining whether psychosocial intervention with spouses and significant others or families can increase abstinence rates, overall social support for individuals who are attempting to stop smoking appears to improve the outcome. Others in the smoker's immediate family or social circle can be involved in their treatment through education about appropriate supportive behaviors. Concerned others can also be engaged in treatment to provide assessment information or to help enhance the individual's motivation.

Hypnosis and acupuncture are two approaches that some individuals believe have helped them in their efforts to quit smoking; however, there is limited research support for these approaches and treatment guidelines still list them as potentially promising approaches. Studies suggest that hypnosis has little more than a weak positive effect on outcome in smoking cessation. Meta-analysis of studies on the effect of acupuncture shows no evidence of efficacy on the outcome of smoking cessation. Positive effects likely represent a placebo effect related to the individual's expectations.

Combined Psychosocial and Psychopharmacological Therapies

All nicotine dependence treatment practice guidelines recommend the integration of nicotine dependence treatment medications (NRT and bupropion) with behavioral and supportive psychosocial treatment approaches. Empirical evidence supports the finding that medications double the quit rate compared to placebo, and face-to-face therapy can double the quit rate compared to minimal psychosocial intervention. Therapy also can increase medication compliance. Integrated treatment further increases the quit rate by another 50% and triples the outcome rate.

Managing Repeated Relapses

The degree of aggressiveness in treating smokers who have repeated relapses will depend in part on the immediacy and seriousness of the consequences of continued smoking. For example, a pregnant woman endangering the health of a developing fetus is a situation that requires immediate intervention. Likewise, a man with severe cardiac or vascular disease in whom continued smoking poses a serious threat to health or life may require immediate aggressive multimodal interventions.

The skills, knowledge, and experience of a nicotine dependence treatment specialist may be required in complex cases in which more intensive or aggressive individualized treatment is indicated or when more complex psychosocial interventions such as relapse prevention are tailored to the individual. Smokers who suffer repeated relapses may require more frequent monitoring as well as coordination of multiple services or interventions that can involve considerable expenditure of clinical time. This is especially true for persons with serious medical or psychiatric problems, or for pregnant women who require careful coordination of treatment through active collaboration with medical caretakers. The person providing or overseeing treatment for smokers who have chronic relapses must accept the reality of an ongoing long-term relationship that may be demanding of her or his time and attention as well as clinical acumen if appropriate support and monitoring are to be available.

Some smokers may not be able to achieve successful abstinence with outpatient treatment despite intensive multiple interventions. Inpatient treatment represents a drastic intervention that should be reserved for the most treatment-resistant individuals who have been completely unsuccessful despite repeated attempts and treatment with a variety of interventions. Inpatient treatment can provide the most intensive and aggressive program of treatment interventions coupled with close monitoring and prevention of access to nicotine. It requires a commitment of both time and money, however, as almost no insurance policies reimburse for such treatment. Inpatient nicotine dependence treatment is usually 1 week in duration. Follow-up data from the few programs in existence suggest that it may be effective for some highly treatment-resistant smokers.

Treatment with Co-Occurring Mental Illness or Other Addictions

Individuals with nicotine dependence and either a co-occurring mental illness, another addiction, or all three are more likely to be seeking treatment and require some modifications in the traditional nicotine treatment approach. A critical issue in the treatment planning is the timing of the nicotine dependence treatment. There is literature supporting treating all together and also in delaying the nicotine dependence treatment until the other problems are stabilized.

Successful nicotine dependence treatment in persons with active alcohol dependence is less likely than in individuals recovering from alcohol dependence; however, a few addiction treatment programs have addressed both problems simultaneously with success. Nicotine replacement appears to be especially beneficial in helping smokers with co-occurring mental illness and addiction. Appropriate treatment of the mental illness or other addiction is also important, including appropriate medications and therapy approaches. These individuals often benefit from clinicians beginning with a motivational enhancement approach that enhances the smoker's readiness to change and self-efficacy.

There is a growing literature supporting that treatment can be effective with these harder-to-treat smokers when motivational enhancement, NRT medications, psychiatric medications, and psychotherapy are integrated.

COMPARISON OF DSM-IV-TR AND ICD-10 DIAGNOSTIC CRITERIA

The DSM-IV-TR and ICD-10 symptom lists for nicotine withdrawal include some different items: the ICD-10 list has craving, malaise, increased cough, and mouth ulceration and does not include the DSM-IV-TR decreased heart rate item.

22 Substance-Related Disorders: Opioids

The term *opioids* describes a class of substances that acts on opioid receptors. Opioids can be naturally occurring substances such as morphine, semisynthetics such as heroin, and synthetics with morphine-like effects such as meperidine. These drugs are prescribed as analgesics, anesthetics, antidiarrheal agents, or cough suppressants. In addition to morphine and heroin, the opioids include codeine, hydromorphone, methadone, oxycodone, and fentanyl, among others. Drugs such as buprenorphine and pentazocine, an agonist–antagonist, are also included in this class because their physiologic and behavioral effects are mediated through opioid receptors (Table 22-1).

Opioids are the most effective medications for relief of severe pain and are widely used for that purpose. The more potent opioids approved for medical use are under DEA schedule II—examples are fentanyl, hydromorphone, methadone, and morphine; others are under schedules III and IV.

DIAGNOSIS

As with other substances, there are two general categories of opioid-related disorders: opioid use disorders and opioid-induced disorders. Opioid use disorders include opioid dependence and opioid abuse. Opioid dependence has two sets of specifiers, the first set being with physiologic features (i.e., tolerance and/or withdrawal), or without physiologic features. The second set consists of course specifiers: early full remission, early partial remission, sustained full remission, sustained partial remission, on agonist therapy, and in a controlled environment. The agonist therapy specifier is used only to note the status of opioid dependence, and not for other opioid-related disorders or substance dependencies.

Opioid-induced disorders include opioid intoxication, opioid withdrawal, opioid intoxication delirium (see the summary of DSM-IV-TR diagnostic criteria for substance-induced disorders in Chapter 13, page 125), opioid-induced psychotic disorder, opioid-induced mood disorder, opioid-induced sexual dysfunction, and opioid-induced sleep disorder.

Opioid Dependence

Opioid dependence is diagnosed by the signs and symptoms associated with compulsive, prolonged self-administration of opioids that are used for no legitimate medical purpose, or if a medical condition exists that requires opioid treatment, are used in doses that greatly exceed the amount needed for pain relief (see generic DSM-IV-TR diagnostic criteria for Substance Dependence in Chapter 13, page 125). Persons with opioid dependence typically demonstrate continued use in spite of adverse physical, behavioral, and psychological consequences. Almost all persons meeting criteria for opioid dependence have significant levels of tolerance and will experience withdrawal upon abrupt discontinuation of opioid drugs. Persons with opioid dependence tend to develop such regular patterns of compulsive use that daily activities are typically planned around obtaining and administering drugs. Unlike cocaine, hallucinogens, solvents, and other substances that do not always produce withdrawal symptoms, opioid dependence is almost always accompanied by significant physiological tolerance and a defined withdrawal–abstinence syndrome.

Opioids are usually purchased on the illicit market, but they can also be obtained by forging prescriptions, faking or exaggerating medical problems, or by receiving simultaneous prescriptions from several physicians. Physicians and other health care professionals who are dependent will often obtain opioids by writing prescriptions or by diverting opioids that have been prescribed for their own patients.

Opioid Abuse

Opioid abuse is a maladaptive pattern of intermittent use in hazardous situations (driving under the influence,

Clinical Guide to the Diagnosis and Treatment of Mental Disorders. M. B. First and A. Tasman
© 2006 John Wiley & Sons, Ltd.   ISBN 0 470 019158

Table 22-1	Opioids*						
Drug	Active Metabolite	Route of Administration	Relative Potency	Medical Use	Plasma Half-Life (Hours)	Duration of Action (Hours)
Morphine		IM	1	Analgesia	2	4–6
Heroin	Morphine	IM	1–2	None	0.5	3–5
Codeine		PO	0.05	Analgesia, antitussive	2–4	4–6
Fentanyl		IM	40–100	Analgesia	3–4	1–2
Hydromorphone		IM	13	Analgesia	2–3	4–6
Oxycodone		PO	0.5–1	Analgesia		4–6
Methadone		PO	0.50	Analgesia, opioid substitution	15–40	18–30
l-α-Acetylmethadol (LAAM)		PO	0.40	Opioid substitution	14–104[†]	48–80
	Nor-LAAM				13–130[†]	
	Dinor-LAAM				97–430[†]	
Buprenorphine		SL	N/A (partial agonist)	Analgesia (opioid substitution, investigational)	6–12	4–6 (for analgesia) 12–48[‡]

*IM, intramuscular; PO, by mouth; SL, sublingual; N/A, not applicable.
[†]At steady state.
[‡]Appears to be dose dependent.

Opioid Intoxication

Opioid intoxication is characterized by maladaptive and clinically significant behavioral changes developing within minutes to a few hours after opioid use. Symptoms include an initial euphoria sometimes followed by dysphoria or apathy. Psychomotor retardation or agitation, impaired judgment, and impaired social or occupational functioning are commonly seen. Intoxication is accompanied by pupillary constriction unless there has been a severe overdose with consequent anoxia and pupillary dilatation. Persons with intoxication are often drowsy (described as being "on the nod") or even obtunded, have slurred speech, impaired memory, and demonstrate inattention to the environment to the point of ignoring potentially harmful events. Dryness of secretions in the mouth and nose,

being intoxicated while using heavy machinery, working in dangerous places, etc.), or periodic use resulting in adverse social, legal, or interpersonal problems (see generic DSM-IV-TR diagnostic criteria for Substance Abuse in Chapter 13, page 125). All of these signs and symptoms can also be seen in persons who are dependent; abuse is characterized by less regular use than dependence (i.e., compulsive use not present) and by the absence of significant tolerance or withdrawal. As with other substance use disorders, opioid abuse and dependence are hierarchical and thus, persons diagnosed as having opioid abuse must never have met criteria for opioid dependence.

slowing of gastrointestinal activity, and constipation are associated with both acute and chronic opioid use. Visual acuity may be impaired as a result of pupillary constriction. The magnitude of the behavioral and physiologic changes depends on the dose as well as individual characteristics of the user such as rate of absorption, chronicity of use, and tolerance. Symptoms

DSM-IV-TR Diagnostic Criteria

292.89 OPIOID INTOXICATION

A. Recent use of an opioid.
B. Clinically significant maladaptive behavioral or psychological changes (e.g., initial euphoria followed by apathy, dysphoria, psychomotor agitation or retardation, impaired judgment, or impaired social or occupational functioning) that developed during, or shortly after, opioid use.
C. Pupillary constriction (or pupillary dilation due to anoxia from severe overdose) and one (or more) of the following signs, developing during, or shortly after, opioid use:

  1. drowsiness or coma
  2. slurred speech
  3. impairment in attention or memory

D. The symptoms are not due to a general medical condition and are not better accounted for by another mental disorder.

Specify if:

With perceptual disturbances

Reprinted with permission from the *Diagnostic and Statistical Manual of Mental Disorders*, 4th ed., Text Rev. Copyright 2000 American Psychiatric Association.

Table 22-2	Signs and Symptoms of Opioid Intoxication

Symptoms
Euphoria, dysphoria, or apathy
Psychomotor retardation or agitation
Impaired judgment, social, or occupational functioning

Signs
Pupillary constriction
Drowsy or obtunded
Slurred speech, impaired memory, and inattention to
   environment
Dryness in mouth or nose
Slowed gastrointestinal activity and constipation
Severe intoxication can lead to coma, respiration
   depression, pupillary dilation, unconsciousness, and
   death.

of opioid intoxication usually last for several hours, but are dependent on the half-life of the particular opioid that has been used. Severe intoxication following an opioid overdose can lead to coma, respiratory depression, pupillary dilatation, unconsciousness, and death (Table 22-2).

Opioid Withdrawal

Opioid withdrawal is a clinically significant, maladaptive behavioral and physiological syndrome associated with cessation or reduction of opioid use

DSM-IV-TR Diagnostic Criteria

292.0 OPIOID WITHDRAWAL

A. Either of the following:

  (1) cessation of (or reduction in) opioid use that has been heavy and prolonged (several weeks or longer)
  (2) administration of an opioid antagonist after a period of opioid use

B. Three (or more) of the following, developing within minutes to several days after Criterion A:

  (1) dysphoric mood
  (2) nausea or vomiting
  (3) muscle aches
  (4) lacrimation or rhinorrhea
  (5) papillary dilation, piloerection, or sweating
  (6) diarrhea
  (7) yawning
  (8) fever
  (9) insomnia

C. The symptoms in Criterion B cause clinically significant distress or impairment in social, occupational, or other important areas of functioning.

D. The symptoms are not due to a general medical condition and are not better accounted for by another mental disorder

Reprinted with permission from the *Diagnostic and Statistical Manual of Mental Disorders*, 4th ed., Text Rev. Copyright 2000 American Psychiatric Association.

that has been heavy and prolonged. It can also be precipitated by administration of an opioid antagonist such as naloxone or naltrexone. Individuals in opioid withdrawal typically demonstrate a pattern of signs and symptoms that are opposite from the acute agonist effects. The first of these are subjective and consist of complaints of anxiety, restlessness, and an "achy feeling" that is often located in the back and legs. These symptoms are accompanied by a wish to obtain opioids (sometimes called "craving") and drug-seeking behavior, along with irritability and increased sensitivity to pain. Additionally, individuals typically demonstrate three or more of the following: dysphoric or depressed mood, nausea or vomiting, diarrhea, muscle aches, lacrimation or rhinorrhea, increased sweating, yawning, fever, insomnia, pupillary dilatation, fever, and piloerection. Piloerection and withdrawal-related fever are rarely seen in clinical settings (other than prison) as they are signs of advanced withdrawal in persons with a very significant degree of physiologic dependence; opioid-dependent persons with "habits" of that magnitude usually manage to obtain drugs before withdrawal becomes so far advanced (Table 22-3).

For short-acting drugs such as heroin, withdrawal symptoms occur within 6 to 24 hours after the last dose in most dependent persons, peak within 1 to 3 days, and gradually subside over a period of 5 to 7 days. Symptoms may take 2 to 4 days to emerge in the case of longer-acting drugs such as methadone or levo-alpha-acetylmethadol (LAAM). Less acute withdrawal symptoms are sometimes present and can last for weeks to months. These more persistent symptoms can include anxiety, dysphoria, anhedonia, insomnia, and drug craving.

Opioid use disorders can occur at any age, including adolescence and the geriatric years, but most affected persons are between 20 and 45 years. There

Table 22-3	Signs and Symptoms of Opioid Withdrawal

Symptoms
Anxiety, irritability, restlessness
Muscle aching
Craving for opioids
Increased pain sensitivity

Signs
Dysphoric or depressed mood
Nausea/vomiting/diarrhea
Lacrimation/rhinorrhea
Sweating
Yawning
Insomnia
Pupillary dilatation
Piloerection
Fever

have recently been increasing numbers of reports of adolescents presenting for treatment with opioid problems, but good data are hard to find. Neonates whose mothers are addicted can also experience opioid withdrawal. Rarely, young children are affected, with some cases of dependence having been reported in persons who are 8 to 10 years of age. Males are more commonly affected, with the male–female ratio typically being 3 or 4 to 1.

A nonjudgmental and supportive yet firm approach to these individuals is especially important. They typically have engaged in antisocial or other forms of problematic behavior. They are often embarrassed or afraid to describe the extent of their behavior, and have extremely low self-esteem. At the same time, they are prone to be impulsive, manipulative, and to act-out when frustrated. Communicating a feeling of nonjudgmental support in the context of setting limits, along with a clear and informed effort to provide appropriate help, will encourage optimum therapeutic opportunities.

On physical examination, sclerosed veins ("tracks") and puncture marks on the lower portions of the upper extremities are common in intravenous users. When these veins become unusable or otherwise unavailable, persons will usually switch to veins in the legs, neck, or groin. Veins sometimes become so badly sclerosed that peripheral edema develops. When intravenous access is no longer possible, persons will often inject directly into their subcutaneous tissue ("skin-popping") resulting in cellulitis, abscesses, and circular-appearing scars from healed skin lesions. Tetanus is a relatively rare but extremely serious consequence of injecting into the subcutaneous tissues. Infections also occur in other organ systems, including bacterial endocarditis, hepatitis B and C, and HIV infection.

Persons who "snort" heroin or other opioids often develop irritation of the nasal mucosa. Difficulties in sexual function are common, as are a variety of sexually transmitted diseases. Males often experience premature ejaculation associated with opioid withdrawal, and impotence during intoxication or chronic use. Females commonly have disturbances of reproductive function and irregular menses.

During dependence, routine urine toxicology tests are often positive for opioid drugs and remain positive for most opioids for 12 to 36 hours. Methadone and LAAM, because they are longer acting, can be identified for several days. Fentanyl is not detected by standard urine tests but can be identified by more specialized procedures. Oxycodone, hydrocodone, and hydromorphone are often not routinely included on urine toxicology tests though they can be identified by gas

chromatography/mass spectrometry. Testing for fentanyl is not necessary in most programs, but needs to be performed in assessing and treating health care professionals such as anesthesiologists who have access to this drug. Concomitant laboratory evidence of other abusable substances such as cocaine, marijuana, alcohol, amphetamines, and benzodiazepines is common.

Hepatitis screening tests are often positive, either for hepatitis B antigen (signifying active infection) or hepatitis B and/or C antibody (signifying past infection). Mild to moderate elevations of liver function tests are common, usually as a result of chronic infection with hepatitis C but also from toxic injury to the liver due to contaminants that have been mixed with injected opioids, or from heavy use of other hepatotoxic drugs such as alcohol. Low platelet count, anemia, or neutropenia, as well as positive HIV tests or low CD-4 cell counts are often signs of HIV infection. HIV is commonly acquired via the practice of sharing injection equipment, or by unprotected sexual activity that may be related to the substance use disorder, for example, exchanging sex for drugs or money to buy drugs.

Course

Opioid dependence can begin at any age, but problems associated with opioid use are most commonly first observed in the late teens or early twenties. Once dependence occurs, it is usually continuous over a period of many years even though periods of abstinence are frequent. Reoccurrence is common even after many years of forced abstinence, such as occurs during incarceration. Increasing age appears to be associated with a decrease in prevalence. This tendency for dependence to remit generally begins after age 40 and has been called "maturing out." Many persons, however, have remained opioid dependent for 50 years or longer. Thus, though spontaneous remission can and does occur, most cases of untreated opioid dependence follow a chronic, relapsing course for many years.

Differential Diagnosis

Individuals who are dependent on "street" opioids are usually easy to diagnose because of the physical signs of intravenous use, drug-seeking behavior, reports from independent observers, the lack of medical justification for opioid use, urine test results, and the signs and symptoms of intoxication or withdrawal.

The signs and symptoms of opioid withdrawal are fairly specific, especially lacrimation and rhinorrhea, which are not associated with withdrawal from any other abusable substances. Other psychoactive substances with sedative properties such as alcohol, hypnotics, or anxiolytics can cause a clinical picture that resembles opioid intoxication. A diagnosis can usually be made by the absence of pupillary constriction, or by the lack of response to a naloxone challenge. In some cases, intoxication is due to opioids along with alcohol or other sedatives. In these cases, the naloxone challenge will not reverse all of the sedative drug effects.

Difficult diagnostic situations are seen among persons who fabricate or exaggerate the signs and symptoms of a painful illness (such as kidney stones, migraine headache, back pain, etc.). Because pain is subjective and difficult to measure, and because some of these individuals can be very skillful and deceptive, diagnosis can be difficult and time-consuming. Persons with opioid dependence will often present with psychiatric signs and symptoms such as depression or anxiety. Such subjective distress often serves to motivate the individual to seek treatment, and thus can be therapeutically useful. These symptoms can be the result of opioid intoxication or withdrawal, or they might result from the pharmacological effects of other substances that are also being abused such as cocaine, alcohol, or benzodiazepines. They may also represent independent, non-substance-induced psychiatric disorders that require long-term treatment. The correct attribution of psychiatric symptoms that are seen in the context of opioid dependence and abuse follows the principles that are outlined in the substance-related section and other relevant parts of DSM-IV-TR.

Opioids are much less likely to produce psychopathology than most other drugs of abuse, and in some instances, they reduce psychiatric symptoms. In these cases, symptoms will emerge not during opioid use, but after it is discontinued. Examples have been observed by clinicians in methadone maintenance programs, who occasionally see an exacerbation of symptoms of schizophrenia, posttraumatic stress disorder (PTSD), or other problems in individuals who discontinue chronic opioid use.

TREATMENT

There are currently a number of effective pharmacological and behavioral therapies for the treatment of opioid dependence, with these two approaches often combined to optimize outcome. There are also some newer treatment options, which may take various forms. For example, methadone maintenance is an established treatment, while the use of buprenorphine/naloxone in an office-based setting represents a new variation on that theme. Clonidine has been used extensively to treat opioid withdrawal while lofexidine is a structural

analog that appears to have less hypotensive and sedating effects. The depot dosage form of naltrexone may increase compliance with a medication that has been an effective opioid antagonist, but which has been underutilized because of poor acceptance by individuals. In almost every treatment episode using pharmacotherapy, it is combined with some type of psychosocial or behavioral treatment. Recent research has documented the value of these additional treatments and provided insight into the ones that are the most effective.

Detoxification: Long-Term, Short-Term, Rapid, and Ultrarapid

Detoxification from opioids, for most individuals, is only the first phase of a longer treatment process. Pharmacological detoxification is generally ineffective in achieving sustained remission unless combined with long-term pharmacologic, psychosocial, or behavioral therapies. Most individuals seeking treatment have been addicted to heroin or other opioids for 2 to 3 years, and some for 30 years or more. Thus, treatment usually involves changes in individuals' lifestyles. Though generally ineffective in achieving sustained remission unless combined with long-term pharmacological, psychosocial, or behavioral therapies, detoxification alone continues to be widely used.

The detoxification process may include use of opioid agonists (e.g., methadone), partial agonists (e.g., buprenorphine), antagonists (e.g., naloxone, naltrexone), or nonopioid alternatives such as clonidine, benzodiazepines, or nonsteroidal anti-inflammatory agents. In many cases, one or more medications are combined, such as naloxone with clonidine and a benzodiazepine (Table 22-4). The choice of detoxification medication and the duration of the process depend on numerous factors, including individual preference, clinician expertise and experience, type of treatment facility, licensing, and available resources. Ultimately, however, the goal of detoxification is the achievement (and maintenance) of a drug-free state while minimizing withdrawal.

Opioid detoxification paradigms are frequently categorized according to their duration: long-term

Table 22-4	Pharmacologic Agents in Opioid Detoxification

Opioid agonists (methadone)
Partial agonists (buprenorphine)
Antagonists (naloxone, naltrexone)
Nonopioid alternatives (clonidine, benzodiazepines, nonsteroidal anti-inflammatory agents)
Combinations of above medications

(typically 180 days), short-term (up to 30 days), rapid (typically 3–10 days), and ultrarapid (1–2 days). These temporal modifiers provide only a coarse description of the paradigm; they do not provide other important information such as the medications used or whether postdetoxification pharmacological, psychosocial, or behavioral therapy is provided. However, some general guidelines typically apply.

The most common detoxification protocols, and those for which the most data are available, are the long-term (typically 180 days) and short-term (up to 30 days) paradigms involving the use of methadone. Unfortunately, these strategies have not generally been associated with acceptable treatment response using relapse to opioid use as an outcome criterion. Results from more rapid detoxification evaluations using short- or even intermediate-term (up to 70 days) medication-tapering protocols are even less encouraging and have an unfortunately low success rate. It should be noted, however, that provision of additional services such as counseling, behavioral therapy, treatment of underlying psychopathologies, job skills training, and family therapy to address concomitant treatment needs can improve outcome though success rates remain low, even with these services.

Rapid detoxification involves the use of an opioid antagonist, typically naltrexone or naloxone, in combination with other medications (such as clonidine and benzodiazepines) to mitigate the precipitated withdrawal syndrome. The procedure is intended to expedite and compress withdrawal in order to minimize discomfort and decrease treatment time. Ultrarapid detoxification also utilizes other medications, along with an opioid antagonist, to moderate withdrawal effects. However, rather than individuals being awake as they are during the rapid detoxification process, they are placed under general anesthesia or alternatively, deeply sedated.

A major concern regarding ultrarapid detoxification is the occurrence of potentially serious adverse effects, such as respiratory distress, or other pulmonary and renal complications during or immediately following the procedure. A high frequency of vomiting has also been reported. The degree to which serious adverse events occur has not yet been determined; however, there have been reports of sudden death occurring shortly after the procedure, which was not caused by relapse to opioid use and overdose.

In spite of the emerging evidence about serious adverse events, ultrarapid detoxification may be appropriate for highly selected individuals based on considerations of previous treatment history, economic factors, and individual choice. However, individuals seeking this treatment must be thoroughly informed that serious adverse events, including sudden unexpected deaths, have occurred in association with this procedure and its use should probably be limited to inpatient settings where monitoring by anesthesiologists and other highly trained staff is available.

Buprenorphine, a μ-opioid partial agonist, has also been used as a detoxification agent. Results from inpatient and outpatient studies have shown that it is safe, well tolerated, and mitigates opioid withdrawal signs and symptoms over a range of doses and detoxification schedules. Clonidine, an alpha-2-adrenergic agonist, has been shown to suppress many of the autonomic signs and symptoms of opioid withdrawal. It can cause sedation and hypotension but has been used with few problems when appropriate monitoring is available. It does not suppress the subjective discomfort of withdrawal, and probably for that reason, is not well accepted by most individuals.

Other alpha-2-adrenergic agonists have also been evaluated in order to find agents that are as or more effective, but less sedating and hypotensive than clonidine. Lofexidine, a medication that was originally promoted as an antihypertensive but was shown to lack clinically significant hypotensive effects, has been the most studied. Lofexidine is likely to be shown to be a useful opioid detoxification agent whose efficacy approximates that of clonidine but with fewer side effects.

Opioid Agonist Pharmacotherapy

Methadone maintenance has become the most commonly used pharmacotherapy for opioid dependence. Methadone suppresses opioid withdrawal for 24 to 36 hours following a single oral dose, making it an ideal medication for this purpose. Another μ-opioid agonist, LAAM, received FDA approval for maintenance treatment in 1993. LAAM is a long-acting congener of methadone, which suppresses withdrawal for 48 to 72 hours, and thus has the advantage of requiring less frequent clinic visits than methadone, which must be taken daily. A third medication, buprenorphine, has unique properties that are likely to result in it being used with fewer regulatory controls than methadone and LAAM.

Both methadone and LAAM are Schedule II controlled substances and can only be used for maintenance and detoxification in programs that are licensed and regulated by the FDA and the Drug Enforcement Administration (DEA).

This combination of FDA and DEA regulations has resulted in a treatment system that is separated from the mainstream of other medical care and that consists almost entirely of specially licensed and inspected clinics.

The appropriate dose of agonist medication has been a subject of both federal and state regulations, although there has been a gradual shift toward allowing more clinical judgment in its determination. A number of studies have been done during the past 25 years to determine the optimal dose and, although it is clear that some individuals do well on low doses of methadone or LAAM (about 20–50 mg), studies have consistently shown that most individuals need higher doses, in the 80–120 mg range, if they are to achieve maximum benefit from agonist treatment. Clear relationships between methadone blood levels and clinical response have not been observed consistently, suggesting that some individuals may be more sensitive to dose changes and that clinical response, including subjective complaints, is a more important guide to adequate dosing than blood levels. No controlled studies have been done examining doses above 120 mg; thus, the upper limits of dosing effectiveness are not well understood.

Physicians who choose to treat persons with opioid dependence under new DEA regulations will need to notify the Secretary of Health and Human Services in writing of their intent and show that they are qualified to provide addiction treatment by virtue of certification or experience. No physician will be allowed to treat more than 30 individuals at one time without special approval according to the proposed legislation.

This change in the regulations is especially important for buprenorphine and the buprenorphine/naloxone combination, as it provides better access to treatment for persons who are unwilling or unable to be treated in the current methadone or LAAM system. The overall intent of the regulatory reform is to better integrate maintenance treatment into the mainstream of medical care, and to make it more available and improve its quality.

The greatest advantage of buprenorphine compared to full agonists such as methadone and LAAM is the plateau effect of its agonist activity. Parenteral doses as high as 12 mg intravenously have been given to individuals who are not tolerant to opioids with only limited adverse effects (e.g., sedation, irritability, nausea, itching). A number of large trials have confirmed the utility of buprenorphine for agonist maintenance therapy.

Buprenorphine has the potential to be abused and can produce addiction; however, most persons who abuse buprenorphine initiated opioid use with other drugs. Abuse may take the form of using greater than prescribed dosages for analgesia, using buprenorphine in place of a more desired but less available opioid, or using buprenorphine for its positive reinforcing effects.

Buprenorphine in combination with naloxone has less potential for abuse than buprenorphine alone. The therapeutic utility of combining naloxone with buprenorphine derives from the low sublingual bioavailability of naloxone as compared to buprenorphine. Parenteral misuse of the combination by persons addicted to opioids would be expected to produce antagonist-like effects; thus, most persons with opioid dependence would be unlikely to inject the combination more than once. The use of the buprenorphine/naloxone combination in an office-based setting represents an innovative alternative to the restrictive methadone or LAAM maintenance paradigm described previously and should expand the availability of agonist maintenance treatment with a relatively low risk for abuse or diversion. In addition, the partial agonist activity of buprenorphine results in a much lower risk for overdose death than is the case with methadone or LAAM.

Antagonist Maintenance

Naltrexone is the prototypical opioid antagonist used in abstinence therapy, blocking the effects of heroin and other opioids through competitive receptor inhibition. Naltrexone has no opioid agonist effects and is a competitive opioid antagonist. It is orally effective and can block opioid effects for 24 hours when administered as a single daily dose of 50 mg; doses of 100–150 mg can block opioid effects for 48–72 hours. Despite a favorable adverse event profile (nausea is typically the most common side effect), naltrexone is generally not favored by opioid addicts because, unlike opioid agonists and partial agonists, it produces no positive, reinforcing effects. Furthermore, it may be associated with the precipitation of an opioid withdrawal syndrome if used too soon after opioid use stops, an effect that can be minimized by administering a naloxone challenge prior to giving the first dose of naltrexone.

While there is a literature spanning more than 25 years on naltrexone treatment, work continues on increasing compliance and improving outcomes. Presently, an individual treated with naltrexone has only to stop the medication for 1 to 3 days in order to experience the full effects of subsequent opioid use. A depot dosage form of naltrexone would provide more time for individuals to overcome ambivalence about stopping opioid use and could result in more long-term success than has currently been the case. Another variant on antagonist treatment is nalmefene, an orally effective but somewhat longer acting (about 48 hours at dosages of 50–100 mg/day) opioid antagonist that has been used for alcohol treatment and shows promise as an alternative to naltrexone for opioid dependence.

Psychosocial Treatments

As in other substance use disorders, most individuals with opioid dependence and abuse are ambivalent about stopping use. This ambivalence presents a challenge as it contributes to varying levels of motivation to enter and remain in treatment, to early dropout, and to partial or (in some cases) nontreatment response. Clinicians must be aware of this "normal" ambivalence, and make reasonable efforts to resolve it in favor of treatment participation and cessation of use. Suggestions that have been made regarding initial steps to maximize the chances for engagement in treatment and cessation of drug use include avoiding unnecessary delays in entering treatment, expressing a hopeful and nonjudgmental attitude, performing a comprehensive evaluation, and developing a treatment plan that is responsive to the individual's self-identified goals.

In addition to challenges related to ambivalence, individuals often have serious problems with nonopioid substance abuse and/or with medical, psychiatric, legal, employment, and family/social issues that preexist or result from the addiction. Addressing these additional problems can be helpful, but is complex and requires coordination between agonist pharmacotherapy staff, and other medical and psychosocial services.

The most common type of psychosocial treatment in opioid agonist maintenance is individual drug counseling. Counselors are typically persons at the masters level or below who deliver a behaviorally focused treatment aimed to identify specific problems, help the individual access services that may not be provided in the clinic (e.g., medical, psychiatric, legal, family/social), stop substance use, and improve overall adjustment. Functions that counselors perform include monitoring methadone and LAAM doses and requesting changes when needed, reviewing urine test results, responding to requests for take-home doses, assisting with family problems, responding to crises, writing letters for court or social welfare agencies, recommending inpatient treatment when necessary, and providing support and encouragement for a drug-free lifestyle.

Other approaches involve group therapy, contingency management techniques, self-help groups, and outpatient-based therapeutic community programs.

Though counseling and other services are effective enhancements of agonist treatment, compliance is often an issue and clinics vary in the way they respond to this problem. Some remind individuals of appointments, others do not permit individuals to be medicated unless they keep appointments, and others suspend individuals who miss appointments. For noncompliant individuals, a powerful contingency is requiring certain behaviors for individuals to remain on the program, a procedure that is often formalized in a "treatment contract." Here, the individual is given the option of stopping heroin and other drug use, keeping regular counseling appointments, looking for work, or correcting other behaviors that need improvement as a condition for remaining in treatment. Individuals who fail are administratively detoxified, suspended for months to years, and referred to another program, although the referrals are not always successful. The long-term effects of this form of contingency management have not been well studied.

Addressing Comorbidity

Individuals seeking treatment for opioid dependence are typically using one or more other substances (cocaine, alcohol, benzodiazepines, amphetamines, marijuana, nicotine), and have additional problems in the psychiatric, medical, family/social, employment, or legal areas. In fact, it is rare to find a person with only opioid dependence and no other substance use, or without a psychiatric, medical, or family/social problem. The presence of these problems, perhaps with the exception of nicotine dependence, tends to magnify the severity of the opioid dependence and makes the individual even more difficult to treat.

Among the mental disorders seen in persons with opioid dependence, antisocial personality disorder is one of the most common. Diagnostic studies of persons with opioid dependence have typically found rates of antisocial personality disorder ranging from 20% to 50%, as compared to less than 5% in the general population. PTSD is also seen with increased frequency.

Opioid-dependent persons are especially at risk for the development of brief depressive symptoms, and for episodes of mild to moderate depression that meet symptomatic and duration criteria for major depressive disorder or dysthymia. These syndromes represent both substance-induced mood disorders as well as independent depressive illnesses. Brief periods of depression are especially common during chronic intoxication or withdrawal, or in association with psychosocial stressors that are related to the dependence. Insomnia is common, especially during withdrawal; sexual dysfunction, especially impotence, is common during intoxication. Delirium or brief, psychotic-like symptoms are occasionally seen during opioid intoxication.

Less than 5% of persons with opioid dependence have psychotic disorders such as bipolar illness or schizophrenia; however, these individuals can present special problems since programs typically have few psychiatric staff. As a result, these individuals are sometimes excluded from methadone treatment because they cannot be effectively managed within the constraints of the available resources. Others are treated with methadone, counseling, and the same medications used for nonaddicted individuals with similar disorders. Though studies evaluating the outcome of combining opioid agonist treatment with antipsychotic or antimanic medications have not been done, there is little controversy that these medications are useful for persons with opioid dependence and psychotic disorders.

Women with opioid dependence can present special challenges because many have been sexually abused as children, have other mental disorders, and are involved in difficult family/social situations. Abusive relationships with addicted males are common, sometimes characterized by situations in which the male exerts control by providing drugs. These complex psychiatric and relationship issues have emphasized the need for comprehensive psychosocial services that include psychiatric assessment and treatment, and access to other medical, family, and social services.

Medical comorbidity is a major problem among persons with opioid dependence; HIV infection, AIDS, and hepatitis B and C have become some of the most common problems. Sharing injection equipment including "cookers" and rinse water, or engaging in high-risk sexual behaviors are the main routes of infection. Sexual transmission appears to be a more common route of HIV transmission among females than males because the HIV virus is spread more readily from males to females than from females to males. Females who are intravenous drug users and also engage in prostitution or other forms of high-risk sex are at extremely high risk for HIV infection. Cocaine use has been found to be a significant risk factor as a single drug of abuse or when used in combination with heroin or other opioids.

After rising rapidly in the late 1970s and early 1980s, the incidence of new HIV infections among intravenous drug users, of whom opioid-dependent individuals constitute a large proportion, has decreased, though still a substantial source of new HIV infections. However, as a result of high levels of needle sharing and other risky behavior in the early phases of the epidemic, HIV infection rates are as high as 60% in some areas of the United States.

Recent studies have identified several important interactions between methadone and drugs to treat HIV. Information is not complete, however, and more studies are needed to map out the full extent of these interactions. One important interaction is that methadone increases plasma levels of zidovudine; the associated symptoms resemble methadone withdrawal. There have been instances in which methadone doses have been increased in response to complaints of withdrawal with increasing doses compounding the problem. Another important interaction involves decreased methadone blood levels secondary to nevirapine that may result in mild to moderate withdrawal. This interaction can be important if the individual is taken off either of these two drugs while on methadone, since the result may be a sudden rise in methadone blood levels with signs and symptoms of over medication.

As mentioned earlier, mortality is high and studies have found annual death rates of approximately 10 per 1000 or greater, which is substantially higher than demographically matched samples in the general population. Common causes of death are overdose, accidents, injuries, and medical complications such as cellulitis, hepatitis, AIDS, tuberculosis, and endocarditis. The cocaine and alcohol dependence that is often seen among opioid-dependent persons contributes to cirrhosis, cardiomyopathy, myocardial infarction, and cardiac arrhythmias.

Tuberculosis has become a particularly serious problem among intravenous drug users, especially heroin addicts. In most cases, infection is asymptomatic and evident only by the presence of a positive tuberculin skin test. However, many cases of active tuberculosis have been found, especially among those who are infected with HIV.

Other medical complications of heroin dependence are seen in children born to opioid-dependent women. Perhaps the most serious is premature delivery and low birth weight, a problem that can be reduced if the mother is on methadone maintenance and receiving prenatal care. Another is physiological dependence on opioids, seen in about half the infants born to women maintained on methadone or dependent on heroin or other opioids. Effective treatments for neonatal withdrawal are available and long-term adverse effects of opioid withdrawal have not been demonstrated. Adverse neonatal effects associated with LAAM or buprenorphine have not been observed, but few studies have been done since neither medication is approved for use in pregnancy.

The comorbidity data have led to research that has demonstrated the positive effects of integrating psychiatric and medical care within agonist and other substance abuse treatment programs. Clinical experience and National Institute on Drug-Abuse demonstration projects have shown that integration of these services can be done, and with very positive results since individuals are seen frequently and treatment retention is high. Related to this line of research are studies that have shown improved compliance with directly observed antituberculosis pharmacotherapy. These findings have important implications for tuberculosis control policies in methadone programs since intravenous drug users are at very high risk for tuberculosis infection and because maintenance programs provide settings in which directly observed therapy can be easily applied. Similar principles apply to administration of psychotropic medication in noncompliant individuals with schizophrenia or other major Axis I disorders.

COMPARISON OF DSM-IV-TR AND ICD-10 DIAGNOSTIC CRITERIA

The DSM-IV-TR and ICD-10 criteria sets for opioid intoxication are almost the same. The DSM-IV-TR and ICD-10 symptom lists for opioid withdrawal include some different items: the ICD-10 list has craving, abdominal cramps, and tachycardia and does not include the fever and dysphoric mood items from the DSM-IV-TR criteria set.

Substance-Related Disorders: Phencyclidine

Phencyclidine (1-(1-phenylcyclohexyl)piperidine, PCP) was developed as a general anesthetic agent in the 1950s under the brand name Sernyl. The drug was considered physiologically promising because of its lack of respiratory and cardiovascular depressant effects. In fact, individuals under PCP anesthesia rather than manifesting a state of relaxed sleep such as that induced by typical anesthetic agents appeared semiconscious with open eyes, fixed staring, flat facies, open mouth, rigid posturing, and waxy flexibility. Because of this apparent sharp dissociation from the environment without true unconsciousness, PCP and the related drug ketamine were classified as dissociative anesthetics.

Approximately 50% of individuals anesthetized with PCP developed behavioral syndromes including agitation and hallucinations during emergence from anesthesia. A substantial number of individuals developed postoperative psychotic reactions, which in some cases persisted up to 10 days. Trials of subanesthetic doses of PCP for treatment of chronic pain led to similar although less severe adverse reactions. As a result, after 1965, PCP was limited to veterinary applications. Ketamine remains available for human anesthesia; side effects are less frequent and less severe owing to the lower potency and shorter duration of ketamine action compared to PCP.

Illicit use of phencyclidine was first noted in 1965 in Los Angeles. The spread of the drug from California throughout the country was facilitated by its ease of synthesis compared to other drugs. At least six synthetic methods, some simple, are published in scientific journals. Surveys of street drug samples indicated that PCP was sold under many street names (Table 23-1) and frequently combined with or misrepresented as other substances.

Despite its well-documented aversive and disruptive behavioral effects, PCP emerged during the 1970s as a popular drug of abuse, increasing in popularity to the point that in 1979, 13% of high school seniors had tried it. Although PCP has never regained that remarkable

Table 23-1	Street Names for Phencyclidine and Mixtures
Phencyclidine	**Phencyclidine Mixtures and Analog**
Angel dust	Beam me up Scottie (crack dipped in PCP)
Animal trank	
Baby doll	Blunt (marijuana and PCP in cigar wrapper)
Black whack	
Butt naked	Love boat (marijuana dipped in PCP)
Devil's dust	Peanut butter (PCP mixed in peanut butter)
Elephant tranquilizer	
Embalming fluid	Special K (ketamine)
Gorilla biscuits	Tragic magic (crack dipped in PCP)
Heaven	Wet
HogJet fuel	Illy (marijuana treated with formaldehyde/formalin and PCP)
Mad dog	Hydro
Peace pill	Fry
Rocket fuel	
Talk to the angels	
Yellow fever	
Zombie weed	

level of popularity, it has remained a significant public health problem among certain populations and in certain geographical areas. Compared to most other drugs of abuse, PCP has more complex and potentially more harmful effects.

DIAGNOSIS

Physicians must be alert to the wide spectrum of PCP effects on multiple-organ systems. Because fluctuations in serum levels may occur unpredictably, an individual being treated for apparently selective psychiatric or behavioral complications of PCP abuse may suddenly undergo radical alterations in medical status; emergency medical intervention may become necessary to avoid permanent organ damage or death. Any individual manifesting significant cardiovascular, respiratory, neurological, or metabolic derangement subsequent to PCP use should be evaluated and treated in a medical

Clinical Guide to the Diagnosis and Treatment of Mental Disorders. M. B. First and A. Tasman
© 2006 John Wiley & Sons, Ltd. ISBN 0 470 019158

service; the mental health professional plays a secondary role in diagnosis and treatment until physiological stability has been reached and sustained.

PCP-intoxicated individuals may come to medical attention on the basis of alterations in mental status, bizarre or violent behavior, injuries sustained while intoxicated, or medical complications, such as rhabdomyolysis, hyperthermia, or seizures. As illicit ketamine use has increased significantly as part of the "club drug" phenomenon, it is important to remember that ketamine can induce the same spectrum of effects and complications, the chief difference from PCP being the much shorter duration of action of ketamine.

The presenting symptoms may be predominantly or exclusively psychiatric, without significant alterations in the level of consciousness, and may closely resemble an acute schizophrenic decompensation with concrete or illogical thinking, bizarre behavior, negativism, catatonic posturing, and echolalia. Subjective feelings and objective signs of "drunkenness" may or may not be present.

In PCP intoxication, the central nervous, cardiovascular, respiratory, and peripheral autonomic systems are affected to degrees ranging from mild to catastrophic (Table 23-2).

The level of consciousness may vary from full alertness to coma. Coma of variable duration may occur

Table 23-2	Nonpsychiatric Findings in Phencyclidine Intoxication

Altered level of consciousness
Central nervous system changes including nystagmus, hyperreflexia, and motor abnormalities
Hypertension
Cholinergic or anticholinergic signs
Hypothermia or hyperthermia
Myoglobinuria

spontaneously or after an episode of bizarre or violent behavior. Prolonged coma due to continued drug absorption from ruptured ingested packages of PCP has been described.

Nystagmus (which may be horizontal, vertical, or rotatory) frequently has been described in individuals with PCP intoxication.. Consequences of PCP-induced central nervous system hyperexcitability may range from mildly increased deep tendon reflexes to grand mal seizures. Other motor signs have been observed, such as generalized rigidity, localized dystonias, facial grimacing, and athetosis.

Hypertension is one of the most frequent physical findings, and is usually mild and self limiting, but some have had severe hypertension, and some remain hypertensive for days. Tachycardia occurs in 30% of individuals with PCP intoxication. PCP-induced tachypnea can progress to periodic breathing and respiratory arrest. Autonomic signs seen in PCP intoxication may be cholinergic (diaphoresis, bronchospasm, miosis, salivation, bronchorrhea) or anticholinergic (mydriasis, urinary retention).

Hypothermia and hyperthermia have been observed. Hyperthermia may reach malignant proportions.

Rhabdomyolysis frequently results from a combination of PCP-induced muscle contractions and trauma occurring in relation to injuries sustained as a result of behavioral effects. Acute renal failure can result from myoglobinuria.

The disruption of normal cognitive and memory function by PCP frequently renders individuals incapable of giving an accurate history, including a history of having used PCP. Therefore, assay of urine or blood for drugs may be the only way to establish the diagnosis. PCP is frequently taken in forms in which it has been used to adulterate other drugs, such as marijuana and cocaine, often without the user's knowledge. One of the most recent and alarming manifestations of this phenomenon is a preparation known variously as *illy*, *hydro*, *wet*, or *fry*, consisting of a marijuana cigarette or blunt containing formaldehyde/formalin (which is advertised) and PCP (which often is not); PCP precursors and synthesis by-products as well as PCP have been detected in toxicological screens of users who have consumed these preparations.

DSM-IV-TR Diagnostic Criteria

292.89 PHENCYCLIDINE INTOXICATION

A. Recent use of phencyclidine (or a related substance).
B. Clinically significant maladaptive behavioral changes (e.g., belligerence, assaultiveness, impulsiveness, unpredictability, psychomotor agitation, impaired judgment, or impaired social or occupational functioning) that developed during, or shortly after, phencyclidine use.
C. Within an hour (less when smoked, "snorted," or used intravenously), two (or more) of the following signs:

 (1) Vertical or horizontal nystagmus
 (2) Hypertension or tachycardia
 (3) Numbness or diminished responsiveness to pain
 (4) Ataxia
 (5) Dysarthria
 (6) Muscle rigidity
 (7) Seizures or coma
 (8) Hyperacusis

D. The symptoms are not due to a general medical condition and are not better accounted for by another mental disorder.

Specify if:

With perceptual disturbances

Reprinted with permission from the *Diagnostic and Statistical Manual of Mental Disorders*, 4th ed., Text Rev. Copyright 2000 American Psychiatric Association.

By disrupting sensory pathways, PCP frequently renders users hypersensitive to environmental stimuli to the extent that physical examination or psychiatric interview may cause severe agitation. If PCP intoxication is suspected, measures should be taken from the outset to minimize sensory input. The individual should be evaluated in a quiet, darkened room with the minimal necessary number of medical staff present. Assessments may need to be interrupted periodically.

Vital signs should be obtained immediately on presentation. Temperature, blood pressure, and respiratory rate are dose-dependently increased by PCP and may be of a magnitude requiring emergency medical treatment to avoid the potentially fatal complications of malignant hyperthermia, hypertensive crisis, and respiratory arrest. In all cases, monitoring of vital signs should continue at 2- to 4-hour intervals throughout treatment, because serum PCP levels may increase spontaneously as a result of mobilization of drug from lipid stores or enterohepatic recirculation.

Analgesic and behavioral changes induced by PCP not only predispose individuals to physical injury but also mask these injuries, which may be found only with careful physical examination.

On neurological examination, nystagmus and ataxia, although not conclusive, are strongly suggestive of PCP intoxication. Examination of deep tendon reflexes helps establish the degree of nervous system hyperexcitability. Crossed or clonic deep tendon reflexes alert the physician to the possibility of subsequent seizures.

Because PCP is usually supplied in combination with other drugs and is often misrepresented, toxicological analysis of urine or blood is essential. However, there may be circumstances in which PCP may not be detected in urine even if it is present in the body, for example, when the urine is alkaline. On the other hand, in chronic PCP users, drug may be detected in urine up to 30 days after the last use.

Blood and urine samples should be sent for toxicological analysis. In addition, serum uric acid, creatine kinase, aspartate transaminase, and alanine transaminase elevations are common findings in PCP intoxication.

Course

As drug levels decline, the clinical picture recedes in 5 to 21 days through periods of moderating neurological, autonomic, and metabolic impairments to a stage at which only psychiatric impairments are apparent. Once the physical symptoms and signs have cleared, the period of simple PCP psychosis may last from 1 day to 6 weeks, whether or not neuroleptics are administered,

during which the psychiatric symptoms and signs abate gradually and progressively. Even after complete recovery, flashbacks may occur if PCP sequestered in lipid stores is mobilized. Any underlying mental disorders can be detected and evaluated only after complete resolution of the drug-induced psychosis. Although systematic studies in humans have not been carried out, clinical experience predicts a high likelihood of resumption of PCP use after recovery from PCP psychosis.

Differential Diagnosis

The presence of nystagmus and hypertension with mental status changes should raise the possibility of PCP intoxication. Because of the close resemblance of both the acute and the prolonged forms of PCP psychosis to schizophrenia, and the increased sensitivity of individuals with schizophrenia to the psychotomimetic effects of the drug, an underlying schizophrenia spectrum disorder should be considered, particularly if paranoia or thought disorder persists beyond 4 to 6 weeks after the last use of PCP. PCP psychosis may also resemble mania or other mood disorders. Therefore in all cases, a detailed psychiatric history should be obtained. Robust response of psychotic symptoms to treatment with neuroleptics would favor a diagnosis other than simple PCP psychosis.

PCP psychosis is readily distinguishable from lysergic acid diethylamide (LSD) psychosis in normal as well as in individuals with schizophrenia by the lack of typical LSD effects, such as synesthesia. The cluster of psychotic symptoms, hypertension, and stereotypy may be seen in both PCP psychosis and chronic amphetamine psychosis; in such cases, accurate histories and toxicological analysis are particularly important.

In cases involving prominent PCP-induced neurological, cardiovascular, or metabolic derangement, encephalitis, head injury, postictal state, and primary metabolic disorders must be ruled out. Either intoxication with or withdrawal from sedative–hypnotics may be associated with nystagmus Neuroleptic malignant syndrome should be ruled out in the differential diagnosis of PCP-induced hyperthermia and muscle rigidity.

TREATMENT

The hierarchy of treatment goals begins with detection and treatment of physical manifestations of PCP intoxication.

Equally important are measures to anticipate PCP-induced impulsive, violent behaviors and provide appropriate protection for the PCP user and others. The individual must then be closely observed during the period of PCP-induced psychosis, which may persist for weeks after resolution of physical symptoms and signs. Finally, the possibly dramatic medical and psychiatric presentation and its resolution must not divert the attention of the clinician from full assessment and treatment of the individual's drug-seeking behavior.

In contrast to psychotic states induced by drugs such as LSD, in which "talking the individual down" (by actively distracting the individual from his LSD-induced sensory distortions and convincing the individual that his or her distress stems from nothing more than the temporary effects of a drug that soon will wear off) may be highly effective, no such effort should be made in the case of PCP psychosis, particularly during the period of acute intoxication, because of the risk of sensory overload that can lead to dramatically increased agitation. The risk of sudden and unpredictable impulsive, violent behavior can also be increased by sensory stimulation.

Somatic Treatments

There is no pharmacological competitive antagonist for PCP, in contrast to opiates and benzodiazepines. Oral or intramuscular benzodiazepines are recommended for agitation. Neuroleptics usually have little or no effect on acute or chronic PCP-induced psychosis or thought disorder. Because they lower the seizure threshold, neuroleptics should be used with caution. Physical restraint may be lifesaving if the individual's behavior poses an imminent threat to his or her safety or that of others; however, such restraint risks triggering or worsening rhabdomyolysis.

Because of the large volume of distribution of PCP, dialysis is ineffective as a means of clearing the drug from circulation. The "trapping" of PCP in acidic body compartments suggests either gastric gavage or urinary acidification as a measure to reduce levels of PCP in the body. However, these should be considered measures of last resort because of the possibility of electrolyte imbalance and additional nephrotoxic effects. Administration of activated charcoal may be useful but is unproved.

Special Features Influencing Treatment

PCP psychosis may be clinically indistinguishable from schizophrenia. It has been suggested that some individuals who remain psychotic for weeks after PCP ingestion may have an underlying predisposition to schizophrenia or mania. In some series, significant percentages of individuals suffering prolonged PCP-induced psychosis are subsequently hospitalized with nondrug-induced schizophrenic disorders. In the case of an individual with schizophrenia, responsiveness to neuroleptic treatment may resume after recovery from prolonged PCP psychosis.

Individuals with preexisting neurological, cardiovascular, respiratory, or renal disorders are at increased risk for complications of PCP intoxication, such as seizures, stroke, hypertensive crisis, respiratory arrest, or renal failure. Abusers of more than one drug may be at increased risk from the presence of other drugs exerting toxic effects on the same organ systems (e.g., cardiovascular effects of cocaine and amphetamine) or because of damage to specific organs secondary to infectious complications of parenteral drug use.

COMPARISON OF DSM-IV-TR AND ICD-10 DIAGNOSTIC CRITERIA

ICD-10 does not have a separate class for PCP-related disorder and instead includes PCP in the hallucinogen class.

24   Substance-Related Disorders: Sedatives, Hypnotics, and Anxiolytics

Sedative–hypnotics and anxiolytics include prescription sleeping medications and most medications used for the treatment of anxiety. The sedative–hypnotics include a chemically diverse group of medications. Pharmacologically alcohol is appropriately included among sedative–hypnotics; however, it is generally considered separately, as it is in DSM-IV-TR and in this book. The medications usually included in the category of sedative–hypnotics are listed in Table 24-1

The sedative–hypnotics include a chemically diverse group of medications. Although buspirone is marketed for the treatment of anxiety, its pharmacological profile is sufficiently different that it is not usually included among the sedative–hypnotics. Antidepressant medications may also have antianxiety properties, and their sedative effects are often of clinical utility in sleep induction; however, they too are usually excluded from the sedative–hypnotic classification.

For treatment of anxiety and insomnia, the benzodiazepines have largely supplanted the older sedative–hypnotics. The benzodiazepines have a major advantage over the older compounds. In an overdose, the older sedative–hypnotics are lethal at 10 to 15 times the usual therapeutic doses. Benzodiazepines, if taken alone, have a therapeutic ratio exceeding 100. In combination with alcohol or other drugs, the benzodiazepines may contribute to the lethality, but death from a benzodiazepine overdose is rare. Some atavistic uses of the older compounds remain driven primarily by economic considerations and misguided attempts to reduce abuse of benzodiazepines by addicts and perceived overprescription of benzodiazepines by physicians.

Most people do not like the subjective effects of benzodiazepines, especially in high doses. Even among drug addicts, the benzodiazepines alone are not common intoxicants. They are, however, widely used by drug addicts to self-medicate opiate withdrawal and

to alleviate the side effects of cocaine and amphetamines. Individuals receiving methadone maintenance use benzodiazepines to boost (enhance) the effects of methadone. Some alcoholic individuals use benzodiazepines either in combination with alcohol or as a second-choice intoxicant, if alcohol is unavailable. Fat-soluble benzodiazepines that enter the central nervous system (CNS) quickly are usually the benzodiazepines preferred by addicts.

Addicts whose urine is being monitored for benzodiazepines prefer benzodiazepines with high milligram potency, such as alprazolam or clonazepam. These benzodiazepines are excreted in urine in such small amounts that they are often not detected in drug screens, particularly with thin-layer chromatography.

DIAGNOSIS

Sedative–hypnotics are among the most commonly prescribed medications. They are also often misused and abused and can produce severe, life-threatening dependence. With the exception of the benzodiazepines and newer hypnotics (e.g., zaleplon, zopiclone and zolpidem), overdose with sedative–hypnotics can be lethal. Benzodiazepines and the newer hypnotics are rarely lethal if taken alone; in combination with alcohol or other drugs, however, they can be lethal.

Sedative–Hypnotic–Anxiolytic Dependence

Sedative–hypnotics can produce tolerance and physiological dependence (see generic DSM-IV-TR diagnostic criteria for Substance Dependence in Chapter 13, page 125). Physiological dependence can be induced within several days with continuous infusion of anesthetic doses. Individuals who are taking barbiturates daily, for example, for a month or more above the upper

Table 24-1	Medications Usually Included in the Category of Sedative–Hypnotics		
Generic Name	**Trade Names**	**Common Therapeutic Use**	**Therapeutic-Dose Range (mg/d)**
Barbiturates			
Amobarbital	Amytal	Sedative	50–150
Butabarbital	Butisol	Sedative	45–120
Butalbital	Fiorinal, Sedapap	Sedative/analgesic	100–300
Pentobarbital	Nembutal	Hypnotic	50–100
Secobarbital	Seconal	Hypnotic	50–100
Benzodiazepines			
Alprazolam	Xanax	Antianxiety	0.75–6
Chlordiazepoxide	Librium	Antianxiety	15–100
Clonazepam	Klonopin	Anticonvulsant	0.5–4
Clorazepate	Tranxene	Antianxiety	15–60
Diazepam	Valium	Antianxiety	5–40
Estazolam	ProSom	Hypnotic	1–2
Flunitrazepam	Rohypnol*	Hypnotic	1–2
Flurazepam	Dalmane	Hypnotic	15–30
Halazepam	Paxipam	Antianxiety	60–160
Lorazepam	Ativan	Antianxiety	1–16
Midazolam	Versed	Anesthesia	–
Oxazepam	Serax	Antianxiety	10–120
Prazepam	Centrax	Antianxiety	20–60
Quazepam	Doral	Hypnotic	15
Temazepam	Restoril	Hypnotic	7.5–30
Triazolam	Halcion	Hypnotic	0.125–0.5
Others			
Chloral hydrate	Noctec, Somnos	Hypnotic	250–1000
Eszopiclone	Lunesta	Hypnotic	1–3
Ethchlorvynol	Placidyl	Hypnotic	200–1000
Glutethimide	Doriden	Hypnotic	250–500
Meprobamate	Miltown, Equanil, Equagesic	Antianxiety	1200–1600
Methyprylon	Noludar	Hypnotic	200–400
Zaleplon	Sonata (Stilnox, other countries)	Hypnotic	5–20
Zolpidem	Ambien	Hypnotic	5–10

*Rohypnol is not marketed in the United States.

therapeutic range listed in Table 24-1 should be presumed to be physically dependent and in need of medically managed detoxification.

Sedative–Hypnotic–Anxiolytic Abuse

Abuse may occur on its own or in conjunction with use of other substances (e.g., while using high doses of sedatives in order to "come down" from a cocaine or amphetamine high). Abuse of sedatives in hazardous situations (e.g., getting "high" and then driving while intoxicated) is among the more common reasons for a diagnosis of Sedative–Hypnotic–Anxiolytic Abuse (see generic DSM-IV-TR diagnostic criteria for Substance Abuse in Chapter 13, page 125).

Sedative–Hypnotic–Anxiolytic Intoxication

The acute toxicity of sedative–hypnotics consists of slurred speech, incoordination, ataxia, sustained nystagmus, impaired judgment, and mood lability. When taken in large amounts, sedative–hypnotics produce progressive respiratory depression and coma. The amount of respiratory depression produced by the benzodiazepines is much less than that produced by the barbiturates and other sedative–hypnotics. Consistent with its general approach, the DSM-IV-TR diagnosis of intoxication requires "clinically significant maladaptive behavioral or psychological changes" developing after drug use in addition to the signs and symptoms of acute toxicity. The DSM-IV-TR criteria for intoxication are shown on page 126.

Sedative–Hypnotic–Anxiolytic Withdrawal

The withdrawal syndrome arising from the discontinuation of short-acting sedative–hypnotics is similar to that from stopping or cutting down on the use of alcohol (see DSM-IV-TR diagnostic criteria, page 137). Signs and symptoms of sedative–hypnotic withdrawal include anxiety, tremors, nightmares, insomnia, anorexia, nausea, vomiting, postural hypotension, seizures,

DSM-IV-TR Criteria

292.89 SEDATIVE, HYPNOTIC, OR ANXIOLYTIC INTOXICATION

A. Recent use of a sedative, hypnotic, or anxiolytic.
B. Clinically significant maladaptive behavioral or psychological changes (e.g., inappropriate sexual or aggressive behavior, mood lability, impaired judgment, impaired social or occupational functioning) that developed during, or shortly after, sedative, hypnotic, or anxiolytic use.
C. One (or more) of the following signs, developing during, or shortly after, sedative, hypnotic, or anxiolytic use:

(1) slurred speech
(2) incoordination
(3) unsteady gait
(4) nystagmus
(5) impairment in attention or memory
(6) stupor or coma.

D. The symptoms are not due to a general medical condition and are not better accounted for by another mental disorder.

Reprinted with permission from the *Diagnostic and Statistical Manual of Mental Disorders*, 4th ed., Text Rev. Copyright 2000 American Psychiatric Association.

Diagnostic Criteria

292.0 SEDATIVE, HYPNOTIC, OR ANXIOLYTIC WITHDRAWAL

A. Cessation of (or reduction in) sedative, hypnotic, or anxiolytic use that has been heavy and prolonged.
B. Two (or more) of the following, developing within several hours to a few days after Criterion A:

(1) autonomic hyperactivity (e.g., sweating or pulse rate greater than 100)
(2) increased hand tremor
(3) insomnia
(4) nausea or vomiting
(5) transient visual, tactile, or auditory hallucinations or illusions
(6) psychomotor agitation
(7) anxiety
(8) grand mal seizures.

C. The symptoms in Criterion B cause clinically significant distress or impairment in social, occupational, or other important areas of functioning.
D. The symptoms are not due to a general medical condition and are not better accounted for by another mental disorder.

Specify if:

With Perceptual Disturbances

Reprinted with permission from the *Diagnostic and Statistical Manual of Mental Disorders*, 4th ed., Text Rev. Copyright 2000 American Psychiatric Association.

delirium, and hyperpyrexia. The syndrome is qualitatively similar for all sedative–hypnotics; however, the time course of symptoms depends on the particular

drug. With short-acting sedative–hypnotics (e.g., pentobarbital, secobarbital, meprobamate, oxazepam, alprazolam, and triazolam), withdrawal symptoms typically begin 12 to 24 hours after the last dose and peak in intensity between 24 and 72 hours (symptoms may develop more slowly in individuals with liver disease or in the elderly because of decreased drug metabolism). With long-acting drugs (e.g., phenobarbital, diazepam, and chlordiazepoxide), withdrawal symptoms peak on the fifth to eighth day.

During untreated sedative–hypnotic withdrawal, the electroencephalogram (EEG) may show paroxysmal bursts of high-voltage, low-frequency activity that precedes the development of seizures. The withdrawal delirium may include confusion, and visual and auditory hallucinations. The delirium generally follows a period of insomnia. Some individuals may have only delirium; others only seizures; and some may have both delirium and convulsions.

Many people who have taken benzodiazepines in therapeutic doses for months to years can abruptly discontinue the drug without developing withdrawal symptoms. But other individuals taking similar amounts of a benzodiazepine develop symptoms ranging from mild to severe when the benzodiapine is stopped or when the dosage is substantially reduced. Characteristically, individuals tolerate a gradual tapering of the benzodiazepine until they are at 10–20% of their peak dose. Further reductions in benzodiazepine dose then cause individuals to become increasingly symptomatic. In addition, in medicine literature, the low-dose withdrawal may be called therapeutic-dose withdrawal, normal-dose withdrawal, or benzodiazepine discontinuation syndrome. The symptoms can ultimately be categorized as symptom reemergence, symptom rebound, or a prolonged withdrawal syndrome.

Many individuals experience a transient increase in symptoms for 1 to 2 weeks after benzodiazepine withdrawal. The symptoms are an intensified return of the symptoms for which the benzodiazepine was prescribed. This transient form of symptoms intensification is called *symptom rebound*. The term comes from sleep research where rebound insomnia is commonly observed after sedative–hypnotic use. Symptom rebound lasts a few days to weeks after discontinuation. Symptom rebound is the most common withdrawal consequence of prolonged benzodiazepine use.

The symptoms for which the benzodiazepine has been taken may return to the same level as before the benzodiazepine therapy. This is called symptom reemergence (or recrudescence). In other words, the individual's symptoms, such as anxiety, insomnia, or muscle tension, that had abated during benzodiazepine treatment return.

The reason for making a distinction between symptom rebound and symptom reemergence is that symptom reemergence suggests that the original symptoms are still present and must be treated. Symptom rebound is a transient withdrawal syndrome that will disappear over time.

Some drugs or medications may facilitate neuroadaptation by increasing the affinity of benzodiazepines for their receptors. Prior treatment with phenobarbital has been found to increase the intensity of chlordiazepoxide (45 mg/day) withdrawal symptoms. Individuals at increased risk for development of the low-dose withdrawal syndrome are those with a family or personal history of alcoholism, those who use alcohol daily, and those who concomitantly use other sedatives. Case–control studies suggest that individuals with a history of addiction, particularly to other sedative–hypnotics, are at high risk for low-dose benzodiazepine dependence. The short-acting, high-milligram-potency benzodiazepines appear to produce a more intense low-dose withdrawal syndrome.

A few individuals experience a severe, protracted withdrawal syndrome that includes symptoms (e.g., paresthesia and psychosis) that were not present before. This withdrawal syndrome has generated much of the concern about the long-term safety of the benzodiazepines. Protracted benzodiazepine withdrawal may consist of relatively mild withdrawal symptoms such as anxiety, mood instability, and sleep disturbance similar to the protracted withdrawal syndrome described for alcohol and other drugs. In some individuals, the protracted withdrawal syndrome from benzodiazepines can be severe and disabling and lasts many months.

There is considerable controversy surrounding even the existence of this syndrome, which evolves primarily from the addiction medicine literature. Many symptoms are nonspecific and often mimic an obsessive–compulsive disorder (OCD) with psychotic features. As a practical matter, it is often difficult in the clinical setting to separate symptom reemergence from protracted withdrawal. New symptoms, such as increased sensitivity to sound, light, and touch and paresthesia, are particularly suggestive of low-dose withdrawal.

The protracted benzodiazepine withdrawal has no pathognomonic signs or symptoms, and the broad range of nonspecific symptoms produced by the protracted benzodiazepine withdrawal syndrome could also be the result of agitated depression, generalized anxiety disorder (GAD), panic disorder, partial complex seizures, and schizophrenia. The time course of symptom resolution is the primary differentiating feature between symptoms generated by withdrawal and symptom reemergence. Symptoms from withdrawal gradually subside with continued abstinence, whereas symptom reemergence and symptom sensitization do not.

The waxing and waning of symptom intensity are characteristic of the low-dose protracted benzodiazepine withdrawal syndrome. Individuals are sometimes asymptomatic for several days, and then, without apparent reason, they become acutely anxious. Often there are concomitant physiological signs (e.g., dilated pupils, increased resting heart rate, and increased blood pressure). The intense waxing and waning of symptoms are important in distinguishing low-dose withdrawal symptoms from symptom reemergence.

Assessment Issues

The individual's drug use history is usually the first source of information that is used in assessing sedative–hypnotic abuse or dependence. If the sedative–hypnotics were being used for treatment of insomnia or anxiety, the history is often best obtained as part of the history of the primary disorder and its response to treatment. A detailed history of use of all sedative–hypnotics, including alcohol, should be elicited from the individual. When framed in terms of the presenting disorder, individuals are generally more candid about their drug use and their relationship with past treating physicians.

For many reasons, individuals may minimize or exaggerate their drug use and not accurately report the behavioral consequences of their use. High doses of benzodiazepines or therapeutic doses of benzodiazepines in combination with alcohol may disrupt memory. Individuals are likely to attribute impairment of function to the underlying disorder rather than to the medication use. Observations of the individual's behavior by family members can be a source of valuable information. Whenever possible, the individual's history should be supplemented by medical records to help piece together as accurate a picture of drug use as possible. Pharmacy records may be helpful in establishing and verifying the individual's drug use history, and urine testing can be useful in verifying recent drug use history.

Individuals who obtain some or all of their medication from street sources may not know what they have been taking, as deception in the street-drug marketplace is common. For example, tablets sold as methaqualone have been found to contain phenobarbital or diazepam.

Sustained horizontal nystagmus is a reliable indicator of sedative–hypnotic intoxication. Onset of tremor, abnormal sweating, and blood pressure or pulse increase may be produced by sedative–hypnotic withdrawal.

Urine toxicology can be useful in monitoring the individual's use of drugs and in confirming a history of drug or medication use. The detection time varies widely for benzodiazepines. Diazepam or chlordiazepoxide may be detected for weeks following chronic or high-dose use, whereas others, such as alprazolam or clonazepam, may not be detectable in routine toxicology urinalysis. Because of the variability in laboratory cut-offs and detection time, and different drugs included in the screening panel, the analytical laboratory should be asked about what they routinely screen for as well as the detection limits.

Patterns of Use/Abuse

Some sedative–hypnotics, such as the short-acting barbiturates, are primary drugs of abuse—that is, they are injected for the "rush" or are taken orally to produce a state of disinhibition similar to that achieved with alcohol. Sedative hypnotics may also be taken in combination with other primary intoxicants, such as alcohol or heroin, to intensify the desired subjective effects.

Drug addicts may also use sedative–hypnotics to self-medicate withdrawal of drugs such as heroin. When the avowed intent is to stop the use of drugs such as heroin, physicians may be lured into thinking that addicts' self-administration of sedative–hypnotics is not an "abuse" but rather a reasonable approximation of medical use. While on occasion this may be the case, often it is not. Addicts' episodic attempts to stop using heroin by self-medicating opiate-withdrawal symptoms with sedative–hypnotics without entering drug abuse treatment are rarely successful, and may result in the secondary development of sedative–hypnotic dependence.

Addicts may also use sedative–hypnotics to reduce unpleasant side effects of stimulants, particularly cocaine or methamphetamine. Impairment of judgment and memory produced by the sedative–hypnotic in combination with wakefulness of a stimulant may result in unpredictable behavior.

Barbiturates. During the late 1960s and early 1970s, the short-acting barbiturates, secobarbital and pentobarbital, were common drugs of abuse. Addicts dissolved the tablets or the contents of capsules in water and injected the solution. The desired effect was the "rush," a dreamy, floaty feeling lasting a few minutes after the injection. After the rush, the addict was intoxicated, but the primary appeal to injection was the rush. The intoxication is not qualitatively different from that produced by oral ingestion of a short-acting barbiturate.

Injection of a barbiturate is associated with the usual infectious risk of injecting street drugs, but the barbiturates are particularly pernicious if inadvertently injected into an artery or if the solution is injected or leaked from a vein or artery into tissue surrounding the vessel. Barbiturates are irritating to the tissue, and the affected tissue becomes indurated and may abscess. In addition, barbiturate solution injected into an artery produces intense vasoconstriction and blockage of the arterioles, resulting in gangrene of areas supplied by the artery.

Methaqualone. Methaqualone (Quaalude) was removed from the US market in 1984 because of its abuse. Subsequently, it has continued to be sold on the street-drug black market. Some tablets sold on the black market as Quaalude contain methaqualone, apparently diverted from countries where methaqualone is still available; others contain diazepam, phenobarbital, or another sedative–hypnotic.

Benzodiazepines. Benzodiazepines are often used or misused by addicts to self-medicate opiate withdrawal, to intensify the CNS effects of methadone, or to ameliorate the adverse effects of cocaine or methamphetamine.

The benzodiazepine, flunitrazepam (Rohypnol, Narcozep), is singled out for additional discussion because of the media and legislative attention it received during the 1990s, and because it is still widely abused in Europe and other areas of the world. Flunitrazepam, a potent benzodiazepine hypnotic, was never marketed in the United States but is widely available by prescription in many other countries in 1- or 2-mg oral dosage forms and for injection.

Flunitrazepam has many street names, including rophies, ropies, roopies, roofies, ruffes, rofinol, loops, and wheels. Tablets of Rohypnol have the name of the manufacturer Roche engraved on them and a number indicating the milligram strength (either 1 or 2). Drug abusers usually prefer the 2-mg tablets, which are often called "Roche dos" or just "Roche" (usually pronounced "row-shay"). Although flunitrazepam is similar in many respects to other benzodiazepines in abuse potential, flunitrazepam is among the benzodiazepines with the highest abuse potential and has considerable appeal among heroin addicts.

In the mid-1990s, Rohypnol achieved notoriety as the "date-rape drug." Subsequently, GHB (gamma-hydroxybutyric acid), which has some properties of a sedative–hypnotic, was also called a "date-rape drug." Because of the media attention, considerable public debate ensued and the US Congress was prompted to pass legislation increasing penalties for rape when Rohypnol or other drugs were used to facilitate it.

Flunitrazepam and other benzodiazepines have also been associated with deaths among opiate addicts taking buprenorphine in France. Although buprenorphine alone or benzodiazepines alone are rarely fatal, the combination appears to increase the risk of overdose. Benzodiazepines and buprenorphine may have synergistic action in suppressing respiration.

Zolpidem. Zolpidem (Ambien) is an imidazopyridine hypnotic, chemically unrelated to the benzodiazepines. However, it binds to a subunit of the same gamma-aminobutyric acid (GABA)–benzodiazepine complex as the benzodiazepines and its sedative effects are reversed by the benzodiazepine antagonist flumazenil. Zolpidem has been available for prescription since 1993 in the United States and in Europe for several years before.

A few case reports of abuse suggest that some individuals increase the dosage many times above what is prescribed and that zolpidem produces a withdrawal syndrome similar to that of other sedative–hypnotics. The case histories also describe significant tolerance to the sedative effects of zolpidem.

Zolpidem is rapidly absorbed and has a short half-life (2.2 hours). Its sedative effects are additive with alcohol.

In addition to dependence, zolpidem has produced idiosyncratic psychotic reactions. A report from Belgium described two cases of transient psychosis after the first dose of 10 mg of zolpidem. Neither individual had a history of drug abuse or misuse nor were they using alcohol at the time. Both individuals experienced a transient psychosis with visual hallucinations beginning 20 to 30 minutes after 10 mg of zolpidem. Both individuals previously used benzodiazepines without difficulty and both were amnestic for the psychotic episode. Additional case reports of psychosis have been reported in the United States.

Zaleplon. Zaleplon (Sonata) is a pyrazolopyrimidine approved by the FDA as a hypnotic in 1999. Like zolpidem, it is chemically unrelated to the benzodiazepines and binds to the omega-1 receptor, which is a subunit of the GABA–benzodiazepine receptor. Peak plasma concentration occurs about 1 hour following oral ingestion. It is rapidly metabolized with a half-life of about 1 hour. Impairment of short-term memory may occur at dosages of 10 to 20 mg.

Course

Once a diagnosis of sedative–hypnotic dependence is manifested, it is unlikely that an individual will be able to return to controlled, therapeutic use of sedative–hypnotics. All sedative–hypnotics, including alcohol, are cross-tolerant, and physical dependence and tolerance are quickly reestablished if an individual resumes use of sedative–hypnotics.

If after sedative–hypnotic withdrawal the individual has another mental disorder, such as GAD, panic attacks, or insomnia, alternate treatment strategies other than sedative–hypnotics should be used if possible. Definitive diagnosis of a mental disorder during early abstinence is often not possible because protracted withdrawal symptoms may mimic anxiety disorders, and disruption of sleep architecture for days to months after drug withdrawal is extremely common.

If the sedative–hypnotic dependence has developed secondary to stimulant or alcohol use, primary treatment of the chemical dependence should be a priority. Often the symptom that was driving the sedative–hypnotic use disappears after the individual is drug-abstinent.

Differential Diagnosis

The diagnosis of sedative–hypnotic abuse and dependence is based primarily on drug use history and the DSM-IV-TR criteria of continuing behavior dysfunction caused by the drug. With dependence developing from prescribed use, the practical difficulty is determining when the dysfunction is a result of the drug use rather than the disorder for which the medication was prescribed.

Long-term use of benzodiazepines can result in physical dependence in nondrug-dependent medical patients. Withdrawal symptoms or return of symptoms suppressed by the benzodiazepines may make discontinuation difficult.

Some individuals who are physically dependent on or unable to discontinue a medication do not necessarily have a substance use disorder. Physical dependence results from neuroadaptive changes resulting from long-term exposure to a medication. Inability to discontinue the medication may simply mean that individuals are unwilling to tolerate the severity of postwithdrawal symptoms that develop. In the absence of medication-produced dysfunction, the continuation of the medication may be an appropriate choice. Individuals who do not have a substance use disorder take medications in the quantity prescribed. They follow their physicians' recommendations, and they do not mix them with drugs of abuse.

Abusers of alcohol and other drugs rarely present for primary treatment of sedative–hypnotic dependency. From the drug-abusing individual's point of view, sedative–hypnotic use is an effort to self-medicate anxiety or insomnia, which is often the result of alcohol or stimulant abuse. Despite their assertion that the medication is being taken for symptom relief, they often take the medication in larger than physician-prescribed doses, combine the medication with intoxicating amounts of alcohol or other drugs, and purchase medications from street sources. They may also use the sedative–hypnotic as an intoxicant when other drugs are not available.

TREATMENT

Treatment of sedative–hypnotic dependence that has developed as a result of treatment of an underlying mental disorder is almost always a lengthy undertaking. The goals of the first phase of treatment are to establish the diagnosis and, to the extent possible, to delineate the comorbid psychiatric diagnoses and to establish a therapeutic relationship with the individual. The art of treatment is to know when the therapeutic alliance is sufficiently established to institute drug withdrawal, and knowing when outpatient treatment is not progressing adequately.

Somatic Treatments

Detoxification. Three general strategies are used for withdrawing individuals from sedative–hypnotics, including benzodiazepines. The first is to use decreasing doses of the agent of dependence. The second is to substitute phenobarbital or some other long-acting barbiturate for the addicting agent, and gradually withdraw the substitute medication. The third, used for individuals with a dependence on both alcohol and a benzodiazepine, is to substitute a long-acting benzodiazepine, such as chlordiazepoxide, and taper it during 1 to 2 weeks.

The withdrawal strategy selected depends on the particular sedative–hypnotic, the involvement of other drugs of dependence, and the clinical setting in which the detoxification program takes place. The gradual reduction of the benzodiazepine of dependence is used primarily in medical settings for dependence arising from treatment of an underlying condition. The individual must be cooperative, must be able to adhere to dosing regimens, and must not be abusing alcohol or other drugs.

Substitution of phenobarbital can also be used to withdraw individuals who have lost control of their benzodiazepine use or who are polydrug-dependent. Phenobarbital substitution has the broadest use for all sedative–hypnotic drug dependencies and is widely used in drug treatment programs.

For high-dose sedative–hypnotic dependence, the pharmacological treatment strategy is the same as that for barbiturates. The phenobarbital conversion equivalents are shown in Tables 24-2 and 24-3. The dose conversions computed using Table 24-2 and 24-3 prevent the emergence of severe withdrawal of the classic sedative–hypnotic type.

For treatment of protracted benzodiazepine withdrawal, the phenobarbital conversions based on Tables 24-2 and 24-3 are not adequate to suppress symptoms. For example, someone discontinuing 20 mg of diazepam would have a computed phenobarbital conversion of 60 mg. In managing low-dose withdrawal, an approach is to begin with about 200 mg/day of phenobarbital and then taper the phenobarbital, slowly as tolerated. If palpitations or other symptoms of autonomic hyperactivity are bothersome, beta-adrenergic blockers, such as propranolol, or alpha-2-adrenergic agonists, such as clonidine, may be useful adjuncts. Reports on the use of clonidine to reduce benzodiazepine withdrawal severity have yielded mixed results.

Stabilization Phase. The individual's history of drug use during the month before treatment is used to compute the stabilization dose of phenobarbital. Although many addicts exaggerate the number of pills they are taking, the individual's history is the best guide to initiating pharmacotherapy for withdrawal. Individuals who have overstated the amount of drug that they have taken will become intoxicated during the first day or two of treatment. Intoxication is easily managed by omitting one or more doses of phenobarbital and reducing the daily dose.

To compute the initial daily starting dose of phenobarbital, the individual's average daily use of each sedative–hypnotic is estimated. Next, the individual's average daily sedative–hypnotic dose for each drug is converted to its phenobarbital withdrawal equivalent by multiplying the average daily dose by the drug's phenobarbital conversion constant shown in both Tables 24-2 and 24-3. Finally, the phenobarbital withdrawal equivalences for each drug are added together. In any case, the maximum daily phenobarbital dose is limited to 500 mg/day. The total daily amount of phenobarbital is divided into three doses per day.

Before receiving each dose of phenobarbital, the individual is checked for signs of phenobarbital toxicity: sustained nystagmus, slurred speech, or ataxia. Of these, sustained nystagmus is the most reliable. If nystagmus is present, the scheduled dose of phenobarbital is withheld. If all three signs are present the next two doses of phenobarbital are withheld, and the daily dosage of phenobarbital for the next day is halved.

Table 24-2	Phenobarbital Withdrawal Equivalents of Benzodiazepines		
Generic Name	Trade Name	Dose Equal to 30 mg of Phenobarbital for Withdrawal* (mg)	Phenobarbital Conversion Constant
Alprazolam	Xanax	1	30
Chlordiazepoxide	Librium	25	1.2
Clonazepam	Klonopin	2	15
Clorazepate	Tranxene	7.5	4
Diazepam	Valium	10	3
Estazolam	ProSom	1	30
Flurazepam	Dalmane	15	2
Halazepam	Paxipam	40	0.75
Lorazepam	Ativan	2	15
Oxazepam	Serax	10	3
Prazepam	Centrax	10	3
Quazepam	Doral	15	2
Temazepam	Restoril	15	2
Triazolam	Halcion	0.25	120

*Phenobarbital withdrawal conversion equivalence is not the same as therapeutic-dose equivalence.

Table 24-3	Phenobarbital Withdrawal Equivalents of Nonbenzodiazepines		
Generic Name	Trade Name	Dose Equal to 30 mg of Phenobarbital for Withdrawal*(mg)	Phenobarbital Conversion Constant
Barbiturates			
Amobarbital	Amytal	100	0.33
Butabarbital	Butisol	100	0.33
Butalbital†	Fiorinal	100	0.33
Pentobarbital	Nembutal	100	0.33
Secobarbital	Seconal	100	0.33
Others			
Chloral hydrate	Noctec, Somnos	500	0.06
Ethchlorvynol	Placidyl	500	0.06
Glutethimide	Doriden	250	0.12
Meprobamate	Miltown	1200	0.025
Methyprylon	Noludar	200	0.15
Zaleplon	Sonata	10	3
Zolpidem	Ambien	5	6

*Phenobarbital withdrawal conversion equivalence is not the same as therapeutic-dose equivalence.

†Butalbital is in combination with opiate or nonopiate analgesics.

If the individual is in acute withdrawal and has had, or is in danger of having, withdrawal seizures, the initial dose of phenobarbital is administered by intramuscular injection. If nystagmus and other signs of intoxication develop 1 to 2 hours after the intramuscular dose, the individual is in no immediate danger from barbiturate withdrawal. Individuals are maintained with the initial dosing schedule of phenobarbital for 2 days. If the individual has neither signs of withdrawal nor phenobarbital toxicity (slurred speech, nystagmus, unsteady gait), phenobarbital withdrawal is begun.

Withdrawal Phase. Unless the individual develops signs and symptoms of phenobarbital toxicity or sedative–hypnotic withdrawal, phenobarbital is decreased by 30 mg/day. Should signs of phenobarbital toxicity develop during withdrawal, the daily phenobarbital dose is decreased by 50% and the 30-mg/day withdrawal is continued from the reduced phenobarbital dose. Should the individual have objective signs of sedative–hypnotic withdrawal, the daily dose is increased by 50% and the individual is restabilized before continuing the withdrawal.

Psychosocial Treatments

Psychotherapy has an important role in motivating an individual for primary treatment of drug dependency.

Therapists can help break down the individual's denial of their drug dependence by helping them see how drug use is interfering with relationships and undermining their ability to function. In some instances, it is desirable to continue the psychotherapeutic relationship while the individual is undergoing treatment for chemical dependence.

Alcoholics Anonymous, Narcotics Anonymous, and Cocaine Anonymous groups are important treatment adjuncts for many people recovering from alcohol and other forms of drug dependence. Although many groups are becoming more tolerant of appropriate use of pharmacotherapies, it is important to be aware that many individuals who attend 12 Step recovery meetings are adamantly opposed to any form of psychotropic medication use and counsel fellow members to stop their use. Individuals with underlying mental disorders and the need for treatment with psychopharmacotherapeutic medications often require ongoing support from their psychotherapist if they must have medication.

Treatment of Individuals with Comorbid Disorders

Most individuals who are being prescribed long-term benzodiazepine therapy have underlying major depressive disorder, panic disorder, or GAD. The clinical dilemma is deciding which individuals are receiving appropriate maintenance therapy for a chronic mental disorder. Long-term use of benzodiazepines may be acceptable if the individual's disabling anxiety symptoms are ameliorated. The reason for the individual's request for benzodiazepine withdrawal from long-term, stable dosing should be carefully explored. Valid reasons to discontinue benzodiazepine treatment include: (1) breakthrough of symptoms that were previously well controlled; (2) impairment of memory or other neurocognitive functions; and (3) abuse of alcohol, cocaine, or other medications.

Individuals with severe underlying mental disorders may have unrealistic hopes of becoming medication-free. Often the origin of request for benzodiazepine withdrawal comes from concerned friends or relatives. The individual's "problems" may be reframed as the use of "addictive medications" or "dependence" rather than the underlying psychopathology. As a practical matter, a trial of medication discontinuation may be undertaken with the understanding that return to a benzodiazepine or use of an antidepressant or other medications may be appropriate.

Many abusers of alcohol or other drugs have symptoms that would reasonably indicate treatment with benzodiazepines or other sedatives if they were not drug abusers. Treating drug abusers with benzodiazepines or other sedatives, while they are still abusing drugs, is, however, generally not helpful. Such individuals are at high risk of misusing or abusing the medications, and the medication may enable them to continue abuse of their primary drug. Drug abusers who are symptomatic because of drug toxicity need hospitalization and detoxification. In individuals with drug dependence disorders, abstinence from all abusable medications is the preferred treatment goal, particularly during the first 6 months of abstinence. In individuals who do not have a drug dependence disorder, return to benzodiazepine use after detoxification may have a different implication than among individuals with a drug dependence disorder. The term *relapse* could reasonably be applied to individuals who self-administer a benzodiazepine when benzodiazepine abstinence is the agreed goal of treatment. The term relapse, however, should not be applied to individuals without a substance abuse disorder who return to prescribed benzodiazepine use because emerging symptoms are not otherwise manageable.

Numerous studies have documented a high prevalence of psychopathological conditions among alcohol and drug abusers. Although the abuse of drugs can induce a psychopathological condition, and there is considerable uncertainty as to the extent to which drug abuse itself contributes to estimates of psychopathology, it is clinically apparent that some drug abusers have severe underlying psychopathological conditions that must be treated if they are to remain abstinent and functional.

COMPARISON OF DSM-IV-TR AND ICD-10 DIAGNOSTIC CRITERIA

The DSM-IV-TR and ICD-10 criteria sets for Sedative, Hypnotic, or Anxiolytic Intoxication are almost equivalent (except that ICD-10 also includes "erythematous skin lesions or blisters"). The DSM-IV-TR and ICD-10 symptom lists for Sedative, Hypnotic, or Anxiolytic Withdrawal include some different items: the ICD-10 list has craving, postural hypotension, headache, malaise or weakness, and paranoid ideation and does not include the DSM-IV-TR anxiety item.

Schizophrenia and Other Psychotic Disorders

Schizophrenia

DIAGNOSIS

Schizophrenia is the most severe and debilitating mental illness, and it has long been the focus of medical, scientific, and societal attention. The term schizophrenia is relatively new to our vocabulary, yet chronic psychotic illnesses have most likely been in existence throughout civilized times. The words used historically to describe psychotic symptoms included madness, folie, insanity, and dementia. They depict a constellation of symptoms that have been poorly understood and shrouded in mystery and fear. Even in the twenty-first century, the layperson's conception of schizophrenia is influenced by these early beliefs. It is only with our modern understanding of the pathophysiology and manifestations of this debilitating illness that the stigmata associated with schizophrenia can be overcome.

In DSM-IV-TR, criterion A of schizophrenia includes delusions, hallucinations, disorganized speech, disorganized or catatonic behavior, and negative symptoms (see DSM-IV-TR diagnostic criteria, page 220). Two or more of these symptoms are required during the active phase of the illness. However, if the individual describes bizarre delusions or auditory hallucinations consisting of a voice commenting on the individual's behavior or voices conversing, only one of these symptoms is required to reach the diagnosis. It is important to distinguish negative symptoms, which are often difficult to appreciate, from the myriad factors that may contribute to the severity and serious morbidity associated with schizophrenia. Individuals who are not motivated to attend to their personal hygiene or suffer from alogia and a flattened affect are sadly at a disadvantage in society. The addition of negative symptoms as a separate criterion in DSM-IV recognizes the prominence of these symptoms in individuals with schizophrenia.

Criterion B addresses loss of social and occupational functioning, not exclusively because of any one of the items in criterion A. Individuals may have difficulties maintaining employment, relationships, or academic achievements. If the illness presents at an early age, rather than as a degeneration or reversal of function, there may be a break from continued academic and social gains that are developmentally appropriate so that the person never achieves what had been expected.

Criterion C eliminates individuals with less than 6 months of continued disturbance and again requires at least 1 month of the symptoms from criterion A. Criterion C allows prodromal and residual periods to include only negative symptoms or a less severely manifested version of the other symptoms of the A criteria.

Criterion D excludes individuals who have a more compelling mood aspect of their illness and therefore their symptoms might instead meet criteria for schizoaffective disorder or a mood disorder. Both of these restrictions force a narrower view of the diagnosis of schizophrenia, which lessens the tendency of clinicians to overdiagnose schizophrenia.

Criterion E clarifies the fact that individuals with schizophrenia are not suffering from other medical illnesses or the physiological effects of substances that might mimic the symptoms of schizophrenia. Finally, criterion F acknowledges that schizophrenia can be diagnosed in individuals with autistic disorder or developmental disorder, as long as there have been prominent delusions or hallucinations that have lasted at least 1 month.

In an attempt to describe schizophrenia in a way that was different from prevailing psychodynamic principles of the day, researchers in the 1960s reported that individuals with schizophrenia demonstrated profound deficits in selective attention. By now, it is widely accepted that individuals with schizophrenia experience neuropsychological deficits that can be characterized by difficulties with attention, information processing, executive function, learning, and memory, which leads to a generalized performance deficit. Typically, there is a wide variance with some aspects of performance being more impaired then others. Interestingly, a small

Clinical Guide to the Diagnosis and Treatment of Mental Disorders. M. B. First and A. Tasman
© 2006 John Wiley & Sons, Ltd. ISBN 0 470 019158

DSM-IV-TR Diagnostic Criteria

295.xx SCHIZOPHRENIA

A. *Characteristic symptoms*: Two (or more) of the following, each present for a significant portion of time during a 1-month period (or less if successfully treated):

(1) delusions
(2) hallucinations
(3) disorganized speech (e.g., frequent derailment or incoherence)
(4) grossly disorganized or catatonic behavior
(5) negative symptoms, i.e., affective flattening, alogia, or avolition

Note: Only one criterion A symptom is required if delusions are bizarre or hallucinations consist of a voice keeping up a running commentary on the person's behavior or thoughts, or two or more voices conversing with each other.

B. *Social/occupational dysfunction*: For a significant portion of the time since the onset of the disturbance, one or more major areas of functioning such as work, interpersonal relations, or self-care are markedly below the level achieved prior to the onset (or when the onset is in childhood or adolescence, failure to achieve expected level of interpersonal, academic, or occupational achievement).

C. *Duration*: Continuous signs of the disturbance persist for at least 6 months. This 6-month period must include at least 1 month of symptoms (or less if successfully treated) that meet criterion A (i.e., active-phase symptoms) and may include periods of prodromal or residual symptoms. During these prodromal or residual periods, the signs of the disturbance may be manifested by only negative symptoms or two or more symptoms listed in criterion A present in an attenuated form (e.g., odd beliefs, unusual perceptual experiences).

D. *Schizoaffective and mood disorder exclusion*: Schizoaffective disorder and mood disorder with psychotic features have been ruled out because either (1) no major depressive, manic, or mixed episodes have occurred concurrently with the active-phase symptoms; or (2) if mood episodes have occurred during active-phase symptoms, their total duration has been brief relative to the duration of the active and residual periods.

E. *Substance/general medical condition exclusion*: The disturbance is not due to the direct physiological effects of a substance (e.g., a drug of abuse, a medication) or a general medical condition.

F. *Relationship to a pervasive developmental disorder*: If there is a history of autistic disorder or another pervasive developmental disorder, the additional diagnosis of schizophrenia is made only if prominent delusions or hallucinations are also present for at least a month (or less if successfully treated).

Reprinted with permission from the *Diagnostic and Statistical Manual of Mental Disorders*, 4th ed., Text Rev. Copyright 2000 American Psychiatric Association.

In contrast, their performance is usually worse even in first-episode individuals. Usually, individuals with schizophrenia underperform relative to estimates of their premorbid functioning. Cognitive impairments involving verbal learning, verbal delayed recall, working memory, vigilance, and executive functioning have a significant negative impact on social and occupational functioning. Meta-analyses of studies suggest that treatment with novel antipsychotic agents improves cognitive function compared to typical antipsychotic agents.

The degree of cognitive deficit appears to be more strongly associated with severity of negative symptoms, symptoms of disorganization, and adaptive dysfunction than with positive symptoms. Verbal fluency is severely impaired in individuals with psychotic disorders and the use of atypical antipsychotic medications results in significant improvement. Motor functions (e.g., reaction time, motor and graphomotor speed) improve with clozapine, olanzapine, and risperidone. Furthermore, motor functions are related to outcome, underscoring the importance of this domain. The digit symbol test has been among the most responsive tests to atypical antipsychotic treatment.

In general, individuals with schizophrenia have impairments in information processing, especially when they are exposed to increasing demands on their attentional capabilities, such as under timed conditions or in stressful situations. Therefore, these deficits are not only viewed as trait linked (i.e., a manifestation of the illness itself) but may also be compounded when state linked (i.e., when there are increases in symptoms). The trait-linked disturbances in neuropsychological parameters are seen in those at high risk for developing schizophrenia, those who have schizophrenia, and relatives who appear clinically unaffected, which may indicate a genetic vulnerability.

Although there are generally no consistent gross deficits of memory in individuals with schizophrenia, close examination of certain aspects of learning and memory has revealed striking abnormalities. Individuals with schizophrenia have been shown to be poorer in recall of word lists if the words are not grouped into categories. Furthermore, unlike normal control subjects, schizophrenic individuals do not seem to show an improvement in memory when asked to recall words with latent positive emotional meaning. These findings have been attributed to poor cognitive organization in individuals with schizophrenia.

Mental Status Examination in Schizophrenia

There is no specific laboratory test, neuroimaging study, or clinical presentation of an individual that yields a

subgroup of individuals with schizophrenia have cognitive functioning within the normal range. Most individuals with schizophrenia have only modest reductions in their IQs with an average of 90 and about 0.67 standard deviation below that of the general population.

definitive diagnosis of schizophrenia. Schizophrenia can present with a wide variety of symptoms, and a longitudinal history of symptoms and comorbid clinical variables such as medical illness and a history of substance abuse must necessarily be reviewed before a diagnosis can be considered. The Mental Status Examination, much like the physical examination, is an additional clinical tool that aids the clinician in generating a differential diagnosis and appropriate treatment recommendations.

Appearance. Although a disheveled look is not pathognomonic for schizophrenia, individuals with this disorder often present, especially acutely, with a disordered appearance. The description of an individual's appearance is an objective verbal sketch, much like the description of a heart murmur, that can uniquely identify a particular individual.

A person with schizophrenia often has difficulty attending to activities of daily living, either because of negative symptoms (apathy, social withdrawal, or motor retardation) or because of the presence of positive symptoms, such as psychosis, disorganization, or catatonia, that interfere with the ability to maintain personal hygiene. Also, schizophrenic individuals often present with odd or inappropriate attire, such as a coat and hat worn during the summer or dark sunglasses worn during an interview. It is generally thought that the inappropriate dress is a manifestation of symptoms such as disorganization or paranoid ideation. It should be noted that some individuals are quite neatly groomed. Thus, appearance is noted but is not diagnostic.

Attitude. Individuals with schizophrenia may be friendly and cooperative, or they may be hostile, annoyed, and defensive during an interview. The latter may be secondary to paranoid symptoms, which can make individuals quite cautious and guarded in their responses to questions.

Behavior. Schizophrenic individuals can have bizarre mannerisms or stereotyped movements that can make them look unusual. Individuals with catatonia can stay in one position for weeks, even to the point of causing serious physical damage to their body; for example, an individual who stands in one place for days may develop stress fractures, peripheral edema, and even pulmonary emboli. Individuals with catatonia may have waxy flexibility, maintaining a position after someone else has moved them into it. Individuals with catatonic excitement exhibit odd posturing or purposeless, repetitive, and often strange movements.

Behaviors seen in schizophrenic individuals include choreoathetoid movements, which may be related to

neuroleptic exposure but have been reported in individuals even before neuroleptic use. Other behaviors or movement disorders may be seen as parkinsonian features, such as a shuffling gait or a pill-rolling tremor.

Psychomotor retardation may be present and may be a manifestation of catatonia or negative symptoms. On close observation, it is usually characterized, in this group of individuals, as a lack of motor movements rather than slowed movements.

Individuals may present with agitation, ranging from minimal to extreme. This agitation is often seen in the acute state and may require immediate pharmacotherapy. However, agitation may be secondary to neuroleptic medications, as in akathisia, which is felt as an internal restlessness making it difficult for the person to sit still. Akathisia can manifest itself in limb shaking, pacing, or frequent shifting of position. Severely agitated individuals may be unresponsive to verbal limits and may require measures to ensure their safety and the safety of others around them.

Eye Contact. Paranoid individuals may look hypervigilant, scanning a room or glancing suspiciously at an interviewer. Psychotic individuals may make poor eye contact, looking away, or appear to stare vacuously at the interviewer, making a conversational connection seem distant. Characteristic responding to internal stimuli is seen when a individual appears to look toward a voice or an auditory hallucination, which the individual may hear. A nystagmus may also be observed. This clinical finding has a large differential diagnosis, including Wernicke–Korsakoff syndrome; alcohol, barbiturate, or phenytoin intoxication; viral labyrinthitis; or brain stem syndromes including infarctions or multiple sclerosis.

Speech. In a mental status examination, one usually comments on the rate, tone, and volume of an individual's speech, as well as any distinct dysarthrias that may be present. Pressured speech is usually thought of in conjunction with mania; however, it can be seen in schizophrenic individuals, particularly on acute presentation. This is often difficult to assess, as it may be a normal variant or a cultural phenomenon, because some languages are spoken faster than others.

Tone refers to prosody, or the natural singsong quality of speech. Negative symptoms may include a lack of prosody, resulting in monotonous speech. Furthermore, odd tones may be consistent with neurological disorders or bizarre behavior.

Speech volume is important for a number of reasons. Loud speech can be a measure of agitation, it can occur in conjunction with psychosis, or it could even be an indication of hearing loss. Speech that is soft may be an indication of guardedness or anxiety.

Dysarthrias are notable because they can be idiopathic and long-standing, or they can be an indication of neurological disturbance. In individuals who have been exposed to neuroleptics, orobuccal tardive dyskinesia should be considered when there is evidence of slurred speech.

Mood and Affect. Affect, which is the observer's objective view of the individual's emotional state, is often constricted or flat in individuals with schizophrenia. In fact, this is one of the hallmark negative symptoms. Flattened affect may also be a manifestation of pseudoparkinsonism, an extrapyramidal side effect of typical neuroleptics.

Inappropriate affect is commonly seen in individuals with more predominant positive symptoms. A smile or a laugh while relating a sad tale is an example. Individuals with catatonic excitement or hebephrenia may have bizarre presentations or affective lability, laughing and crying out of context with the situation. Emotional reactivity must alert the clinician to the possibility of neurological impairment as well, as in the case of pseudobulbar palsy.

Mood is based on an individual's subjective report of how he or she feels, emotionally, at the time of the interview. It is not uncommon for individuals with schizophrenia to be depressed (especially individuals with history of higher premorbid functioning who may have some insight into the losses they are facing) or to be indifferent, with seemingly no emotional awareness of their situation.

Thought Process. Because actual thoughts cannot be measured, thought processes are assessed by extrapolation from the organization of speech. Thought disorders can be more or less obvious, and a trained listener, much like a cardiologist who listens for heart murmurs or a neurologist who detects aphasias, is one who appreciates the normal logical pattern of flow of words and ideas in speech and can thus sense abnormalities.

There are many different versions of thought disorders: lack of logical connections of ideas (looseness of associations); shift of the original theme because of weak connections of ideas (tangentiality); overinclusiveness to the point of loss of the theme (circumstantiality); use of words and phrases with no relation to grammatical rules (word salad); repetition of words spoken by others (echolalia); use of sounds of other words, such as "yellow bellow, who is this fellow?" (clang associations); use of made-up words (neologisms); and repetition of

a particular word or phrase, such as "this and that, this and that" (perseveration).

Other thought disorders are part of a constellation of negative symptoms. Examples would be thoughts that appear to stop abruptly, either because of interruption by an auditory hallucination or because the thought is lost (thought blocking); absence of thoughts (paucity of thought content); and a delayed response to questions (increased latency of response).

Thought Content. Although not necessarily present in every individual, characteristic symptoms of schizophrenia include the belief that outside forces control a person's thoughts or actions. An individual might report that others can insert thoughts into her or his head (thought insertion), broadcast them to others (thought broadcasting), or take thoughts away (thought withdrawal). Other delusions, or fixed false beliefs, may also be prominent. Individuals may describe ideas of reference, which is the phenomenon of feeling that some external event or report relates to oneself specifically; for example, an individual may infer special meaning from an image seen on television or a broadcast heard on the radio.

Paranoid ideation may be manifested as general suspiciousness or frank, well-systematized delusions. The themes may be considered bizarre, such as feeling convinced that aliens are sending signals through wires in the individual's ear, or nonbizarre, such as being watched by the Central Intelligence Agency or believing that one's spouse is having an affair. These symptoms can be quite debilitating and lead to a great deal of personal loss, which individuals may not understand because the ideas are so real to them.

Individuals with schizophrenia commonly express an abundance of vague somatic concerns, and a particular individual might develop a delusion around a real physiological abnormality. Therefore, somatic symptoms should be evaluated appropriately in their clinical context without automatically dismissing them as psychotic. Preoccupations and obsessions are also seen commonly in this population, and certain individuals have comorbid obsessive–compulsive disorder.

The mortality rate for suicide in schizophrenia is approximately 10%. It is therefore imperative to evaluate an individual for both suicidal and homicidal ideation. Individuals with mental disorders, and particularly those with schizophrenia, may not spontaneously articulate suicidal or homicidal ideation and must therefore be asked directly about such feelings. Moreover, psychotic individuals may feel compelled by an auditory hallucination telling them to hurt themselves.

Perceptions. Perceptual disturbances involve illusions and hallucinations. Hallucinations may be olfactory, tactile, gustatory, visual, or auditory, although hallucinations of the auditory type are more typical of schizophrenia. Hallucinations in the other sensory modalities are more commonly seen in other medical or substance-induced conditions. Auditory hallucinations can resemble sounds, background noise, or human voices. Auditory hallucinations that consist of a running dialogue between two or more voices or a commentary on the individual's behavior are typical of schizophrenia. These hallucinations are distinct from verbalized thoughts that most humans experience. They are often described as originating from outside the individual's head, as if they were emanating from the walls or the radiators in the room. Less commonly, an individual with schizophrenia describes illusions or misperceptions of a real stimulus, such as seeing demons in a shadow.

Consciousness and Orientation. One of the observations that struck Kraepelin in his first descriptions of dementia praecox was that individuals did not have clouding of consciousness. Individuals with schizophrenia most likely have a clear sensorium unless there is some comorbid medical illness or substance-related phenomenon. A schizophrenic individual may be disoriented, but this could be a result of inattentiveness to details or distraction secondary to psychotic preoccupation. In fact, there is some literature suggesting that a subgroup of individuals may present as disoriented to temporal relations such as the date or their own age.

Attention and Concentration. Studies utilizing continuous performance task paradigms have demonstrated repeatedly that individuals with schizophrenia have pervasive deficits in attention in both acute and residual phases. On a mental status examination, these deficits may present themselves as the inability to perform mental exercises, such as spelling the word "earth" backward or serial subtractions.

Memory. Careful assessment of memory in individuals with schizophrenia may yield some deficits. Acquisition of new information, immediate recall, and recent and remote memory may be impaired in some individuals. Furthermore, answers to questions regarding memory may lead to idiosyncratic responses related to delusions, thought disorder, or other overriding symptoms of the illness. In general, individuals with schizophrenia do not show gross deficits of memory such as may be seen in individuals with dementia or head trauma.

Fund of Knowledge. Schizophrenia is not the equivalent of mental retardation, although these syndromes can coexist in some individuals. Individuals with schizophrenia generally experience a slight shift in intellectual functioning after the onset of their illness, yet they typically demonstrate a fund of knowledge consistent with their premorbid level. Schizophrenic individuals manifest a characteristic discrepancy on standardized tests of intelligence, with the nonverbal scores being lower than the verbal scores. Furthermore, some reports suggest that individuals who have been chronically hospitalized or those with some cerebral atrophy may evidence diminished intellectual function.

Abstraction. A classical aberration of mental function in an individual with schizophrenia involves the inability to utilize abstract reasoning, which is similar to metaphorical thinking, or the ability to conceptualize ideas beyond their literal meaning. For example, when the individual is asked what brought him or her to the hospital, a typical answer might be "an ambulance." On a mental status examination, this concrete thinking is best elicited by asking an individual to interpret a proverb or state the similarities between two objects. For example, "a rolling stone gathers no moss" may mean, to the individual with schizophrenia, that "if a stone just stays in one place, the moss won't be able to collect." More profound difficulties in abstraction and executive function, often seen in schizophrenia, such as inability to shift cognitive focus or set, may be assessed by neuropsychological tests.

Judgment and Insight. Individuals suffering from schizophrenia often display a lack of insight regarding their illness. Whether it is a reflection of a negative symptom, such as apathy, or a constricted display of emotion, individuals often appear to be emotionally disconnected from their illness and may even deny that anything is wrong. Poor judgment, which is also characteristic and may be related to lack of insight, may lead to potentially dangerous behavior. For example, an individual walking barefoot in the snow because of the feeling that her or his shoes could be traced by surveillance cameras would be displaying both poor judgment and poor insight. On a formal mental status examination, judgment is commonly assessed by asking individuals what they would do if they saw a fire in a movie theater or if they saw a stamped, addressed envelope on the street. Insight can be ascertained by asking individuals about their understanding of why they are being evaluated by a mental health professional or why they are receiving a certain medication.

Physical Examination

Although there are no pathognomonic physical signs of schizophrenia, some individuals have neurological "soft" signs on physical examination. The neurological deficits include nonspecific abnormalities in reflexes, coordination (as seen in gait and finger-to-nose tests), graphesthesia (recognition of patterns marked out on the palm), and stereognosis (recognition of three-dimensional pictures). Other neurological findings include odd or awkward movements (possibly correlated with thought disorder), alterations in muscle tone, an increased blink rate, a slower habituation of the blink response to repetitive glabellar tap, and an abnormal pupillary response.

The exact etiology of these abnormalities is unknown, but they have historically been associated with minimal brain dysfunction and may be more likely in individuals with poor premorbid functioning and a chronic course. These neurological abnormalities have been seen in neuroleptic-naive individuals as well as those with exposure to traditional antipsychotic medication. Overall, the literature suggests that these findings may be associated with the disease itself, although further research is needed to determine the role of neuroleptic exposure in the manifestation of neurological signs and the extent to which schizophrenia is itself associated with neurological abnormalities.

Neuroophthalmological investigations have shown that individuals with schizophrenia have abnormalities in voluntary saccadic eye movements (rapid eye movement toward a stationary object) as well as in smooth pursuit eye movements. The influence of attention and distraction, neuroleptic exposure, and the specificity of smooth pursuit eye movements for schizophrenia have raised criticisms of this area of study, and further investigation is necessary to determine its potential as a putative genetic marker for schizophrenia.

Clinical Subtypes of Schizophrenia

In DSM-IV-TR, schizophrenia has been divided into clinical subtypes based on the most prominent symptoms, although it is acknowledged that the specific subtype may exist simultaneously with or change over the course of the illness. DSM-IV-TR also includes an optional dimensional descriptor (included in the appendix for criteria sets and axes provided for further study), which allows the condition to be characterized by the presence or absence of a psychotic, disorganized, or negative symptom dimension over the entire course of the illness.

DSM-IV-TR Diagnostic Criteria

295.30 PARANOID TYPE

A type of schizophrenia in which the following criteria are met:

A. Preoccupation with one or more delusions or frequent auditory hallucinations.
B. None of the following is prominent: disorganized speech, disorganized or catatonic behavior, or flat or inappropriate affect.

Reprinted with permission from the *Diagnostic and Statistical Manual of Mental Disorders*, 4th ed., Text Rev. Copyright 2000 American Psychiatric Association.

Paranoid Type. In DSM-IV-TR, paranoid-type schizophrenia is marked by hallucinations or delusions in the presence of a clear sensorium and unchanged cognition. Disorganized speech, disorganized behavior, and flat or inappropriate affect are not present to any significant degree. The delusions (usually of a persecutory or grandiose nature) and the hallucinations most often revolve around a particular theme or themes. Because of their delusions, these individuals may attempt to keep the interviewer at bay, and thus they may appear hostile or angry during an interview. This type of schizophrenia may have a later age of onset and a better prognosis than the other subtypes.

Disorganized Type. Disorganized schizophrenia, historically referred to as hebephrenic schizophrenia, presents with the hallmark symptoms of disorganized speech and/or behavior, along with flat or inappropriate (incongruent) affect. Any delusions or hallucinations, if present, also tend to be disorganized and are not related to a single theme. Furthermore, these individuals would not be classified as having catatonic schizophrenia. These individuals in general have more

---

DSM-IV-TR Diagnostic Criteria

295.10 DISORGANIZED TYPE

A type of schizophrenia in which the following criteria are met:

A. All of the following are prominent:

(1) disorganized speech
(2) disorganized behavior
(3) flat or inappropriate affect

B. The criteria are not met for catatonic type.

Reprinted with permission from the *Diagnostic and Statistical Manual of Mental Disorders*, 4th ed., Text Rev. Copyright 2000 American Psychiatric Association.

DSM-IV-TR Diagnostic Criteria

295.20 CATATONIC TYPE

A type of schizophrenia in which the clinical picture is dominated by at least two of the following:

A. motoric immobility as evidenced by catalepsy (including waxy flexibility) or stupor
B. excessive motor activity (that is apparently purposeless and not influenced by external stimuli)
C. extreme negativism (an apparently motiveless resistance to all instructions or maintenance of a rigid posture against attempts to be moved) or mutism
D. peculiarities of voluntary movement as evidenced by posturing (voluntary assumption of inappropriate or bizarre postures), stereotyped movements, prominent mannerisms, or prominent grimacing
E. echolalia or echopraxia

Reprinted with permission from the *Diagnostic and Statistical Manual of Mental Disorders*, 4th ed., Text Rev. Copyright 2000 American Psychiatric Association.

severe deficits on neuropsychological tests. According to DSM-IV-TR, these individuals tend to have an earlier age at onset, an unremitting course, and a poor prognosis.

Catatonic Type. Catatonic schizophrenia has unique features that distinguish it from the other subtypes of schizophrenia. During the acute phase of this illness, individuals may demonstrate marked negativism or mutism, profound psychomotor retardation or severe psychomotor agitation, echolalia (repetition of words or phrases in a nonsensical manner), echopraxia (mimicking the behaviors of others), or bizarreness of voluntary movements and mannerisms. Some individuals demonstrate a waxy flexibility, which is seen when a limb is repositioned on examination and remains in that position as if the individual were made of wax. Individuals with catatonic stupor must be protected against bodily harm resulting from the profound psychomotor retardation. They may remain in the same position for weeks at a time. Because of extreme mutism or agitation, individuals may not be able to report any difficulties. Some individuals may experience extreme psychomotor agitation, with grimacing and bizarre postures. These individuals may require careful monitoring to safeguard them from injury or deterioration in nutritional status or fluid balance.

Undifferentiated Type. There is no hallmark symptom of undifferentiated schizophrenia; thus, it is the subtype that meets the criterion A for schizophrenia but does not fit the profile for paranoid, disorganized, or catatonic schizophrenia.

DSM-IV-TR Diagnostic Criteria

295.90 UNDIFFERENTIATED TYPE

A type of schizophrenia in which symptoms that meet criterion A are present, but the criteria are not met for the paranoid, disorganized, or catatonic type.

Reprinted with permission from the *Diagnostic and Statistical Manual of Mental Disorders*, 4th ed., Text Rev. Copyright 2000 American Psychiatric Association.

Residual Type. The diagnosis of residual schizophrenia, according to DSM-IV-TR, is appropriately used when there is a past history of an acute episode of schizophrenia but at the time of presentation, the individual does not manifest any of the associated psychotic or positive symptoms. However, there is continued evidence of schizophrenia manifested in either negative symptoms or low-grade symptoms of criterion A. These may include odd behavior, some abnormalities of thought processes, or delusions or hallucinations that exist in a minimal form. This type of schizophrenia has an unpredictable, variable course.

Late-Onset Schizophrenia

The phenomenology of late-onset compared with early-onset schizophrenia may be distinct, with later-onset cases having a higher level of premorbid social functioning and exhibiting paranoid delusions and hallucinations more often than formal thought disorder, disorganization, and negative symptoms. Studies have also shown a high comorbid risk of sensory deficits, such as loss of hearing or vision, in individuals with late-onset schizophrenia. Specifically, late-onset individuals are more likely to report visual, tactile, and olfactory hallucinations and are less likely to display

DSM-IV-TR Diagnostic Criteria

295.60 RESIDUAL TYPE

A type of schizophrenia in which the following criteria are met:

A. Absence of prominent delusions, hallucinations, disorganized speech, and grossly disorganized or catatonic behavior.
B. There is continuing evidence of the disturbance, as indicated by the presence of negative symptoms or two or more symptoms listed in criterion A for schizophrenia, present in an attenuated form (e.g., odd beliefs, unusual perceptual experiences).

Reprinted with permission from the *Diagnostic and Statistical Manual of Mental Disorders*, 4th ed., Text Rev. Copyright 2000 American Psychiatric Association.

affective flattening or blunting. For individuals over the age of 65, community prevalence estimates range from 0.1% to 0.5%. One of the most robust findings among the late-onset cases is the higher prevalence seen in women. This does not appear to be due to sex differences in seeking care, societal role expectations, or delay between emergence of symptoms and service contact.

Prevalence

Lifetime prevalence rates of schizophrenia, based on the ECA data, were approximately 1% (range across three sites, 1–1.9%). Point prevalence rates based on International Pilot Study of Schizophrenia data showed no significant differences across study centers: schizophrenia was found universally with relatively equal frequencies in a wide variety of cultures, with a range of point prevalence between 0.6 and 8.3 cases of schizophrenia per 1000 persons in the population.

Interestingly, smaller studies have found specific populations with either a higher or a lower prevalence of schizophrenia. For example, a higher rate of schizophrenia has been found in a specific community in the north of Sweden, in northeastern Finland, in northwestern Croatia, and in western Ireland. Lower rates of schizophrenia have been found in, for example, parts of Tonga, Papua New Guinea, Taiwan, and Micronesia. In the United States, schizophrenia was almost nonexistent in the Hutterite community, a Protestant sect living in South Dakota. Epidemiologists generally agree that these communities may represent aberrant findings. However, if these differences in prevalence rates are accurate, several theories have been offered as explanations, including genetic preloading, differences in diet, or even differences in factors such as maternal age.

Sex Differences

A large body of data suggests that although men and women have an equivalent lifetime risk, the age at onset varies with sex. Although some sites showed different prevalence rates of schizophrenia in men and women, the overall prevalence rates, as reported in the ECA survey, did not differ significantly between sexes. However, there is strong evidence that onset of schizophrenia is on average 3.5 to 6 years earlier in men than in women. The WHO 10-country study observed this phenomenon in most cultures studied. Therefore, incidence and prevalence rates of schizophrenia across sexes may vary according to age. Interestingly, in some cultural populations (e.g., West Ireland, Micronesia),

the ratio of prevalence of schizophrenia for men could be as high as 2 : 1

Race and Ethnicity

The ECA data have shown that there is no significant difference in the prevalence of schizophrenia between black and white persons when corrected for age, sex, socioeconomic status, and marital status.. This finding is significant because it refutes prior studies that have shown the prevalence of schizophrenia to be much greater in the black population than in the white population. Several factors have been proposed to explain these discrepancies, including racial differences in help-seeking behavior, research populations, commitment status, and treatment.

Socioeconomic Status

For many years, epidemiological studies revealed a higher incidence and prevalence of schizophrenia in groups with lower socioeconomic status. With these findings came the hypothesis that lower social class could be considered a plausible risk factor for schizophrenia, possibly because of a higher risk of obstetrical complications, poorer nutrition, increased exposure to environmental toxins or infectious disease, or exposure to greater life stressors. In the past half century, studies have found that the actual incidence of schizophrenia does not vary with social class, based on first admission rates, adoption studies, and a series of studies examining the social class of the fathers of people with schizophrenia.

When these findings did not validate the original theory, it became clear that lower socioeconomic status was more a result than a cause of schizophrenia. This led to the acceptance of the downward drift hypothesis, which stated that because of the nature of schizophrenic symptoms, people who develop schizophrenia are unable to attain employment and positions in society that would allow them to achieve a higher social status. Thus, these individuals drift down the socioeconomic ladder, and because of the illness itself they may become dependent on society for their well-being.

Course

The natural couse of schizophrenia can be divided into three phases: an early phase marked by deterioration from premorbid levels of functioning; a middle phase characterized by a prolonged period of little change termed the stabilization phase; and the last period, which is called the improving phase.

An enormous clinical and research effort is directed internationally toward individuals in very early stages of their illness and especially during their first psychotic break with a focus on early and effective intervention. First episode provides a unique opportunity to intervene early and effectively and possibly change the course of illness. It is well known that there is a delay of 1 to 2 years on an average between onset of psychosis and starting of treatment. This duration of untreated psychosis (DUP) is recognized by many, though not all, as an important indicator of subsequent clinical outcome. Clinical deterioration appears to be correlated with the duration of psychosis and number of episodes of psychosis. The deterioration usually occurs during the first 5 years after onset and then stabilizes at a level where the individual has persistent symptoms and is impaired in social and vocational function. After that point, additional exacerbations may occur, but they are not usually associated with further deterioration.

Long-term studies of schizophrenia suggest that negative symptoms tend to be less common and less severe in the early stages of the illness but increase in prevalence and severity in the later stages. Positive symptoms such as delusions and hallucinations are more common earlier on while thought disorganization, inappropriate affect, and motor symptoms occur more commonly in the later stages of illness. A possible decline in the prevalence of the hebephrenic and catatonic subtypes of schizophrenia may be attributed to effective treatment and possible arrest of the progression of illness. Thus with effective treatment, and with long-term compliance, it is possible to produce favorable outcomes.

Following onset of the illness, individuals experience substantial decline in cognitive functions from their premorbid levels. However, it is unclear whether, after the first episode, there is further cognitive decline due to the illness. Some studies even suggest a slight and gradual improvement. Increased number of episodes and the longer DUP are associated with greater cognitive dysfunction.

Individuals with first-episode psychosis usually have excellent clinical response to antipsychotic treatment early in their course of illness when compared to individuals with chronic multiple episodes. *Effective and early intervention does help achieve clinical remission and good outcome.* Some suggest that atypical antipsychotic medication should be used preferentially in the treatment of individuals with first-episode psychosis as they are a highly treatment-responsive group, and may be best able to optimize the outcome. In addition, individuals with first-episode psychosis are sensitive to side effects, especially extrapyramidal and weight gain

side effects. They require lower doses of medication to achieve therapeutic responses. The issue of treatment adherence is of critical importance in individuals in their first episode of psychosis. Although these individuals respond very well with 1-year remission rates of greater than 80%, the 1-year attrition rates are as high as 60%. This important issue undermines management of individuals with first episode psychosis during this critical period of their illness.

The mortality rate of schizophrenia is estimated to be twice that of the general population. Approximately 10% of the mortality is secondary to suicide. Young men with schizophrenia are most likely to complete suicide attempts, especially early in their illness. Degree of social isolation, agitation, depression, a sense of hopelessness, a history of prior suicide attempts, and recent loss may be associated with increased risk of suicide among schizophrenic individuals. There is also some evidence that an increased number of relapses, rehospitalizations, and discharges lead to an increased risk of suicide. There have been observations that suicide rates of individuals with schizophrenia may be increasing in the era of shorter hospital stays and community treatment. However, with the advent of the novel antipsychotic medications and especially with clozapine use, it is possible that this risk of suicide may even out or decrease owing to their possible protective effects against suicide. Other factors leading to increased mortality rates in schizophrenic individuals include an increased incidence of accidents as well as a more frequent association with other medical illnesses (including cardiovascular disease), comorbid substance abuse, a general neglect of health, an increased rate of damaging behaviors such as smoking and poor diet, decreased access to health services, and depression.

Differential Diagnosis

Making an accurate diagnosis of schizophrenia requires high levels of clinical acumen, extensive knowledge of schizophrenia, and sophisticated application of the principles of differential diagnosis. It is unfortunately common for individuals with psychotic disorders to be misdiagnosed and consequently treated inappropriately. The importance of accurate diagnosis is underlined by an emerging database indicating that early detection and prompt pharmacological intervention may improve the long-term prognosis of the illness.

Possibly the most difficult diagnostic dilemma in cases in which an individual has both psychotic symptoms and affective symptoms is in the differentiation between schizophrenia and schizoaffective disorder. In

DSM-IV-TR, an individual with schizoaffective disorder must have an uninterrupted period of illness during which, at some time, they have symptoms that meet the diagnostic criteria for a major depressive episode, manic episode, or a mixed episode concurrently with the diagnostic criteria for the active phase of schizophrenia (criterion A for schizophrenia). Additionally, *the individual must have had delusions or hallucinations for at least 2 weeks in the absence of prominent mood disorder symptoms* during the same period of illness. The mood disorder symptoms must be present for a substantial part of the active and residual psychotic period. The essential features of schizoaffective disorder must occur within a single uninterrupted period of illness where the "period of illness" refers to the period of active or residual symptoms of psychotic illness, and this can last for years and decades. The total duration of psychotic symptoms must be at least 1 month to meet the criterion A for schizophrenia and thus, the minimum duration of a schizoaffective episode is also 1 month.

The criterion for major depressive episode requires a minimum duration of 2 weeks of either depressed mood or markedly diminished interest or pleasure. As the symptoms of loss of pleasure or interest commonly occur in nonaffective psychotic disorders, to meet the criteria for schizoaffective disorder criterion A, the major depressive episode must include pervasive depressed mood. Presence of markedly diminished interest or pleasure is not sufficient to make a diagnosis as it is possible that these symptoms may occur with other conditions too.

The distinctions among brief psychotic disorder, schizophreniform disorder, and schizophrenia are based on duration of active symptoms. DSM-IV-TR has a requirement of 6 months of active, prodromal, and/or residual symptoms for a diagnosis of schizophrenia. Brief psychotic disorder is a transient psychotic state, not caused by medical conditions or substance use, which lasts for at least 1 day and up to 1 month. Schizophreniform disorder falls in between and requires symptoms for at least 1 month and not exceeding 6 months, with no requirement for loss of functioning.

If the delusions that an individual describes are not bizarre (e.g., examples of bizarre delusions include the belief that an outside force or person has taken over one's body or that radio signals are being sent through the caps in one's teeth), it is wise to consider delusional disorder in the differential diagnosis. Delusional disorder is usually characterized by specific types of false fixed beliefs such as erotomanic, grandiose, jealous, persecutory, or somatic types. Delusional disorder, unlike schizophrenia, is not associated with a marked so-cial impairment or odd behavior. Moreover, individuals with delusional disorder do not experience hallucinations or typically have negative symptoms.

If the individual experiences psychotic symptoms solely during times when affective symptoms are present, the diagnosis is more likely to be mood disorder with psychotic features. If the mood disturbance involves both manic and depressive episodes, the diagnosis is bipolar disorder. According to DSM-IV-TR, affective disorders that are seen in individuals with schizophrenia may fall in the category of depressive disorder not otherwise specified or bipolar disorder not otherwise specified.

Psychotic disorders, delirium, and dementia that are caused by substance use, in DSM-IV-TR, are distinguished from schizophrenia by virtue of the fact that there is clear-cut evidence of substance use leading to symptoms. Examples of psychotomimetic properties of substances include a phencyclidine psychosis (PCP) that can resemble schizophrenia clinically, chronic alcohol intoxication (Korsakoff's psychosis), and chronic amphetamine administration, which can lead to paranoid states. Therefore, individuals who have symptoms that meet criterion A of schizophrenia in the presence of substance use must be reevaluated after a significant period away from the suspected substance, and proper toxicology screens must be performed to rule out recent substance abuse.

General medical conditions ranging from vitamin B_{12} deficiency to Cushing's syndrome have been associated with a clinical presentation resembling that of schizophrenia. The most common neurological disorder appearing clinically similar to schizophrenia is epilepsy, particularly of the temporal lobe. Other medical illnesses with symptoms similar to those of schizophrenia include basal ganglia calcifications and acute intermittent porphyria. Imbalances of endocrine function as well as certain infectious diseases can present with symptoms that mimic schizophrenic psychosis. Because the prognosis for the associated medical condition is better than that for schizophrenia and the stigma attached to schizophrenia is significant, it is imperative to provide individuals with a thorough medical workup before giving a diagnosis of schizophrenia. This includes a physical examination; laboratory analyses including thyroid function tests, syphilis screening, and folate and vitamin B_{12} levels; a CT or MRI scan; and a lumbar puncture when indicated in new-onset cases.

TREATMENT

It could be argued that the successful treatment of schizophrenia requires a greater level of clinical knowledge and sophistication than the treatment of most other mental disorders and medical illnesses. It begins with the formation of a therapeutic relationship between the clinician and the individual with schizophrenia and must combine the latest developments in pharmacological and psychosocial therapeutics and interventions.

The relationship between the clinician and the patient is the foundation for treating individuals with schizophrenia. Because of the clinical manifestations of the illness, the formation of this relationship is often difficult. Paranoid delusions may lead to mistrust of the clinician. Conceptual disorganization and cognitive impairment make it difficult for individuals with schizophrenia to attend to what the clinician is saying and to follow even the simplest directions. Negative symptoms result in lack of emotional expression and social withdrawal, which can be demoralizing for the clinician who is attempting to "connect" with the individual.

It is important for the clinician to understand the ways in which the psychopathology of the illness affects the therapeutic relationship. The clinician should provide constancy to the individual with schizophrenia, which helps "anchor" individuals in their turbulent world. The qualities of the relationship should include consistency, acceptance, appropriate levels of warmth that respect the individual's needs for titrating emotional intensity, nonintrusiveness, and, most important, caring. "Old-fashioned" family doctors who know their patients well, are easily approachable, have a matter-of-fact style, attend to a broad range of needs, and are available and willing to reach out during crises provide a useful model for the relationship between the clinician and the patient in the treatment of schizophrenia.

Psychopharmacological Treatment

Although chlorpromazine had been around since the late 1800s, it was not until 1952 that it was first used to treat psychosis. The implementation of chlorpromazine became the turning point for psychopharmacology. Individuals who had been institutionalized for years were able to receive treatment as outpatients and live in community settings. The road was paved for the deinstitutionalization movement, and scientific understanding of the pathophysiology of schizophrenia burgeoned.

The discovery of chlorpromazine led to the development of other phenothiazines and new classes of antipsychotic medications, now totaling 11 different classes available in the US today. The word *neuroleptic*, literally "nerve cutting," was used to describe the tranquilizing effects of these medications. The enormous

efforts to understand the mechanism of action of typical antipsychotics uncovered the intimate association of dopamine D_2 receptor blockade to the antipsychotic effects. This formed the basis of the hypothesis suggesting that symptoms of schizophrenia were possibly related to the hyperactivity of the (mesolimbic and mesocortical) dopaminergic systems in the brain. Antipsychotics developed subsequent to chlorpromazine such as haloperidol, thiothixene, and so on, were modeled on the (misguided) belief that induction of extrapyramidal symptoms (EPS) was an integral part of having an antipsychotic efficacy. Over the years, another belief developed that all antipsychotics were similar in their efficacy and varied only in their side effects. However, clozapine challenged these beliefs by being significantly superior in efficacy than the existing antipsychotics and having minimal to no EPS! This started the era of antipsychotic agents being referred to as either *typical (conventional or traditional)* or *atypical (or novel)* antipsychotic drugs. If chlorpromazine started the first revolution in the psychopharmacological treatment of schizophrenia, then clozapine ushered in the second and more profound revolution, whose impact is felt beyond schizophrenia and whose full extent is yet to be realized. Moreover, clozapine has invigorated the psychopharmacology of schizophrenia and rekindled one of the most ambitious searches for new antipsychotic compounds by the pharmaceutical industry. Following approval of clozapine in 1990, FDA has already approved five novel antipsychotics—risperidone, olanzapine, quetiapine, ziprasidone, and aripiprazole.

Though clozapine, a dibenzodiazepine compound, was approved for use in the US in 1990, it had been available in European markets during the 1970s but had been found to be associated with agranulocytosis, a potentially fatal side effect, which led to its removal from clinical trials. The need for improved treatment of schizophrenia, particularly for individuals who do not respond to traditional neuroleptics, generated interest in resuming investigations of clozapine's clinical efficacy.

Double-blind, controlled studies demonstrated the superior clinical efficacy of clozapine compared to standard neuroleptics, without the associated EPS. It is clearly superior to traditional neuroleptics for psychosis. A summary of the US studies of individuals with chronic and treatment-resistant schizophrenia suggests that approximately 50% of individuals derive a better response from clozapine than from traditional neuroleptics. Its effect on negative symptoms is somewhat controversial and has started an intense and a passionate debate as to whether the efficacy of the medication is with primary or secondary negative symptoms or both. There is substantial evidence that clozapine decreases relapses, improves stability in the community, and diminishes suicidal behavior. There have also been reports that clozapine may cause a gradual reduction in preexisting tardive dyskinesia.

Unfortunately, clozapine is associated with agranulocytosis, and because of this risk, it requires weekly white blood cell testing. Approximately 0.8% of individuals taking clozapine and receiving weekly white blood cell monitoring develop agranulocytosis. Women and the elderly are at higher risk than other groups. The period of highest risk is the first 6 months of treatment. These data have led to monitoring of white cell counts less frequently after the first 6 months to every other week if a person has a history of white cell counts within normal range in the preceding 6 months. Current guidelines state that the medication must be held back if the total white blood cell count is 3000/mm^3 or less or if the absolute polymorphonuclear cell count is 1500/mm^3 or less. Individuals who stop clozapine treatment continue to require blood monitoring for at least 4 weeks after the last dose according to current guidelines. Other side effects of clozapine include orthostatic hypotension, tachycardia, sialorrhea, sedation, elevated temperature, and weight gain. Furthermore, clozapine can lower the seizure threshold in a dose-dependent fashion, with a higher risk of seizures seen particularly at doses greater than 600 mg/day.

Clozapine has an affinity for dopamine receptors (D_1, D_2, D_3, D_4, and D_5), serotonin receptors (5-HT$_{2A}$, 5-HT$_{2C}$, 5-HT$_6$, and 5-HT$_7$), alpha-1- and alpha-2-adrenergic receptors, nicotinic and muscarinic cholinergic receptors, and H$_1$ histaminergic receptors. As clozapine has a relatively shorter half-life, it is usually administered twice a day.

Following clozapine, risperidone was the first novel antipsychotic medication approved by FDA in 1994. Risperidone is a benzisoxazol compound with a high affinity for 5-HT$_{2A}$ and D$_2$ receptors and has a high serotonin–dopamine receptor antagonism ratio. It has high affinity for alpha-1-adrenergic and H$_1$ histaminergic receptors and moderate affinity for alpha-2-adrenergic receptors. Risperidone is devoid of significant activity against the cholinergic system and the D$_1$ receptors. The efficacy of this medication is equal to that of other first-line atypical antipsychotic agents, and it is well tolerated and can be given once or twice a day. It is available in a liquid form and as a long-acting injectable form. The most common side effects reported are drowsiness, orthostatic hypotension, lightheadedness, anxiety, akathisia, constipation, nausea, nasal congestion, prolactin elevation, and weight gain. At doses above 6 mg/day, EPS can become a significant issue.

The risk of tardive dyskinesia at the regular therapeutic doses is low.

Olanzapine is a thienobenzodiazepine compound approved in 1996. It has antagonistic effects at dopamine D$_1$ through D$_5$ receptors and serotonin 5-HT$_{2A}$, 5-HT$_{2C}$, and 5-HT$_6$ receptors. The antiserotonergic activity is more potent than the antidopaminergic one. It also has affinity for alpha-1-adrenergic, M$_1$ muscarinic acetylcholinergic, and H$_1$ histaminergic receptors. It differs from clozapine by not having high affinity for the 5-HT$_7$, alpha-2-adrenergic, and other cholinergic receptors. It has significant efficacy against positive and negative symptoms and also improves cognitive functions. EPS is minimal when used in the therapeutic range with the exception of mild akathisia. As the compound has a long half-life, it is used once a day and as it is well tolerated, it can be started at a higher dose or rapidly titrated to the most effective dose. It is available as a rapidly disintegrating wafer form (Zyprexa Zydis), which dissolves immediately in the mouth. An intramuscular form has also been approved by FDA for agitation. The major side effects of olanzapine include weight gain, sedation, dry mouth, nausea, lightheadedness, orthostatic hypotension, dizziness, constipation, headache, akathisia, and transient elevation of hepatic transaminases. The risk of tardive dyskinesia and neuroleptic malignant syndrome (NMS) is low. Though used as a once-a-day medication, it is often administered twice a day with an average dose of 15–20 mg/day. However, doses higher than 20 mg/day are often used clinically and are thus being evaluated in clinical trials.

Quetiapine, a dibenzothiazepine compound approved in 1997, has a greater affinity for serotonin 5-HT$_2$ receptors than for dopamine D$_2$ receptors; it has considerable activity at dopamine D$_1$, D$_5$, D$_3$, D$_4$, serotonin 5-HT$_{1A}$, and alpha-1-, alpha-2-adrenergic receptors. Unlike clozapine, it lacks affinity for the muscarinic cholinergic receptors. It is usually administered twice a day due to a short half-life. Quetiapine is as effective as typical agents and also appears to improve cognitive function. Among 2035 individuals enrolled in seven controlled studies, quetiapine at all doses used did not have an EPS rate greater than a placebo. This is in contrast to olanzapine, risperidone, and ziprasidone, where there were dose-related effects on EPS levels. The rate of treatment-emergent EPS was very low even in high at-risk populations such as adolescents, parkinsonian individuals with psychosis, and geriatric individuals. There was no elevation of prolactin. Major side effects include somnolence, postural hypotension, dizziness, agitation, dry mouth, and weight gain. Akathisia occurs on rare occasions. The package insert warns about developing lenticular opacity or cataracts and advises periodic eye examination based on data from animal studies. However, recent data suggest that this risk may be minimal.

Ziprasidone, approved by FDA in 2001, has the strongest $5\text{-}HT_{2A}$ receptor binding relative to D_2 binding among the atypical agents currently in use. Interestingly, ziprasidone has $5\text{-}HT_{1A}$ agonist and $5\text{-}HT_{1D}$ antagonist properties with a high affinity for $5\text{-}HT_{1A}$, $5\text{-}HT_{2C}$, and $5\text{-}HT_{1D}$ receptors. As it does not interact with many other neurotransmitter systems, it does not cause anticholinergic side effects and produces little orthostatic hypotension and relatively little sedation. Just like some antidepressants, ziprasidone blocks presynaptic reuptake of serotonin and norepinephrine. Ziprasidone has a relatively short half-life and thus it should be administered twice a day and along with food for best absorption. Ziprasidone is not completely dependent on CYP3A4 system for metabolism, thus inhibitors of the cytochrome system do not significantly change the blood levels. Ziprasidone at doses between 80 and 160 mg/day is probably the most effective for treating symptoms of schizophrenia. To assess the cardiac risk of ziprasidone and other antipsychotic agents, Pfizer and FDA designed a landmark study to evaluate the cardiac safety of the antipsychotic agents, given at high doses alone and with a known metabolic inhibitor in a randomized study involving individuals with schizophrenia. This was done to replicate the possible worst-case scenario (overdose or dangerous combination treatment) in the real world. All antipsychotic agents studied caused some degree of QTc prolongation. Oral form of haloperidol was associated with the least and thioridazine with the greatest change. Major side effects reported with the use of ziprasidone are somnolence, nausea, insomnia, dyspepsia, and prolongation of QTc interval. Dizziness, weakness, nasal discharge, orthostatic hypotension, and tachycardia occur less commonly.

Ziprasidone should not be used in combination with other drugs that cause *significant* prolongation of the QTc interval. It is also contraindicated for individuals with a known history of significant QTc prolongation, recent myocardial infarction, or symptomatic heart failure. Ziprasidone has low EPS potential, does not elevate prolactin levels, and causes approximately 1 lb weight gain in short-term studies.

Aripiprazole was approved by the FDA for the treatment of schizophrenia in 2003. It has a unique pharmacodynamic profile compared to the other atypical neuroleptics—partial agonist activity (rather than full antagonist activity) at both dopaminergic (D_2) and serotonergic ($5\text{-}HT_{1A}$) receptors and full antagonist activity at ($5\text{-}HT_{2A}$) receptions. The recommended starting

and target dose is 10–15 mg a day. The most commonly reported adverse events from a pooled analysis of safety and tolerability data were headache, insomnia, agitation, and anxiety, but these were also the most frequently reported events in the placebo, haloperidol, and risperidone comparison groups. The incidence of adverse events was similar in the aripiperazole and placebo groups. There was also a similar incidence of EPS-related adverse events in the aripiperazole and placebo groups. There were also only minimal changes in mean body weight and no increases in prolactin level.

At present, with respect to efficacy, it does not appear that any one of the novel antipsychotic agents (except clozapine) is better than another one in treating schizophrenia. The randomized controlled trials suggest that, on average, these antipsychotic agents are each associated with 20% improvement in symptoms. However, clozapine is the only new antipsychotic agent that is more effective than haloperidol in managing treatment-resistant schizophrenia. Unfortunately, its potential for treatment-emergent agranulocytosis, seizures, and the new warning of myocarditis precludes its use as a first-line agent for schizophrenia. A major difference among the newer antipsychotic agents is the side-effect profile and its effect on the overall quality of life of the individual.

Acute Treatment. Until recently, the typical antipsychotics were the mainstay of the treatment for acute episodes of psychosis. In the past few years, the use of novel antipsychotics has surpassed the use of typical ones in the management of acute phase symptoms of schizophrenia, except for the use of parenteral and liquid forms of antipsychotics where typical antipsychotic agents still hold an upper hand. However, this trend will most likely change once the injectable preparations of the novel antipsychotics (olanzapine, ziprasidone, aripiprazole) become more widely used. The primary goal of acute treatment is the amelioration of any behavioral disturbances that would put the individual or others at risk of harm. Acute symptom presentation or relapses are heralded by the recurrence of positive symptoms, including delusions, hallucinations, disorganized speech or behavior, severe negative symptoms, or catatonia. Quite frequently, a relapse is a result of antipsychotic discontinuation, and resumption of antipsychotic treatment aids in the resolution of symptoms. There is a high degree of variability in response rates among individuals. When treatment is initiated, improvement in clinical symptoms can be seen over hours, days, or weeks of treatment.

Studies have shown that although typical neuroleptics are undoubtedly effective, a significant percentage (between 20% and 40%) of individuals show only a poor or partial response to traditional agents. Furthermore, there is no convincing evidence that one typical antipsychotic is more efficacious as an antipsychotic than any other, although a given individual may respond better to a specific drug. Once an informed choice has been made between using a novel or a typical antipsychotic medication by the patient and the clinician, selection of a specific antipsychotic agent should be based on efficacy, side-effect profile, history of prior response (or nonresponse) to a specific agent, or history of response of a family member to a certain antipsychotic agent. (For a pharmacotherapy decision tree based on Texas Medication Algorithm Project, see Figure 25-1.) Among the typical antipsychotic medications, low-potency, more sedating agents, such as chlorpromazine, were long thought to be more effective for agitated individuals, yet there are no consistent data proving that high-potency agents are not equally useful in this context. The low-potency antipsychotics, however, are more associated with orthostatic hypotension and lowered seizure threshold and are often not as well tolerated at higher doses. Higher potency neuroleptics, such as haloperidol and fluphenazine, are safely used at higher doses and are effective in reducing psychotic agitation and psychosis itself. However, they are more likely to cause EPS than the low-potency agents.

The efficacy of novel antipsychotic drugs on positive and negative symptoms is comparable to or even better than that of the typical antipsychotic drugs. The significantly low potential to cause EPS or dystonic reaction and thus the decreased long-term consequences of TD has made the novel agents more tolerable and acceptable in acute treatment of schizophrenia. Other significant advantages adding to the popularity of novel antipsychotics include their beneficial impact on mood symptoms, suicidal risk, and cognition. Except for clozapine, which is not considered first-line treatment because of substantial and potentially life-threatening side effects, there is no convincing data supporting the preference of one atypical antipsychotic over the other. However, if the individual does not respond to one, a trial with another atypical antipsychotic is reasonable and may produce response.

Once the decision is made to use an antipsychotic agent, an appropriate dose must be selected. Initially, higher doses or repeated dosing may be helpful in preventing grossly psychotic and agitated individuals from doing harm. In general, there is no clear evidence that higher doses of neuroleptics (more than 2000 mg

chlorpromazine equivalents per day) have any advantage over standard doses (400–600 chlorpromazine equivalents per day).

Some individuals who are extremely agitated or aggressive may benefit from concomitant administration of high-potency benzodiazepines such as lorazepam, at 1 to 2 mg, until they are stable. Benzodiazepines rapidly decrease anxiety, calm the person, and help with sedation to break the cycle of agitation. They also help decrease agitation due to akathisia. The use of these medications should be limited to the acute stages of the illness to prevent tachyphylaxis and dependency. Benzodiazepines are quite beneficial in the treatment of catatonic or mute individuals but the results are only temporary, though of enough duration to help with body functions and nutrition.

Maintenance Treatment. There is by now a great deal of evidence from long-term follow-up studies that individuals with schizophrenia have a higher risk of relapse and exacerbations if not maintained with adequate antipsychotic regimens. Noncompliance with medication, possibly because of intolerable neuroleptic side effects, may contribute to increased relapse rates. In a double-blind placebo-controlled study of relapse rates, 50% of patients in a research ward demonstrated clinically significant exacerbation of their symptoms within 3 weeks of stopping neuroleptic treatment. Furthermore, in a comprehensive review of the literature on neuroleptic withdrawal examining 4365 subjects, 53.2% of individuals withdrawn from neuroleptics relapsed, compared with 15.6% of control subjects who were maintained with neuroleptic treatment. The length of follow-up was related to the risk of relapse. Long-term outcome studies show that persistent symptoms that do not respond to standard neuroleptic therapy are associated with a greater risk of rehospitalization. Nonpharmacological interventions may help decrease relapse rates.

Long-term treatment of schizophrenia is a complex issue. It is clear that the majority of individuals require maintenance medication. Some individuals do well with stable doses of neuroleptics for years without any exacerbations. However, many individuals who are maintained with a stable neuroleptic dose have episodic breakthroughs of their psychotic symptoms. In a 1974 study, schizophrenic individuals were followed up for 2 years after hospitalization and randomized to receive placebo alone, placebo and sociotherapy, chlorpromazine alone, or chlorpromazine and sociotherapy. In this study, the placebo-only group had a relapse

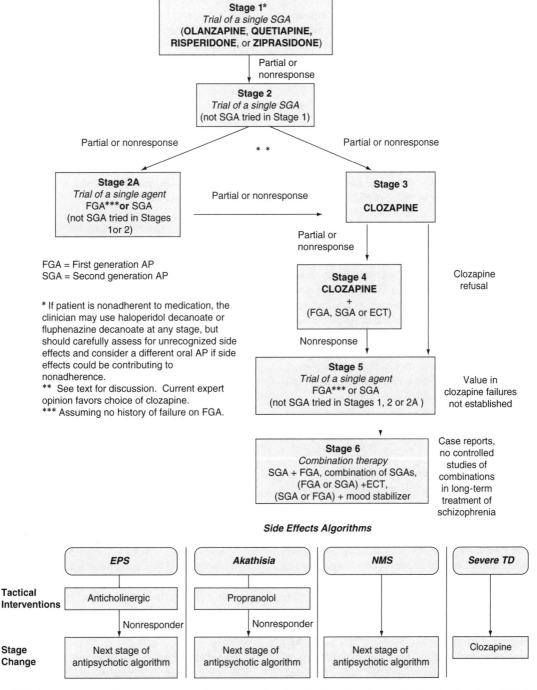

Figure 25-1 *Selecting antipsychotic treatment using Texas medication algorithm for schizophrenia. Choice of antipsychotic (AP) should be guided by considering the clinical characteristics of the patient and the efficacy and side effect profiles of the medication. Any stage(s) can be skipped depending on the clinical picture or history of antipsychotic failures. Texas Medication Algorithm Project for choosing antipsychotic treatment, managing side effects, and coexisting symptoms. This project is a public–academic collaborative effort to develop, implement, and evaluate medication treatment algorithms for public sector patients. For more information or to view the most current version of the algorithm, visit www.mhmr.state.tx.us/centraloffice/medicaldirector/tmaptoc.html).*

rate that was almost twice that of the chlorpromazine-treated group. Unfortunately, the difficulty in tolerating neuroleptic side effects often results in noncompliance with medication. Furthermore, intensive case management and rehabilitation counseling did prevent relapse but only after a delayed period. Sociotherapy and drug treatment were found to have additive effects in preventing relapse.

Given these findings, it would be prudent to assess individuals for medication compliance when signs of relapse are suspected. Prodromal cues may be present before an exacerbation of psychotic symptoms. For example, any recent change in sleep, attention to activities of daily living, or disorganization may be a warning sign of an impending increase in psychosis.

For individuals for whom compliance is a problem, long-acting, depot neuroleptics are available in the US for fluphenazine, haloperidol, and risperidone. The antipsychotic drug is is injected every 1 to 6 weeks to circumvent the need for daily oral antipsychotic medications in most cases (although some individuals benefit from adjuvant oral medication). This form of medication delivery guarantees that the medication is in the system of the person taking it and eliminates the need to monitor daily compliance. This alternative should be considered if noncompliance with oral agents has led to relapses and rehospitalization. With these individuals, maintenance treatment using long-acting preparations should begin as early as possible.

Depression and Schizophrenia. Symptoms of depression occur in a substantial percentage of individuals with schizophrenia, with a wide range of 7% to 75% and a modal rate of 25%, and is associated with poor outcome, impaired functioning, suffering, higher rates of relapse or rehospitalization, and suicide. It is important to distinguish depression as a symptom or as a syndrome when it occurs. There is an important overlap of symptoms of depression with the negative symptoms. Differentiating these states can sometimes be difficult, especially in individuals who lack the interpersonal communication skills to articulate their internal subjective states well. A link between typical antipsychotic use and depression has been suggested, with some considering depression to be a form of medication-induced akinesia. Many individuals have a reaction of disappointment, a sense of loss or powerlessness, or awareness of psychotic symptoms or psychological deficits that contributes to depression. Depression in schizophrenia is heterogeneous and requires careful diagnostic clarification. DSM-IV-TR

suggests that the term *postpsychotic depression* be used to describe depression that occurs at any time after a psychotic episode of schizophrenia, even after a prolonged interval. The atypical antipsychotic medications, with less potential to cause motor side effects and different mechanisms of action at receptor levels, themselves may contribute substantially towards a decrease in the rate of depression. Moreover, the atypical antipsychotic medications appear to be superior to standard neuroleptics in treatment of negative symptoms. The impact of clozapine on the rate of suicide is significantly superior compared to the conventional agents. However, a large number of individuals still end up with a depression that will require treatment with an antidepressant.

Risks and Side Effects of Typical Neuroleptics. Extrapyramidal symptoms (EPS) are side effects of typical antipsychotic medications that include dystonias, oculogyric crisis, pseudoparkinsonism, akinesia, and akathisia. They are referred to collectively as EPS because they are mediated at least in part by dopaminergic transmission in the extrapyramidal system. Prevalence rates vary among the different types of EPS. When present, they can be uncomfortable for the individual and a reason for noncompliance.

Dystonias are involuntary muscular spasms that can be brief or sustained, involving any muscle group. They can occur with even a single dose of medication. When they develop suddenly, these spasms can be quite frightening to the individual and potentially dangerous, as in the case of laryngeal dystonias. They are more likely to be seen in young individuals. Studies differ as to whether the prevalence is higher in males or females. Prevalence rates for dystonias secondary to typical neuroleptic exposure range from 2% to 20%.. Pseudoparkinsonism and akinesia are characterized by muscular rigidity, tremor, and bradykinesia, much as in Parkinson's disease. On examination, individuals typically have masked facies, cogwheel rigidity, slowing, and decreased arm swing with a shuffling gait. This condition is reported to be more prevalent than the dystonias, presenting with a frequency ranging from 15% to 35%.

Akathisia is more common, affecting more than 20% of individuals taking neuroleptic medications. This clinical entity presents as motor restlessness or an internal sense of restlessness. Often, individuals experiencing akathisia are unable to sit still during an interview. Akathisia is difficult to differentiate from agitation. The tendency to treat agitation with neuroleptics may exacerbate akathisia, making treatment decisions challenging.

Treatment of EPS can be difficult but usually involves administration of anticholinergic medications. Some advocate the use of prophylactic anticholinergic agents when beginning typical neuroleptic treatment to decrease the incidence of EPS. This option may be appropriate, but it should be used with caution, considering the side effects associated with anticholinergic agents and their potential for abuse.

Treatment of acute dystonic reactions usually involves acute intramuscular administration of either an anticholinergic or diphenhydramine. Akathisia may not respond to anticholinergic medications. Both neuroleptic dosage reduction and the use of beta-blocking agents such as propranolol have been found to be efficacious in the treatment of akathisia.

Nonextrapyramidal side effects of the typical antipsychotic agents include those that are secondary to blockade of muscarinic, histaminic, and alpha-adrenergic receptors. These side effects, which are more commonly seen with the low-potency neuroleptics, include sedation, tachycardia, and anticholinergic side effects such as urinary hesitancy or retention, blurred vision, or constipation. Other nonextrapyramidal side effects include some cardiac conduction disturbances, retinal changes, sexual dysfunction, weight gain, lowered seizure threshold, and a risk of agranulocytosis.

Neuroleptic Malignant Syndrome (NMS) is a relatively rare but serious phenomenon seen in approximately 1% of individuals taking neuroleptics. It can be fatal in 15% of cases if not properly recognized and treated. Because the symptoms of NMS may reflect multiple etiologies, making diagnosis difficult, clinical guidelines have been proposed. According to these guidelines, three or two major and four minor manifestations are indicative of a high probability of NMS. Major manifestations of NMS comprise fever, rigidity, and increased creatine kinase levels, and minor manifestations include tachycardia, abnormal blood pressure, tachypnea, altered consciousness, diaphoresis, and leukocytosis. Others do not subscribe to the major–minor manifestation distinctions. In general, NMS is considered to be a constellation of symptoms that usually develops during 1 to 3 days. Although its pathogenesis is poorly understood, it has been associated with all antidopaminergic neuroleptic agents and presents at any time during treatment. It must be distinguished from other clinical entities, including lethal catatonia and malignant hyperthermia.

The mainstay of treatment is cessation of neuroleptic treatment and supportive care, including intravenous hydration, reversal of fever with antipyretics and cooling blankets, and careful monitoring of vital signs because of the risk of cardiac and respiratory disturbance.

Rhabdomyolysis is one of the most serious sequelae of NMS; it can lead to renal failure unless individuals are well hydrated. In some cases, dantrolene and bromocriptine have been reported to be effective pharmacological treatments. Though quite rare, NMS has been reported even with the use of novel antipsychotic agents. The decision to rechallenge the individual with neuroleptics after an episode of NMS must be made with caution.

One of the major risks of neuroleptic treatment with the traditional antipsychotic agents is that of tardive dyskinesia, a potentially irreversible syndrome of involuntary choreoathetoid movements and chronic dystonias associated with long-term neuroleptic exposure. These buccal, orofacial, truncal, or limb movements can be exacerbated by anxiety and disappear during sleep. They can present with a range of severity, from subtle tongue movements to truncal twisting and pelvic thrusting movements and even possible respiratory dyskinesias. The prevalence rates for this syndrome range from less than 10% to more than 50% but it is generally accepted that the risk increases 3% to 5% per year for each year the individual is treated with typical neuroleptics. Older age is a considerable risk factor for tardive dyskinesia, and there is some evidence that women are at increased risk for the development of this condition. Of note, a withdrawal dyskinesia that resembles tardive dyskinesia may appear on cessation of the neuroleptic. The specific mechanism involved in tardive dyskinesia remains unclear, although supersensitivity of dopaminergic receptors has been implicated.

All individuals receiving traditional neuroleptic treatment should be monitored regularly for any signs of a movement disorder. If tardive dyskinesia is suspected, the benefits of antipsychotic treatment must be carefully weighed against the risk of tardive dyskinesia. This should be discussed with the individual, and the antipsychotic should be removed if clinically feasible or at least maintained at the lowest possible dose that provides antipsychotic effect. This would also be an indication to switch to the novel antipsychotic agents with significantly reduced risk of TD or in the case of clozapine no risk of TD. In many instances, clozapine (and possibly quetiapine or olanzapine) may be the best treatment that can be offered for the TD itself. Unfortunately, there is no specific treatment of tardive dyskinesia, although some investigators have proposed the use of adrenergic agents such as clonidine, calcium channel blockers, vitamin E, benzodiazepines, valproic acid, or reserpine to reduce the spontaneous movements.

Sudden death in individual treated with typical antipsychotic drugs has been reported for a long time.

Sudden cardiac deaths probably occur from prolongation of the ventricular action potential duration represented as the QT interval (or QTc when corrected for heart rate) on the electrocardiogram, resulting in a polymorphic ventricular tachycardia termed *torsades des pointes* that can degenerate into ventricular fibrillation. The incidence of *torsades des pointes* is unknown and the specific duration of the QTc interval at which the risk of an adverse cardiac event is greatest has not been established. QTc prolongation alone does not appear to explain *torsades des pointes*; several other risk factors must be present simultaneously with QT prolongation before *torsades des pointes* occurs. These risk factors may include hypokalemia, hypomagnesemia, hypocalcemia, bradycardia, preexisting cardiac diseases (life-threatening arrhythmias, cardiac hypertrophy, heart failure, and congenital QT syndrome), female gender, advancing age, baseline QTc interval of more than 460 m/s and a long list of medications. In some instances, *torsades des pointes* may be associated with an increase in drug plasma concentrations (e.g., combination with drugs that inhibit the cytochrome P450 systems). Thus, the increase in polypharmacy in psychiatry is especially of concern. The frequency of ECG abnormalities in individuals treated with antipsychotic drugs is unclear. QTc prolongation has been reported with virtually all antipsychotic drugs. QTc prolongation by more than 2 standard deviations was reported in 8% of individuals treated with antipsychotics and especially in those receiving thioridazine. Of the typical antipsychotic drugs, haloperidol, chlorpromazine, trifluoperazine, mesoridazine, prochlorperazine, droperidol, and fluphenazine have all been reported to cause QTc prolongation and *torsades des pointes*, but thioridazine may be the worst offender. Pimozide, another typical antipsychotic, has also been associated with QTc prolongation, *torsades des pointes*, and deaths. A reevaluation by the FDA of the cardiac safety parameters of thioridazine, mesoridazine, and droperidol resulted in a black box warning due to significant QTc prolongation. Thus, it is important to monitor QTc interval in the high-risk population to prevent this rare but potentially fatal side effect.

Side Effects of Atypical Antipsychotic Agents. One of the most significant advantages of the newer antipsychotic agent is the relatively less risk of developing EPS and TD. However, treatment-emergent substantial weight gain is a harbinger for long-term health consequences and frequently an important reason for noncompliance with medication. According to a meta-analysis, clozapine and olanzapine are associated with a weight gain of about 10 lb over 10 weeks, and ziprasidone

was among the agents with the lowest weight gain at an average of 1 lb over the same period. Risperidone and quetiapine are intermediate with approximately 5 lb. Individuals with schizophrenia, independent of the use of antipsychotic agents, are at higher risk of developing diabetes mellitus relative to the general population. The data from Patient Outcome Research Team (PORT) suggest that the rate of diabetes mellitus and obesity among individuals with major mental illness was substantially higher even before the advent of the novel antipsychotic drugs. This was more so in women and nonwhite populations. The risk of antipsychotic-induced weight gain and secondary diabetes with clozapine and olanzapine may result from changes in glucose metabolism and insulin resistance induced by these agents. In approximately 40% of the cases of hyperglycemia, insulin resistance appears to occur even in the absence of significant weight gain, raising some interesting questions about how these medications may interact with the insulin-glycemic control. Unfortunately, in the case of clozapine, the risk of developing abnormal glucose tolerance and diabetes mellitus appears to be cumulative over the years. There are no effective countermeasures available to help with weight gain and hyperglycemia. The substantial increased risk to the health of individuals with schizophrenia due to these effects is worrisome and an important shortcoming of these efficacious and important medications.

Among the novel agents, risperidone, due to its potent dopamine D_2 blockade, removes the inhibitory dopaminergic tone in the tuberoinfundibular neurons resulting in significant increase in prolactin levels. This increase in prolactin is significantly more than usually seen with the typical antipsychotic agents. It is likely that the serotonin system is also involved along with dopamine in raising the prolactin levels. Clozapine and quetiapine, on the other hand, are less potent at the D_2 receptors and thus are unlikely to cause prolactin elevations. In some individuals, these elevations of prolactin lead to amenorrhea, galactorrhea, gynecomastia, and may possibly decrease bone mineral density. Ziprasidone and olanzapine within the therapeutic dose range do not cause significant increases in prolactin levels.

Cases of sudden death while receiving clozapine therapy (in physically healthy young adults with schizophrenia) from myocarditis and cardiomyopathy led to a black box warning from FDA.

Treatment Resistance and Negative Symptoms. The concept of treatment resistance has entered into common clinical judgment with the burgeoning interest in atypical antipsychotics, particularly clozapine. Treatment resistance was originally defined for research purposes. Individuals who had failed to respond to or could not tolerate adequate trials of standard neuroleptics from three different biochemical classes and who had a clinically significant psychopathology rating based on the Brief Psychiatric Rating Scale qualified as treatment resistant. However, this research definition did not necessarily encompass individuals who, by clinical standards, would meet the definition of treatment resistance (e.g., backward schizophrenic individuals, who are severely symptomatic or with severe tardive dyskinesia or EPS). One might also think of clinical treatment resistance as seen in individuals who had an early age of illness onset with subsequent repeated hospitalizations and neuroleptic trials and who cannot achieve a level of social and occupational function commensurate with their age and level of education.

The concept of treatment resistance has undergone significant modification in recent years. The original concept of treatment refractory applied to the use of typical antipsychotic agents. With the advent of the novel agents, which are generally more effective than the traditional ones, the individual should fail at least one novel antipsychotic agent before initiating a trial of clozapine mainly to avoid its side effects. The definition of the duration of a drug trial has also evolved over the years. It is increasingly appreciated that a 4- to 6-week duration of treatment with an antipsychotic agent at therapeutic doses can be considered an adequate trial. The recommended dosing has also undergone changes. The original recommendation considered a trial of 1000 mg equivalent of chlorpromazine as a necessary minimum requirement, but this threshold has now been reduced to 400–600 mg/day equivalent on the basis of the knowledge that these doses block enough dopamine D_2 receptors with higher doses providing no additional benefit. Thus, a 4- to 6-week trial of 400–600 mg of chlorpromazine equivalent is accepted as an adequate antipsychotic trial.

In treatment-refractory individuals, typical antipsychotic use results in less than 5% response rate. Clozapine is the only antipsychotic drug proven more efficacious in rigorously defined treatment-refractory groups.

Negative symptoms, such as apathy, amotivational syndrome, flattened affect, and alogia, are often the most problematic for individuals with schizophrenia, accounting for much of the morbidity associated with this illness. In addition, these symptoms are often the most difficult to treat and do not respond well to traditional neuroleptics. The atypical antipsychotic agents are more effective against the negative symptoms than the typical agents. However, the magnitude of the effect

of these compounds on primary negative symptoms is not clear.

Augmentation of Typical Neuroleptics. When an individual has shown an inadequate response to traditional neuroleptic agents from different classes and there is a good reason for not switching to a novel antipsychotic drug, other strategies may be necessary to ameliorate residual symptoms. Adding a different type of psychotropic medication may augment the neuroleptic response in some individuals. Several neuroleptic augmentation strategies have been studied, including the addition of beta-blockers, thyrotropin-releasing hormone, clonidine, and valproic acid, with mixed results. Carbamazepine was initially shown to be effective when added to neuroleptic treatment for schizophrenic individuals with electroencephalographic abnormalities and violent outbursts. Later investigation showed that carbamazepine provided adjunctive amelioration of psychotic and affective symptoms when combined with neuroleptics. Another study reported a significant antipsychotic effect of the addition of carbamazepine to neuroleptics in only one of six treatment-resistant individuals. However, the group as a whole improved significantly in terms of anxiety, withdrawal, and depression.

Lithium has been evaluated extensively for its efficacy as an additional treatment of schizophrenia. In one study, lithium seemed to improve psychotic symptoms of individuals who had not adequately responded to neuroleptics alone. Although lithium does not seem to affect positive or negative symptoms specifically, it may be beneficial for individuals who present at the depressed end of the spectrum.

The use of benzodiazepines as augmenting agents in the treatment of schizophrenia has also been extensively studied. There may be some individuals who show improvement in psychotic symptoms, and others who show improvement in negative symptoms. Interestingly, there has been a suggestion that the triazolobenzodiazepines may be more effective than other types of benzodiazepines in augmenting the neuroleptic response.

Antidepressant medications have also been considered in the treatment of depression associated with schizophrenia. Although there is some evidence that typical neuroleptics themselves cause depression, there undoubtedly are schizophrenic individuals who have primary depressive symptoms. Negative symptoms are often difficult to distinguish from depression (both have features of amotivation, apathy, and social withdrawal), but those that are secondary to depression may respond to the addition of an antidepressant to the individual's medication regimen. One study reported that fluoxetine as an adjuvant agent was effective in treating both positive and negative symptoms in individuals, although other reports of selective serotonin reuptake inhibitors have been less encouraging.

The use of electroconvulsive therapy with concomitant neuroleptic treatment has also been evaluated. With electroconvulsive therapy as an adjuvant treatment, it appears that the individual may improve initially, but relapse is likely. However, individuals with comorbid affective symptoms may have some increased benefit. In general, however, this option should be considered only if the individual is not a candidate for a trial with an atypical antipsychotic agent and only if the individual has severe persistent symptoms.

Nonpharmacological Treatment of Schizophrenia

Although psychopharmacological intervention has proved to be the foundation on which the treatment of schizophrenia depends, other approaches to the management of these individuals serve a critical function. Studies have shown repeatedly that symptoms of schizophrenia have not only a genetic component but also an environmental aspect, and interactions with family and within the community can alter the course of the illness.

For many years, a dichotomous view of treatment options was tenaciously debated as dynamic psychiatry was challenged by developments in the neurosciences. A more unified view is now accepted as it has become clear that psychopharmacological treatment strategies are most efficacious if combined with some type of psychosocial intervention and vice versa. It can be said that because of the chronic nature of schizophrenia, one or more treatments may be required throughout the illness and they are likely to have to be modified as symptoms change over time.

Psychosocial Rehabilitation. Psychosocial rehabilitation is a therapeutic approach that encourages an individual with a severe mental disorder to develop his or her fullest capacities through learning and environmental supports. The rehabilitation process should appreciate the unique life circumstances of each person and respond to the individual's special needs while promoting both the treatment of the illness and the reduction of its attendant disabilities. The treatment should be provided in the context of the individual's unique environment, taking into account social support network, access to transportation, housing, work opportunities, and so on. Rehabilitation should exploit

the individual's strengths and improve his/her competencies. Ultimately, rehabilitation should focus on the positive concept of restoring hope to those who have suffered major setbacks in functional capacity and their self-esteem due to major mental illness. To have this hope grounded in reality, it requires promoting acceptance of one's illness and the limitations that come with it. While work offers the ultimate in sense of achievement and mastery, it must be defined more broadly for the mentally ill and should include prevocational and nonvocational activities along with independent employment. It is extremely important that work is individualized to the talents, skills, and abilities of the individual concerned. However, psychosocial rehabilitation has to transcend work to encompass medical, social, and recreational themes. Psychosocial treatment's basic principle is to provide comprehensive care through active involvement of the individual in his or her own treatment. Thus, it is important that a holding environment be created where individuals can safely express their wishes, aspirations, frustrations, and reservations such that they ultimately mold the rehabilitation plan. Clearly, to achieve these goals, the intervention has to be ongoing.

Given the chronicity of the illness, the process of rehabilitation must be enduring to encounter future stresses and challenges. These goals cannot be achieved without a stable relationship between the individual and the rehabilitation counselor, which is central to an effective treatment and positive outcome. Thus, psychosocial rehabilitation is intimately connected to the biological intervention and forms a core component of the biopsychosocial approach to the treatment of schizophrenia. In the real world, programs often deviate from the aforementioned principles and end up putting excessive and unrealistic expectations on individuals, thus achieving exactly the opposite of the intended values of the program.

Psychodynamic Approach. This psychotherapeutic technique held promise for many years as a potential for unraveling the mystery of individuals' symptoms, with the hope of improvement in course and symptoms and even cure. On the basis of derivations of the classical analytical school, symptoms of schizophrenia were thought of in terms of conflict and defense mechanisms. For example, when paranoid individuals believe that they are being preyed on, they are projecting onto others their own internal, unconscious wish to kill. Thus, unconscious conflicts became manifest as psychotic symptoms. To the psychodynamic therapist then, affectively laden material elicits an increase in thought disorder or psychotic responses, as it touches on the individual's unconscious feelings. These conceptualizations of schizophrenia influenced early work with these individuals.

Although the psychodynamic understanding of intrapsychic events has been of historical interest, the application of traditional psychodynamic principles as primary treatment modalities is not recommended. One of the first studies that compared outcomes between medication-treated individuals and psychotherapy-treated individuals was conducted at the Camarillo State Hospital in 1968. This study found that the group of individuals who received neuroleptic medication showed greater improvement than those who received psychotherapy alone. Subsequent studies have replicated these findings even when different types of therapy are examined. Evidence suggests that insight-oriented individual psychotherapy may not be as helpful for individuals with schizophrenia as supportive, goal-directed individual therapy combined with medication treatment and social skills training.

Individual Psychotherapy. Individual therapy in a nontraditional sense can begin on meeting the individual with schizophrenia. Even the briefest of normalizing contacts with an agitated, acutely psychotic individual can have therapeutic value. Psychodynamic interpretations are not helpful during the acute stages of the illness and may actually agitate the individual further. The clinician using individual psychotherapy should focus on forming and maintaining a therapeutic alliance (which is also a necessary part of psychopharmacological treatment) and providing a safe environment in which the individual is able to discuss symptoms openly. A sound psychotherapist provides clear structure about the therapeutic relationship and helps the individual to focus on personal goals.

Often, an individual is not aware of or does not have insight into the fact that some beliefs are part of a specific symptom. A psychotherapist helps an individual to check whether his or her reality coincides with that of the therapist. The therapeutic intervention then becomes a frank discussion of what schizophrenia is and how symptoms may feel to the individual. This objectifying of psychotic or negative symptoms can prove of enormous value in allowing the individual to feel more in control of the illness. A good analogy is to diabetic individuals, who know they have a medical illness and are educated about the symptoms associated with exacerbation. Just as these individuals can check blood glucose levels, schizophrenic individuals can discuss with a therapist their sleep patterns, their interpersonal relationships, and their internal thoughts, which may lead to earlier detection of relapses.

Schizophrenia often strikes just as a person is leaving adolescence and entering young adulthood. The higher the premorbid level of social adjustment and functioning, the more devastating and confusing the onset of symptoms becomes. Young males with a high level of premorbid function are at increased risk of suicide, presumably in part because of the tremendous loss they face. These feelings can continue for years, with schizophrenic individuals feeling isolated and robbed of a normal life. Therefore, a component of individual work (which can also be achieved to some degree in a group setting) with these individuals is a focus on the impact schizophrenia has had on their lives. Helping individuals to grieve for these losses is an important process that may ultimately help them achieve a better quality of life.

Group Psychotherapy. Acutely psychotic individuals do not benefit from group interaction. In fact, a quiet place with decreased social contact is most useful until medications have controlled acute symptoms. It is common in inpatient settings to slowly integrate individuals into the ward community only as they appear less agitated and are able to remain in good behavioral control with improvement in psychotic symptoms. As their condition improves, inpatient group therapy prepares individuals for interpersonal interactions in a controlled setting. After discharge, individuals may benefit from day treatment programs and outpatient groups, which provide ongoing care for individuals with schizophrenia living in the community.

Because one of the most difficult challenges of schizophrenia is the inherent deficits in relatedness, group therapy is an important means of gathering individuals with schizophrenia together and providing them with a forum for mutual support. Insight-oriented groups may be disorganizing for individuals with schizophrenia, but task-oriented, supportive groups provide structure and a decreased sense of isolation for this population of individuals. Keeping group focus on structured topics, such as daily needs or getting the most out of community services, is useful for these individuals. In the era of community treatment and brief hospitalizations, many individuals are being seen in medication groups, which they attend regularly to discuss any side effects or problems and to get prescriptions.

Psychoeducational Treatment. One of the inherent deficits from which schizophrenic individuals suffer is an inability to engage appropriately in social or occupational activities. This debilitating effect is often a lasting feature of the illness, despite adequate psychopharmacological intervention. This disability often isolates individuals and makes it difficult for them to advocate appropriate social support or community services. Furthermore, studies have found that there is a correlation between poor social functioning and incidence of relapse. One of the challenges of this area of study is the great deal of variability in each individual. However, standardized measures have been developed to ascertain objective ratings of social deficits. These assessments have become important tools in the determination of effective nonpharmacological treatment strategies.

The literature suggests that schizophrenic individuals can benefit from social skills training. This model is based on the idea that the course of schizophrenia is, in part, a product of the environment, which is inherently stressful because of the social deficits from which these individuals suffer. The hypothesis is that if individuals are able to monitor and reduce their stress, they could potentially decrease their risk of relapse.

For this intervention to be successful, individuals must be aware of and set their own goals. Goals such as medication management, activities of daily living, and dealing with a roommate are achievable examples. Social skills and deficits can be assessed by individuals' self-report, observation of behavioral patterns by trained professionals, or a measurement of physiological responses to specific situations (e.g., increased pulse when asking someone to dinner). Individuals can then begin behavioral training in which appropriate social responses are shaped with the help of instructors.

In a large number of individuals, deficits in social competence persist despite antipsychotic treatment. These deficits can lead to social distress, whereas social competence can alleviate distress related to social discomfort. The "token economy" programs with operant conditioning paradigms were used in the past to discourage undesirable behavior. However, nowadays there are better ways to deal with these behaviors. Paradigms using instruction, modeling, role-playing, and positive reinforcement are helpful. Controlled studies suggest that individuals with schizophrenia are able to acquire lasting social skills after attending such programs and apply these skills to everyday life. Besides reducing anxiety, social skills training also improve the level of social activity and foster new social contacts. This in turn improves the quality of life and significantly shortens the duration of inpatient care. However, their impact on symptom resolution and relapse rates is unclear.

Individuals with schizophrenia generally demonstrate poor performance in various aspects of information processing. Cognitive dysfunction can be a rate-limiting factor in learning and social functioning.

Additionally, impaired information processing can lead to increased susceptibility to stress and thus to an increased risk of relapse. Practice appears to improve some of the cognitive dysfunction. Remediation of cognitive dysfunctions with social skills training has been reported to have positive impact. Social skills training programs, cognitive training programs to improve neurocognitive functioning, and cognitive–behavioral therapy approaches are oriented toward coping with symptoms, the disorder, and everyday problems.

Cognitive adaptation training (CAT) is a novel approach to improve adaptive functioning and compensate for the cognitive impairments associated with schizophrenia. A thorough functional needs assessment is done to measure current adaptive functioning. Besides measuring adaptive functioning and quantifying apathy and disinhibition, a neurocognitive assessment using tests to measure executive function, attention, verbal and visual memory, and visual organization is also completed. Treatment plans are adapted to the individual's level of functioning, which includes the individual's level of apathy. Interventions include removal of distracting stimuli, and use of reminders such as checklists, signs, and labels.

Family Therapy. A large body of the literature explores the role of familial interactions and the clinical course of schizophrenia. Many of these studies have examined the outcome of schizophrenia in relation to the degree of expressed emotion (EE) in family members. EE is generally defined as excessive criticism and overinvolvement of relatives. Schizophrenic individuals have been found to have a higher risk of relapse if their relatives have high EE levels. Clearly, an individual's disturbing symptoms at the time of relapse may affect the level of criticism and overinvolvement of family members, but evidence suggests that preexisting increased EE levels in relatives predict increased risk of schizophrenic relapse and that interventions that decrease EE levels can decrease relapse rates.

Specifically, studies have demonstrated that effective strategies lower the risk of relapse with the use of family intervention and measurements of EE levels. For example, in a study conducted in the early 1980s, 37 individuals were randomly assigned to one of two treatment groups. One group received family therapy, the other received individual therapy. In both groups, the individuals were maintained with appropriate neuroleptic doses. Family therapy was done in the home, with a focus on education about schizophrenia and ways in which families could achieve lowered stress levels and improved problem-solving skills. Specific problem-solving mechanisms were rehearsed and modeled by trained therapists. The individual treatment was supportive psychotherapy, which was conducted at the clinic. At the end of 9 months, family therapy was found to be a more effective means of preventing relapse (1 relapsed out of 18) than individual therapy (8 relapsed out of 19). Moreover, the advantages of the family therapy persisted after a second year of less intensive follow-up

A review of family interventions in 25 randomized studies involving 1744 individuals showed that the efficacy of family intervention on relapse rate is fairly well supported. This efficacy was particularly evident when contrasted with low quality or uncontrolled individual treatments. The addition of family intervention to standard treatment of schizophrenia has a positive impact on outcome to a moderate extent. Family intervention effectively reduces the short-term risk of clinical relapse after remission from an acute episode. The elements common to most effective interventions are inclusion of the individual in at least some phases of the treatment, long duration, and information and education about the illness provided within a supportive framework. There is sufficient data only for males with chronic schizophrenia living with high EE parents. Evidence is limited for recent onset individuals, women, people in different family arrangements and families with low EE. Research in family intervention is still a growing field. Thus, at present it is unclear if the effect seen with family therapy is due to family treatment or more intensive care.

On the basis of these findings, it is clear that there is a significant interaction between the level of emotional involvement and criticism of relatives of probands with schizophrenia and the outcome of their illness. Identifying the causative factors in familial stressors and educating involved family members about schizophrenia lead to long-term benefits for individuals. Future work in this field must examine these interactions with an understanding of modern sociological and biological advances in genetics, looking at trait carriers, social skills assessments, positive and negative symptoms, and medication management with the novel antipsychotic agents.

Case Management. Assertive Community Treatment (ACT) is a community care model with a caseload per worker of 15 individuals or fewer in contrast to standard case management (SCM) with a caseload of 30 to 35 individuals. Intensive clinical case management (ICCM) differs from ACT by the case manager not sharing the caseload. In the ACT model, most services are provided in the community rather than in

the office; the caseloads are shared across clinicians rather than individual caseloads. These are time unlimited services provided directly by the ACT team and not brokered out, and 24-hour coverage is provided. Research on the ACT model confirms that it is successful in making individuals comply with treatment and leads to fewer inpatient admissions. ACT also improves housing conditions (fewer homeless individuals, more individuals in stable housing), employment, quality of life, and patient satisfaction. No clear differences between ACT and standard or intensive clinical case management are reported with mental condition, social functioning, self-esteem, or number of deaths.

Combining Pharmacological and Psychosocial Treatments

The combination of pharmacological and psychosocial interventions in schizophrenia can have complex interactions. For example, psychotherapies improve medication compliance on the one hand and are more effective in the presence of antipsychotic treatment on the other. Family psychoeducation has been reported to decrease the level of EE in the family, resulting in better social adjustment and a need for lower doses of antipsychotic medications. The qualitative differences in the interactions between the newer antipsychotic agents and psychotherapy suggest a hopeful trend of better utilization of psychosocial treatments.

Self-Directed Treatment

Groups such as the National Alliance for Mentally Ill (NAMI) and the Manic–Depressive Association offer tremendous resources to individuals with psychiatric problems and their relatives. They provide newsletters, neighborhood meetings, and support groups to interested persons. These nonprofessional self-help measures may feel less threatening to individuals and their families and provide an important adjunct to professional settings.

Structured self-help clubs have also been effective means of bolstering individuals' social, occupational, and living skills. The Fountain House was the first such club aimed at social rehabilitation. Individuals who are involved are called members of the club, giving them a sense of belonging to a group. They are always made to feel welcome, useful, and productive members of the club community.

The clubhouse model has expanded to provide services such as transitional employment programs, apartment programs, outreach programs, and medication management and consultation services, to name a few. A self-supportive rehabilitation program for mentally ill individuals is an important option for many schizophrenic individuals who might otherwise feel isolated and out of reach.

Schizoaffective Disorder

Kraepelin's landmark classification at the dawn of the twentieth century could not accurately classify those individuals who manifested both psychotic (schizophrenia-like) and affective symptoms and had a better course of illness then schizophrenia. It was Kasanin in 1933, who coined the term *schizoaffective disorder* to describe some of these individuals. However, over the decades, these individuals were often classified as having atypical schizophrenia, good prognosis schizophrenia, remitting schizophrenia, or cycloid psychosis. Inherent within these diagnoses was the implication that they shared similarities to schizophrenia and also appeared to have a relatively better course of illness. With the advent of effective treatment of bipolar disorder with lithium salts, some of these individuals started responding to lithium, and the term *schizoaffective disorder* gained further momentum and evolved in the direction of bipolar disorder. Unfortunately, this lack of diagnostic clarity has plagued the diagnosis of schizoaffective disorder such that there is much that is unknown about the illness.

DIAGNOSIS

Schizoaffective disorder criteria have evolved over the years and undergone major changes. According to the DSM-IV-TR, an individual with schizoaffective disorder must have an uninterrupted period of illness during which, at some time, they meet the diagnostic criteria for a major depressive episode, manic episode, or a mixed episode concurrently with the diagnostic criteria for the active phase of schizophrenia (criterion A for schizophrenia). Additionally, "the individual must have had delusions or hallucinations for at least 2 weeks in the absence of prominent mood disorder symptoms" during the same period of illness. The mood disorder symptoms must be present for a substantial part of the active and residual psychotic period. The essential features of schizoaffective disorder must occur within a single uninterrupted period of illness where the "period of illness" refers to the period of active or residual symptoms of psychotic illness, and this can last for years and decades. The total duration of psychotic symptoms must be at least 1 month

---

DSM-IV-TR Diagnostic Criteria

295.70 SCHIZOAFFECTIVE DISORDER

A. An uninterrupted period of illness during which, at some time, there is either a major depressive episode, a manic episode, or a mixed episode concurrent with symptoms that meet criterion A for schizophrenia.

Note: The major depressive episode must include criterion A1: depressed mood.

B. During the same period of illness, there have been delusions or hallucinations for at least 2 weeks in the absence of prominent mood symptoms.

C. Symptoms that meet criteria for a mood episode are present for a substantial portion of the total duration of the active and residual periods of the illness.

D. The disturbance is not due to the direct physiological effects of a substance (e.g., a drug of abuse, a medication) or a general medical condition.

Specify type:

Bipolar type: if the disturbance includes a manic or a mixed episode (or a manic or a mixed episode and major depressive episodes)

Depressive type: if the disturbance only includes major depressive episodes

Reprinted with permission from the *Diagnostic and Statistical Manual of Mental Disorders*, 4th ed., Text Rev. Copyright 2000 American Psychiatric Association.

---

to meet the criterion A for schizophrenia and thus, the minimum duration of a schizoaffective episode is also 1 month.

The criterion for major depressive episode requires a minimum duration of 2 weeks of either depressed mood or markedly diminished interest or pleasure. As the symptoms of loss of pleasure or interest commonly occur in nonaffective psychotic disorders, to meet the criterion A for schizoaffective disorder the major depressive episode must include pervasive depressed mood. Presence of markedly diminished interest or pleasure is not sufficient to make a diagnosis as it is possible that these symptoms may occur with other conditions too.

The clinical signs and symptoms of schizoaffective disorder include all the signs and symptoms of schizophrenia, and a manic episode and/or a major depressive episode. The schizophrenia and mood symptoms may occur together or in an alternate sequence. The clinical course can vary from one of exacerbations and remissions to that of a long-term deterioration. Presence of mood-incongruent psychotic features—where the psychotic content of hallucinations or delusions is not consistent with the prevailing mood—more likely indicates a poor prognosis.

The DSM-IV-TR diagnosis of schizoaffective disorder can be further classified as schizoaffective disorder bipolar type or schizoaffective disorder *depressive type*. For a person to be classified as having the bipolar subtype, he/she must have a disorder that includes a manic or mixed episode with or without a history of major depressive episodes. Otherwise, the person is classified as having depressive subtype having had symptoms that meet the criterion for a major depressive episode with no history of having had mania or mixed state.

As discussed earlier, the diagnosis of schizoaffective disorder has undergone numerous changes through the decades, making it difficult to get reliable epidemiology information. When data was pooled together from various clinical studies, approximately 2–29% of those individuals diagnosed as having mental illness at the time of the study were suffering from schizoaffective disorder, with women having a higher prevalence. This could possibly be explained by a higher rate of depression in women. Relatives of women suffering from schizoaffective disorder have a higher rate of schizophrenia and depressive disorders compared to relatives of male schizoaffective subjects. The estimated lifetime prevalence of schizoaffective disorder is possibly in the range of 0.5–0.8%. In the inpatient settings of New York State psychiatric hospitals, approximately 19% of 6000 individuals had a diagnosis of schizoaffective disorder.

The depressive type of schizoaffective disorder appears to be more common in older people while the bipolar type probably occurs more commonly in younger adults. The higher prevalence of the disorder in women appears to occur particularly among those who are married. As in schizophrenia, the age of onset for women is later than that for men. Depression tends to occur more commonly in women.

Course

Owing to the evolving nature of the diagnosis and limited studies done thus far, much remains unknown. However, to the extent that this illness has symptoms from both a major mood disorder and schizophrenia, theoretically one can confer a relatively better prognosis than schizophrenia and a relatively poorer prognosis than bipolar disorder. In one study in which individuals with DSM-III and DSM-IV schizoaffective disorder were followed for 8 years, the outcome of these individuals more closely resembled schizophrenia than mood disorder with psychosis. Some data indicate that individuals with a diagnosis of schizoaffective disorder bipolar type have a 2- to 5-year course similar to that of bipolar disorder, while individuals diagnosed as having schizoaffective disorder depressive type have a

course similar to schizophrenia on outcome measures such as occupational and social functioning after the index episode. Regardless of the subtype, the following variables are harbingers of a poor prognosis:

(a) a poor premorbid history
(b) an insidious onset
(c) absence of precipitating factors
(d) a predominance of psychotic symptoms, especially deficit or negative ones
(e) an early age of onset
(f) an unremitting course, and
(g) a family history of schizophrenia.

The corollary would be that the opposite of each of these characteristics would suggest a better prognosis. Interestingly, the presence or the absence of Schneiderian first-rank symptoms does not seem to predict the course of illness. The incidence of suicide in individuals with schizoaffective disorder is at least 10%. Some data indicate that the suicidal behavior may be more common in women then men.

Differential Diagnosis

The possible differential diagnosis consists of bipolar disorder with psychotic features, major depressive disorder with psychotic features, and schizophrenia. Clearly, substance-induced states and symptoms caused by coexisting medical conditions should be carefully ruled out. All conditions listed in the differential diagnosis of schizophrenia, bipolar disorder, and major depressive disorder should be considered including but not limited to those individuals undergoing treatment with steroids, those abusing substances such as PCP, and medical conditions such as temporal lobe epilepsy. In circumstances where there is ambiguity, it may be prudent to delay making a final diagnosis until the most acute symptoms of psychosis have subsided and time is allowed to establish a course of illness and collect collateral information.

TREATMENT

With the shifting definitions of schizoaffective disorder, evaluating the treatment of schizoaffective disorder is not easy. Mood stabilizers, antidepressants, and antipsychotic medications clearly have a role in the management of these individuals. The presenting symptoms, their duration and intensity, and the choices of the individual need to be incorporated into deciding what treatment(s) to choose.

Atypical antipsychotic medications are reported to be more effective than the typical ones in the treatment of schizoaffective disorder. They appear to have a more broad-spectrum effect than the typical agents. Optimizing antipsychotic treatment, especially with the novel agents, is more likely to be effective than the routine use of adjunctive antidepressants or mood stabilizers. However, when indicated, the use of antidepressants is well supported in schizoaffective individuals who present with a full depressive syndrome after stabilization of psychosis.

Two small open label studies suggest that valproic acid is effective in treating the manic symptoms associated with schizoaffective disorder bipolar type, with 65.2% reduction in manic episodes in 5 individuals after 29 to 51 months.

Three double-blind, parallel-group studies examined the efficacy of lithium carbonate in schizoaffective mania. One study found that chlorpromazine alone was as effective as the combination of chlorpromazine and lithium. Another study with a small sample found that the combination of lithium and haloperidol was more effective than haloperidol itself in individuals with predominantly affective symptoms compared to those with predominantly psychotic symptoms. Reports of carbamazepine use is sparse and difficult to draw conclusions from. Lamotrigine was also reported to be useful in three cases of schizoaffective disorder.

The novel antipsychotic agents are often efficacious against depression in individuals who suffer from both depression and psychosis, negating the need for routine use of antidepressants. However, there are individuals who remain depressed even with optimal antipsychotic and mood stabilizer treatment. SSRIs are widely used in individuals who present with schizoaffective disorder with depression. If the SSRIs and newer antidepressants do not show efficacy, tricyclic antidepressants do have a role. Many studies suggest that addition of antidepressants helps in effective treatment of depression in schizoaffective disorder. Occasionally, antidepressants may worsen the course. For individuals suffering from depression where they are not responding adequately and are at risk for suicide, ECT is an effective alternative.

To the extent that schizoaffective disorder shares symptoms with schizophrenia, most of the psychosocial treatments used in the treatment of schizophrenia are likely to be useful in the treatment of schizoaffective disorder. Specifically, individuals benefit from individual supportive therapy, family therapy, group therapy, cognitive–behavioral therapy, and social skills training. Many individuals would be suitable candidates for assertive community therapy (ACT).

Depending on the level of recovery, some of the individuals may need rehabilitation services to assist them with either developing skills for some form of employment or assistance to maintain a job. Family members benefit from support groups such as NAMI or MDA groups.

Brief Psychotic Disorder

DIAGNOSIS

Brief psychotic disorder is defined by DSM-IV-TR as a psychotic disorder that lasts more than 1 day and less than a month. Moreover, the disorder may develop in response to severe psychosocial stressors or group of stressors.

European and Scandinavian countries have traditionally diagnosed this type of psychosis as *psychogenic psychosis*, *reactive psychosis*, or *brief reactive psychosis*. Some have also referred to this condition as *hys-*

DSM-IV-TR Diagnostic Criteria

298.8 BRIEF PSYCHOTIC DISORDER

A. Presence of one (or more) of the following symptoms:
   (1) delusions
   (2) hallucinations
   (3) disorganized speech (e.g., frequent derailment or incoherence)
   (4) grossly disorganized or catatonic behavior

Note: Do not include a symptom if it is a culturally sanctioned response pattern.

B. Duration of an episode of the disturbance is at least 1 day but less than 1 month, with eventual full return to premorbid level of functioning.
C. The disturbance is not better accounted for by a mood disorder with psychotic features, schizoaffective disorder, or schizophrenia and is not due to the direct physiological effects of a substance (e.g., a drug of abuse, a medication) or a general medical condition.

Specify if:

With marked stressor(s) (brief reactive psychosis): if symptoms occur shortly after and apparently in response to events that, singly or together, would be markedly stressful to almost anyone in similar circumstances in the person's culture

Without marked stressor(s): if psychotic symptoms do not occur shortly after, or are not apparently in response to events that, singly or together, would be markedly stressful to almost anyone in similar circumstances in the person's culture

With postpartum onset: if onset within 4 weeks postpartum

Reprinted with permission from the *Diagnostic and Statistical Manual of Mental Disorders*, 4th ed., Text Rev. Copyright 2000 American Psychiatric Association.

terical psychosis. These terms are probably more commonly used in Scandinavian countries due to Langfeldt and Leonhard's contributions to the classification of psychosis that does not have a course like schizophrenia. In the United States, brief reactive psychosis was formally included as a diagnostic category in DSM-III. Subsequently, it has undergone a change in its name to *brief psychotic disorder.*

The DSM-IV-TR diagnostic criteria specify the presence of at least one clear psychotic symptom lasting a minimum of 1 day to a maximum of 1 month. Furthermore, DSM-IV-TR allows the specification of two additional features: the presence or the absence of one or more marked stressors and a postpartum onset. DSM-IV-TR describes a continuum of diagnosis for psychotic disorder based primarily on the duration of the symptoms. Once the duration criteria are met, other conditions such as etiological medical illnesses and substance-induced psychosis need to be excluded. In those cases where the duration of psychosis lasts more than 1 month, appropriate diagnoses to be considered are other psychotic conditions based on reevaluation of the clinical features, duration of psychosis, and presence of mood symptoms.

People suffering from this disorder usually present with an acute onset, manifest at least one major symptom of psychosis, and do not always include the entire symptom constellation seen in schizophrenia. Affective symptoms, confusion, and impaired attention may be more common in brief psychotic disorders than in chronic psychotic conditions. Some of the characteristic symptoms include emotional lability, outlandish behavior, screaming or muteness, and impaired memory for recent events. Some of the symptoms suggest a diagnosis of *delirium* and may warrant a more complete medical workup. The symptom patterns include acute paranoid reactions, reactive confusions, excitations, and depressions. In French psychiatry, *bouffée délirante* is similar to brief psychotic disorder.

The precipitating stressors most commonly encountered are major life events that would cause any person significant emotional turmoil. Such events include the death of a close family member or severe accidents. Rarely, it could be accumulation of many smaller stresses.

Course

As defined by DSM-IV-TR, the duration of the disorder is less than 1 month. Nonetheless, the development of such a significant mental disorder may indicate an individual's mental vulnerability. An unknown percentage of individuals who are first classified as having brief psychotic disorder later display chronic mental disorder such as schizophrenia and bipolar disorder. Individuals with brief psychotic disorders generally have good prognosis, and European studies indicate that 50–80% of all individuals have no further major psychiatric problems.

The length of the acute and residual symptoms is often just a few days. Occasionally, depressive symptoms follow the resolution of the psychosis. Suicide is a concern during both the psychotic phase and the postpsychotic depressive phase. Indicators of good prognosis are good premorbid adjustment, few premorbid schizoid traits, severe precipitating stressors, sudden onset of symptoms, confusion and perplexity during psychosis, little affective blunting, short duration of symptoms, and absence of family history of schizophrenia.

Differential Diagnosis

Although the classical presentation may be short in duration and associated with stressors, a thorough and careful evaluation is necessary. Additional information is critical to rule out other major psychotic conditions as temporal association of stressors to the acute manifestation of symptoms may be coincidental and thus misleading. Other conditions to be ruled out include psychotic disorder due to a general medical condition, substance-induced psychosis, factitious disorder with predominantly psychological signs and symptoms, and malingering. Individuals with epilepsy and delirium may also present with similar symptoms. Additional conditions to be considered are dissociative identity disorder and psychotic episodes associated with borderline and schizotypal personality disorder that may last for less than a day.

TREATMENT

These individuals may require short-term hospitalizations for a comprehensive evaluation and safety. Antipsychotic drugs are often most useful along with benzodiazepines. Long-term use of medication is often not necessary and should be avoided. If maintenance medications are necessary, the diagnosis may need to be revised. Clearly, the newer antipsychotic agents have a better neurological side effect profile and would be preferred over the typical agents.

Psychotherapy is necessary to help the person reintegrate the experience of psychosis and possibly the precipitating trauma. Individual, family, and group therapies may be necessary in some individuals. Many individuals need help to cope with the loss of self-esteem and confidence.

Schizophreniform Disorder

DIAGNOSIS

Schizophreniform disorder shares a majority of the DSM-IV-TR diagnostic features with schizophrenia except the following two criteria: (1) the total duration of the illness which includes the prodrome, active, and residual phases is at least 1 month but less than 6 months in duration; and (2) though impairment in social and occupational functioning may occur during the illness, it is not required or necessary. Thus, the duration of more than 1 month eliminates brief psychotic disorder as a possible diagnosis; if the illness lasts or has lasted for more than 6 months, the diagnosis has to be reevaluated for other possible conditions including schizophrenia. Therefore, the diagnosis of schizophreniform disorder is intermediate between brief psychotic disorder and schizophrenia. Hence, those individuals whose duration of episode lasted more than a month and less than 6 months, and have recovered would be diagnosed as having schizophreniform disorder. On the other hand, those individuals who have not recovered from an episode, which is less than 6 months but more than one month in duration, and are likely to have schizophrenia would be diagnosed to have schizophreniform disorder until the 6 months criterion is met for schizophrenia. The diagnosis of 'provisional' schizophreniform disorder is made while the clinician monitors the evolving course of the illness, waits for the symptoms to resolve, or when the clinician cannot obtain a reliable history from an individual about the duration of the symptoms.

DSM-IV-TR has specifiers for the presence or absence of good prognostic features. These features include a rapid onset (within 4 weeks) of prominent psychotic symptoms, presence of (psychogenic) confusion or perplexity at the height of the psychotic episode, good premorbid adjustment as evidenced by social and occupational functioning, and the absence of deficit symptoms such as blunted or flat affect.

Course

The course is, as anticipated, variable. The DSM-IV-TR specifiers "with good prognostic features" and "without good prognostic features," though helpful in guiding the clinician, require further validation. However, confusion or perplexity at the height of the psychotic episode is the feature best correlated with good outcome. Also, the shorter the period of illness, the better the prognosis is likely to be. There is a significant risk of suicide in these individuals. Postpsychotic depression is quite likely and should be addressed in psychotherapy. Psychotherapy may help speed up the recovery and improve the prognosis. By definition, schizophreniform disorder resolves within 6 months with a return to baseline mental functioning.

Differential Diagnosis

This is similar to schizophrenia. Psychotic disorder caused by a general medical condition and substance-induced psychotic disorder must be ruled out. General medical conditions to be considered are HIV infection, temporal lobe epilepsy, CNS tumors, and cerebrovascular disease, all of which can also be associated with relatively short-lived psychotic episodes. The increasing number of reports of psychosis associated with the use of anabolic steroids by young men who are attempting to build up their muscles to perform better in athletic activities require careful history. Factitious disorder with predominantly psychological signs and symptoms and malingering may need to be ruled out in some instances.

TREATMENT

Hospitalization is often necessary and allows for effective assessment, treatment, and supervision of an individual's behavior. The psychotic symptoms, usually treated with a 3- to 6-month course of antipsychotic drugs, respond more rapidly than in individuals with

---

DSM-IV-TR Diagnostic Criteria

295.40 SCHIZOPHRENIFORM DISORDER

A. Criteria A, D, and E of schizophrenia are met.
B. An episode of the disorder (including prodromal, active, and residual phases) lasts at least 1 month but less than 6 months. (When the diagnosis must be made without waiting for recovery, it should be qualified as "provisional.")

Specify if:

Without good prognostic features

With good prognostic features: as evidenced by two (or more) of the following:

(1) onset of prominent psychotic symptoms within 4 weeks of the first noticeable change in usual behavior or functioning
(2) confusion or perplexity at the height of the psychotic episode
(3) good premorbid social and occupational functioning
(4) absence of blunted or flat affect

Reprinted with permission from the *Diagnostic and Statistical Manual of Mental Disorders*, 4th ed., Text Rev. Copyright 2000 American Psychiatric Association.

schizophrenia. One study found that 75% of the individuals with schizophreniform psychosis compared to 20% of those with schizophrenia responded to antipsychotic agents within 8 days. ECT may be indicated for some individuals, especially those with marked catatonic features or depression. If an individual has recurrent episodes, trials of lithium carbonate, valproic acid, or carbamazepine may be warranted for prophylaxis. Psychotherapy is usually necessary to help individuals integrate the psychotic experience into their understanding of their minds, brains, and lives.

Delusional Disorder

DIAGNOSIS

Delusional disorder refers to a group of disorders, the chief feature of which is the presence of *nonbizarre* delusions. People suffering from this illness generally do not regard themselves as mentally ill and actively oppose psychiatric referral. Because they may experience little impairment, they generally remain outside hospital settings, appearing reclusive, eccentric, or odd, rather than ill. They are more likely to have contacts with professionals such as lawyers and other medical specialists for health concerns. The current shift in diagnosis from *paranoid* to *delusional* helps avoid the ambiguity around the term "paranoid." This also emphasizes that other delusions besides the paranoid ones are included in this diagnosis. It is important to understand the definition of nonbizarre delusion so as to reach an unambiguous diagnosis. Nonbizarre delusions typically involve situations or circumstances that can occur in real life (e.g., being followed, infected, or deceived by a lover) and are believable.

According to DSM-IV-TR, the diagnosis of delusional disorder can be made when a person exhibits nonbizarre delusions of at least 1 month's duration that cannot be attributed to other mental disorders. Nonbizarre delusions must be about phenomena that, although not real, are within the realm of being possible. In general, the individual's delusions are well systematized and have been logically developed. If the person experiences auditory or visual hallucinations, they are not prominent except for tactile or olfactory hallucinations where they are tied in to the delusion (e.g., a person who believes that he emits a foul odor might experience an olfactory hallucination of that odor). The person's behavioral and emotional responses to the delusions appear to be appropriate. Usually, the person's functioning and personality are well preserved and show minimal deterioration if at all.

DSM-IV-TR Diagnostic Criteria

297.10 DELUSIONAL DISORDER

A. Nonbizarre delusions (i.e., involving situations that occur in real life, such as being followed, poisoned, infected, loved at a distance, or deceived by spouse or lover, or having a disease) of at least 1 month's duration.
B. Criterion A for schizophrenia has never been met.

Note: Tactile and olfactory hallucinations may be present in delusional disorder if they are related to the delusional theme.

C. Apart from the impact of the delusion(s) or its ramifications, functioning is not markedly impaired and behavior is not obviously odd or bizarre.
D. If mood episodes have occurred concurrently with delusions, their total duration has been brief relative to the duration of the delusional periods.
E. The disturbance is not due to the direct physiological effects of a substance (e.g., a drug of abuse, a medication) or a general medical condition.

Specify type (the following types are assigned based on the predominant delusional theme):

Erotomanic type: delusions that another person, usually of higher status, is in love with the individual

Grandiose type: delusions of inflated worth, power, knowledge, identity, or special relationship to a deity or famous person

Jealous type: delusions that the individual's sexual partner is unfaithful

Persecutory type: delusions that the person (or someone to whom the person is close) is being malevolently treated in some way

Somatic type: delusions that the person has some physical defect or general medical condition

Mixed type: delusions characteristic of more than one of the above types but no one theme predominates

Unspecified type

Reprinted with permission from the *Diagnostic and Statistical Manual of Mental Disorders*, 4th ed., Text Rev. Copyright 2000 American Psychiatric Association.

Subtypes

Persecutory Type. This is the most common form of delusional disorder. Here, the person affected believes that he or she is being followed, spied on, poisoned or drugged, harassed, or conspired against. The person affected may get preoccupied by small slights that can become incorporated into the delusional system. These individuals may resort to legal actions to remedy perceived injustice. Individuals suffering from these delusions often become resentful and angry with a potential to get violent against those believed to be against them.

Jealous Type. Individuals with this subtype have the delusional belief that their spouses/lovers are unfaithful.

This is often wrongly inferred from small bits of benign evidence, which is used to justify the delusion. Delusions of infidelity have also been called *conjugal paranoia*. The term *Othello syndrome* has been used to describe morbid jealousy. This delusion usually affects men with no history of prior psychiatric problems. The condition is difficult to treat and may diminish only on separation, divorce, or death of the spouse. Marked jealousy (pathological jealousy or morbid jealousy) is a symptom of many disorders including schizophrenia and is not unique to delusional disorder. Jealousy is a powerful emotion and when it occurs in delusional disorder or as part of another condition, it can be potentially dangerous and has been associated with violence, including suicidal and homicidal behavior.

Erotomanic Type. These individuals have delusions of secret lovers. Most frequently, the individual is a woman, though men are also susceptible to these delusions. The individual believes that a suitor, usually more socially prominent than herself, is in love with her. This can become the central focus of the individual's existence and the onset can be sudden. Erotomania is also referred to as *de Clerambault's syndrome*. Again, these delusions can occur as part of other disorders too. Generally women (but not exclusively so), unattractive in appearance, working at a lower-level jobs, who lead withdrawn, lonely single lives with few sexual contacts are reported to be more prone to develop this condition. They select lovers who are substantially different from them. They exhibit what has been called paradoxical conduct, the delusional phenomenon of interpreting all denials of love no matter how clear as secret affirmations of love. Separation from the love object may be the only satisfactory means of intervention. When it affects men, it can manifest with more aggressive and possibly violent pursuit of love. Thus, such people are often in the forensic system. The object of aggression is often companions or protectors of the love object who are viewed as trying to come between the lovers. However, resentment and rage in response to an absence of reaction from all forms of love communication may escalate to a point that the love object may be in danger too.

Somatic Type. Delusional disorder with somatic delusions has been called *monosymptomatic hypochondriacal psychosis*. This disorder differs from other conditions with hypochondriacal symptoms in degree of reality impairment. The frequency of these conditions is low, but cases may be underdiagnosed because individuals present to dermatologists, plastic surgeons, and infectious disease specialists more often than to mental health professionals. Individuals with these conditions

do sometimes to pimozide, a typical antipsychotic medication, and also to SSRIs. Usually prognosis is poor without treatment. It affects both sexes equally. Suicide apparently motivated by anguish is not uncommon.

Grandiose Type. This is also referred to as *megalomania*. In this subtype, the central theme of the delusion is the grandiosity of having made some important discovery or having great talent. Sometimes there may be a religious theme to the delusional thinking such that the person believes that he or she has a special message from God.

Mixed Type. This subtype is reserved for those with two or more delusional themes. However, it should be used only where it is difficult to clearly discern one theme of delusion.

Unspecified Type. This subtype is used for cases in which the predominant delusion cannot be subtyped within the above-mentioned categories. A possible example is certain delusions of misidentification, for example, *Capgras's syndrome*, named after the French psychiatrist who described the "illusions of doubles." The delusion here is the belief that a familiar person has been replaced by an imposter. A variant of this is *Fregoli's syndrome* where the delusion is that the persecutors or familiar persons can assume the guise of strangers and the very rare delusion that familiar persons could change themselves into other persons at will (intermetamorphosis). Each disorder is not only a rare delusion but is highly associated with other conditions such as schizophrenia and dementia.

Though the existence of delusional disorder has been known for a long time, relatively little is known about the demographics, incidence, and prevalence. People suffering from this illness function reasonably well in the community and lack insight, resulting in minimal or no contact with the mental health system. However, the crude incidence is roughly 0.7 to 3.0 per 100,000 with a more frequent occurrence in females. Some have associated this condition with widowhood, celibacy, and history of substance abuse. In one study, 1.2% of 4144 consecutively attending subjects in an outpatient clinic were diagnosed to have delusional disorder. Half of the subjects were diagnosed to have *persecutory* type of delusional disorder. Females suffering from this disorder were significantly older than males.

Course

Though the onset can occur in adolescence, generally it begins from middle to late adulthood with variable patterns of course, including lifelong disorder in some cases. Delusional disorder does not lead to severe impairment or change in personality, but rather to a gradual, progressive involvement with the delusional concern. Suicide has often been associated with this disorder. The base rate of spontaneous recovery may not be as low as previously thought, especially because only the more severely afflicted are referred for a treatment. The more chronic forms of the illness tend to have their onset early in the fifth decade. Onset is acute in nearly two-thirds of the cases and gradual in the remainder. In almost half of the cases, the delusion disappears at follow-up, improves in 10%, and is unchanged in about a third. In the more acute forms of the illness, the age of onset is in the fourth decade, a lasting remission occurs in over half of the individuals, and a pattern of chronicity develops in only 10%; a relapsing course has been observed in a third. Thus, the more acute and earlier the onset of the illness, the more favorable the prognosis. The presence of precipitating factors, married status, and female gender are associated with better outcome. The persistence of delusional thinking is most favorable for cases with persecutory delusions and somewhat less favorable for delusions of grandeur and jealousy. However, the outcome in terms of overall functioning appears somewhat more favorable for the jealous subtype.

TREATMENT

Though generally considered resistant to treatment and interventions, the management is focused on managing the morbidity of the disorder by reducing the impact of the delusion on the individual's (and family's) life. However, in recent years, the outlook has become less pessimistic or restricted in planning effective treatment for these conditions. An effective and therapeutic clinician–patient relationship is important but difficult to establish.

Overall, treatment results suggest that 80.8% of cases recover either fully or partially. Pimozide, the most frequently reported treatment, produced full remission in 68.5% and partial recovery in 22.4% ($N = 143$). There are reports of treatment with other typical antipsychotic agents with variable success in a small number of subjects. SSRIs have been used and reported to be helpful. The newer atypical antipsychotic agents have been used in a small number of cases with success but the data is anecdotal.

As mentioned earlier, developing a therapeutic relationship is very important and yet significantly difficult, and requires a frank and supportive attitude. Supportive therapy is very helpful in dealing with emotions of

anxiety and dysphoria generated because of delusional thinking. Cognitive therapy, when accepted and implemented, is helpful. Confrontation of the delusional thinking usually does not work and can further alienate the individual.

Shared Psychotic Disorder

DIAGNOSIS

Shared psychotic disorder is a rare disorder, which is also referred to as *shared paranoid disorder, induced psychotic disorder, folie à deux,* and *double insanity.* Jules Baillarger, in 1860, first described the syndrome and called it *folie à communiquée,* while Lasegue and Falret, in 1877, first described *folie à deux.* In this disorder, the transfer of delusions takes place from one person to another. Both persons are closely associated for a long time and typically live together in relative social isolation. In its more common form, *folie imposée,* the individual who first has the delusion is often chronically ill and typically is the influential member of the close relationship with another individual, who is more suggestible and who develops the delusion too. The second individual is frequently less intelligent, more gullible, more passive, or more lacking in self-esteem than the primary case. If the two people involved are separated, the second individual may abandon the delusion. However, this is not seen consistently. Other forms of shared psychotic disorder reported are *folie simultanée,* where similar delusional systems develop independently in two closely associated people. Occasionally, more than two individuals are involved (e.g. *folie à trois, quatre, cinq;* also *folie à famille*) but such cases are very rare.

An important feature in the diagnosis is that the person with shared psychotic disorder does not have a pre-

---

DSM-IV-TR Diagnostic Criteria

297.3 SHARED PSYCHOTIC DISORDER

A. A delusion develops in an individual in the context of a close relationship with another person(s), who has an already-established delusion.
B. The delusion is similar in content to that of the person who already has the established delusion.
C. The disturbance is not better accounted for by another Psychotic Disorder (e.g., Schizoprenia) or a Mood Disorder with Psychotic Features and is not due to the direct physiological effects of a substance (e.g., a drug of abuse, a medication) or a general condition.

Reprinted with permission from the *Diagnostic and Statistical Manual of Mental Disorders,* 4th ed., Text Rev. Copyright 2000 American Psychiatric Association.

existing psychotic disorder. The delusions arise in the context of a close relationship with a person who suffers from delusional thinking and resolve on separation from that person. The key symptom of shared psychosis is the unquestioning acceptance of another person's delusions. The delusions themselves are often in the realm of possibility and usually not as bizarre as those seen in individuals with schizophrenia. The content of the delusion is often persecutory or hypochondriacal. Symptoms of a coexisting personality disorder may be present, but signs and symptoms that meet criteria for schizophrenia, mood disorders, and delusional disorder are absent. The individual may have ideation about suicide or pacts about homicide; clinicians must elicit this information during the interview.

More than 95% of all cases of shared psychotic disorder involve two members of the same family. About a third of the cases involve two sisters, another one-third involve husband and wife or a mother and her child. The dominant person is usually affected by schizophrenia or a similar psychotic disorder. In 25% of all cases, the submissive person is usually affected with physical disabilities such as deafness, cerebrovascular diseases, or other disability that increases the submissive person's dependence on the dominant person. This condition is more common in people from low socioeconomic groups and in women.

Course

Though separation of the submissive person from the dominant person should resolve the psychosis, this probably occurs only in 10–40% of the cases. Unfortunately, when these individuals are discharged from hospital, they usually move back together.

Differential Diagnosis

Malingering, factitious disorder with predominantly psychological sign and symptoms, psychotic disorder due to a general medical condition, and substance-induced psychotic disorder must be considered.

TREATMENT

The initial step in treatment is to separate the affected person from the source of the delusions, the dominant individual. Antipsychotic agents may be used if the symptoms have not abated in a week after separation. Psychotherapy with the nondelusional members of the individual's family should be undertaken, and psychotherapy with both the individual and the person sharing the

delusion may be indicated later in the course of treatment. To prevent redevelopment of the syndrome, the family may need family therapy and social support to modify the family dynamics and to prevent redevelopment of the syndrome. Steps to decrease the social isolation may also help prevent the syndrome from reemerging.

COMPARISON OF DSM-IV-TR AND ICD-10 DIAGNOSTIC CRITERIA

The ICD-10 and DSM-IV-TR criteria sets for schizophrenia are similar in many important ways although not identical. The ICD-10 Diagnostic Criteria for Research provide two ways to satisfy the criteria for schizophrenia: having one Schneiderian first-rank symptom or having at least two of the other characteristic symptoms (hallucinations accompanied by delusions, thought disorder, catatonic symptoms, and negative symptoms). In contrast to DSM-IV-TR, which requires 6 months of symptoms (including prodromal, active, and residual phases), the ICD-10 definition of schizophrenia requires only a 1-month duration, thereby encompassing the DSM-IV-TR diagnostic categories of both schizophrenia and schizophreniform disorder. Thus, cases of DSM-IV-TR schizophreniform disorder are diagnosed in ICD-10 as schizophrenia.

The DSM-IV-TR and ICD-10 definitions of schizoaffective disorder differ with regard to the relationship of the Schizoaffective Disorder category with the category Mood Disorder with Psychotic Features. In DSM-IV-TR, the differentiation depends on the temporal relationship between the mood and psychotic symptoms (i.e., Mood Disorder with Psychotic Features is diagnosed whenever the psychotic symptoms occur only in the presence of a mood episode, regardless of the characteristics of the psychotic symptoms). In contrast, the ICD-10 definition of schizoaffective disorder is much broader. It includes situations in which certain specified psychotic symptoms (i.e., thought echo, insertion, withdrawal, or broadcasting; delusions of control or passivity; voices giving a running commentary; disorganized speech, catatonic behavior) occur even if they are confined to a mood episode. Therefore, many cases of DSM-IV-TR mood disorder with mood-incongruent psychotic features would be considered to be schizoaffective disorder in ICD-10. Furthermore, the ICD-10 definition suggests that there should be an "approximate balance between the number, severity, and duration of the schizophrenic and affective symptoms." For delusional disorder, the ICD-10 Diagnostic Criteria for Research specify a minimum 3-month duration in contrast to the 1-month minimum duration in DSM-IV-TR.

In contrast to the single DSM-IV-TR category Brief Psychotic Disorder, ICD-10 has a much more complex way of handling brief psychotic disorders. It includes criteria sets for four specific brief psychotic disorders that differ on the basis of types of symptoms (i.e., with or without symptoms of schizophrenia) and course

(i.e., whether they change rapidly or not). Furthermore, the maximum duration of these brief psychotic episodes varies depending on the type of symptoms (i.e., 1 month for schizophrenia-like symptoms and 3 months for predominantly delusional). In contrast, DSM-IV-TR has a single criteria set and a maximum 1-month duration.

Finally, the ICD-10 and DSM-IV-TR definitions of shared psychotic disorder are almost identical.

26 Mood Disorders: Depressive Disorders

Major depressive disorder (MDD), dysthymic disorder (DD), and depressive disorder not otherwise specified (DDNOS) are the group of clinical conditions in the DSM-IV-TR characterized by depressive symptomatology. These conditions specifically exclude a history of manic, mixed, or hypomanic episodes, and are not due to the physiologic effects of substances of abuse, other medications, or toxins. MDD is characterized by episodes of depression, each lasting at least 2 weeks. DD is characterized by at least 2 years of depressed mood accompanied by two or three depressive symptoms that fall short of threshold criteria for a major depressive episode. Depressive disorder not otherwise specified includes a set of conditions that do not meet criteria for MDD, DD, or adjustment disorder with depressed mood. These syndromes include premenstrual dysphoric disorder, minor depressive disorder, recurrent brief depressive disorder, and postpsychotic depressive disorder occurring during the residual phase of schizophrenia. In DSM-IV-TR, two other depressive disorders are diagnosed on the basis of etiology: mood disorder due to a general medical condition and substance-induced mood disorder.

Major Depressive Disorder

DIAGNOSIS

The depressive disorders are characterized by lifelong vulnerability to episodes of disease, involving depressed mood or loss of interest and pleasure in activities. Individuals may demonstrate ongoing potential for cycling of mood from euthymia to depression to recovery and sometimes to hypomania or mania. When individuals cycle to hypomania or mania, then a diagnosis of bipolar II (in the case of hypomania) or bipolar I (in the case of mania) is made (see Chapter 28, page 279). When the mood disorder is severe, assessment for psychosis is essential.

The detection of major depressive episodes in both primary care settings and mental health settings requires the presence of mood disturbance or loss of interest and pleasure in activities for 2 weeks or more accompanied by at least four other symptoms of depression. There are problems in differential diagnosis because depressive experiences vary from individual to individual. One or more depressive episodes, occurring in the absence of a lifetime history of mania, hypomania, or intraepisode psychotic symptoms, warrants a DSM-IV-TR diagnosis of Major Depressive Disorder (see DSM-IV-TR diagnostic criteria for Major Depressive Disorder, page 253). If the individual has had only one episode, then subtype "Single Episode" is noted. Often, however, individuals suffer from multiple major depressive episodes during their lifetime. If the major depressive episodes have been recurrent, the subtype "Recurrent" is noted. Remission of depression requires a 2-month interval in which the full criteria are not met for a major depressive episode.

The core symptoms comprising a major depressive episode are illustrated in the DSM-IV-TR criteria. Each symptom is critical to evaluate in an individual with depressive symptomatology since each represents one of the essential features of a major depressive episode. Their persistence for much of the day, nearly every day for at least 2 weeks, is the criterion for diagnosis. The clinical syndrome is associated with significant psychological distress or impairment in psychosocial or work functioning.

The clinical observation of mood reveals variations in presentation. An individual may have depressed symptomatology and experience typical sadness. Another individual may deny sadness and experience internal agitation and dysphoria. Another individual with depression may experience no feelings at all, and the depressed mood is inferred from the degree of psychological pain that is exhibited. Some individuals experience irritability, frustration, somatic preoccupation, and the sensation of being numb.

An equally important aspect of the depressive experience involves loss of interest or pleasure, when an

Clinical Guide to the Diagnosis and Treatment of Mental Disorders. M. B. First and A. Tasman
© 2006 John Wiley & Sons, Ltd. ISBN 0 470 019158

<table>
</table>

DSM-IV-TR Diagnostic Criteria

MAJOR DEPRESSIVE DISORDER

A. Presence of a single Major Depressive Episode (296.2x Major Depressive Disorder, Single Episode) or two or more Major Depressive Episodes (296.3x Major Depressive Disorder, Recurrent).

Note: To be considered separate episodes, there must be an interval of at least 2 Consecutive month in which criteria are not met for a Major Depressive Episode.

B. The Major Depressive Episodes are not better accounted for by Schizoaffective Disorder and are not superimposed on Schizophrenia, Schizophreniform Disorder, Delusional Disorder, or Psychotic Disorder Not Otherwise Specified.
C. There has never been Manic Episode, a Mixed Episode, or a Hypomanic, Episode.

Note: This exclusion does not apply if all of the manic-like, mixed-like, or hypomanic-like episodes are substance or treatment induced or are due to the direct physiological effects of a general medical condition.

Code in fifth digit: 1 = Mild; 2 = Moderate; 3 = Severe Without Psychotic Features; 4 = Sever With Psychotic Features (Specify Mood-Congruent/Mood-Incongruent); 5 = In Partial Remission; 6 = In Full Remission; 0 = Unspecified

If the full criteria are currently met for a Major Depressive Episode, *specify* is current clinical status and/or features:

Mild Moderate, Severe Without Psychotic Features/ Severe With Psychotic Features
Chronic
With Catatonic Features
With Melancholic Features
With Atypical Features
With Postpartum Onset

If the full criteria are not currently met for a Major Depressive Episode, *specify* the current clinical status of the Major Depressive Disorder or features of the most recent episode:

In Partial Remission, In Full Remission
Chronic
With Catatonic Features
With Melancholic Features
With Atypical Features
With Postpartum Onset

Specify (for Major Depressive Disorder, Recurrent):

Longitudinal Course Specifiers (With and Without Interposed Recovery)
With Seasonal Pattern

Note: This is a summary of two criteria sets.

Reprinted with permission from *DSM-IV-TR Guidebook*. Copyright 2004, Michael B First, Allen Frances, and Harold Alan Pincus.

DSM-IV-TR Diagnostic Criteria

MAJOR DEPRESSIVE EPISODE

A. Five (or more) of the following symptoms have been present during the same 2-week period and represent a change from previous functioning; at least one of the symptoms is either (1) depressed mood or (2) loss of interest or pleasure.

Note: Do not include symptoms that are clearly due to a general medical condition, or mood-incongruent delusions or hallucinations.

(1) Depressed mood most of the day, as indicated by either subjective report (e.g., feels sad or empty) or observation made by others (e.g., appears tearful).

Note: In children and adolescents, can be irritable mood.

(2) Markedly diminished interest or pleasure in all, or almost all, activities most of the day, nearly every day (as indicated by either subjective account or observation made by others).
(3) Significant weight loss when not dieting or weight gain (e.g., a change of more than 5% of body weight in a month), or decrease or increase in appetite nearly every day.

Note: In children, consider failure to make expected weight gains.

(4) Insomnia or hypersomnia nearly every day.
(5) Psychomotor agitation or retardation nearly every day (observable by others, not merely subjective feelings of restlessness or being slowed down).
(6) Fatigue or loss of energy nearly every day.
(7) Feelings of worthlessness or excessive or inappropriate guilt (which may be delusional) nearly every day (not merely self-reproach or guilt about being sick).
(8) Diminished ability to think or concentrate, or indecisiveness, nearly every day (either by subjective account or as observed by others).
(9) Recurrent thoughts of death (not just fear of dying), recurrent suicidal ideation without a specific plan, or a suicide attempt or a specific plan for committing suicide.

B. The symptoms do not meet criteria for a mixed episode.
C. The symptoms cause clinically significant distress or impairment in social, occupational, or other important areas of functioning.
D. The symptoms are not due to the direct physiological effects of a substance (e.g., a drug of abuse, a medication) or a general medical condition (e.g., hypothyroidism).
E. The symptoms are not better accounted for by bereavement, i.e., after the loss of a loved one, the symptoms persist for longer than 2 months or are characterized by marked functional impairment, morbid preoccupation with worthlessness, suicidal ideation, psychotic symptoms, or psychomotor retardation.

Reprinted with permission from the *Diagnostic and Statistical Manual of Mental Disorders*, 4th ed., Text Rev. Copyright 2000 American Psychiatric Association.

individual feels no sense of enjoyment in activities that were previously considered pleasurable. There is associated reduction in all drives including energy and alteration in sleep, interest in food, and interest in sexual activity.

A common experience of insomnia or hypersomnia is noted in individuals with persistent depression. Observations of psychomotor activity include profound psychomotor retardation leading to stupor in more

severe cases or alternatively significant agitation leading to inability to sit still and profound pacing in agitated forms of depression.

The complaint of guilt or guilty preoccupation is a common aspect of the depressive syndrome. Delusional forms of guilt are a common presentation of depressive disorder with psychotic features.

The loss of ability to concentrate, to focus attention, and to make decisions is a particularly distressing symptom for individuals. One may experience a loss of memory that simulates dementia. Loss of concentration is reflected in an inability to perform both complicated and simple tasks. The loss of ability to perform in school may be a symptom of a major depressive episode in children, and memory difficulties in the older adult may be mistaken for a primary dementia. In some older adults, a depressive episode with memory difficulties occurs in the early phase of an evolving dementia.

The most common psychiatric syndrome associated with thoughts of death, suicidal ideation, or completed suicide is a major depressive episode. The experience of hopelessness is commonly associated with suicidal ideation. The preoccupation with suicide in major depressive disorder requires that the assessment always includes careful monitoring of suicidality. Suicidality is the feature of depressive disorder that poses substantial risk of mortality in the disease. Prevention of suicide, more than any other treatment goal, requires immediate intervention and may require hospitalization. The risk for subsequent completed suicide for an individual hospitalized for an episode of severe MDD is estimated to be 15%. To assess risk for suicide, one inquires about the presence of active suicidal ideation in relation to the current episode of depression and a history of prior suicide attempts. The occurrence of significant life events such as separation, divorce, and death of significant others may precipitate the episode. It is also necessary to review onsets of other medical conditions that may precipitate a new episode of depression. When alcohol or other drug use co-occurs with such significant life events, the risk of suicidal behavior during an episode of depression increases. The presence of a recent suicide attempt may suggest the need for immediate hospitalization and treatment.

Familiarity with risk factors for major depressive disorder may help the clinician recognize or diagnose this common and serious psychiatric illness. Accordingly, the following 10 primary risk factors for depression have been identified: (1) history of prior episodes of depression; (2) family history of depressive disorder especially in first-degree relatives; (3) history of suicide attempts; (4) female gender; (5) age of onset before age 40; (6) postpartum period; (7) comorbid medical illness; (8) absence of social support; (9) negative, stressful life events; and (10) active alcohol or substance abuse.

The assessment of MDD involves the specific identification of 5 of 9 criterion symptoms that would constitute a diagnosis of MDD. A careful general medical assessment to ascertain the presence of an etiologic general medical condition is required. After the assessment for general medical conditions, one examines the individual for the presence of alcohol or drug dependence. Then the clinician is required to assess retrospectively the occurrence of prior episodes of mood disorder, either depression or mania. It is necessary to examine for other comorbid mental disorders as well. Depressive illnesses are very common and recurrent, but an individual with MDD may or may not recall prior episodes. It is therefore essential to interview a significant other or family member in addition to the individual with depression to identify prior manic, hypomanic, or depressive episodes. Family inquiry allows one to elicit the family history of addiction, anxiety, depressive disorder, mania, psychosis, trauma, or neurologic disorders in first-degree relatives.

The individual who presents for outpatient or hospital treatment for a primary depressive disorder will require general medical examination, including a physical examination and laboratory testing to rule out an associated medical condition. Clinical assessment, including the cognitive mental status examination, will direct the extent of the general medical examination.

Traditional psychological testing may complement structured diagnostic instruments developed to ascertain the presence or absence of depressive disorders according to DSM-IV-TR criteria. Psychological testing such as the Rorschach Inkblot Test are sensitive to the degree of affective lability, intensity of suicidality, and impulse control in individuals with depression. In addition, inventories are commonly used in outpatient and inpatient settings to establish scores of clinical severity of depressive symptoms. Self-administered scales include the Beck Depression Inventory. the Zung Self-Rating Depression Scale, and the Inventory for Depressive Symptomatology (self-report). Clinician-administered scales used for assessment of depressive symptoms include the Hamilton Rating Scale for Depression, the Montgomery Asberg Depression Rating Scale, and the Inventory for Depressive Symptomatology (clinician rated). It is essential to recognize that a cross-sectional assessment is only one component of the total assessment. Corroborative family data and longitudinal assessment and reassessment of mood disorder symptoms are crucial in following the natural history and course of MDD.

Laboratory studies in the management of the individual with MDD includes complete blood count with differential, electrolytes, chemical screening for renal and liver function as well as thyroid function studies. More detailed evaluation will depend upon the nature of the clinical presentation as well as neuropsychological examination. These studies may identify cerebral vulnerability factors that would complicate the treatment for MDD.

When clinical signs suggest cognitive disruption or cognitive impairment, the clinician may also consider administering neuropsychological tests or conducting more focused neurologic examination to explore cognitive, behavioral, and neurological correlates of brain function. Neuropsychological assessment may help clarify the relative contribution of depression or another disease process to the individual's clinical presentation. Further, neuropsychological assessment will provide a functional analysis of the individual's cognitive and behavioral strengths and limitations. Neurological examination may reveal minor neurological abnormalities suggesting early neurodevelopmental vulnerability.

Individuals with MDD report health difficulties and actively use health services. Studies have indicated that as many as 23% of depressed individuals report health difficulties severe enough to keep them bedridden. The Medical Outcomes Study examined role functioning, social functioning, and number of days in bed secondary to poor health, and compared the degree of impact of depression and other chronic medical conditions. Depression was associated with more impairment in occupational and interpersonal functioning, and more days in bed, in comparison to several common medical illnesses.

A significant relationship exists between MDD and mortality, characterized by suicide and accidents. Therefore, an accurate diagnosis of MDD, early appropriate intervention, and specific assessment of suicidality is essential. Fifteen percent of individuals with MDD who require hospitalization owing to severe depression will die by committing suicide. Approximately 10% of individuals with MDD who attempt suicide will eventually succeed in killing themselves. Roughly 50% of individuals who have successfully committed suicide carried a primary depressive diagnosis. Individuals with MDD who were admitted to nursing homes were found to have a 59% greater likelihood of death within the first year of admission in comparison with nondepressed admissions. The epidemiologic catchment area (ECA) study indicated that individuals with MDD 55 years of age and older evidence a mortality rate over the next 15 months four times higher than nondepressed controls matched for age.

Subtyping of MDD

The current subtyping of MDD is based on severity, cross-sectional features, and course features.

Severity/Psychotic/Remission. The rating of severity is based on a clinical judgment of the number of criteria present, the severity of the symptomatology, and the degree of functional distress. The ratings of current severity are classified as *mild, moderate, severe without psychotic features, severe with psychotic features, in partial remission*, or in *full remission* (see DSM-IV-TR diagnostic criteria, page 256). The definition of "mild" refers to an episode that results in only mild impairment in occupational or psychosocial functioning or mild disability. "Moderate" implies a level of severity that is intermediate between mild and severe and is associated with moderate impairment in psychosocial functioning. The definition of "severe" describes an episode that meets several symptoms in excess of those required to make a diagnosis of major depressive episode and is associated with marked impairment in occupational or psychosocial functioning and definite disability characterized by inability to work or perform basic social functions. "Severe with psychotic features" indicates the presence of delusions or hallucinations, which occur in the context of the major depressive episode. Since the introduction of DSM-III, the categories of mood-congruent versus mood-incongruent psychotic features are made in the context of a psychotic depressive disorder. When the content of delusions or hallucinations is consistent with depressive themes, a mood-congruent psychotic diagnosis is made. When the psychotic features are not related to depressive themes or include symptoms such as thought insertion, broadcast, or withdrawal, the modifier of mood-incongruent psychotic features is used. Mood-incongruent psychosis in MDD may be associated with a poorer prognosis. For depression with psychotic features, whether they are mood-congruent or mood-incongruent, antipsychotic medication in combination with antidepressant medication or electroconvulsive therapy (ECT) is required to treat the disorder.

Partial remission indicates that the episode no longer meets full criteria for major depressive episode but that some symptoms are still present or the period of remission has been less than 2 months. In full remission, the individual has no significant symptoms of depression for a period of at least 2 months.

Cross-Sectional Features. The assessment of cross-sectional features involves the presence or absence of catatonic, melancholic, or atypical features during an

DSM-IV-TR Diagnostic Criteria

SEVERITY/PSYCHOTIC/REMISSION SPECIFIERS

Note: Code in fifth digit. Mild, Moderate, Severe Without Psychotic Features, and Severe With Psychotic Features can be applied only if the criteria are currently met for a Major Depressive Episode. In Partial Remission and In Full Remission can be applied to the most recent Major Depressive Episode in Major Depressive Disorder and to a Major Depressive Episode in Bipolar I or II Disorder only if it is the most recent type of mood episode.

.x1—Mild: Few, if any, symptoms in excess of those required to make the diagnosis and symptoms result in only minor impairment in occupational functioning or in usual social activities or relationships with others.

.x2—Moderate: Symptoms or functional impairment between "mild" and "severe."

.x3—Severe Without Psychotic Features: Several symptoms in excess of those required to make the diagnosis, and symptoms markedly interfere with occupational functioning or with usual social activities or relationships with others.

.x4—Severe With Psychotic Features: Delusions or hallucinations. If possible, specify whether the psychotic features are mood-congruent or mood-incongruent:

Mood-Congruent Psychotic Features: Delusions or hallucinations whose content is entirely consistent with the typical depressive themes of personal inadequacy, guilt, disease, death, nihilism, or deserved punishment.

Mood-Incongruent Psychotic Features: Delusions or hallucinations whose content does not involve typical depressive themes of personal inadequacy, guilt, disease, death, nihilism, or deserved punishment. Included are such symptoms as persecutory delusions (not directly related to depressive themes), thought insertion, thought broadcasting, and delusions of control.

.x5—In Partial Remission: Symptoms of a Major Depressive Episode are present but full criteria are not met, or there is a period without any significant symptoms of a Major Depressive Episode lasting less than 2 months following the end of the Major Depressive Episode. (If the Major Depressive Episode was superimposed on Dysthymic Disorder, the diagnosis of Dysthymic Disorder alone is given once the full criteria for a Major Depressive Episode are no longer met.)

.x6—In Full Remission: During the past 2 months, no significant signs or symptoms of the disturbance were present.

.x0—Unspecified.

Reprinted with permission from the *Diagnostic and Statistical Manual of Mental Disorders*, 4th ed., Text Rev. Copyright 2000 American Psychiatric Association.

DSM-IV-TR Diagnostic Criteria

WITH CATATONIC FEATURES

Specify if:

With Catatonic Features (can be applied to the current or most recent Major Depressive Episode, Manic Episode, or Mixed Episode in Major Depressive Disorder, Bipolar I Disorder, or Bipolar II Disorder)

The clinical picture is dominated by at least two of the following:

A. Motoric immobility as evidenced by catalepsy (including waxy flexibility) or stupor
B. Excessive motor activity (that is apparently purposeless and not influenced by external stimuli)
C. Extreme negativism (an apparently motiveless resistance to all instructions or maintenance of a rigid posture against attempts to be moved) or mutism
D. Peculiarities of voluntary movement as evidenced by posturing (voluntary assumption of inappropriate or bizarre postures), stereotyped movements, prominent mannerisms, or prominent grimacing
E. Echolalia or echopraxia

Reprinted with permission from the *Diagnostic and Statistical Manual of Mental Disorders*, 4th ed., Text Rev. Copyright 2000 American Psychiatric Association.

cation-induced movement disorder leading to catatonic features, or neuroleptic malignant syndrome.

The specifier *with melancholic features* is applied when the depressive episode is characterized by profound loss of interest or pleasure in activities and lack of reactivity to external events as well as usual pleasurable stimuli (see DSM-IV-TR diagnostic criteria, page 257). In addition, at least three of the following melancholic features must be present: depression is typically worse in the morning, early morning awakening, psychomotor change with marked retardation or agitation, significant weight loss, or profound and excessive guilt. A major depressive episode with melancholic features is particularly important to diagnose because of the prediction that it is more likely to respond to somatic treatment, including electroconvulsive therapy. Individuals with melancholic features experience more recurrence of MDD. The findings of hypercortisolism following dexamethasone as well as reduced rapid eye movement (REM) latency is associated with the melancholic episodes of MDD.

Finally, the category of major depressive episode *with atypical features* was previously called "atypical depression." This syndrome is characterized by prominent mood reactivity in which there is responsiveness of the depressed mood to external events and at least two of the following associated features: increased appetite or weight gain, hypersomnia, leaden paralysis (a feeling of profound anergia or heavy feeling), and in-

episode of depression. The specifier *with catatonic features* is used when profound psychomotor retardation, prominent mutism, echolalia, echopraxia, or stupor dominates the clinical picture. The presentation of catatonia requires a differential diagnosis that includes schizophrenia, catatonic type, bipolar I disorder, catatonic disorder due to a general medical condition, medi-

DSM-IV-TR Diagnostic Criteria

WITH MELANCHOLIC FEATURES

Specify if:

With Melancholic Features (can be applied to the current or most recent Major Depressive Episode in Major Depressive Disorder and to a Major Depressive Episode in Bipolar I or Bipolar II Disorder only if it is the most recent type of mood episode)

A. Either of the following, occurring during the most severe period of the current episode:

(1) loss of pleasure in all, or almost all, activities
(2) lack of reactivity to usually pleasurable stimuli (does not feel much better, even temporarily, when something good happens)

B. Three (or more) of the following:

(1) distinct quality of depressed mood (i.e., the depressed mood is experienced as distinctly different from the kind of feeling experienced after the death of a loved one)
(2) depression regularly worse in the morning
(3) early morning awakening (at least 2 hours before usual time of awakening)
(4) marked psychomotor retardation or agitation
(5) significant anorexia or weight loss
(6) excessive or inappropriate guilt.

Reprinted with permission from the *Diagnostic and Statistical Manual of Mental Disorders*, 4th ed., Text Rev. Copyright 2000 American Psychiatric Association.

DSM-IV-TR Diagnostic Criteria

WITH ATYPICAL FEATURES

Specify if:

With Atypical Features (can be applied when these features predominate during the most recent 2 weeks of a current Major Depressive Episode in Major Depressive Disorder or in Bipolar I or Bipolar II Disorder when a current Major Depressive Episode is the most recent type of mood episode, or when these features predominate during the most recent 2 years of Dysthymic Disorder; if the Major Depressive Episode is not current, it applies if the feature predominates during any 2-week period)

A. Mood reactivity (i.e., mood brightens in response to actual or potential positive events)
B. Two (or more) of the following features:

(1) significant weight gain or increase in appetite
(2) hypersomnia
(3) leaden paralysis (i.e., heavy, leaden feelings in arms or legs)
(4) long-standing pattern of interpersonal rejection sensitivity (not limited to episodes of mood disturbance) that results in significant social or occupational impairment

C. Criteria are not met for With Melancholic Features or With Catatonic Features during the same episode.

Reprinted with permission from the *Diagnostic and Statistical Manual of Mental Disorders*, 4th ed., Text Rev. Copyright 2000 American Psychiatric Association.

terpersonal hypersensitivity (rejection sensitivity). Depressive episodes with atypical features are also common in individuals with bipolar I or II disorder as well as seasonal affective disorder.

Course Features. MDD is diagnosed with certain course features such as postpartum onset, seasonal pattern, recurrent, chronic, and with or without full interepisode recovery. Depression *with postpartum onset* has been the subject of increasing attention in psychiatric consultation to obstetrics and gynecology. The specifier applies only to the current or most recent major depressive episode in MDD (or bipolar disorder). The presence of a major depressive episode may occur from 2 weeks to 12 months after delivery, beyond the usual duration of postpartum "blues" (3–7 days). Postpartum blues are brief episodes of labile mood and tearfulness that occur in 50–80% of women within 5 days of delivery. However, depression is seen in 10–20% of women after childbirth, which is higher than rates of depression found in matched controls. There is greater vulnerability in women with prior episodes of major mood disorder, particularly bipolar disorder, and there is a high risk of recurrence with subsequent deliveries after an MDD with postpartum onset. The postpar-

tum onset episodes can present either with or without psychosis. Postpartum psychotic episodes occur in 0.1–0.2% of deliveries. Depression in postpartum psychosis is associated with prominent guilt and may involve individuals with a prior history of bipolar I disorder. If an episode of postpartum psychosis occurs, there is a high risk of recurrence with subsequent deliveries. Heightened attention to identification of postpartum episodes is required because of potential risk of morbidity and mortality to mother and newborn child.

The specifier *with seasonal pattern* is diagnosed when episodes of MDD occur regularly in fall and

DSM-IV-TR Diagnostic Criteria

POSTPARTUM ONSET

Specify if:

With Postpartum Onset (can be applied to the current or most recent Major Depressive, Manic, or Mixed Episode in Major Depressive Disorder, Bipolar I Disorder, or Bipolar II Disorder; or to Brief Psychotic Disorder)
Onset of episode within 4 weeks postpartum.

Reprinted with permission from the *Diagnostic and Statistical Manual of Mental Disorders*, 4th ed., Text Rev. Copyright 2000 American Psychiatric Association.

DSM-IV-TR Diagnostic Criteria

SEASONAL PATTERN

Specify if:

With Seasonal Pattern (can be applied to the pattern of Major Depressive Episodes in Bipolar I Disorder, Bipolar II Disorder, or Major Depressive Disorder, Recurrent)

A. There has been a regular temporal relationship between the onset of Major Depressive Episodes in Bipolar I or Bipolar II Disorder or Major Depressive Disorder, Recurrent, and a particular time of the year (e.g., regular appearance of the Major Depressive Episode in the fall or winter). Note: Do not include cases in which there is an obvious effect of season-related psychosocial stressors (e.g., regularly being unemployed every winter).
B. Full remissions (or a change from depression to mania or hypomania) also occur at a characteristic time of the year (e.g., depression disappears in the spring).
C. In the last 2 years, two Major Depressive Episodes have occurred that demonstrate the temporal seasonal relationships defined in Criteria A and B, and no nonseasonal Major Depressive Episodes have occurred during that same period.
D. Seasonal Major Depressive Episodes (as described above) substantially outnumber the nonseasonal Major Depressive Episodes that may have occurred over the individual's lifetime.

Reprinted with permission from the *Diagnostic and Statistical Manual of Mental Disorders*, 4th ed., Text Rev. Copyright 2000 American Psychiatric Association.

DSM-IV-TR Diagnostic Criteria

WITH AND WITHOUT INTEREPISODE RECOVERY

Specify if (can be applied to Recurrent Major Depressive Disorder or Bipolar I or II Disorder):

With Full Interepisode Recovery: if full remission is attained between the two most recent Mood Episodes
Without Full Interepisode Recovery: if full remission is not attained between the two most recent Mood Episodes

Reprinted with permission from the *Diagnostic and Statistical Manual of Mental Disorders*, 4th ed., Text Rev. Copyright 2000 American Psychiatric Association.

---

winter seasons and subsequently remit during spring and summer. When the pattern of onset and remission occurs for the last 2 years, one diagnoses an MDD with seasonal pattern. Often, this pattern is characterized by atypical features, including low energy, hypersomnia, weight gain, and carbohydrate craving. Although the predominant pattern is fall–winter depression, a minority of individuals show the reverse seasonal pattern with spring–summer depression. Specific forms of light therapy with 2500 lux exposure has been shown to be effective in MDD with seasonal pattern. Because seasonal depression has clinical features that are similar to atypical features, the risk of a possible bipolar II disorder must be considered since atypical features are more common in depressive episodes occurring as part of bipolar II. These individuals, when exposed to antidepressant medication or bright light therapy, may evolve a switch into hypomanic or manic episode.

Clinical and scientific attention to the course of MDD focuses upon the depiction of longitudinal course. Life charting of MDD involves the use of several course specifiers. Each episode is denoted with or without full recovery (see DSM-IV-TR diagnostic criteria, page •••). The specifier chronic MDD involves the persistence of a major depressive episode continually, satisfying full MDD criteria for at least 2 years.

Across epidemiologic studies, MDD is found to be a common psychiatric disorder. The lifetime risk for MDD in community samples varies from 10% to 25% for women and from 5% to 12% for men. The point prevalence of MDD (proportion of the individuals that have the disorder being studied at a designated time) for adults in community samples has varied from 5% to 9% for women and from 2% to 3% for men. The point prevalence of MDD in primary care outpatient settings ranges from 4.8% to 8.6%. In hospitalized individuals for all medical conditions, more than 14% had MDD. While the incidence rates of MDD in prepubertal boys and girls are equal, women over the course of their lifetime are 2 to 3 times more likely to have MDD after puberty.

For preschool children, the point prevalence is thought to be 0.8%. Point prevalences of major and minor depressive disorder of 1.8% and 2.5%, respectively, were found in a 1983 sample of 9-year-old children from the general population, based upon the use of a semistructured diagnostic instrument. A semistructured diagnostic instrument was used to find a 4.7% point prevalence rate of major depressive disorder in a community sample of 150 adolescents. Those adolescents diagnosed with MDD had symptoms that met criteria for dysthymic disorder as well. A point prevalence rate of 3.3% was found for dysthymic disorder.

Changing rates of MDD for recent birth cohorts have been found in North America, Puerto Rico, Western Europe, Middle East, Asia, and the Pacific Rim. Specifically, an earlier age of onset and increased rate of depression occur in individuals born in more recent decades. Historical, social, economic, or biological events most likely account for the variability in the rate of depression noted in different countries included in the study. However, an overall increase in the rate of depression has been noted across many of the geographic locations.

Older adults continue to manifest a higher suicide rate than in younger age groups. However, suicide rates have increased in younger age groups as the changing rate of MDD is observed in younger cohorts. In keeping with the birth cohort effect, recurrences of MDD in late life may become a significant health concern as the population ages.

Course

The mean age of onset of major depression is 27 years of age, although an individual can experience the onset of MDD at any age. New symptoms of MDD often develop over several days to several weeks. Early manifestations of an episode of MDD include anxiety, sleeplessness, worry, and rumination prior to the experience of overt depression. Over a lifetime, the presence of one major depressive episode is associated with a 50% chance of a recurrent episode. A history of two episodes is associated with a 70–80% risk of a future episode. Three or more episodes are associated with extremely high rates of recurrence. Because the majority of cases of MDD recur, continuation treatment and ongoing education regarding warning signs of relapse or recurrence are essential in ongoing clinical care.

In comparison to individuals who develop a single episode (many of whom return to premorbid functioning), individuals with recurrent episodes of depression are at greater risk to manifest bipolar disorder. Individuals who experience several recurrent episodes of depression may develop a hypomanic or manic episode requiring rediagnosis to bipolar disorder. In children and adolescents, the transformation of a diagnosis of depression to a diagnosis of bipolar disorder is higher. Approximately 40% of adolescents who are depressed evolve into a bipolar course. Because bipolar disorder is initiated with a depressive episode in at least 4 of 5 cases, it is important to identify those individuals who are most likely to develop a bipolar disorder. Therefore, the clinician is confronted with significant diagnostic and treatment challenges when called upon to evaluate an individual, particularly an adolescent, who presents with depression and has no previous history of mania. Several risk factors have been identified which predict when a first episode of MDD will evolve into bipolar disorder: (1) the first episode of depression emerges during adolescence; (2) the depression is severe and includes psychotic features; (3) psychomotor retardation and hypersomnia are present; (4) a family history of bipolar disorder exists, particularly across two to three generations; and (5) the individual experiences hypomania induced by antidepressant medication.

Recurrent MDD requires longitudinal observation because of its highly variable course. Generally, complete remission of an episode of MDD heralds a return to premorbid levels of social, occupational, and interpersonal functioning. Therefore, the goal of treatment is in achieving full remission of depressive symptoms and recovery. Untreated episodes of depression last 6 to 24 months. Symptom remission and a return to premorbid level of functioning characterize approximately 66% of depressed individuals. By comparison, roughly 5–10% of individuals continue to experience a full episode of depression for greater than 2 years and approximately 20–25% of individuals experience partial recovery between episodes. Furthermore, 25% of the individuals manifest "double depression," characterized by the development of MDD superimposed upon a mild, chronic dysthymic disorder (DD). Individuals with double depression often demonstrate poor interepisode recovery. The following four characteristics are seen in a partial remission of an episode: (1) increased likelihood of a subsequent episode; (2) partial interepisode recovery following subsequent episodes; (3) possible requirement of longer-term treatment; and (4) treatment with a combination of pharmacotherapy and psychotherapy may be indicated.

Follow-up naturalistic studies have indicated that 40% of individuals with MDD carry the same diagnosis 1 year later, 3% evidence DD, 17% manifest incomplete recovery, and 40% do not meet criteria for MDD. A significant percentage of individuals with MDD have persist chronic symptoms of MDD. A 5-year follow-up study of MDD indicated that 50% of the individuals showed recovery by 6 months but 12% of the sample continued to be depressed for the entire 5-year period. The authors of this study noted that inadequate treatment may have contributed to the chronicity.

Poor outcome and likelihood of recurrent episodes is associated with comorbid conditions such as personality disorder, active substance or alcohol abuse, organicity, or medical illness. Recurrence and outcome may be affected by the rapidity of clinical intervention. Inadequate treatment (e.g., insufficient dosing or duration of pharmacotherapy) contributes to poor outcome, including chronic MDD. Early treatment intervention in an episode of MDD may be relatively more effective than later intervention in an episode.

Depression in the Medically Ill

Whereas a 4–5% current prevalence rate of MDD exists in community samples, symptoms of depression are found in 12–36% of individuals with a general medical condition. The rate of depression may be higher in individuals with a specific medical condition. MDD is identified as an independent condition and calls for specific treatment when it occurs in the presence of a general medical condition.

Four possible relationships have been identified between depression and a general medical condition: (1) depression is biologically caused by the general medical condition, (2) an individual who carries a genetic vulnerability to MDD manifests the onset of depression triggered by the general medical condition, (3) depression is psychologically caused by the general medical condition, and (4) no causal relationship exists between the general medical condition and mood disorder. The first two cases warrant initial treatment directed at the general medical condition. Treatment is advocated for persistent depression upon stabilization of the general medical condition. When the general medical condition causes depression, specific treatment for the former condition is optimized, while psychiatric management, education, and antidepressant medication are administered to treat the depression. In cases where the two conditions are not etiologically related, appropriate treatment is indicated for each disorder.

Stroke. Some poststroke patients manifest depression owing to cerebrovascular disease related to cerebral infarction in left frontal and left subcortical brain regions. Mood disorder due to cerebrovascular disease is diagnosed when an individual manifests a recent stroke and has significant symptoms of depression. A point prevalence of mood disorder due to cerebrovascular disease in poststroke patients between 10% and 27% has been documented, with an average duration of depression lasting approximately 1 year. Case reports of mood disorder due to cerebrovascular disease in poststroke individuals suggest poor treatment compliance, irritability, and personality change.

Alzheimer's Disease. According to DSM-IV-TR, when symptoms of clinically significant depressed mood accompany dementia of the Alzheimer's type, and in the clinician's judgment, the depression is due to the direct physiological effects of the Alzheimer's disease, mood disorder due to Alzheimer's disease is diagnosed. When dementia consistent with cerebrovascular disease leads to prominent cognitive deficits, focal neurological signs and symptoms, significant impairment in functioning as well as predominant depressed mood, vascular dementia with depressed mood is diagnosed. The distinction between depressive disorders and dementia is often complicated because depression and dementia commonly co-occur. Treatment of co-occurring depressive features may relieve symptoms and improve overall quality of life.

Parkinson's Disease. Fifty percent of individuals with Parkinson's disease experience an MDD during the course of the illness. When depression occurs in this context, one diagnoses mood disorder due to Parkinson's disease. Active treatment of the depressive disorder may result in improvement in the signs and symptoms of depression without alleviation of the involuntary movement disorder or cognitive changes associated with subcortical brain disease. The underlying etiology of associated dementia and depressive disorder in Parkinson's disease appears to involve physiologic changes in subcortical brain regions.

Diabetes. It is estimated that the prevalence of depression in treated individuals with diabetes is three times as frequent than in the general population. Further, there is no difference in the prevalence rate of depression in individuals with insulin-dependent diabetes mellitus (Type I) in comparison with individuals with noninsulin-dependent mellitus (Type II). The symptomatic presentation of MDD in individuals with diabetes is similar to individuals without diabetes. Consequently, full assessment of and treatment for MDD is recommended in individuals who become depressed during the course of diabetes. The relatively high point prevalence rate may be due to higher detection rate in this treated population having a chronic illness as well as metabolic and endocrine factors.

Coronary Artery Disease. When MDD is present, increased morbidity and mortality is reported in postmyocardial infarction patients as well as in individuals having coronary artery disease without myocardial infarction (MI). Therefore, treatment of MDD in individuals with coronary artery disease is indicated. Prevalence estimates of MDD in postmyocardial infarction range from 40% to 65%. Over a 15-month period, individuals 55 years or older who had mood disorder evidenced a mortality rate four times higher than expected, and coronary heart disease or stroke accounted for 63% of the deaths. Depression may promote poor adherence to cardiac rehabilitation and worse outcome. During the first year following MI, depression is considered to be associated with a three- to fourfold increase in subsequent cardiovascular morbidity and mortality. Depression in individuals with coronary artery disease is associated with more social problems, functional impairment, and increased health care utilization.

Cancer. MDD occurs in 25% of individuals with cancer at some time during the illness. MDD should be assessed and treated as an independent disorder. The intense reaction in individuals diagnosed with cancer may lead to dysphoria and sadness without evolving a full syndrome of MDD. The consulting clinician must evaluate the individual's response to chemotherapy, side effects of the treatment, and medication interactions in the overall assessment of the individual. Among individuals with cancer, MDD is typically characterized by heightened distress, impaired functioning, and decreased capacity to adhere to treatment. Treating comorbid MDD with psychotherapy or pharmacotherapy may improve the overall outcome in individuals with cancer and mitigate complications of MDD.

Chronic Fatigue Syndrome. Lifetime rates of MDD in individuals with chronic fatigue syndrome range from 46% to 75%. Comorbid anxiety and somatization disorders are also common in individuals with chronic fatigue. According to the Centers for Disease Control (CDC) criteria, the diagnosis of chronic fatigue syndrome is excluded in individuals whose symptoms meet criteria for a formal mental disorder, such as MDD or DD. Individuals whose symptoms meet criteria for both a mood disorder and a chronic fatigue syndrome should be maximally treated for the mood disorder with appropriate pharmacotherapy and cognitive–behavioral psychotherapy. The etiological relationship between mood disorder and chronic fatigue syndrome is unclear.

Fibromyalgia. In comparison with other general medical conditions, little is known about the relationship between fibromyalgia and MDD. Two studies have found higher lifetime rates of major mood disorder in fibromyalgia patients in comparison with rheumatoid arthritis patients.

Depression due to Medications

If MDD is judged to be a direct physiologic effect of a medication, then substance-induced mood disorder is diagnosed. Medications reported to cause depression involve several drugs from the associated groups listed in Table 26-1.

Among antihypertensive treatment, beta-adrenergic blockers have been studied regarding the risk of depression. No significant differences are found between individuals treated with beta-blockers and those treated with other antihypertensives regarding the propensity to develop depressive symptoms. Lethargy is the most common side effect reported. No significant depressive complications are reported with calcium channel

Table 26-1	Medications Associated with Depression	
Cardiovascular Drugs	Hormones	Psychotropics
Methyldopa	Oral contraceptives	Benzodiazepines
Reserpine	Corticotropin and glucocorticoids	Neuroleptics
Propranolol	Anabolic steroids	
Guanethidine		
Clonidine		
Thiazide diuretics		
Digitalis		
Anticancer Agents	Anti-inflammatory and anti-infective agents	Others
Cycloserine	Nonsteroidal anti-inflammatory agents	Cocaine (withdrawal)
	Ethambutol	Amphetamines (withdrawal)
	Disulfiram	Levodopa
	Sulfonamides	Cimetidine
	Baclofen	Ranitidine
	Metoclopramide	

blockers or angiotensin converting enzyme (ACE) inhibitors.

Hormonal treatments, such as corticosteroids and anabolic steroids, can elicit depression, mania, or psychosis. Oral contraceptives require monitoring regarding the possible precipitation of depressive symptoms.

Because individuals with seizure disorders and Parkinson's disease are at high risk for concomitant MDD, it is difficult to establish a link between anticonvulsant or anti-Parkinsonian treatment and the precipitation of depression. Nevertheless, individuals require close monitoring and evaluation for evolution of depressive symptomatology.

Comorbid Depression with Other Mental Disorders

More than 40% of individuals with MDD have additional symptoms that meet criteria during their lifetime for one or more additional mental disorders. In a recent community sample, assessing both pure and comorbid MDD, the current prevalence of major depression was 4.9%. Of the sample with current MDD, 56.3% also had another mental disorder. The presence of a comorbid mental disorder may alter the course of major mood disorder in a dramatic fashion and is identified as a primary risk factor for poor treatment response. Therefore, proper assessment, preferably with the use of a semistructured diagnostic instrument, additional informants, and longitudinal observation, will identify comorbid conditions.

Alcohol/Drug Dependence. Results of family and twin studies in a population-based female sample are consistent with a modest correlation of the liability between alcohol dependence and MDD. It is common for individuals with alcohol dependence to evidence signs of depression or MDD, but alcoholism is not thought to be a common consequence of mood disorder. Between 10% and 30% of individuals with alcoholism manifest depression, whereas alcoholism is thought to occur in under 5% of depressed individuals.

Depressed women are more likely to self-medicate their mood disorder with alcohol than are depressed men. The effect of comorbid alcoholism on the course of major mood disorder is unclear. Some evidence suggests that remission of depression occurs within the first month of sobriety. The effect of comorbid depression requires further attention in relation to the course of drug dependence. Drug dependence is often associated with major mood disorder and the presence of associated comorbid personality disorder.

Panic/Phobias/GAD. The co-occurrence of symptoms of anxiety and depression is very common. Very high genetic correlations between MDD and generalized anxiety disorder have been found in contrast to only a modest overlap between phobic disorders and MDD. Anxiety symptoms commonly appear in depressive syndromes and MDD is frequently comorbid with anxiety disorders. From a longitudinal perspective, either symptom constellation can be a precursor to the development of the other disorder. The combination of anxiety and depression predicts greater severity and impairment than the presence of each syndrome in isolation. The association of severe panic and MDD is one of the predictors of suicidal risk. The clinician is advised to assess for symptoms of each disorder and to obtain a thorough family history. Individuals with anxiety disorders often experience prior episodes of MDD or have relatives who suffer from mood disorder.

Of outpatients with MDD, 10–20% evidence comorbid panic disorder while 30–40% of depressed outpatients have had symptoms that met criteria for generalized anxiety disorder during the course of the mood disorder. In both cases, the anxiety disorder has preceded the major mood disorder about 50% of the time.

The clinician is advised to evaluate three factors in order to determine treatment approaches when MDD co-occurs with panic disorder or social phobia: (1) the individual's family history, (2) the constellation of symptoms that were first evident in the current episode, and (3) the symptoms that cause the individual the most distress.

Recovery is less likely and symptomatology more severe in individuals with comorbid MDD and panic disorder than in cases with a single diagnosis. Lifetime suicide rate is twice as high for individuals with comorbid panic disorder and MDD than in panic disorder alone. It is imperative to assess for the presence of mood disorder and suicidality among individuals who present with symptoms of anxiety.

Obsessive–Compulsive Disorder. The occurrence of symptoms of depression is very common in individuals with obsessive–compulsive disorder (OCD), although full symptom criteria may not be reached to warrant a formal diagnosis of MDD. Of individuals with OCD, 10–30% have mood symptoms that meet full criteria for MDD. The relationship between OCD and schizophrenia is less clear. Individuals with OCD are at an increased risk to develop MDD but not schizophrenia. It is important to distinguish between obsessive–compulsive personality features that can accompany, and can exacerbate during, an episode of depression and OCD itself. Symptoms of depression often diminish with successful initial treatment of OCD, since biological treatments typically involve use of selective serotonergic antidepressant medications such as clomipramine, fluoxetine, or fluvoxamine.

Posttraumatic Stress Disorder. Individuals with PTSD often experience co-occurring depressive disorders, anxiety disorders, and substance use disorders. The range of reported rates of concurrent depressive disorder in individuals with PTSD is 30–50%. Many of the symptoms of PTSD overlap with signs and symptoms of depression such that both PTSD and MDD can be considered to be the result of traumatic events. In addition, depressive disorder may be associated with worse outcome in individuals with co-occurring PTSD.

Somatization Disorder. It is common for individuals with MDD to experience somatic symptoms including pain, although the intensity and frequency of the somatic complaints and the range of body systems affected do not usually meet criteria for somatization disorder. Individuals who have mood symptoms that meet criteria for MDD evidence more complaints of pain, experience more physical, interpersonal, and occupational limitations, and perceive their overall health as worse than individuals with chronic medical illness. The clinician should carefully evaluate for the presence of MDD in cases where the individual reports unexplained pain. Typically, pain complaints are relieved upon successful treatment of the MDD. However, somatoform disorders, as outlined in DSM-IV-TR, may be associated with demoralization and depression.

Eating Disorders. There are little data available regarding prevalence of eating disorders in individuals with MDD. However, 33–50% of individuals with anorexia nervosa or bulimia nervosa experience a comorbid mood disorder. Between 50% and 75% of individuals with an eating disorder have a history of an MDD over a lifetime. Initial treatment is aimed at the eating disorder. If depression continues after proper nourishment has been reestablished in anorexia nervosa, treatment is directed at the primary mood disorder.

Personality Disorders. High rates of personality disorders are found in depressed inpatients and outpatients. Most studies report a rate of co-occurrence between 30% and 40% in outpatients and between 50% and 60% in inpatient samples. Several studies have found that individuals with comorbid MDD and personality disorder evidence an earlier age of onset for the first episode of depression, increased severity of depressive symptoms, more episodes, longer duration of episodes, poorer response to both pharmacotherapy and psychotherapy, and increased risk for self-injury.

Grief and Bereavement. Depressive symptoms associated with normal grieving usually begin within 2 to 3 weeks of the loss and resolve spontaneously over 6 to 8 weeks. If full symptom criteria for MDD persist for more than 2 months beyond the death of a loved one, then an episode of MDD can be diagnosed. Specific treatment for a major depressive episode such as short-term psychotherapy focusing on unresolved grief or pharmacotherapy is indicated.

Depression in Children and Adolescents

In prepubertal children, MDD occurs equally among boys and girls. MDD in childhood is considered to have high recurrence rates with up to 70% recurrence in 5 years. After puberty, girls experience an increased rate of depression as compared to boys. There is an increased risk of depressive disorder in children and adolescents when one or more of the parents are depressed. The earlier the age of onset of depression, the higher the familiar loading. In addition, a number of childhood psychosocial risk factors have been identified to be associated with juvenile-onset MDD. These risk factors include more perinatal insults, motor skill abnormalities, instability in caregivers, and psychopathology in the first-degree relatives. Adolescent-onset depression often takes on a more chronic course associated with dysthymic symptoms. In adolescence, MDD appears to be associated with greater fatigue, worthlessness, and more prominent vegetative signs, while DD has more prominent changes in mood, irritability, anger, and hopelessness. The signs and symptoms used for diagnosis in children and adolescents are identical to those used for diagnosis in adults except that irritable mood can substitute for depressed mood. The sequelae of depression in children and adolescents is often characterized by disruption in school performance, social withdrawal, increased behavioral disruption, and substance abuse. Differential diagnosis among children and adolescents with MDD include behavioral disorders such as conduct disorder, attention deficit hyperactivity disorder, and bipolar disorder.

Later-onset MDD in adolescents is also associated with decline in school performance, social withdrawal, or disruptive behavior. The critical differential diagnostic consideration in adolescents with MDD is the misdiagnosis of depression when the clinical presentation will evolve into a diagnosis of bipolar disorder. When depression occurs during adolescence, it often heralds a severe disorder with recurrent course, and a family history of MDD is often noted. An additional psychosocial risk factor in later-onset depression in adolescence is childhood sexual abuse.

Major Depressive Disorder in the Older Adult

Older adults with depression often experience cognitive impairment as part of the clinical syndrome. Symptoms of depression may simulate dementia with concentration difficulties, memory loss, and distractibility. Commonly, MDD and dementia co-occur. It is less frequent that findings of dementia are fully explained on the basis of depression (pseudodementia). The prevalence of MDD in older adults residing in nursing homes is estimated to be approximately 30%. MDD in the elderly often co-occurs in the presence of medical conditions, which complicates the treatment for both the depression and the primary medical condition. Careful evaluation of medications may also reveal explanations for associated symptoms of depression. Older adults with first onset of depression must be carefully evaluated for co-occurring medical conditions. Among the common disorders to be considered are silent cerebral ischemic events, undiagnosed cancer, or complications of metabolic conditions such as adult-onset diabetes mellitus and thyroid dysfunction.

TREATMENT

The goals of treatment in MDD are full remission of symptoms of depression with restoration of optimal work and social functioning. During the course of treatment, ongoing education of the individual and family regarding remission, relapse, and recurrence is critical. This education alerts both those affected by the illness and their families to the early signs of relapse and can assist in prevention of recurrence. Improved social and work functioning following an episode of depression is an important associated goal of treatment. Many studies have demonstrated the benefit of depression-specific psychotherapy as an important aspect of maintaining remission and improving work and social functioning. The establishment of a collaborative working relationship among the individual with depression, the family, and the clinician is an essential aspect of recovery.

All treatment, whether pharmacotherapy or psychotherapy or the integration of pharmacotherapy and psychotherapy, first requires a well-established diagnostic formulation in order to achieve optimal response to treatment. As the diagnostic process is undertaken, an ongoing therapeutic alliance must be established. In the treatment of MDD, an understanding of the clinical history of each individual's distress is necessary. As the clinical history is elicited, the appropriate target signs and symptoms of MDD are obtained and the individual is educated as to the nature of the symptom patterns that represent his or her unique form of depressive disorder.

The phases of treatment include:

1. An acute phase directed at reduction and elimination of depressive signs and symptoms, and active restoration of psychosocial and work functioning.
2. A continuation phase directed at prevention of relapse and reduction of recurrence through ongoing education, pharmacotherapy, and depression-specific psychotherapy.
3. A maintenance phase of treatment directed at prevention of future episodes of depression based upon the individual's personal history of relapse and recurrence.

Acute phase treatment may involve all interventions that are directed toward decreasing signs and symptoms of depression and maintaining the individual's capacity to work and interact with others in a manner consistent with premorbid levels of social and work functioning. The acute phase treatments may include supportive psychotherapy focusing on resolution of current disputes. A form of supportive therapy may be combined with recommendations for pharmacotherapy. The standard pharmacotherapies that are available for treatment of depression have increased dramatically in the past two decades. In mild to moderate depressive disorder, more depression-specific forms of psychotherapy have been established, including cognitive–behavioral

psychotherapy, interpersonal psychotherapy, or short-term dynamic psychotherapy. In these forms of psychotherapy, which have been studied to address mild to moderate nonbipolar depressive disorder, the focus of the psychotherapy is very clearly explicated to the individual before the initiation of the psychotherapy. For severe depressive disorder with melancholic or psychotic features, these specific forms of short-term psychotherapy may not be as effective as focused pharmacotherapy. Pharmacotherapy, in these conditions, is associated with more rapid treatment response than is psychotherapy.

During the acute phase of treatment for depressive disorder, the optimal treatment should result in resolution of depressive signs and symptoms any time between week 8 and week 16 of treatment. If resolution of depressive signs and symptoms does not occur during the first 2 to 4 months, then the initial diagnostic formulation must be reviewed and alternative treatment strategies must be introduced. Some of the factors associated with lack of complete treatment response include the presence of co-occurring personality disorders, concurrent alcohol or substance abuse, a poor therapeutic alliance leading to lack of adherence to treatment recommendations, and persistent or unfavorable side effects of treatment.

When acute phase treatment does lead to remission of signs and symptoms, then the next phase of treatment begins. This phase of treatment is termed continuation treatment and its goal is prevention of relapse. It is often necessary to maintain ongoing pharmacotherapy for 6 to 12 months after an acute episode of depression during this continuation phase, because there is substantial vulnerability to relapse if medication treatment is prematurely interrupted. During the continuation phase, ongoing psychotherapy may be particularly important to address residual symptoms of depression and to alert the individual to a depressive response to subsequent traumatic circumstances; ongoing clinical interaction with significant others is required as well in order to address persisting interpersonal conflicts, and may promote even more complete recovery from the depressive episode. The continuation phase of treatment typically lasts 9 to 12 months to minimize the risk of recurrent episode. If this represents the initial episode of depression, then medication treatment may be carefully withdrawn at the end of the continuation phase. However, if this represents a history of recurrence of depression (particularly two or more episodes in the preceding 3 years), maintenance treatment may well be recommended. In addition, maintenance treatment is recommended if two prior episodes have occurred within one's lifetime.

Maintenance treatment of MDD is focused on prevention of future episodes of depression, after a recent recurrence of MDD and a prior history of two or more episodes of MDD. Often, the maintenance phase of treatment involves ongoing treatment with antidepressants or alternatively mood-stabilizing treatment (particularly lithium carbonate), or a combination to sustain recovery from depression. When there is early onset (adolescent onset) of depressive symptoms with associated psychosocial impairment, then ongoing maintenance treatment along with rehabilitative psychotherapy may be most critical. During maintenance treatment, continuing education of the individual and family, identification of prodromal symptoms, and continuing efforts at work and psychosocial rehabilitation are indicated. Often, the trials of maintenance pharmacotherapy in depression demonstrate the preventive benefit of maintenance medication. In the study quoted most often, recurrence rates of 20–25% were found in individuals maintained with full dose of imipramine, while the recurrence rate was 80–100% in those individuals treated with placebo. The advantage of ongoing maintenance medicine has also been demonstrated at 5 to 10 years. With tricyclic antidepressants, maintenance medication is likely more effective at full dose rather than lower doses. Limited data exists as to the dosing of SSRIs or other types of antidepressants in maintenance treatment.

The site of treatment for MDD is based upon the severity of the acute episode and the clinician's judgment of the individual's potential for suicide. Individuals with mild to moderate depression are often treated in primary care or specialty office settings. Acute phase pharmacotherapy involving antidepressant medication is often initiated by a primary care physician. However, the overall longitudinal care of MDD in primary care is the subject of increasing attention. Typically, individuals do not receive treatment for long enough periods and there is limited attention to the domains of social or work functioning. The referral to a psychiatrist may include a request for more expertise regarding medication as well as the need for depression-specific psychotherapy. In addition, there has been a lack of focused attention to the role of integrated psychotherapy and pharmacotherapy in primary care. Inpatient treatment for depression is recommended when there is an immediate risk for suicide or recent suicide attempt. In these settings, safety of the individual is the primary concern and often, more intensive treatments including electroconvulsive therapy may be initiated. When there are comorbid general medical conditions and mental disorders, inpatient psychiatric hospitalization may be useful in stabilizing both the general medical condition as well as the associated mental disorder.

Pharmacotherapy and Other Somatic Treatment

Treatment during the acute phase with medication is highly efficacious in reducing signs and symptoms of MDD. Antidepressant medication has the most specific effect on reduction of symptoms and is often associated with improved psychosocial functioning. When symptoms of depression are mild to moderate, a course of depression-specific psychotherapy without medicine may also be effective. If symptoms of depression are moderate to severe, acute phase treatment with medications is often indicated. A wide variety of antidepressant medications have been documented as effective in moderate to severe MDD.

The range of treatments available in the United States has included the tricyclic antidepressants available since the 1960s, MAOIs available since the late 1950s, heterocyclic antidepressants available since the 1970s, and between 1989 and until the present, newer SSRIs have been available. In addition, antidepressants with both serotonergic and noradrenergic activity or noradrenergic activity alone have become available in the 1990s. Clearly, clinical trials comparing the efficacy of newer treatments with standard tricyclic antidepressants have shown equal efficacy with improvement in overall tolerance to side effects with newer treatments.

Antidepressant medications that are currently available for acute treatment of MDD are listed in (Table 26-2).

Choice of treatment with a specific antidepressant treatment in a given clinical situation is based on prior treatment response to medication, consideration of potential side effects, history of response to medicines in first-degree relatives, and the associated presence of co-occurring mental disorders that may lead to a more specific choice of antidepressant treatment. Table 26-3 illustrates an algorithm developed for pharmacotherapy of MDD, which includes a staged trial of newer medications (because of their superior side-effect profiles) followed by treatments with older medicines available for the treatment of MDD. The ultimate goal of pharmacotherapy is complete remission of symptoms during a standard 6- to 12-week course of treatment.

Selective Serotonin Reuptake Inhibitors. The most commonly prescribed antidepressant medicines in the past 10 years are SSRIs. They are selectively active at serotonergic neurochemical pathways and are

Table 26-2   Antidepressant Medications Category

Category			Side Effects			
Trade Name	Compound	Usual Therapeutic Dose (mg)	Sedation	Hypotension (Decreased Blood Pressure)	Anticholinergic (i.e., Dry Mouth, Constipation)	Cardiac (Slowed Heart Rate)
Tricyclics						
Tertiary amines						
Anafranil	Clomipramine	150–300	High	High	High	Yes
Elavil	Amitriptyline	150–300	High	High	High	Yes
Sinequan	Doxepin	150–300	High	Moderate	Moderate	Yes
Surmontil	Trimipramine	150–300	High	Moderate	Moderate	Yes
Tofranil	Imipramine	150–300	Moderate	High	Moderate	Yes
Norpramine	Desipramine	100–300	Low	High	Low	Yes
Pamelor	Nortriptyline	50–150	Moderate	Low	Low	Yes
Vivactil	Protriptyline	20–60	Low	Low	High	Yes
Monoamine Oxidase inhibitors						
Marplan	Isocarboxazid	30–60	Low	Moderate	Low	Low
Nardil	Phenelzine	45–90	Low	Moderate	Low	Low
Parnate	Tranylcypromine	30–90	Low	Moderate	Low	Low
Atypical agents						
Ascendin	Amoxapine	200–300	Low	Moderate	Low	Yes
Desyrel	Trazodone	300–600	High	High	Minimal	Low
Ludiomil	Maprotiline	150–200	Moderate	Moderate	Low	Low
Wellbutrin	Bupropion	150–450	Minimal	Low	Minimal	Yes
Selective serotonin reuptake inhibitors						
Paxil	Paroxetine	20–50	Low	Minimal	Minimal	Low
Prozac	Fluoxetine	20–100	Minimal	Minimal	Minimal	Low
Zoloft	Sertraline	50–300	Minimal	Minimal	Minimal	Low
Luvox	Fluvoxamine	150–400	Low	Low	Low	Low
Celexa	Citalopram	20–50	Minimal	None	None	Minimal
Lexapro	Escitalopram	10–30	Minimal	None	None	Minimal
Serotonin/ norepinephrine reuptake inhibitors						
Effexor	Venlafaxine	75–450	Low	None	None	Minimal
Cymbalta	Duloxetine	30–60	Low	None	None	Minimal
Alpha-2- adrenergic antagonist						
Remeron	Mirtazapine	30–60	Moderate	Low	Minimal	Minimal

effective in mild to moderate nonbipolar depression. They may also be particularly effective in MDD with atypical features as well as DD. Often, these treatments are well tolerated and involve single daily dosing for MDD. Because of selective serotonergic activity, these treatments have also been demonstrated to be effective with co-occurring OCD, panic disorder, generalized anxiety disorder, PTSD, premenstrual dysphoric disorder, bulimia nervosa, and social anxiety disorder as well as MDD. They tend to be reasonably well tolerated in individuals with comorbid medical conditions. There are particular medication-specific interactions based on inhibition of cytochrome P-450 liver enzyme systems that require attention if an individual

is taking other medications for primary medical conditions or associated mental disorders. The currently available SSRIs in the United States include fluoxetine (Prozac), paroxetine (Paxil), sertraline (Zoloft), fluvoxamine, citalopram (Celexa), and escitalopram (Lexapro).

Other Newer Antidepressants. In addition to SS-RIs, greater attention has been brought to medicines with dual noradrenergic and serotonergic pathways, including venlafaxine (Effexor XR) and duloxetine (Cymbalta). In addition, an alpha-2-adrenergic agonist, mirtazapine (Remeron) has become available. A predominantly noradrenergic and dopaminergic agonist,

Table 26-3	Pharmacotherapy Algorithm in Major Depressive Disorder

Major Depressive Disorder, Single or Recurrent Episode, without Psychotic Features
Begin effective monotherapy with bupropion SR, citalopram, escitalopram, fluoxetine, nefazodone, paroxetine, sertraline, venlafaxine XR, or duloxetine (augment with lithium carbonate 600–900 mg).

or

Begin effective monotherapy with alternative antidepressant from list above (augment with bupropion SR, mirtazapine, or tricyclic antidepressant, either nortriptyline or desipramine, recognizing important drug interactions.
If ineffective, consider tranylcypromine, augmented with lithium carbonate, if necessary, for anergic features.

or

Consider phenelzine, augmented with lithium carbonate, if necessary, for anxious, dependent, and phobic features.
Augment with atypical antipsychotics for agitation, rumination, or suspicion.

or

Offer electroconvulsive therapy to remission (ECT).

Major Depressive Disorder, Single or Recurrent Episode, with Psychotic Features
Begin typical or atypical antipsychotic to adequate doses in order to interrupt delusional features, augmented with SSRI, venlafaxine XR, or tricyclic antidepressants, either nortriptyline or desipramine, recognizing important drug interactions.

or

Begin amoxapine as alternative.

or

Begin electroconvulsive therapy as alternative, in context of immediate suicide risk, physical deterioration, or prior response to electroconvulsive therapy

Major Depressive Disorder with Atypical Features
Begin SSRI starting at low dose to minimize early side effects.

or

Begin MAOI, either phenelzine or tranylcypromine, to therapeutic doses.

Major Depressive Disorder with Catatonic Features
Begin lorazepam 1–3 mg/d, to interrupt catatonic symptoms; evaluate for presence of psychotic features or longitudinal history of bipolar disorder.
Add antipsychotic medication to therapeutic doses or lithium carbonate to therapeutic doses, if bipolar or schizoaffective disorder emerges from the longitudinal history.

bupropion (Wellbutrin), is also available in an immediate release, sustained release (SR), and extended release (XL) preparation.

Tricyclic Antidepressants. Tricyclic antidepressants have been best studied in individuals with MDD with melancholic features and with psychotic features. The combination of typical antipsychotic pharmacotherapy in association with tricyclic antidepressants has been recommended. The side-effect profile of tricyclic antidepressants has included moderate to severe sedation, anticholinergic effects including constipation, and cardiac effects, which has made these medicines less popular in typical primary care or psychiatric practice. Nevertheless, the secondary amines that are metabolites of imipramine and amitriptyline, specifically desipramine and nortriptyline, have continued to be useful agents in more refractory depression.

Monoamine Oxidase Inhibitors. There continues to be a role for the use of MAOIs in individuals with MDD with atypical features. These agents may be particularly useful in intervention in depressive episodes with atypical features, characterized by prominent mood reactivity, reverse neurovegetative symptom patterns (i.e., overeating and oversleeping), and marked interpersonal rejection sensitivity. MAOIs continue to have a significant role in treatment of comorbid panic disorder, social phobia, and agoraphobia if individuals are not responsive to SSRIs. The ongoing prescription of phenelzine (Nardil) or tranylcypromine (Parnate) requires continued education of the individual regarding standard food interactions involving tyramine as well as specific drug–drug interactions involving sympathomimetic medications. These cautions regarding diet and drug interaction make MAO inhibitors less attractive to primary care physicians and most psychiatrists. However, they continue to be effective treatments that may be useful in depression with atypical features as well as anergic bipolar depression.

General Recommendations. Increasingly, a trial of one class of antidepressants may be associated with incomplete response, leading to a question of augmenting a treatment with another medicine versus switching from one medicine to another within the same class or to a different class altogether.

All of the antidepressant medications used in the treatment of MDD must be prescribed in the context of an overall clinical relationship characterized by supportive interaction with the individual and family and ongoing education about the nature of the disorder and its treatment. Clinical management optimally involves careful monitoring of symptoms using standardized instruments and careful attention to side effects of medication in order to promote treatment adherence. Outpatient visits, which may be scheduled weekly at the outset of treatment, and subsequently biweekly, encourage and sustain collaborative treatment relationships. These office consultations allow the clinician to make dosage adjustments as indicated, monitor side effects, and measure clinical response to treatment.

For the majority of individuals with MDD, a course of 6 to 8 weeks of acute treatment with weekly outpatient visits is indicated. Subsequent office visits may be scheduled every 2 to 4 weeks during the continuation phase of treatment. Appropriate adjustments of dose are determined by the psychiatrist as indicated by best clinical judgments of medication effect. Optimal dosing ranges of SSRIs, tricyclics, and MAOIs are noted in Table 26-2. Because of the early anxiety, agitation, and occasional insomnia associated with SSRIs, somewhat lower doses may be initiated early in the course before achieving the typical standard therapeutic dose.

Incomplete response, which entails the failure to respond to acute treatment with an antidepressant medication at 6 to 8 weeks, requires reassessment of diagnosis and determination of adequacy of dosing. Ongoing substance abuse, associated general medical condition, or concurrent mental disorder may partially explain a lack of complete response. If substance dependence is present, a full substance-free interval (preferably 4 weeks or longer) with appropriate detoxification and rehabilitation may be indicated. If a reassessment discloses an associated mental disorder, then more specific treatment of that associated disorder, whether it be bipolar disorder or concurrent posttraumatic disorder, is necessary. If the reassessment suggests an associated comorbid personality disorder, then appropriate and more specialized psychotherapy may be necessary in order to achieve a complete response to treatment. As indicated before, if the MDD has psychotic features, then antipsychotic pharmacotherapy to adequate doses must be initiated prior to initiating a course of standard tricyclic antidepressants or a combined serotonin norepinephrine uptake inhibitor such as venlafaxine or duloxetine. If MDD is associated with severe personality disorder (e.g., borderline personality disorder), then adjunctive psychotherapy and low dose antipsychotic medications may be necessary. If the individual has severe melancholic, delusional, or catatonic features, a course of electroconvulsive therapy may be necessary to achieve remission of symptoms.

There is also evidence that continuation of treatment beyond 6 to 12 weeks may convert some partial responders to responders if drug treatment is increased to full doses. This time allows for evaluation of the role of focused psychotherapy to address residual interpersonal disputes, loss or grief, or ongoing social deficits. The associated augmentation strategies to standard treatments include lithium carbonate augmentation, tricyclic antidepressant augmentation of SSRIs, thyroid hormone augmentation, and bupropion augmentation of SSRIs.

Electroconvulsive Therapy. Electroconvulsive therapy (ECT) remains an effective treatment in individuals with severe MDD and those individuals with psychotic MDD. Many individuals who have responded to ECT do not respond to pharmacotherapy. There is increased need for understanding the role of maintenance ECT in those individuals who respond to ECT because ongoing pharmacotherapy does not always prevent recurrence of depression after ECT is successful. ECT can be particularly useful in interrupting acute suicidality for those individuals who may require rapid resolution of symptoms. ECT may be indicated in older adults when lack of self-care and weight loss may represent a greater risk. The most common side effect associated with ECT is amnesia for the period of treatment. There is no consistent evidence to suggest chronic cognitive or memory impairment as a result of ECT.

Other Somatic Treatments. Light therapy investigators have continued to demonstrate benefit in individuals with seasonal MDD by providing greater than 2500 lux light therapy for 1 to 2 hours/day. Many of these individuals experience recurrent winter depression in the context of a recurrent MDD or bipolar II disorder. Bright light exposure has been associated with favorable response within 4 to 7 days. As with ECT, light therapy is best prescribed by specialists who have experience in its use and can appropriately evaluate the indication for light therapy and monitor carefully the response to treatment.

Ongoing investigation of alternative brain stimulation techniques have been the subject of recent investigation. The use of a powerful magnet to provide transcranial magnetic stimulation has been the subject of several open trials. It is not yet determined whether the repetitive transcranial magnetic stimulation demonstrates its effectiveness through reduction of inhibitory neurotransmission or other mechanisms.

Vagus nerve stimulation (VNS), which has been found to be effective in epilepsy, has been approved by the FDA for the treatment of recurrent MDD that has not responded adequately to four or more antidepressant treatments. This procedure requires the implantation of a stimulating device in the chest with the capacity to stimulate the vagus nerve at regular intervals through the course of the day. The most common side effects from VNS therapy include hoarseness, a prickling feeling on the skin, and increased coughing. These side effects tend to diminish over time. Although only a third of patients responded to VNS (i.e., at least a 50% improvement in their depression after a year of use), the fact that these patients responded to VNS and to no other treatments persuaded the FDA to grant approval after initially rejecting the treatment.

Psychosocial Treatment

The past decade has also led to the development of more specific depression-based treatment for MDD. These treatments have included supportive psychiatric management techniques during pharmacotherapy, interpersonal psychotherapy, cognitive–behavioral therapy, brief dynamic psychotherapy, and marital and family therapy.

Clinical management and supportive psychotherapy is the standard in office practice. The clinician focuses on establishing a positive therapeutic relationship in the course of diagnosis and initiation of treatment of depression. The clinician is attentive to all signs and symptoms of the disorder, particularly suicidality. The clinician provides ongoing education, collaboration with the individual, and supportive feedback to the individual regarding ongoing response and prognosis. The supportive psychotherapeutic management of depression facilitates the ongoing pharmacologic response. Brief supportive psychotherapy in individuals with mild to moderate depression is indicated to improve medication compliance, to facilitate reduction of active depressive signs and symptoms, and to provide education regarding relapse and recurrence.

Interpersonal Psychotherapy. Interpersonal psychotherapy in nonhospitalized individuals with nonbipolar MDD has been demonstrated to be effective in acute treatment trials. Interpersonal psychotherapy of depression addresses four areas of current interpersonal difficulties: (1) interpersonal loss or grieving; (2) role transitions; (3) interpersonal disputes; and (4) social deficits. This type of treatment, like other psychotherapies for depression, also involves education about the nature of MDD and the relationship between symptoms of depressive disorder and current interpersonal difficulties.

Prior studies demonstrated efficacy of interpersonal psychotherapy for outpatients with depression. Interpersonal psychotherapy, cognitive–behavioral

psychotherapy, and medication treatment were comparable on several outcome measures and superior to placebo. Medication treatment was associated with the most rapid response and was superior to both interpersonal psychotherapy and cognitive–behavioral therapy in more severely depressed individuals. Continuation studies with interpersonal psychotherapy offered monthly as well as during maintenance treatment have demonstrated response in prevention of recurrence, and was superior to placebo treatment. Those individuals who received ongoing interpersonal psychotherapy and medication had the longest intervals without recurrence of depressive symptoms.

Cognitive–Behavioral Therapy. Cognitive–behavioral therapy for depression is a form of treatment aimed at symptom reduction through the identification and correction of cognitive distortions. These involve negative views of the self, one's current world, and the future. Several controlled studies have demonstrated the efficacy of cognitive therapy in resolution of MDD in adults. Cognitive–behavioral therapy as well as interpersonal psychotherapy is generally considered to be somewhat less effective than medication treatment in moderate to severe MDD. However, some investigators have suggested a relatively equal response to cognitive–behavioral therapy and medication in more severely depressed outpatients.

Brief Dynamic Psychotherapy. Brief dynamic psychotherapy addresses current conflicts as manifestations of difficulty in early attachment and disruption of early object relationships. Brief dynamic psychotherapy was not specifically designed for treatment of MDD and is currently the subject of ongoing studies as well as controlled clinical trials in comparison with medication treatment. The results of these trials will allow us to address the appropriate role of brief dynamic psychotherapy in outpatients with mild to moderate depression. In addition, it will be important to understand whether dynamic psychotherapy may address demoralization or response to traumatic circumstances.

Martial and Family Therapy. It has been difficult to assess the specific efficacy of marital or family therapy in individuals with MDD based on current studies to date. There is substantial evidence that marital distress is a major event associated with the development of a depressive episode. Marital discord often will persist after the remission of depression and subsequent relapses are frequently associated with disruptions of marital relationships. Both acute and continuation phase treatment of MDD will require ongoing attention to marital and family issues to prevent recurrence of depression.

Factors Influencing Treatment Response

There are a number of factors that influence ultimate treatment response in MDD, including individual characteristics, diagnostic issues, comorbidity, treatment-related complications including side effects, and demographic factors. Reevaluation of diagnosis, comorbidity, and the clinician–patient relationship itself is often critical.

Suicide Risk. Individuals with MDD are often at increased risk for suicide. Suicidal risk assessment is especially indicated as individuals begin to recover from depression with increased energy and simultaneous continued despair. Persistent suicidal ideation coupled with increased energy can often lead to impulsive suicidal acts. The careful attention to the clinician–patient relationship can mediate suicidal urges through availability and accessibility. Outpatients and inpatients with MDD and melancholic features will often require antidepressant therapy addressing multiple neurotransmitter systems, or ECT as well.

Psychotic Features. MDD with psychotic features requires careful assessment to rule out comorbid mental disorders. The combined treatment with antipsychotic as well as antidepressant medication is indicated. In addition, ECT is an effective intervention in psychotic depression and may be considered as a first-line alternative.

Catatonic Features. MDD with catatonic features can be associated with significant morbidity owing to the individual's refusal to eat or drink. Active treatment with a benzodiazepine such as lorazepam 1 to 3 mg daily may offer short-term treatment response. Subsequent treatment with lithium alone or in association with antidepressants may be indicated given the possible link between catatonic features and bipolar vulnerability. If psychosis is associated with catatonia, then atypical antipsychotic medication or a course of ECT may be indicated as well.

Atypical Features. Atypical features are associated with significant comorbid anxiety disorders, reverse neurovegetative symptoms such as hypersomnia, increased appetite, and weight gain, as well as fatigue and leaden paralysis. SSRIs are likely to be effective in individuals with MDD with atypical features as well as MAOIs. Conversely, tricyclic antidepressants,

in particular, are unlikely to be effective in such individuals.

Severity. Individuals with mild to moderate depression may be effectively treated with psychotherapy, pharmacotherapy, or the combination. Individuals with severe MDD almost always require somatic intervention with antidepressant medication or electroconvulsive therapy.

Recurrence. Because MDD is a recurrent disorder, current treatment guidelines suggest maintenance antidepressant treatment at full therapeutic doses if there is a history of more than two prior episodes of MDD.

History of Hypomania or Mania. Any of the antidepressant treatments including medication, ECT, light therapy, or newer somatic interventions may induce hypomania or mania in individuals who are vulnerable to bipolar disorder. Individuals who may have a family history of bipolar disorder should be carefully evaluated for treatment with lithium carbonate or other anticonvulsant mood stabilizers before antidepressant treatment because they are at particular risk for antidepressant-induced mania. Attention to this history of prior hypomania or mania as well as family history may promote treatment response if such individuals have mood-stabilizing treatment offered initially.

Comorbidity with Alcohol or Substance Dependence. The comorbidity of MDD and alcohol or other substance dependence requires careful attention to both diagnoses. The first priority in treatment is abstinence from alcohol or substance use. Co-occurring addiction will complicate depressive disorders and increases risk for suicide. If detoxification from alcohol or other substance abuse is required, this should be undertaken before initiation of any somatic antidepressant therapy. Individuals who have a family history of depression or bipolar disorder are likely to require early initiation of appropriate mood disorder treatment following detoxification.

Comorbidity with Obsessive–Compulsive Disorder. In individuals with OCD, lifetime risk of MDD approaches 70%. The use of higher dose SSRI treatment is often indicated to treat both conditions. Alternatively, the tricyclic antidepressant, clomipramine (Anafranil), may be effective for those individuals with both OCD and MDD who do not respond to SSRIs.

Comorbidity with Panic Disorder. Lifetime risk of MDD approaches 50% in individuals with panic

Table 26-4	Staging Criteria for Treatment-Resistant Depression
Stage	**Description**
1.	Failure of at least one adequate trial of an antidepressant
2.	Stage 1 resistance plus failure of adequate trial of an antidepressant from a distinctly different class than in Stage 1
3.	Stage 2 resistance plus failure of an adequate trial of a tricyclic antidepressant (TCA)
4.	Stage 3 resistance plus failure of an adequate trial of a monoamine oxidase inhibitor (MAOI)
5.	Stage 4 resistance plus failure of a course of bilateral electroconvulsive therapy (ECT)

disorder. Because many of the SSRIs and other antidepressants are effective treatments to treat panic as well as depression, these treatments have gained increasing popularity. One may continue to prescribe short-term courses of benzodiazepines, including lorazepam or clonazepam to alleviate acute symptoms of panic, as low doses of antidepressant treatments are introduced into the treatment for comorbid panic and MDD. In addition, MAOIs continue to be effective treatments for both panic and MDD.

Refractory Major Depressive Disorder

A staging system for treatment-resistant depression (TRD) has been proposed, ranging from failure to respond to a single agent (Stage 1) to failure of multiple treatments and ECT (Stage 5), and is presented in Table 26-4. The term refractory depression has been proposed to describe individuals who have Stage 5 TRD.

Refractory MDD or Stage 5 in this table is estimated to occur in up to 20% of individuals. A larger percentage of individuals with MDD, up to 30%, may show only partial improvement. The concept of treatment-resistant depression or refractory depression describes this lack of response to a number of clinical trials using optimal dosing and duration of antidepressant medication. One must typically offer the individual a rational series of treatment trials using optimal dosing and duration of each antidepressant. An individual is considered refractory if a course of three, four, or five treatments is offered without substantial clinical response. The standard approach to the management of refractory depression includes increasing the antidepressant dose and monitoring for a full 8- to 12-week course, augmenting the treatment with several augmentation strategies using an adequate combination of antidepressant drug treatment and psychotherapy and

switching to alternative somatic treatments including ECT when indicated.

Refractory MDD is ameliorated in the context of a caring and collaborative treatment relationship based on a favorable therapeutic alliance. Sometimes, individuals will undermine treatment through their own persistent use of substances such as alcohol or lack of adherence to specific pharmacotherapy recommendations. In this context, the attention to the therapeutic alliance is particularly critical. In assessing an individual with refractory symptoms, pharmacologic factors, including pharmacokinetic considerations, drug–drug interactions, and extreme sensitivity to antidepressant drugs, must be considered.

Despite many alternative strategies, substantial morbidity and occasional mortality are associated with refractory MDD. In addition, careful attention to psychosocial factors associated with refractoriness is critical. These psychosocial factors include early childhood adversity and abuse, early family dysfunction, increased neuroticism, and marked disruption in the development of a stable sense of self.

Dysthymic Disorder

DIAGNOSIS

Dysthymic disorder is defined by the presence of chronic depressive symptoms most of the day, more days than not, for at least 2 years (see DSM-IV-TR diagnostic criteria for Dysthymic Disorder, page 272). While chronic depressive conditions were traditionally conceptualized as characterological and amenable to psychotherapy and resistant to pharmacotherapy, recent pharmacologic trials of antidepressants as well as depression-specific psychotherapy have demonstrated effectiveness in the overall treatment of DD. Both focused interpersonal and variations of cognitive–behavioral psychotherapy have demonstrated response in dysthymia. Individuals with DD have a substantial risk for the development of MDD. This highlights the importance of early assessment and treatment to minimize subsequent long-term complications.

If signs and symptoms of DD follow an MDD, then a diagnosis of MDD, in partial remission, is made. A diagnosis of DD can be made if the individual develops full remission of MDD for 6 months and subsequently develops signs and symptoms of DD, which then last a minimum of 2 years. In contrast, the diagnosis of chronic MDD is made when an episode of MDD meets full criteria for MDD continuously for at least 2 years. If DD has been present for at least 2 years in adults (or 1 year in children and adolescents) and is subsequently

DSM-IV-TR Diagnostic Criteria

300.4 DYSTHYMIC DISORDER

A. Depressed mood for most of the day, for more days than not, as indicated either by subjective account or by observation by others, for at least 2 years.

Note: In children and adolescents, mood can be irritable and duration must be at least 1 year.

B. Presence, while depressed, of two (or more) of the following:

    (1) poor appetite or overeating
    (2) insomnia or hypersomnia
    (3) low energy or fatigue
    (4) low self-esteem
    (5) poor concentration or difficulty making decisions
    (6) feelings of hopelessness

C. During the 2-year period (1 year for children or adolescents) of the disturbance, the person has never been without the symptoms in Criteria A and B for more than 2 months at a time.

D. No major depressive episode has been present during the first 2 years of the disturbance (1 year for children and adolescents); i.e., the disturbance is not better accounted for by chronic major depressive disorder or major depressive disorder, in partial remission.

Note: There may have been a previous major depressive episode provided there was a full remission (no significant signs or symptoms for 2 months) before development of the dysthymic disorder. In addition, after the initial 2 years (1 year in children or adolescents) of dysthymic disorder, there may be superimposed episodes of major depressive disorder, in which case both diagnoses may be given when the criteria are met for a major depressive episode.

E. There has never been a manic episode, a mixed episode, or a hypomanic episode, and criteria have never been met for cyclothymic disorder.

F. The disturbance does not occur exclusively during the course of a chronic psychotic disorder, such as schizophrenia or delusional disorder.

G. The symptoms are not due to the direct physiological effects of a substance (e.g., a drug of abuse, a medication) or a general medical condition (e.g., hypothyroidism).

H. The symptoms cause clinically significant distress or impairment in social, occupational, or other important areas of functioning.

Specify if:

Early onset: if onset is before age 21 years
Late onset: if onset is age 21 years or older

Specify (for most recent 2 years of dysthymic disorder):

With atypical features

Reprinted with permission from the *Diagnostic and Statistical Manual of Mental Disorders*, 4th ed., Text Rev. Copyright 2000 American Psychiatric Association.

followed by a superimposed MDD, then both DD and MDD are diagnosed, which is often referred to as "double depression." The following specifiers apply to DD as noted in DSM-IV-TR: *Early onset*—if the onset of dysthymic symptoms occurs before age 21; and *Late*

onset—if the onset of dysthymic symptoms occurs at age 21 or older, and *With Atypical Features*.

Atypical features refer to a pattern of symptoms that include mood reactivity and two of the additional atypical symptoms (i.e., weight gain or increased appetite, hypersomnia, leaden paralysis, or interpersonal rejection sensitivity). Early-onset DD is usually associated with subsequent episodes of MDD. DD with atypical features may herald a bipolar I or II course.

The diagnosis of DD cannot be made if depressive symptoms occur exclusively during the course of a nonaffective psychosis such as schizophrenia, schizoaffective disorder, or delusional disorder. Diagnosis of depressive disorder NOS is made if there are symptoms that meet criteria for MDD during the residual phase of a psychotic disorder. If DD is determined to be etiologically related to a chronic medical condition, then one diagnoses mood disorder due to the general medical condition. If substance use is judged to be the etiologic factor, then a substance-induced mood disorder is diagnosed. Individuals with DD often have co-occurring personality disorders and in these situations, separate diagnoses on Axes I and II are made.

Ongoing studies have not completely clarified the distinction between DD and depressive personality disorder. Depressive temperaments may predispose an individual to a condition within the spectrum of Axis I mood disorders. However, it may not be specifically associated with MDD. This depressive temperament may also be associated with vulnerability to bipolar disorder.

Individuals with early-onset DD are at substantial risk for development of other mental disorders, including alcohol or substance dependence, MDD, and personality disorders. Up to 15% of individuals with DD may also have a substance use pattern that meets criteria for comorbid alcohol or substance dependence diagnosis. The most common associated personality disorders include mixed, dependent, and borderline personality. Childhood and adolescent-onset DD is associated with a substantial risk for later occurrence of both MDD and bipolar disorder.

A lifetime prevalence of 4.1% for women and 2.2% for men has been reported for DD. In adults, DD is more common in women than in men. In children, DD occurs equally in both sexes. Across both women and men, DD has a 2.5% 12-month prevalence.

Course

Dysthymic disorder often begins in late childhood or early adolescence and by definition takes a chronic course. The risk for development of MDD among children who have DD is significant because childhood onset of DD is an early marker for recurrent mood disorder, both recurrent MDD and bipolar disorder.

The course of DD suggests impairment in functional status, including social and occupational and physical functioning. Individuals who have both DD and MDD have more severe functional impairment. Untreated DD contributes to significant occupational and financial burden. There is substantial reduction in activity, more days spent in bed, more complaints of poor general medical health, and more disability days than reported in the general population.

TREATMENT

The treatment goals in DD are similar to those in MDD. They include full remission of symptoms and full psychosocial recovery. Many individuals who have been enrolled in clinical trials for MDD have an associated history of DD. Randomized controlled trials of pharmacotherapy and cognitive–behavior therapy suggest a favorable response to active treatments. The most favorable response occurred in those individuals treated with both active medication and specific cognitive–behavioral treatments.

COMPARISON OF DSM-IV-TR AND ICD-10 DIAGNOSTIC CRITERIA

The criteria set for a major depressive episode in ICD-10 contains 10 items, in contrast to the nine DSM-IV-TR items (loss of self-esteem has been separated from inappropriate guilt). Furthermore, ICD-10 provides separate criteria sets for each level of severity of a major depressive episode: a threshold of 4 out of 10 symptoms defines mild, 6 out of 10 symptoms defines moderate, and 8 out of 10 symptoms defines severe. Furthermore, the ICD-10 diagnostic algorithm differs by requiring that there be at least two of the following three symptoms—depressed mood, loss of interest, and decreased energy—for mild and moderate depressive episodes and all three for severe episodes. ICD-10 episodes with psychotic features exclude first-rank symptoms and bizarre delusions, which if present would shift the diagnosis to schizoaffective disorder.

The ICD-10 Diagnostic Criteria for Research and DSM-IV-TR also differ on the threshold for defining when major depressive disorder is characterized as single episode versus recurrent. ICD-10 specifies that there be a period of at least two months free from any significant mood symptoms between mood episodes, whereas DSM-IV-TR requires an interval of at least two consecutive months in which full criteria for a major depressive episode have not been met.

The ICD-10 definition of dysthymic disorder specifies that three items from a list of 11 symptoms (which include 5 of the 6 DSM-IV-TR items) must accompany the depressed mood. Furthermore, ICD-10 restricts co-occurring major depressive episodes to "none or very few" and specifies that dysthymic disorder may follow a depressive episode without a period of full remission.

27 Mood Disorders: Premenstrual Dysphoric Disorder

DIAGNOSIS

Premenstrual syndrome (PMS) is a combination of emotional, behavioral, and physical symptoms that occur in the premenstrual or luteal phase of the menstrual cycle. Diagnostic criteria for PMS often require a minimum of one premenstrual symptom, such as the criteria proposed in the *American College of Obstetrics and Gynecology Practice Guidelines* or in the *International Classification of Diseases*, 10th Revision. Approximately 80% of women report at least mild premenstrual symptoms, 20–50% report moderate to severe premenstrual symptoms, and approximately 5% of women report severe symptoms for several days with impairment of role and social functioning. The 5% of women with the severest form of PMS generally have symptoms that meet the diagnostic criteria for premenstrual dysphoric disorder (PMDD).

Research diagnostic criteria for PMDD are listed in the appendix of DSM-IV-TR. A clinician can indicate that a woman has symptoms that meet the diagnostic criteria for PMDD by recording the DSM-IV-TR diagnosis 311, depressive disorder not otherwise specified. To meet the PMDD criteria, at least five out of the eleven possible symptoms must be present in the premenstrual phase; these symptoms should be absent shortly following the onset of menses; and at least one of the five symptoms must be depressed mood, anxiety, lability, or irritability. The PMDD criteria require that role functioning be impaired as a result of the premenstrual symptoms. The functional impairment reported by women with PMDD is similar in severity to the impairment reported in major depressive disorder and dysthymic disorder. Unlike the functional impairment reported in depressive disorders, women with severe PMS and PMDD report more disruption in their relationships and parenting roles than in their work roles.

The PMDD criteria require that a woman prospectively rate her emotional, behavioral, and physical

---

DSM-IV-TR Research Criteria

PREMENSTRUAL DYSPHORIC DISORDER

A. In most menstrual cycles during the past year, five (or more) of the following symptoms were present for most of the time during the last week of the luteal phase, began to remit within a few days after the onset of the follicular phase, and were absent in the week postmenses, with at least one of the symptoms being either (1), (2), (3), or (4):

   (1) markedly depressed mood, feelings of hopelessness, or self-deprecating thoughts
   (2) marked anxiety, tension, feelings of being "keyed up," or "on edge"
   (3) marked affective lability (e.g., feeling suddenly sad or tearful or increased sensitivity to rejection)
   (4) persistent and marked anger or irritability or increased interpersonal conflicts
   (5) decreased interest in usual activities (e.g., work, school, friends, hobbies)
   (6) subjective sense of difficulty in concentrating
   (7) lethargy, easy fatigability, or marked lack of energy
   (8) marked change in appetite, overeating, or specific food cravings
   (9) hypersomnia or insomnia
   (10) a subjective sense of being overwhelmed or out of control
   (11) other physical symptoms, such as breast tenderness or swelling, headaches, joint or muscle pain, a sensation of "bloating," weight gain

B. The disturbance markedly interferes with work or school or with usual social activities and relationships (e.g., avoidance of social activities, decreased productivity and efficiency at work or school).

C. The disturbance is not merely an exacerbation of the symptoms of another disorder such as major depressive disorder, panic disorder, dysthymic disorder, or a personality disorder (although it may be superimposed on any of these disorders).

D. Criteria A, B, and C must be confirmed by prospective daily ratings during at least two consecutive symptomatic cycles. (The diagnosis may be made provisionally prior to this confirmation.)

Reprinted with permission from the *Diagnostic and Statistical Manual of Mental Disorders*, 4th ed., Text Rev. Copyright 2000 American Psychiatric Association.

---

symptoms over two menstrual cycles to confirm the diagnosis. Several studies have reported that retrospective reports of premenstrual symptoms may inaccurately identify the timing or amplify the severity of symptoms compared to prospective reporting. Charting two menstrual cycles is advantageous, since some women have variability of symptom severity from cycle to cycle due to factors such as seasonal worsening, or a woman might have the unusual presence of follicular phase psychological symptoms due to a transient stressor. Studies of PMDD tend to utilize visual analog scales, or Likert scale daily rating forms such as the Daily Record of Severity of Problems, with a scoring method that compares the average of symptom scores during the premenstrual days to the average of symptom scores postmenses.

A woman presenting with PMS should ideally bring to her clinician two cycles of an established daily rating form, or alternatively ratings of her most problematic symptoms, rated with anchor points ranging from "not present" to "severe." The clinician should review the daily ratings to confirm that the symptoms are in fact confined largely to the premenstrual phase, with the relative absence of symptoms in the follicular phase, and

the clinician should also assess premenstrual functional impairment (Figure 27-1). Ratings that demonstrate follicular symptoms with increased symptom severity in the premenstrual phase suggest "premenstrual exacerbation" of an underlying disorder rather than PMDD. The DSM-IV-TR PMDD criteria state that the premenstrual symptoms should not be an exacerbation of an underlying disorder, but that PMDD could be superimposed on another disorder, like panic disorder. No formal guidelines exist on how to apply this criterion clinically.

Irritability has been identified as the most common premenstrual symptom in US and European samples. Studies have suggested some genetic liability for PMS, but the overlap with genetic liability for major depression or personality characteristics has received mixed reports. Elevated lifetime prevalence of major depressive disorder in women with PMDD has been reported in several studies, as well as an elevated lifetime prevalence of postpartum depression. Even though premenstrual symptoms are described in women from menarche to menopause, it is unclear if symptoms remain stable or increase in severity with age. PMS has been described in several countries and cultures and some cultures have a preponderance of somatic rather than emotional symptoms.

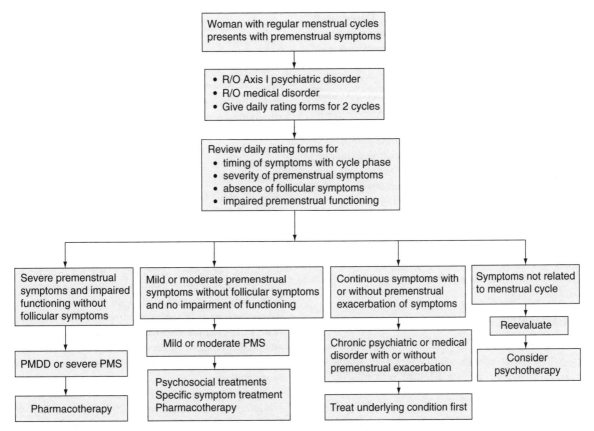

Figure 27-1 *Diagnosis and initial treatment algorithm of premenstrual symptoms.*

Differential Diagnosis

Depression and anxiety disorders are the most common Axis I mental disorders that may be concurrent and exacerbated premenstrually, with less clear evidence for bipolar disorder, eating disorders, and substance abuse. Since most PMDD symptoms are affective or anxiety-related, "pure PMS" or PMDD is generally not diagnosed when an underlying depression or anxiety disorder is present; these women would be considered to have premenstrual exacerbation of their underlying depression or anxiety disorder. Personality disorders are not elevated in prevalence in women with PMDD, but women with PMDD and a personality disorder may demonstrate premenstrual phase amplification of personality dysfunction. Schizophrenia may be an example of a disorder that does not have premenstrual exacerbation of psychotic symptoms but may have the superimposition of affective and anxiety symptoms of PMDD. The prevalence of premenstrually exacerbated disorders is unknown, but women with these conditions present frequently to their primary care clinician or gynecologist. Since most recent treatment studies have been conducted on women with PMS and PMDD without follicular symptomatology, this literature is not particularly informative on how to treat women with premenstrually exacerbated disorders. The general guideline is to treat the underlying disorder first and see if subsequent daily ratings suggest persistence of premenstrual symptoms that might meet the criteria for PMDD.

Several medical conditions should also be considered when evaluating a woman with premenstrual complaints. Symptoms of endometriosis, polycystic ovary disease, thyroid disorders, disorders of the adrenal system, hyperprolactinemia, and panhypopituitarism may mimic symptoms of PMS. Several general medical conditions may demonstrate a premenstrual increase in symptoms without accompanying emotional symptoms, such as migraines, asthma, epilepsy, irritable bowel syndrome, diabetes, allergies, and autoimmune disorders. It is presumed that the menstrual cycle fluctuations of gonadal hormones influence some of the symptoms of these medical conditions.

TREATMENT

The treatment studies of SSRIs in PMDD have suggested a similar efficacy rate to treatment studies of SSRIs in major depressive disorder, with 60–70% of women responding to SSRIs compared to approximately 30% of women responding to placebo. In general, the effective SSRI doses are similar to the doses recommended for the treatment of major depressive disorder (Figure 27-2). The efficacy of the continuous (daily) dosing and intermittent dosing (SSRI administered during the luteal phase only from ovulation to menses) is considered to be equivalent. There have not been reports of discontinuation symptoms from doses of fluoxetine (10 mg/day during luteal phase) and sertraline (50–100 mg/day during luteal phase) when they were abruptly stopped from the first day of menses. The efficacy of intermittent dosing, as well as the findings from most SSRI trials that efficacy is achieved by the first treatment cycle, has suggested a more rapid and different mechanism of action of SSRIs in PMDD compared to its effect in major depressive disorder that typically takes two to six weeks. Studies have also shown that venlafaxine, an antidepressant with both serotonergic and noradrenergic action, reduces emotional and physical symptoms of PMDD. Efficacy has also been reported with clomipramine, a tricyclic antidepressant with largely serotonergic action, with the doses of clomipramine reported to be effective for PMS (25–75 mg q.d.) lower than expected effective doses for major depressive disorder (see Figure 27-2). Since most SSRI trials have been six months or less in duration, long-term treatment recommendations do not exist. Clinically, many women note the recurrence of premenstrual symptoms after SSRI discontinuation and many clinicians treat women over a long period of time.

Gonadotropin releasing hormone (GnRH) agonists suppress ovulation by downregulating GnRH receptors in the hypothalamus, leading to decreased follicle-stimulating hormone and luteinizing hormone release from the pituitary, resulting in decreased estrogen and progesterone levels. GnRH agonists are administered parenterally (e.g., subcutaneous monthly injections of goserelin, intramuscular monthly injections of leuprolide, and daily intranasal buserelin) (see Figure 27-2). GnRH agonists lead to improvement in most emotional and physical premenstrual symptoms, with possible decreased efficacy for premenstrual dysphoria and severe premenstrual symptoms or for the exacerbation of chronic depression. After relief of PMS is achieved with a GnRH agonist, "add-back" hormone strategies have been investigated due to the undesirable medical consequences of the hypoestrogenic state resulting from prolonged anovulation. The addition of estrogen and progesterone to goserelin and leuprolide, however, may lead to the reappearance of mood and anxiety symptoms.

Danazol, a synthetic steroid, alleviates premenstrual symptoms when administered at 200–400 mg q.d. doses that induce anovulation. A recent study with danazol

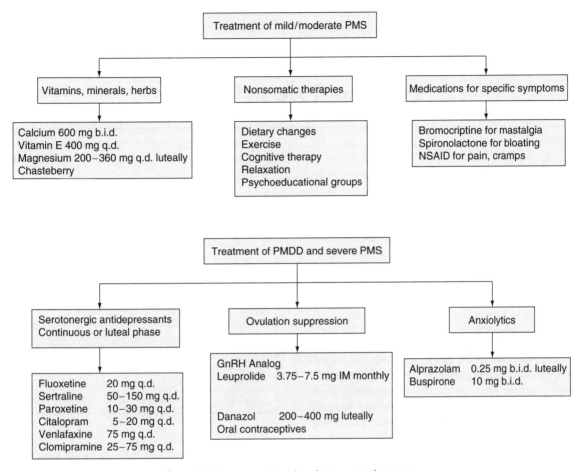

Figure 27-2 *Treatment algorithm of premenstrual symptoms.*

200 mg/day administered during the luteal phase only, not causing anovulation, reported that breast tenderness but not other premenstrual symptoms were reduced. Oophorectomy should be reserved for women with severe PMS and PMDD, unresponsive to antidepressants or hormonal treatment. In addition, the small literature with estrogen and progesterone administered most of the cycle has yielded mixed reports.

Even though oral contraceptives (OCs) are a commonly prescribed treatment for PMS, there is minimal literature endorsing its efficacy. Anecdotally, women report that OCs may benefit, worsen, or not affect their premenstrual symptoms.

Alprazolam (administered during the luteal phase) may be effective for premenstrual emotional symptoms, although it has a lower efficacy rate than SSRIs. Alprazolam should be tapered over the first few days of menses each cycle.

Many lifestyle modifications and psychosocial treatments have been suggested for PMS. Lifestyle modifications are often suggested through self-help materials or in an individual or group psychoeducation format. Weekly peer support and a professional guidance group for four sessions has been shown to reduce premenstrual symptoms. The treatment consisted of diet and exercise regimens, self-monitoring and other cognitive techniques, and environment modification.

COMPARISON OF DSM-IV-TR AND ICD-10 DIAGNOSTIC CRITERIA

Premenstrual Dysphoric Disorder is not included in ICD-10. A related condition "premenstrual tension syndrome" is included in Chapter 14 for diseases of the genitourinary system.

28 Mood Disorders: Bipolar Disorders

DIAGNOSIS

The cardinal symptoms of bipolar disorder are discrete periods of abnormal mood and activation that define depressive and manic or hypomanic episodes. Diagnosis of such episodes is based exclusively on *phenomenology*, the descriptive appearance of the syndrome of interest. One may conceive of phenomenological data for the diagnosis of bipolar disorder as being of two types: *cross-sectional* and *longitudinal*. Cross-sectional data refer to descriptive aspects of a syndrome that occur at a particular point in time, such as the number and type of depressive symptoms that occur during an episode of depression. Longitudinal data refer to the course of symptoms over time, such as the timing, duration, and recurrence of depressive episodes. Both cross-sectional and longitudinal data are essential for the definition of mood disorders and the proper diagnosis of bipolar disorder. It is not infrequent that diagnostic errors occur when longitudinal data are neglected as the clinician focuses solely on cross-sectional presentation: "This must be bipolar disorder because the individual appears manic at the present time," or "This cannot be bipolar disorder because the individual is depressed now."

The DSM-based definition of bipolar disorder is built on the identification of individual mood *episodes* (Table 28-1). It is important to understand that the diagnosis of bipolar disorder derives from the occurrence of individual episodes over time. Persons who experience a manic, hypomanic, or mixed episode, virtually all of whom also have a history of one or more major depressive episodes, are diagnosed with bipolar disorder. Those who experience major depressive and manic episodes are diagnosed with *bipolar I* disorder (see DSM-IV-TR diagnostic criteria, pages 279), and those with major depressive and hypomanic (milder manic) episodes are diagnosed with *bipolar II* disorder (see DSM-IV-TR diagnostic criteria, page 279). Persons who experience subsyndromal bipolar mood fluctuations over an extended

Table 28-1	Summary of Mood Episodes and Mood Disorders	
Episode	**Disorder**
Major depressive episode	Major depressive disorder, single episode
Major depressive episode + major depressive episode	Major depressive disorder, recurrent
Major depressive episode + manic/mixed episode	Bipolar I disorder
Manic/mixed episode	Bipolar I disorder
Major depressive episode + hypomanic episode	Bipolar II disorder
Chronic subsyndromal depression	Dysthymic disorder
Chronic fluctuations between subsyndromal depression and hypomania	Cyclothymic disorder

period without major mood episodes are diagnosed with *cyclothymic disorder* (see DSM-IV-TR diagnostic criteria, page 279).

Mood episodes are discrete periods of altered feeling, thought, and behavior. Typically, they have a distinct onset and offset, beginning over days or weeks and eventually ending gradually after several weeks or months. As noted earlier, bipolar disorder is defined by the occurrence of depressive plus manic, hypomanic, or mixed episodes, or the occurrence of only manic or mixed episodes.

Major depressive episodes are defined by discrete periods of depressed or blue mood or loss of interest or pleasure in life, which typically endures for weeks but must last for at least 2 weeks (see Chapter 26). These symptoms are often accompanied by changes in sleep, appetite, energy, cognition, and judgment. Depressive episodes in bipolar disorder are indistinguishable from those in major depressive disorder. About half of persons with bipolar disorder experience depressive episodes characterized by decreased sleep and appetite, whereas about half experience more "atypical" symptoms of in-

DSM-IV-TR Diagnostic Criteria

BIPOLAR I DISORDER, MOST RECENT EPISODE [INDICATE HYPOMANIC, MANIC, MIXED, DEPRESSED, OR UNSPECIFIED]

A. Currently (or most recently) in a Hypomanic (296.40), Manic (296.4x), Mixed (296.6x), or Major Depressive Episode (296.5x). If the criteria except for duration are met for one of these episodes, the episode is considered unspecified (296.7).

Note: An x in the diagnostic code indicates that a fifth digit indicating severity is required.

B. There has previously been at least one Manic, Mixed, or Major Depressive Episode.

C. The mood episodes in Criteria A and B are not better accounted for by Schizo-affective Disorder and are not superimposed on Schizophrenia, Schizophreni-form Disorder, Delusional Disorder, or Psychotic Disorder Not Otherwise Specified.

If the full criteria are currently met for a Manic or Mixed Episode, specify its current clinical status and/or features:

Mild, Moderate, Severe Without Psychotic Features/Severe With Psychotic

Features

With Catatonic Features

With Postpartum Onset

Reprinted with permission from *DSM-IV-TR Guidebook.* Copyright 2004, Michael B First, Allen Frances, and Harold Alan Pincus.

DSM-IV-TR Diagnostic Criteria

296.89 BIPOLAR II DISORDER

A. Presence (or history) of one or more Major Depressive Episodes.
B. Presence (or history) of at least one Hypomanic Episode.
C. There has never been a Manic Episode or a Mixed Episode.
D. The mood symptoms in Criteria A and B are not better accounted for by Schizoaffective Disorder and are not superimposed on Schizophrenia, Schizophreniform Disorder, Delusional Disorder, or Psychotic Disorder Not Otherwise Specified.
E. The symptoms cause clinically significant distress or impairment in social, occupational, or other important areas of functioning.

Specify current or most recent episode:

Hypomanic: if currently (or most recently) in a Hypomanic Episode

Depressed: if currently (or most recently) in a Major Depressive Episode

If the full criteria are currently met for a Major Depressive Episode, specify its current clinical status and/or features:

Mild, Moderate, Severe Without Psychotic Features/Severe With Psychotic

Features

Chronic

With Catatonic Features

With Melancholic Features

With Atypical Features

With Postpartum Onset

If the full criteria are not currently met for a Hypomanic or Major Depressive Episode, specify the clinical status of the Bipolar II Disorder and/or features of the most recent Major Depressive Episode (only if it is the most recent type of mood episode):

In Partial Remission, In Full Remission

Chronic With Catatonic Features

With Melancholic Features

With Atypical Features

With Postpartum Onset

Specify:

Longitudinal Course Specifiers (With and Without Interepisode Recovery)

With Seasonal Pattern (applies only to the pattern of Major Depressive Episodes)

With Rapid Cycling

Reprinted with permission from the *Diagnostic and Statistical Manual of Mental Disorders*, 4th ed., Text Rev. Copyright 2000 American Psychiatric Association.

creased sleep and appetite. Recall that the differential diagnosis between major depressive and bipolar disorders is made not by cross-sectional symptom analysis but by longitudinal course. The diagnostic decision tree for bipolar disorder is given in Figure 28-1.

Manic episodes are defined by discrete periods of abnormally elevated, expansive, or irritable mood accompanied by marked impairment in judgment and social and occupational function. These symptoms are frequently accompanied by unrealistic grandiosity, excess energy, and increases in goal-directed activity that frequently have a high potential for damaging consequences.

Hypomanic and manic symptoms may be identical, but hypomanic episodes are less severe (see DSM-IV-TR diagnostic criteria for hypomanic episode, page 282). A person is "promoted" from hypomania to mania (type II to type I bipolar disorder) by the presence of one of three features: psychosis during the episode, sufficient severity to warrant hospitalization, or marked social or occupational role impairment.

It is important to note that the phenomenologic differentiation between hypomania and mania is

not as cut-and-dried as one would hope. Of the three characteristics by which one is "promoted" from

---

DSM-IV-TR Diagnostic Criteria

301.13 Cyclothymic Disorder

A. For at least 2 years, the presence of numerous periods with hypomanic symptoms and numerous periods with depressive symptoms that do not meet criteria for a major depressive episode.

Note: In children and adolescents, the duration must be at least 1 year.

B. During the above 2-year period (1 year in children and adolescents), the person has not been without the symptoms in criterion A for more than 2 months at a time.

C. No major depressive episode, manic episode, or mixed episode has been present during the first 2 years of the disturbance.

D. The symptoms in criterion A are not better accounted for by Schizoaffective Disorder and are not superimposed on Schizophrenia, Schizophreniform Disorder, Delusional Disorder, or Psychotic Disorder Not Otherwise Specified.

E. The symptoms are not due to the direct physiological effects of a substance (e.g., a drug of abuse, a medication) or a general medical condition (e.g., hyperthyroidism).

F. The symptoms cause clinically significant distress or impairment in social, occupational, or other important areas of functioning.

Reprinted with permission from the *Diagnostic and Statistical Manual of Mental Disorders*, 4th ed., Text Rev. Copyright 2000 American Psychiatric Association.

DSM-IV-TR Diagnostic Criteria

Manic Episode

A. A distinct period of abnormally and persistently elevated, expansive, or irritable mood, lasting at least 1 week (or any duration if hospitalization is necessary).

B. During the period of mood disturbance, three (or more) of the following symptoms have persisted (four if the mood is only irritable) and have been present to a significant degree:

(1) inflated self-esteem or grandiosity
(2) decreased need for sleep (e.g., feels rested after only 3 hours of sleep)
(3) more talkative than usual or pressure to keep talking
(4) flight of ideas or subjective experience that thoughts are racing
(5) distractibility (i.e., attention too easily drawn to unimportant or irrelevant external stimuli)
(6) increase in goal-directed activity (either socially, at work or school, or sexually) or psychomotor agitation
(7) excessive involvement in pleasurable activities that have a high potential for painful consequences (e.g., engaging in unrestrained buying sprees, sexual indiscretions, or foolish business investments)

C. The symptoms do not meet criteria for a mixed episode.

D. The mood disturbance is sufficiently severe to cause marked impairment in occupational functioning or in usual social activities or relationships with others, or to necessitate hospitalization to prevent harm to self or others, or there are psychotic features.

E. The symptoms are not due to the direct physiological effects of a substance (e.g., a drug of abuse, a medication, or other treatment) or a general medical condition (e.g., hyperthyroidism).

Note: Manic-like episodes that are clearly caused by somatic antidepressant treatment (e.g., medication, electroconvulsive therapy, light therapy) should not count toward a diagnosis of manic–depressive I disorder.

Reprinted with permission from the *Diagnostic and Statistical Manual of Mental Disorders*, 4th ed., Text Rev. Copyright 2000 American Psychiatric Association.

---

hypomania to mania, only the presence of psychosis is firmly grounded in the characteristics of the individual. The other two characteristics, marked social or occupational role impairment or hospitalization, clearly have components that are primarily external to the individual. If for instance, one individual has relatively mild manic symptoms but is living with a family who is unable to tolerate the behavior, he or she is more likely to be hospitalized. Similarly, the comorbid presence of a severe disorder is more likely to result in hospitalization and a "promotion" from type II to type I disorder. Contrarily, limited insurance benefits, or a more tolerant family increase the probability that a manic syndrome of a given severity will be managed without hospitalization and thus be diagnosed as "hypomania" rather than "mania."

Classically, mania has been considered to be the opposite of depression: manic individuals were said to be cheery, optimistic, and self-confident. Hence the name bipolar disorder. However, in most descriptive studies of mania, substantial proportions of hypomanic and manic individuals actually exhibit substantial dysphoric symptoms. Mixed episodes, defined as the simultaneous occurrence of full-blown manic and depressive episodes, are the most prominent example

of dysphoria during mania (see DSM-IV-TR diagnostic criteria, page 282).

Rapid cycling is defined by the occurrence of four or more mood episodes within 12 months (see DSM-IV-TR diagnostic criteria, page 282). It should be noted that, despite the name, the episodes are not necessarily or even commonly truly cyclical; the diagnosis is based simply on episode counting. This subcategory is of significance because it predicts a relatively poorer outcome and worse response to lithium and other treatments. Although rapid cycling has been considered by some to be an "end stage" of the disorder, empirical evidence indicates that it may have its onset at any time during the disorder and may come and go during

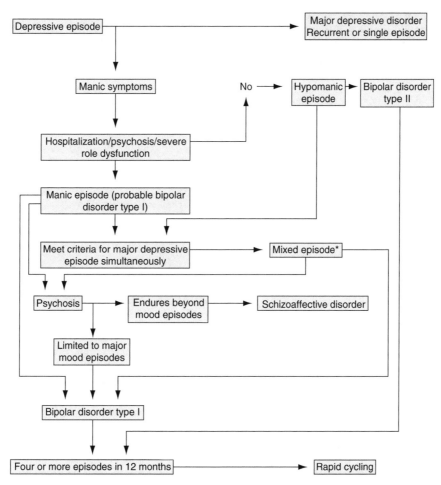

Figure 28-1 *Diagnostic decision tree for bipolar disorder. The building blocks for a diagnosis of bipolar disorder are individual episodes and their characteristics, as summarized in Table 28-1. This decision tree helps the psychiatrist through the steps that lead to diagnosis of manic–depressive disorder and identification of its subtypes. *Does not apply to hypomanic episode as per DSM-IV-TR. Reprinted with permission of American Journal of Psychiatry,* **149,** *1633–1644. McElroy S, Keck P, Pope H et al (1992) Clinical and research implication of the diagnosis of dyphoric or mixed mania or hypomania. Copyright American Psychiatric Publishing Inc.*

the course of illness. Several specific risk factors may be associated with rapid cycling, each of which may give clues to its pathophysiology. These include female gender, antidepressant use, and prior or current hypothyroidism.

Although the diagnosis of bipolar disorder is made on the basis of phenomenology, there are several reasons to conduct a thorough medical history and physical examination. First, there are several general medical or substance-related causes of mania and/or depression that, if treated, may lead to the resolution of the mood episode (see later). Similarly, mania may be the first sign of a general medical illness that will be progressive and serious in its own right. Second, medical evaluation is necessary before starting medications used in the treatment of bipolar disorder. Finally, for many

individuals with mental disorders, particularly chronic or severe illnesses, their first contact with medical care as an adult is during the psychiatric interview—often under inpatient or even involuntary conditions.

The overall approach to evaluating persons with bipolar disorder for medical problems may be generalized as follows. Persons with mental disorders, including bipolar disorder, should have regular screening for disease detection and health maintenance purposes as recommended for the general population. However, it should also be kept in mind that individuals with bipolar disorder, by virtue of having an often severe and disabling behavioral disorder, are less likely than the general population *to have had adequate medical screening and treatment*. Thus, special care must be made to ensure that health problems are not overlooked

DSM-IV-TR Diagnostic Criteria

HYPOMANIC EPISODE

A. A distinct period of persistently elevated, expansive, or irritable mood, lasting throughout at least 4 days, that is clearly different from the usual nondepressed mood.
B. During the period of mood disturbance, three (or more) of the following symptoms have persisted (four if the mood is only irritable) and have been present to a significant degree:

(1) inflated self-esteem or grandiosity
(2) decreased need for sleep (e.g., feels rested after only 3 hours of sleep)
(3) more talkative than usual or pressure to keep talking
(4) flight of ideas or subjective experience that thoughts are racing
(5) distractibility (i.e., attention too easily drawn to unimportant or irrelevant external stimuli)
(6) increase in goal-directed activity (either socially, at work or school, or sexually) or psychomotor agitation
(7) excessive involvement in pleasurable activities that have a high potential for painful consequences (e.g., the person engages in unrestrained buying sprees, sexual indiscretions, or foolish business investments)

C. The episode is associated with an unequivocal change in functioning that is uncharacteristic of the person when not symptomatic.
D. The disturbance in mood and the change in functioning are observable by others.
E. The episode is not severe enough to cause marked impairment in social or occupational functioning, or to necessitate hospitalization, and there are no psychotic features.
F. The symptoms are not due to the direct physiological effects of a substance (e.g., a drug of abuse, a medication, or other treatment) or a general medical condition (e.g., hyperthyroidism).

Note: Hypomanic-like episodes that are clearly caused by somatic antidepressant treatment (e.g., medication, electroconvulsive therapy, light therapy) should not count toward a diagnosis of manic–depressive II disorder.

Reprinted with permission from the *Diagnostic and Statistical Manual of Mental Disorders*, 4th ed., Text Rev. Copyright 2000 American Psychiatric Association.

DSM-IV-TR Diagnostic Criteria

MIXED EPISODE

A. The criteria are met both for a manic episode and for a major depressive episode (except for duration) nearly every day during at least a 1-week period.
B. The mood disturbance is sufficiently severe to cause marked impairment in occupational functioning or in usual social activities or relationships with others, or to necessitate hospitalization to prevent harm to self or others, or there are psychotic features.
C. The symptoms are not due to the direct physiological effects of a substance (e.g., a drug of abuse, a medication, or other treatment) or a general medical condition (e.g., hyperthyroidism).

Note: Mixed-like episodes that are clearly caused by somatic antidepressant treatment (e.g., medication, electroconvulsive therapy, light therapy) should not count toward a diagnosis of manic–depressive I disorder.

Reprinted with permission from the *Diagnostic and Statistical Manual of Mental Disorders*, 4th ed., Text Rev. Copyright 2000 American Psychiatric Association.

general medical condition, more intensive testing is warranted. A clear example of the last situation is when a person with bipolar disorder who has extensive exposure to lithium presents for treatment; such persons, particularly the elderly, require laboratory testing for renal and thyroid abnormalities that can be caused by lithium treatment.

Alcohol and drug abuse and dependence represent the most consistently described and most clinically important mental disorder comorbidities with bipolar disorder. Whereas rates of alcohol abuse combined with alcohol dependence are from 3% to 13% in the general population, lifetime rates for alcohol dependence from Epidemiological Catchment Area (ECA) data indicate that they are greater than 30% in persons with bipolar I

DSM-IV-TR Diagnostic Criteria

RAPID-CYCLING SPECIFIER

Specify if:

With rapid cycling (can be applied to manic–depressive I disorder or manic–depressive II disorder). At least four episodes of a mood disturbance in the previous 12 months that meet criteria for a major depressive, manic, mixed, or hypomanic episode.

Note: Episodes are demarcated by either partial or full remission for at least 2 months or a switch to an episode of opposite polarity (e.g., major depressive episode to manic episode).

Reprinted with permission from the *Diagnostic and Statistical Manual of Mental Disorders*, 4th ed., Text Rev. Copyright 2000 American Psychiatric Association.

and that appropriate treatment or referral is effected. Unfortunately, it is the exception rather than the rule to have well-integrated medical and mental health systems, so that the mental health provider can assume that some effort will need to be expended to ensure adequate care is delivered for individuals with bipolar disorder.

All newly identified individuals with bipolar disorder should undergo a history and if indicated a physical examination. If results of the history or physical examination reveal abnormalities, or if the individual has a mental disorder that is associated with a particular disorder. Further, ECA lifetime rates for drug dependence in individuals with bipolar I disorder are greater than 25% and rates for any substance abuse or dependence are above 60%. Comparable rates for alcohol, drug, or any substance abuse or dependence in major depressive disorder in ECA data are, respectively, 12%, 11%, and 27%. Thus, bipolar disorder represents an enriched sample for substance use disorders, with substantially greater rates than for the general population or even those with unipolar depression.

The reasons for the co-occurrence of bipolar disorder and substance dependence are not clear. One hypothesis suggests that persons with bipolar disorder self-medicate with drugs or alcohol. According to this hypothesis, individuals blunt the painful symptoms of depression with drugs, similarly, they may heighten the manic energy with stimulants. Contrarily, they may also use substances to decrease manic symptoms, particularly if the symptoms are predominantly irritable or dysphoric. Alternatively, chronic substance use may convert otherwise unipolar depression into bipolar disorder by inducing substance-induced manic episodes (according to DSM-IV-TR, such persons would not be classified as having bipolar disorder but would be considered to have a substance-induced mood disorder) or by causing chronic central nervous system changes that change the course of the illness irreversibly.

Finally, it is possible that some common genetic predisposition for mood instability is associated with both bipolar mood phenomenology and increased craving for substances, and the predominant phenotypic expression is then determined by other genetic or environmental factors. According to this hypothesis, some persons possessing the gene develop bipolar disorder, some develop substance dependence, and some develop both. Regardless of the mechanism, comorbid substance dependence represents an important clinical challenge for clinicians treating persons with bipolar disorder.

Among children and adolescents, the diagnosis of bipolar disorder is often complicated by less consistent mood and behavior baseline than occurs in adults. Little evidence is available regarding course and outcome in children. Available data indicate that, as with adults, mixed or cycling episodes predict more recurrences; unlike in adults, manic and mixed presentations may be associated with relatively shorter episodes compared to depressive presentations.

Estimates of the lifetime risk for bipolar I disorder from epidemiological studies have ranged from 0.2% to 0.9%. The ECA study found a lifetime prevalence rate of 1.2% for combined type I and type II variants. These rates are approximately tenfold greater than the

prevalence rate for schizophrenia and about one-fifth that for major depressive disorder. Little is known regarding the prevalence of cyclothymic disorder.

Unlike major depressive disorder, bipolar disorder has an approximately equal gender distribution. Few consistent data are available regarding differences in prevalence across ethnic, cultural, or rural–urban settings. However, one of the more intriguing puzzles is the tendency of bipolar disorder to occur in higher socioeconomic strata than schizophrenia, which tends to aggregate in lower socioeconomic strata. Although many theories have been advanced to explain this phenomenon, no certain mechanism has been identified. However, several issues are clear. First, the finding is most likely not exclusively due to diagnostic bias (i.e., overdiagnosing persons of lower socioeconomic class with schizophrenia more frequently than bipolar disorder and the converse in persons of higher socioeconomic class). Second, the upward socioeconomic "drift" is not due to highly impaired individuals "dragged" upward by higher functioning family members who are normal or who have adaptive subsyndromal bipolar spectrum characteristics; rather, individuals themselves, at least those with type II disorder, are in many cases highly successful and occupy higher socioeconomic levels. Third, the findings are not limited to the United States but have been replicated in European samples as well.

Of particular interest in regard to the epidemiology of bipolar disorder is that the incidence of bipolar disorder (and depressive disorders) appears to have increased since the 1940s. Reasons for this are not clear, although environmental factors, either physiological or psychosocial, may be responsible. For instance, exposure to increasingly severe social stressors, or the breakdown of cultural supports that may buffer stresses, may contribute; increases in exposure to putative environmental toxins might also be considered. In addition, in those families afflicted with bipolar disorder across generations, those in later generations tend to have earlier onset.

Course

Outcome in bipolar disorder can be conceptualized according to three separate but interrelated domains: *clinical outcome, functional outcome*, and *illness costs*. Clinical outcome consists of parameters that measure the illness itself, such as symptom severity, episode number, and duration. Functional outcome consists of social and occupational status and subjective quality of life. Illness costs consist of both direct (treatment) costs and indirect illness costs, which include lost productivity, necessary nontreatment social supports, and nontreatment interventions such as jail and the legal system.

Bipolar disorder has its onset in most persons in adolescence and young adulthood, between the ages of 15 and 30. However, prepubertal mania and first-onset disease in the ninth decade of life also occur. Once developed, multiple episodes are the rule—the majority of individuals with bipolar disorder have four or more episodes in a lifetime. Among rapid-cycling individuals, the basis for the diagnosis is four or more episodes in a year with an average of more than 50 lifetime episodes. There is no typical pattern to episode recurrence, with some individuals having isolated manic, hypomanic, or depressive episodes, others switching from one pole to the other in linked episodes, and still others switching continually from one pole to the other in quasi-cyclical fashion. However, even among rapid-cycling individuals, episodes are rarely periodic. Rather, the pattern is more accurately described by chaotic dynamics.

Episode length typically ranges from 4 to 13 months, with depressive episodes typically longer than manic or hypomanic episodes. Women appear to have more depressive relapses than manic ones, whereas men have a more even distribution. Women predominate among rapid-cycling individuals, representing 70–90% in most studies.

Longitudinal studies conducted in the past three decades suggest an overall guarded prognosis. In early studies conducted in the 1960s, 62% of bipolar individuals had equivocal to poor outcome and 45% of manic individuals were chronically ill 6 years after hospitalization. Another study found only 14.3% to be "well in every way." Although these studies include data from the prelithium era, more recent studies from the lithium era are not terribly reassuring. Approximately 20–40% of individuals with bipolar disorder do not respond well to lithium, and that proportion may increase to as much as 80% for certain subgroups such as individuals who experience rapid-cycling pattern or mixed manic and depressive episodes. When assessed 1.5 years after index hospitalization, between 7% and 32% of bipolar individuals remain chronically ill, depending on polarity of index episode. Only 26% of one sample had good outcome after hospitalization for mania, whereas 40% had moderate and 34% had poor outcome. The probabilities of remaining ill at 1, 2, 3, and 4 years after hospitalization for mania were, respectively, 51%, 44%, 33%, and 28%.

Relatively little is known regarding clinical outcome in bipolar II individuals, although they appear to be at least as impaired in terms of relapse as bipolar I individuals. For instance, one study found that 70% of bipolar II individuals followed up for 5 years, experienced multiple relapses, whereas only 11% were episode free.

Subsyndromal affective symptoms may remain in up to 13–34% and substantial interepisode morbidity may remain despite adequate treatment with lithium. It is not clear whether such interepisode pathology represents incompletely resolved major affective episodes, medication side effects, demoralization due to functional impairment, or a combination of these factors. It should be noted here that side effects are more than a trivial issue, as they may lead to medication discontinuation in 18–53%, a figure that is greater in lower socioeconomic classes. Thus, clinical outcome in bipolar disorder is heterogeneous, and lithium has not proved to be a panacea.

Differential Diagnosis

Psychosis can occur in either pole of the disorder. If psychotic symptoms are limited to the major mood episode, the individual is considered to have bipolar disorder with psychotic features. On the other hand, if psychotic symptoms endure significantly into periods of normal mood, the diagnosis of schizoaffective disorder is made.

Secondary mania is conceptualized as mania occurring close on the heels of a specific known physiological insult, such as general medical illness or exposure to mania-inducing pharmacological agents. Which general medical illnesses may cause symptoms of bipolar disorder? Most medical illnesses that affect brain function have been described in case reports or small case series to cause one or another mental disorder. Several general medical illnesses have been associated with the development of bipolar disorder (Table 28-2), although none can be considered specific risk factors. Furthermore, administration of medications has been observed frequently in clinical practice to be associated with the onset of mania, particularly in individuals with preexisting depression. Such medications are listed in

Table 28-2	Medical Disorders Commonly Associated with Mania	
Neurologic Disorders	**Endocrine**
Stroke	Hyperthyroidism (in those with preexisting manic–depressive disorder)
Head trauma	Postpartum status
Dementia	
Brain tumors	
Infection (including HIV)	
Multiple sclerosis	
Huntington's disease	

Table 28-3	Treatments and Drugs Commonly Associated with Mania	
Antidepressants	**Dopaminergic Agents**	
Medications	Levodopa	
Bright visible spectrum light treatment		
Electroconvulsant therapy	**Drugs of Abuse**	
	Alcohol	
Adrenergic Agents	Cocaine	
Decongestants	Hallucinogens	
Bronchodilators	Amphetamines	
Stimulants	Caffeine	
Other Agents		
Isoniazid		
Corticosteroids		
Anabolic steroids		
Disulfiram		

Table 28-5	Treatments and Drugs Commonly Associated with Depression	
High Blood Pressure Medications	**Hormones**	
Alphamethyldopa	Corticosteroids	
Clonidine	Oral contraceptives	
	Anabolic steroids	
Ulcer Medications		
Cimetadine	**Psychotropic Agents**	
Ranitidine	Benzodiazepines	
	Neuroleptics	
Drugs of Abuse		
Alcohol		
Sedatives		
Amphetamine (withdrawal)		
Cocaine (withdrawal)		
Nicotine (withdrawal)		

Table 28-3. Depressive symptoms may also be associated with certain medical conditions (Table 28-4) and medications or drugs (Table 28-5).

All efficacious antidepressant treatments have been suspected to cause the induction of mania, with the exception of lithium and the possible exception of psychotherapy. Occasionally, when a new antidepressant is developed, hope is raised that it will be the agent that will not induce mania. Clinical experience has not borne out these early hopes. This caveat for antidepressants also includes nonpharmacological antidepressants such as light and electroconvulsive therapy (ECT). The latter effect is paradoxical, as ECT is also used successfully to treat mania.

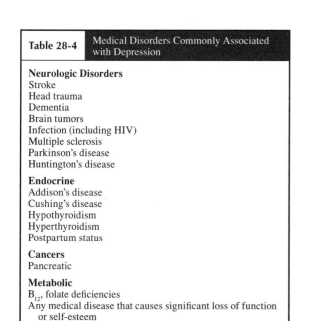

Table 28-4	Medical Disorders Commonly Associated with Depression
Neurologic Disorders	
Stroke	
Head trauma	
Dementia	
Brain tumors	
Infection (including HIV)	
Multiple sclerosis	
Parkinson's disease	
Huntington's disease	
Endocrine	
Addison's disease	
Cushing's disease	
Hypothyroidism	
Hyperthyroidism	
Postpartum status	
Cancers	
Pancreatic	
Metabolic	
B_{12}, folate deficiencies	
Any medical disease that causes significant loss of function or self-esteem	

TREATMENT

Traditionally, treatment for bipolar disorder has been categorized as acute versus prophylaxis, or maintenance; that is, treatment geared toward resolution of a specific episode versus continued treatment to prevent further symptoms. Treatment can also be considered along several other lines (Table 28-6). For instance, interventions can be categorized as somatotherapy (pharmacotherapy, ECT, and light treatment) and psychotherapy. In addition, treatment can be categorized according to intensity. The division into inpatient versus outpatient treatment is becoming more and more blurred as partial or day hospital programs and intensive ambulatory treatment coupled with night hospital programs or respite beds become more popular.

In general, more structured treatment settings, such as full or partial hospitalization, are indicated if individuals are likely to endanger self or others, if bipolar disorder is complicated by other mental disorders or general medical conditions that make ambulatory management particularly dangerous, or if more aggressive management is desired than is easily available on an ambulatory basis (e.g., intensive psychosocial intervention

Table 28-6	Classification Schemata for Bipolar Disorder Treatment and Its Goals
1. Acute versus maintenance	
2. Somatic versus psychotherapeutic	
3. The intensity-of-care continuum*	
(a) Full hospitalization	
(b) Partial or day hospitalization	
(c) Night hospitalization or respite beds	
(d) Ambulatory care	
4. Categorization by goal	
(a) Improve clinical outcome	
(b) Improve functional outcome	
(c) Improve host factors	
(i) Illness management skills	
(ii) Medical and psychiatric comorbidities	

or rapid dosage titration of psychotropic agents). In addition, although it is frequently an afterthought in textbooks, social factors play an important role in the decision to hospitalize in the real world. Such reasons may include lack of social support to ensure medication compliance during acute illness, social stresses aggravating symptoms and making treatment compliance difficult (e.g., manipulative or hostile living situation), or lack of transportation to accommodate frequent ambulatory appointments during acute illness. Unfortunately, it is sometimes the case, although less frequent in this era of managed care, that a person's insurance plan covers inpatient but not ambulatory mental health treatment, forcing expensive inpatient care when less costly, time-limited, intensive ambulatory care would suffice.

Finally, treatment can be categorized according to its goals. Treatment can be focused on improving clinical outcome (episodes and symptoms) or functional outcome (social and occupational function and health-related quality of life). Although this categorization appears straightforward, clinical practice reveals many subtleties. For instance, it is erroneous to assume that clinical outcome is the domain of pharmacotherapy and that functional outcome is the domain of psychotherapy. In actuality, most psychotherapies by design focus on improving symptoms. Likewise, pharmacotherapeutic stabilization of symptoms clearly contributes to improved role function. Further, treatments that improve one domain may cause decrements in another. For instance, effective maintenance treatment with lithium may come at the cost of hand tremor, which interferes with work function and causes embarrassment in social situations.

Balancing the costs and benefits of various specific treatments—and every somatic and psychotherapeutic treatment has both costs and benefits—requires active participation of the person with bipolar disorder and, if available, his or her family. Compassionate psychoeducation and alliance building are integral goals of each form of treatment. In analogy to infectious disease treatment, attention to such host factors can often make the difference between success and failure of treatment.

Somatotherapy

The introduction of lithium for the treatment of bipolar disorder in the 1960s revolutionized management of the illness. Before that, bipolar disorder was managed with treatment targeted only toward resolution of individual episodes: antidepressants and ECT for depressive episodes, and neuroleptics and occasionally ECT

for mania. In contrast, not only did lithium provide an additional treatment for acute mania and depression in bipolar disorder, it was also demonstrated to have substantial prophylactic, or preventive, effects on both manic and depressive episodes.

In evaluating the effectiveness of the various treatments for bipolar disorder, we have found it useful to propose an explicit definition for the term "mood stabilizer" and evaluate the role of various medications against this definition. The US Food and Drug Administration (FDA) does not formally define the term, but it stands to reason that an agent would be optimally useful for treatment of bipolar disorder if it had efficacy in four roles: (a) treatment of acute manic symptoms, (b) treatment of acute depressive symptoms, (c) prophylaxis of manic symptoms, and (d) prophylaxis of depressive symptoms. This approach leads to the conceptual 2×2 table illustrated in Table 28-7. Agents used in bipolar disorder can be listed in any or all of the four boxes in the table in which they have proven efficacy, and according to this schema, an agent may be categorized as a mood stabilizer if it can be listed as having efficacy in each of the four boxes.

Following the FDA lead of considering an agent to have efficacy with at least two such positive trials, we have listed the agents according to the 2×2 table in Table 28-7. As can be seen, at least two placebo-controlled randomized controlled trials support the antimanic efficacy of lithium, carbamazepine, valproate, verapamil, olanzapine, risperidone, ziprasidone, quetiapine, and aripirazole. There are additional randomized controlled trials (nonplacebo-controlled) that support efficacy for multiple older, typical neuroleptics as well as the benzodiazepines, lorazepam, and clonazepam.

In contrast to evidence regarding acute mania, evidence is scarce concerning efficacy of specific agents

Table 28-7	Summary of Efficacy Data from Randomized Controlled Trials for Treating the Various Phases of Bipolar Disorder (At Least Two Placebo-Controlled Trials)	
	Mania	**Depression**
Acute	Lithium	Lithium
	Carbamazepine	Lamotrigine
	Valproate	Quetiapine
	Verapamil	
	Olanzapine	
	Risperidone	
	Ziprasidone	
	Quetiapine	
	Aripiprazole	
Prophylaxis	Lithium	Lithium
	Lamotrigine	Lamotrigine

for acute depressive episodes. Most treatment is undertaken primarily by extension from treatment experience in unipolar depression. Efficacy data from two or more randomized controlled studies exist only for lithium, lamotrigine, and quetiapine. Support for the efficacy of valproate and carbamazepine in acute depressive episodes in bipolar disorder is notably lacking.

In reviewing studies of agents for the prophylaxis of manic or depressive symptoms, we discovered that most of the studies reported recurrence rates without distinguishing between manic and depressive symptoms. For instance, some studies reported such statistics as time-to-first-episode without specifying whether the first episode was manic or depressed. Other studies reported summary statistics for affective symptoms without separating manic or depressive symptoms. We found that when studies did report specific polarity of symptoms during recurrence, it was infrequent that they reported impact of treatment on recurrence of depressive symptoms. Far and away, the most placebo-controlled support for any prophylactic agent comes from studies of lithium, including studies of relapse prevention for depression. There is also support from placebo-controlled trials for lamotrigine, and some support from controlled trials that are not placebo-controlled for carbamazepine. The one prophylaxis study of valproate showed no difference from placebo (lithium was also found to be no different from placebo in this study, although the study was under-powered to make definitive conclusions about this comparison).

Thus, in summary, this standardized evidence-based review of available treatments for bipolar disorder indicates that, to date, only lithium fulfills the stringent definition of a mood stabilizer. It is hoped that additional agents soon take their place in the ranks based on high quality data.

It may be surprising that, given the paucity of data on treatment of acute depression and prophylaxis of bipolar disorder, we frequently encounter many other medications used chronically in this illness, sometimes as first-time agents, for instance, valproate and carbamazepine. Although neuroleptics have acute antimanic evidence, despite the fact that there is little evidence for prophylactic efficacy, they are often used chronically. This is because these agents are typically started during the course of an acute manic episode and clinicians are loathe to stop them and switch to a different agent such as lithium. In addition, many individuals have failed or have been intolerant of treatment with lithium and they are therefore treated using the "next best thing." This is not necessarily suboptimal treatment. However, it is important that the clinician recognize that data on long-term prophylactic efficacy

is quite scanty for these agents—as it is for many other agents used in clinical practice.

Several additional issues in prophylaxis of bipolar disorder deserve comment. First, when is lifetime, or at least long-term, prophylaxis warranted? After one manic episode? One hypomanic episode? One depressive episode with a strong family history of bipolar disorder? There is insufficient empirical evidence with which to make strong recommendations. In clinical practice without clear guidelines, such decisions need to take into account the capability of the individual and family in reporting symptoms, rapidity of onset of episodes, episode severity, and associated morbidity. Clearly, the risks of a wait-and-see strategy would be different in a person who had a psychotic manic episode than in a person who had mild hypomania.

Second, can lithium ever be discontinued? Again, there are no solid data on which to base this decision. However, if lithium discontinuation is contemplated, there is evidence that rapid discontinuation (in less than 2 weeks) is more likely to result in relapse than slow taper (2–4 weeks), with relapse rates higher in type I individuals than in type II individuals. In type I individuals, relapse rates for rapid discontinuation versus slow taper were, respectively, 96% and 73%, whereas in type II individuals they were 91% and 33%. There is some theoretical concern, based on a report of four individuals, that individuals in whom lithium has been discontinued may not be recaptured by resumption of lithium but these were preliminary observations on a sample from the NIMH that may not be representative of persons with bipolar disorder seen in general clinical practice.

Third, a set sequence of treatment for refractory bipolar disorder has yet to be established. In particular, persons with rapid cycling represent a treatment dilemma. Although antidepressants may induce rapid cycling, they often leave the person in a protracted, severe depression. Switching from one antimanic agent to another often results in resumption of cycling. Complex treatment strategies may be required, such as anticonvulsants plus lithium, combinations of anticonvulsants, or adjuvant treatment with high doses of the thyroid hormone thyroxine.

All psychotropic medications have side effects. Some are actually desirable (e.g., sedation with some antidepressants in persons with prominent insomnia), and specific medications are often chosen on the basis of desired side effects. However, side effects usually represent factors that decrease an individual's quality of life and compromise compliance. Furthermore, all antidepressants can cause rapid cycling and mixed states in persons with bipolar disorder. These effects

Table 28-8	Side Effects of Lithium and Commonly Used Anticonvulsants I: Life-Threatening			
I: Life-Threatening				
	At Therapeutic Levels		**At Toxic Levels**	
	Idiopathic	**Dose-Related**	**Dose-Related**	
Lithium			Renal failure Encephalopathy	
CBZ	Agranulocytosis* Aplastic anemia* Stevens–Johnson*			
VPA	Hepatic necrosis	Thrombocytopenia	Thrombocytopenia	
LMT	Stevens–Johnson*			
II: Clinically Significant Side Effect				
	Lithium	**CBZ**	**VPA**	**LMT**
Neurologic/muscular	Lethargy Memory (anomia) Tremor[†] Myoclonus	Lethargy Blurred vision Ataxia[†]	Lethargy Depression Tremor[†] Ataxia	Lethargy Ataxia Blurred vision Headache
Endocrine/metabolic	Weight gain[†] Hypothyroidism		Weight gain[†]	
Cardiopulmonary				
Hematologic			Thrombocytopenia	
Renal	Polyuria			
Hepatic		Jaundice	Jaundice	
Gastrointestinal	Nausea[†] Diarrhea[†]	Nausea[†]	Nausea[†]	Nausea[†]
Dermatologic	Maculopapular rash Psoriasis Acne	Maculopapular rash Alopecia	Maculopapular rash	Maculopapular rash
Other			Back pain	
III: Subclinical Laboratory Abnormalities				
	Lithium	**CBZ**	**VPA**	**LMT**
Neurologic/muscular				
Endocrine/metabolic	Increased TSH	Decreased FTI		
Cardiopulmonary	EKG T-wave depression			

Hematologic	Leukocytosis
	    (to 20,000)
		Leukopenia	Thrombocytopenia
			    (OK > 20,000)	

Renal	Decreased urine specific gravity, GFR			
Hepatic		Increased LFTs	Increased LFTs	

*Typically during first 1–6 months of treatment.
†Most common reasons in our experience for noncompliance.

are not uncommonly encountered in clinical practice and should be watched for, even in persons taking mood-stabilizing agents.

A brief overview of the most frequent or important side effects of lithium, carbamazepine, and valproic acid can be found in Table 28-8. Note that some side effects may be encountered at any serum level of the drug, even within the therapeutic range. Some side effects may be dose related even within that range and may respond to dosage reduction. Others are more idiosyncratic and may need other management. Note that not all laboratory findings represent pathological processes that are associated with or presage morbidity for the individual; that is, not all are clinically significant.

Note also that the concept of the "therapeutic level" is not as straightforward as we would like to assume. The lower limit is usually established by the lowest level necessary for therapeutic effect, whereas the upper limit is set by the lowest level associated with regular, significant toxicity. This range is never established with complete precision. For some medications such as lithium, the therapeutic window is actually quite narrow, with toxic effects developing with some regularity after the upper limit of the therapeutic range is surpassed and with serious toxicity developing at only modestly higher serum levels. As a further complication, for many persons, the minimum level of lithium for good response may be substantially above the 0.5 to 0.8 mEq/L that is usually set as the lower therapeutic limit, but this is reached only at the cost of increased incidence of side effects. On the other hand, experience with valproic acid shows that the upper limit of the therapeutic range for mood stabilization may actually be 125 mg/dL rather than the listed range of 100 mg/dL usually accepted for antiepileptic effect, and this level may be reached without undue side effects.

Thus, established therapeutic levels should be used as important guidelines, and exceeding therapeutic levels should be done only with careful monitoring. However, one must not be falsely reassured that reaching the lower level of a therapeutic range is equally effective for all individuals, while taking with a grain of salt the upper limits of the therapeutic range in drugs with a wider therapeutic window.

Another important issue to consider is drug–drug interactions that may lead to side effects. Such interactions are often associated with increases in serum levels of the drug of interest. For example, addition of thiazide diuretics, or nonsteroidal antiinflammatory agents, the latter available over the counter, is a common reason for increase in lithium level and development of toxicity. However, at other times the drug–drug interactions may not be reflected in an increased serum level if the main interaction is displacement of protein-bound drug. Because free drug concentrations are usually 1–10% of total serum drug, a displacement of even 50% of bound drug may be associated with negligible if any changes in total serum level. However, since both therapeutic and toxic effects are due to free, not bound, drug, unwanted side effects may develop despite total drug levels measured in the therapeutic range.

As noted previously, some side effects may be desirable. However, in many cases they are impediments to treatment, frequently of sufficient importance to lead to noncompliance. As clinicians, however, we might reframe the noncompliance issue more appropriately as "insufficient provider–patient cost-benefit analysis." Stressing compliance when a person suffers from significant side effects is usually much less effective than working to set appropriate expectations of the individual and to find a regimen of minimal toxicity.

Nonetheless, the astute clinician does have several strategies available to improve individuals' tolerance of medications. First, dose reduction may be achieved without compromising efficacy in some individuals. Some side effects, such as lithium-induced nausea,

usually respond well to this, whereas others, such as lithium-induced memory loss, improve less reliably.

Second, simple changes in preparation may be helpful, such as using enteric-coated lithium. Uncoated valproic acid causes nausea so frequently that only the coated forms are routinely used; however, the pediatric "sprinkle" preparation may be of some benefit in persons with nausea even with enteric-coated valproic acid.

Third, changing the administration schedule may ameliorate side effects. Commonsense strategies such as taking nausea-inducing medications after a meal should not be overlooked. Single daily dosing of lithium, carbamazepine, or valproic acid may decrease daytime sedation without compromising efficacy. For more obscure reasons, single daily dosing of lithium appears to decrease polyuria quite effectively.

Fourth, addition of medications to counteract side effects can sometimes be the only way to continue treatment. Addition of beta-blockers can reduce lithium- or valproic acid-induced tremors. Judicious use of thiazide diuretics, often in conjunction with potassium-sparing diuretics or potassium supplements, can reduce lithium-induced polyuria.

Finally, change to another drug may be the only alternative. This is clearly indicated in the case of serious allergic reactions. Polypharmacy should be avoided wherever possible.

Psychotherapies

One of the fastest moving areas of research in bipolar disorder has been psychotherapy. It is important to note that psychotherapy has been studied almost exclusively in the context of ongoing medication management, rather than as a substitute for, or alternative to, medication treatment. Rather, psychotherapy has been utilized as an adjuvant treatment to optimize outcome in the illness. Psychotherapy has been viewed as having one or more of several roles in the management of the disorder.

Recall that both somatic therapies and psychotherapies to date have been predominantly oriented toward improving clinical outcome. Under this conceptualization, psychotherapy has been thought to directly address symptoms, such as cognitive therapy for depressive symptoms. Less frequently has psychotherapy been developed with an explicit component geared toward addressing the functional deficits in bipolar disorder. However, functional outcome has often been measured in formal trials of various types of psychotherapy. A third conceptualization has been to use psychotherapy as a predominantly educative method to assist individuals

Table 28-9	Basics of Education to Improve Disease Management Skills

1. Principles
A. Gear education to educational, cultural, motivational factors of individuals and their families.
B. Include both knowledge about the disorder in general and exploration of the individual's specific form of illness and how it affects their own life.
C. Pay close attention to opportunities for destigmatization and demystification.
D. Emphasize the role of the person in treatment and his/her family as comanagers of the illness, including judging costs and benefits of specific treatment options according to the individual's priorities.

2. Components of Psychoeducation
A. The disorder
  (1) Biological basis
    (a) Genetic factors (especially for persons of childbearing age)
    (b) Possible brain mechanisms
  (2) Environmental components
    (a) Psychosocial factors
    (b) Physical environmental factors
  (3) Course and outcome
    (a) Prevalence
    (b) Episode types and patterns
    (c) Potential triggers for episodes
    (d) Comorbidities and complications
B. Treatment
  (1) Somatic therapies: somatic and psychosocial
    (a) Goals
    (b) Side effect recognition and management
    (c) Costs and benefits of individual treatment options
  (2) Coping skills
    (a) Recognition of early warning signs of relapse
    (b) Avoidance/management of triggers for episodes
    (c) Activation of adaptive coping behaviors and avoidance of maladaptive responses

in participating more effectively in treatment. In this latter regard, treatment is geared toward improving "host factors," that is, those factors not directly due to the disease but that have an impact on its course or treatment, through education, support, and problem solving. Such host factors include illness management skills, which may be improved through psychoeducation and attention to building the therapeutic alliance. Basics of education are summarized in Table 28-9.

Five main types of psychotherapy have been studied in bipolar disorder: couples–partners, group interpersonal or psychoeducative, cognitive–behavioral, family, and interpersonal and social rhythms. Couples–partners, cognitive–behavioral, and family methods all have some randomized clinical trials data supporting a role in improving clinical outcome or functional outcome or the intermediate outcome variable of improving illness management skills. The degree of convergent validity across interventions regarding agenda for disease management information and skills to be imparted is quite

striking. Specifically, imparting education, focusing on early warning symptoms and triggers of episodes, and developing detailed and individual-specific action plans are found across most of the other interventions as well.

Treatment of Bipolar Disorder across the Life Cycle

Although the somatotherapeutic and psychotherapeutic mainstays of treatment endure across the life cycle, several phases of life present particular challenges. There exist few data on treatment of bipolar disorder in childhood. Treatments are chosen by extension from the adult literature, with the one caveat that there have been rare cases of liver failure in conjunction with valproic acid use in children younger than 10 years of age who have been exposed to multiple anticonvulsants.

In pregnancy, there is some evidence that lithium may be teratogenic, associated with increased rates of cardiac abnormalities, although more recent data indicate that this risk may be overestimated. Valproic acid and perhaps carbamazepine have been associated with neural tube defects, leaving the neuroleptics, antidepressants, and ECT as the preferable management strategies during pregnancy, particularly during the first trimester. It should be kept in mind, however, that treatment decisions are based on *risk*, not *certainty*. Risk of fetal malformation, parental attitude toward raising children with birth defects, severity of illness, and ease of management with alternative therapies all need to be considered in conjunction with the woman and her partner.

Aging also presents certain treatment concerns. Tricyclic antidepressants may be associated with clinically significant cardiac conduction abnormalities, hypotension, sedation, glaucoma, and urinary retention, particularly in the presence of prostatic hypertrophy. These are of even greater concern in the elderly. The risk of sedation due to neuroleptics and benzodiazepines, and of hypotension due to low-potency neuroleptics can also particularly complicate treatment of elderly persons with bipolar disorder. Such side effects can cause far-reaching and serious complications, such as hip fracture, which is not infrequently the initial event in a cascade of complications that can be terminal.

By contrast, lithium, carbamazepine, and valproic acid are relatively well tolerated in the elderly once attention is given to the slower clearance of drugs in general in this population group. The risk of clinically significant renal toxicity with appropriately dosed lithium is not great. Although glomerular filtration rate decreases with age in persons treated with lithium, the rate of decline does not appear to be accelerated by lithium treatment. Nonetheless, careful monitoring of renal function is needed in the elderly.

In addition, increasing age is clearly a risk factor for hypothyroidism, as is lithium use. Thus, elderly persons taking lithium should be followed up carefully for decrements in thyroid function, although hypothyroidism is not an indication for lithium discontinuation but rather simply for thyroid hormone supplementation.

COMPARISON OF DSM-IV-TR AND ICD-10 DIAGNOSTIC CRITERIA

The ICD-10 item set for a manic episode contains nine items in contrast to the seven items in the DSM-IV-TR criteria set, the two additional items being marked sexual energy or indiscretions and loss of normal social inhibitions. However, the number of items required by ICD-10 Diagnostic Criteria for Research remains the same as the number in DSM-IV-TR (i.e., three items if mood is euphoric, four items if mood is irritable), which is likely to result in a more inclusive diagnosis of a manic episode in ICD-10. Furthermore, the duration of mixed episodes differs, with DSM-IV-TR requiring a duration of 1 week (as is the case for a manic episode), whereas the ICD-10 Diagnostic Criteria for Research require a duration of at least 2 weeks.

The criteria sets for hypomanic episode differ as well. The ICD-10 Diagnostic Criteria for Research contain several additional items (increased sexual energy and increased sociability) and do not include the DSM-IV-TR items, inflated self-esteem and flight of ideas. Furthermore, ICD-10 does not require that the change in mood be observed by others.

Regarding the definition of bipolar I disorder, in addition to differences in the diagnostic criteria for a manic and major depressive episode, the ICD-10 definition of "Bipolar Affective Disorder" (i.e., any combination of hypomanic, manic, mixed, and depressive episodes) does not distinguish between bipolar I and bipolar II disorder (i.e., cases of DSM-IV-TR Bipolar II

Disorder are diagnosed as Bipolar Affective Disorder in ICD-10). However, ICD-10 Diagnostic Criteria for Research does include diagnostic criteria for bipolar II in its appendix, which are identical to the criteria set in DSM-IV-TR.

For cyclothymic disorder, the ICD-10 Diagnostic Criteria for Research provides list of symptoms that must be associated with the periods of depressed mood and hypomania, which differ from the ICD-10 item sets for dysthymic disorder and hypomania. In contrast, the DSM-IV-TR definition of cyclothymic disorder just refers to numerous periods of hypomania and depressive symptoms.

DSM-IV-TR Diagnostic Criteria

BIPOLAR I DISORDER, MOST RECENT EPISODE [*INDICATE* HYPOMANIC, MANIC, MIXED, DEPRESSED, OR UNSPECIFIED]

A. Currently (or most recently) in a Hypomanic (296.40), Manic (296.4x), Mixed (296.6x), or Major Depressive Episode (296.5x). If the criteria except for duration are met for one of these episodes, the episode is consider is considered unspecified (296.7).

   Note: An x in the diagnostic code indicates that a fifth digit indicating severity is required.

B. There has previously been at least one Manic, Mixed, or Major Depressive Episode.
C. The mood episodes in Criteria A and B are not better accounted for by Schizoaffective Disorder and are not superimposed on Schizophrenia, Schizophreni-form Disorder, Delusion Disorder, or Psychotic Disorder Not Otherwise Specified.

If the full criteria are currently met for a Manic or Mixed Episode, *specify* its current clinical status and/or features:

Mild, Moderate, Severe Without Psychotic Features/ Sever With Psychotic Features
With Catatonic Features
With Postpartum Onset

Reprinted with permission from *DSM-IV-TR Guidebook*. Copyright 2004, Michael B First, Allen Frances, and Harold Alan Pincus.

Anxiety Disorders: Panic Disorder with and without Agoraphobia

DIAGNOSIS

According to the DSM-IV-TR, panic disorder is defined by recurrent and unexpected panic attacks. At least one of these attacks must be followed by 1 month or more of (1) persistent concern about having more attacks, (2) worry about the implications or consequences of the attack, or (3) changes to typical behavioral patterns (e.g., avoidance of work or school activities) as a result of the attack. In addition, the panic attacks must not stem solely from the direct effects of illicit substance use, medication, or a general medical condition (e.g., hyperthyroidism, vestibular dysfunction) and are not better explained by another mental disorder (such as social phobia for attacks that occur only in social situations). A diagnosis of panic disorder with agoraphobia is warranted when the criteria for panic disorder are satisfied and accompanied by agoraphobia.

Although panic attacks are a cardinal feature of panic disorder and in combination with agoraphobia (i.e., anxiety about being in a place or a situation that is not easily escaped or where help is not easily accessible if panic occurs) are essential to a diagnosis of panic disorder with agoraphobia, the criteria sets for panic attacks (see DSM-IV-TR diagnostic criteria for Panic Attack, page 293) and for agoraphobia (see DSM-IV-TR diagnostic criteria for Agoraphobia, page 293) are listed separately as stand-alone, noncodable conditions that are referred to by the diagnostic criteria for panic disorder and agoraphobia without history of panic disorder. Notwithstanding, accurate diagnosis is difficult without a proficient understanding of these features. While the criteria for agoraphobia are generally straightforward, panic attacks can be difficult to understand.

Many people report having what they consider to be a panic attack during or in association with actual physical threat (i.e., a true alarm situation). It is, however, important to distinguish between a fear reaction

---

DSM-IV-TR Diagnostic Criteria

300.01 PANIC DISORDER WITHOUT AGORAPHOBIA AND 300.21 PANIC DISORDER WITH AGORAPHOBIA

A. Both (1) and (2):

  (1) recurrent unexpected Panic Attacks
  (2) at least one of the attacks has been followed by 1 month (or more) of one (or more) of the following:

    (a) persistent concern about having additional attacks
    (b) worry about the implications of the attack or its consequences (e.g., losing control, having a heart attack, "going crazy")
    (c) a significant change in behavior related to the attacks

B. This criterion differs for Panic Disorder With and Without Agoraphobia as follows:

  For 300.21 Panic Disorder With Agoraphobia: the presence of Agoraphobia
  For 300.01 Panic Disorder Without Agoraphobia: absence of Agoraphobia

C. The Panic Attacks are not due to the direct physiological effects of a substance (e.g., a drug of abuse, medication) or a general medical condition (e.g., hyperthyroidism).

D. The Panic Attacks are not better accounted for by another mental disorder, such as Social Phobia (e.g., occurring on exposure to feared social situations), Specific Phobia (e.g., on exposure to the phobic situation), Obsessive-Compulsive Disorder (e.g., on exposure to dirt in someone with an obsession about contamination), Posttraumatic Stress Disorder (e.g., in response to stimuli associated with a severe stressor), or Separation Anxiety Disorder (e.g., in response to being away from home or close relatives).

Note: This is a summary of two criteria sets.

Reprinted with permission from *DSM-IV-TR Guidebook*. Copyright 2004, Michael B First, Allen Frances, and Harold Alan Pincus.

Clinical Guide to the Diagnosis and Treatment of Mental Disorders. M. B. First and A. Tasman
© 2006 John Wiley & Sons, Ltd.   ISBN 0 470 019158

DSM-IV-TR Diagnostic Criteria

PANIC ATTACK

A panic attack is a discrete period of intense fear or discomfort in the absence of real danger that develops abruptly, reaches a peak within 10 min, and is accompanied by four (or more) of the following symptoms:

A. palpitations, pounding heart, or accelerated heart rate
B. sweating
C. trembling or shaking
D. sensations of shortness of breath or smothering
E. feeling of choking
F. chest pain or discomfort
G. nausea or abdominal distress
H. feeling dizzy, unsteady, light-headed, or faint
I. derealization (feelings of unreality) or depersonalization (being detached from oneself)
J. fear of losing control or going crazy
K. fear of dying
L. paresthesias (numbness or tingling sensations)
M. chills or hot flushes

Reprinted with permission from the *Diagnostic and Statistical Manual of Mental Disorders*, 4th ed., Text Rev. Copyright 2000 American Psychiatric Association.

in response to actual threat and a panic attack. In an attempt to do so, the DSM-IV-TR has clarified that panic attacks occur "in the absence of real danger" (page 430). Such attacks involve a paroxysmal occurrence of intense fear or discomfort accompanied by a minimum of 4 of the 13 symptoms shown in the diagnostic criteria for Panic Attack. The DSM-IV-TR recognizes three characteristic types of panic attacks, including those that are *unexpected* (i.e., not associated with an identifiable internal or external trigger and appear to occur "out of the blue"), *situationally bound*

DSM-IV-TR Diagnostic Criteria

AGORAPHOBIA

A. Agoraphobia is characterized by anxiety about being in places or situations from which escape might be difficult (or embarrassing) or in which help may not be available in the event of having an unexpected or situationally predisposed panic attack or panic-like symptoms. Agoraphobic fears typically involve characteristic clusters of situations, such as being outside the home alone, being in a crowd, standing in a line, being on a bridge, or traveling in a motor vehicle.
B. The situations are avoided or are endured with marked distress or worry about having a panic attack or panic-like symptoms. Confronting situations is aided by the presence of a companion.
C. The anxiety or avoidance is not better accounted for by another mental disorder.

Reprinted with permission from the *Diagnostic and Statistical Manual of Mental Disorders*, 4th ed., Text Rev. Copyright 2000 American Psychiatric Association.

(i.e., almost invariably occur when exposed to a situational trigger or when anticipating it), and *situationally predisposed* (i.e., usually, but not necessarily, occur when exposed to a situational trigger or when anticipating it). The term *limited symptom attacks* is used to refer to panic-like episodes comprising fewer than four symptoms.

Although unexpected panic attacks are required for a diagnosis of panic disorder, not all panic attacks that occur in panic disorder are unexpected. The occurrence of unexpected attacks can wax and wane and over the developmental course of the disorder; they tend to become situationally bound or predisposed. Moreover, unexpected panic attacks as well as those that are situationally bound or predisposed can occur in the context of other mental disorders, including all of the other anxiety disorders (e.g., a person with social phobia might have an occasional unexpected panic attack without the other features required to diagnose panic disorder; a dog phobic might panic whenever a large dog is encountered) and some general medical conditions. A clear understanding of the distinction between types of panic attacks outlined in the DSM-IV-TR provides a foundation for diagnosis and differential diagnosis.

Panic disorder with or without agoraphobia is associated with impaired occupational and social functioning and poor overall quality of life. People with panic disorder, compared to people in the general population, report poorer physical health. Panic disorder is a leading reason for seeking emergency department consultations and a leading cause for seeking mental health services, surpassing both schizophrenia and mood disorders. Panic disorder exceeds the economic costs associated with many other anxiety disorders such as social phobia, generalized anxiety disorder, and obsessive–compulsive disorder. The high medical costs are partly because individuals with panic disorder quite often present to their primary care physician or hospital emergency departments, thinking they are in imminent danger of dying or "going crazy." In these settings, individuals may undergo a series of extensive medical tests before panic disorder is, if ever, finally diagnosed. Ruling out general medical conditions is good clinical practice but the process contributes substantially to the costs that panic disorder places on health care systems.

When assessing for the presence of panic disorder, the most comprehensive and accurate diagnostic information emerges when the clinician uses open-ended questions and empathic listening, combined with structured inquiry about specific events and symptoms. To gain more detailed information on panic attacks, clinicians and clinical researchers are increasingly including some form of prospective monitoring in their assessment batteries. The most widely used are the *panic attack records*. The individual is provided with a definition of a panic attack and then given a pad of panic attack records that can be readily carried in a purse or pocket. The individual is instructed to carry the records at all times and to complete one record (sheet) for each full-blown or limited symptom attack, soon after the attack occurs.

Consider the application of the panic attack record to the following case vignette. Sandra B. was a 20-year-old college student who presented to a student health clinic reporting recurrent panic attacks. Her first attack occurred seven months earlier while smoking marijuana at an end-of-term party. At the time, she felt depersonalized, dizzy, short of breath, and her heart was beating wildly. Sandra had an overwhelming fear that she was going crazy. Friends took her to a nearby hospital emergency department where she was given a brief medical evaluation, reassured that she was simply experiencing anxiety and given a prescription for lorazepam. In the following months, Sandra continued to experience unexpected panic attacks and became increasingly convinced that she was losing control of her mind. Most of her panics occurred unexpectedly during the day, although they sometimes also occurred at night, wrenching her out of a deep sleep. An example of how Sandra B. might complete the panic attack record for one of her panic attacks is shown in Figure 29-1. These records are then reviewed during treatment sessions to glean information about the links among beliefs, bodily sensations, and safety behaviors, and to assess treatment progress.

Sandra B. reported that the panic attack summarized in Figure 29-1 occurred when she was in a neighborhood

PANIC ATTACK RECORD

NAME: **Sandra.B.**

DATE: **Oct 2** TIME: **4pm** DURATION (min): **15**

WITH: SPOUSE ____ FRIEND ____ STRANGER ____ ALONE ✓

STRESSFUL SITUATION: YES / (NO) EXPECTED: YES / (NO)

MAXIMUM ANXIETY (CIRCLE)

0 -------- 1 -------- 2 -------- 3 -------- 4 -------- (5) -------- 6 -------- 7 -------- 8
NONE MODERATE EXTREME

SENSATIONS (CHECK):

POUNDING HEART	✓	SWEATING	✓	HOT/COLD FLASH	✓
TIGHT/PAINFUL CHEST	✓	CHOKING	____	FEAR OF DYING	____
BREATHLESS	✓	NAUSEA	____	FEAR OF GOING CRAZY	✓
DIZZY	✓	UNREALITY	✓	FEAR OF LOSING CONTROL	✓
TREMBLING	____	NUMB/TINGLE	✓		

THOUGHTS OR MENTAL IMAGES AT THE TIME (DESCRIBE):

I'm losing contact with reality

Figure 29-1 *A completed panic attack record for Sandra B.*

supermarket. As she walked down the aisle, she looked at the long rows of fluorescent lights and then began to feel mildly depersonalized. Upon noticing this sensation, she began to increasingly worry that the depersonalization might become so intense that she would lose all contact with reality, to the point that she would be permanently insane. This greatly frightened her and led to an increase in the intensity of arousal sensations. In an effort to reduce the intensity of the feared depersonalization, she averted her gaze from the lights and began studying the list of ingredients on cereal boxes. This distracting safety behavior calmed her down and reduced the feared depersonalization to the point that she was able to make her way to the express checkout counter and leave with the grocery items she had collected.

Lifetime comorbidity in panic disorder is common, with over 90% of community-dwelling and treatment-seeking individuals having had symptoms meeting diagnostic threshold for at least one other disorder. Epidemiological studies indicate that major depressive disorder occurs in up to 65% of individuals with panic disorder at some point in their lives. In approximately two-thirds of these cases, the symptoms of depression develop along with, or secondary to, panic disorder. However, since depression precedes panic disorder in the remaining third, depressive symptoms co-occurring with panic disorder cannot be considered simply as a demoralized response to paroxysms of anxiety. While the risk of developing secondary depression appears to be more closely associated with the severity of agoraphobia than with the severity or frequency of panic attacks, this may be a confound of misdiagnosing of some behavioral manifestations of depression as agoraphobia. Panic disorder and depression do not appear to be identical disorders and their co-occurrence may be due to a shared diathesis or mutual exacerbation of symptoms.

As illustrated in the case of Sandra B., panic disorder can be precipitated by the use of psychotropic drugs. Risk is higher with chronic use. Alcohol has been identified as playing a precipitating, maintaining, and aggravating role in panic disorder. The 6-month prevalence of alcohol abuse or dependence in panic disorder has been reported to be 40% in men and 13% in women. These rates are higher than those observed in people with other anxiety disorders and those with no anxiety disorder. Although alcohol problems have been reported to precede panic disorder in a majority of cases, most reports indicate that alcohol problems develop secondary to panic disorder, often as a means of self-medication. Those having panic disorder with agoraphobia appear to be at greater risk for comorbid alcohol abuse or dependence than those without agoraphobia.

The 1-year prevalence for any panic attack, whether unexpected or situationally cued, is approximately 28%. Lifetime prevalence rates for unexpected panic attacks and agoraphobia are approximately 4% and 9%, respectively. Investigations of unexpected panic attacks in college student samples using self-report methodology have revealed similar rates, ranging from approximately 5% to 11%.

The National Comorbidity Study has reported the lifetime prevalence of panic disorder (with or without agoraphobia) in the general population to be 3.5%. However, despite uncertainty as to the reason, this rate is somewhat of an anomaly in the literature. Most epidemiological studies, including those based on Epidemiologic Catchment Area and other data sources, have consistently shown lifetime rates between 1% and 2%. Despite some minor variation, lifetime prevalence rates are generally consistent around the world. One-year prevalence rates in the general community also vary slightly from lifetime rates, being between 0.2% and 1.7%. In treatment-seeking individuals, the prevalence of panic disorder is considerably higher. Approximately 10% of individuals in mental health clinics and between 10% and 60% in various medical specialty clinics (e.g., cardiology, respiratory, vestibular) have panic disorder. Panic disorder with agoraphobia is more common than panic disorder without agoraphobia in clinical samples.

The clinical features of panic disorder such as number and severity of symptoms are much the same across the sexes. However, women are diagnosed with panic disorder more than twice as often as men. Recent research indicates that women are more likely to have panic disorder with agoraphobia and that they are more likely to have recurrence of symptoms after remission of their panic attacks than are men. Men, on the other hand, are more likely to have panic disorder without agoraphobia and are more likely to self-medicate with alcohol than are women. The literature remains unclear as to why these sex differences exist but alludes to the possible role of biological and/or socialization factors.

Course

Age of onset for panic disorder is distributed bimodally, typically developing between 15 and 19 or 25 and 30 years. Panic disorder symptoms may wax and wane but, if left untreated, the typical course is chronic. Data from a sample of individuals assessed and treated through the Harvard/Brown Anxiety Disorders Research Program and followed prospectively over a 5-year period indicated remission rates in both men and women to be 39%. In general, among those receiving tertiary treatment, approximately 30% of individuals have symptoms that are in remission, 40–50% are improved but still have significant symptoms, and 20–30% are unimproved or worse at 6 to 10 years follow-up.

Differential Diagnosis

A complete assessment for panic disorder includes a general medical evaluation, consisting of a medical history, review of organ systems, physical examination, and blood tests. A general medical evaluation is important for identifying general medical conditions that mimic or exacerbate panic attacks or panic-like symptoms (e.g., seizure disorders, cardiac conditions, pheochromocytoma). These disorders should be investigated and treated before contemplating a course of panic disorder treatment. It is also important to rule out the other anxiety disorders and major depressive disorder as primary factors in the person's panic attacks and avoidance prior to initiating treatment for panic disorder. See Figure 29-2 for a decision tree outlining the differential diagnosis for a panic attack.

TREATMENT

There are a number of approaches that can be taken in treating panic disorder with and without agoraphobia (see Figure 29-3).

Somatic Treatment

Controlled studies show that effective antipanic medications include tricyclic antidepressants (e.g., imipramine), monoamine oxidase inhibitors (MAOIs; e.g., phenelzine), high-potency benzodiazepines (e.g., alprazolam), and SSRIs (e.g., fluoxetine). These treatments have broadly similar efficacy, although there is some evidence that SSRIs tend to be most effective. The classes of medication differ in their side effects and their contraindications. Anticholinergic effects (e.g., blurred vision, dry mouth) are common problems with tricyclics. They are also contraindicated in individuals with particular comorbid cardiac disorders. Dietary restrictions (i.e., abstaining from foods containing tyramine) are a limitation of many MAOIs. Sedation, impaired motor coordination, and addiction are concerns with benzodiazepines.

When efficacy and side effects are considered together, SSRIs emerge as the most promising drug treatments for panic disorder. However, even SSRIs have side effects, with the most problematic being a short-term increase in arousal-related sensations. To overcome this problem, SSRIs can be started at a low dose (e.g., 5–10 mg/d for paroxetine; 12.5–25 mg/d for sertraline) and then increased gradually (e.g., up to 10–50 mg/d for paroxetine; up to 25–200 mg/d for sertraline). The choice of SSRI is determined on the basis of several factors, including side effects, individual preference, and the individual's history of responding (or not responding) to particular agents.

For drug refractory individuals, or individuals who are unable to tolerate SSRI side effects, combination medications are sometimes used. For example, SSRIs can be augmented with benzodiazepines. The latter are used to dampen the side effects of SSRIs. Despite some positive preliminary reports supporting this strategy, its value in the treatment of panic disorder remains to be properly evaluated. An alternative strategy is to change the individual's medication. Some of the newer, non-SSRI antidepressants could be considered, such as venlafaxine, duloxetine, buproprion, or gabapentin. A concern with using these medications to treat panic disorder is that there are fewer data to guide the clinician. Another approach to the drug refractory individual is to use a psychosocial treatment such as cognitive–behavioral therapy (CBT), as an alternative or adjunctive intervention.

Psychosocial Treatments

CBT treatment packages include a number of components, such as psychoeducation (e.g., information about the cognitive model of panic), breathing retraining, cognitive restructuring, relaxation exercises, interoceptive exposure, and situational exposure. Breathing retraining involves teaching the individual to breathe with the diaphragm rather than with the chest muscles. Cognitive restructuring focuses on challenging individual's beliefs about the dangerousness of bodily sensations (e.g., challenging the belief that palpitations lead to heart attacks).

Interoceptive exposure involves inducing feared bodily sensations to further teach individuals that the sensations are harmless. For example, Sandra B.'s treatment involved interoceptive exposure exercises that induced depersonalization. Several tasks were used, including (1) staring at a ceiling fluorescent light for 1 minute, (2) staring at her reflection in the mirror for 2 minutes, and (3) staring at a spot on the wall for 3 minutes. Multiple tasks were used in order to promote the generalization of treatment effects (i.e., to help her learn that depersonalization was harmless regardless of how it arises).

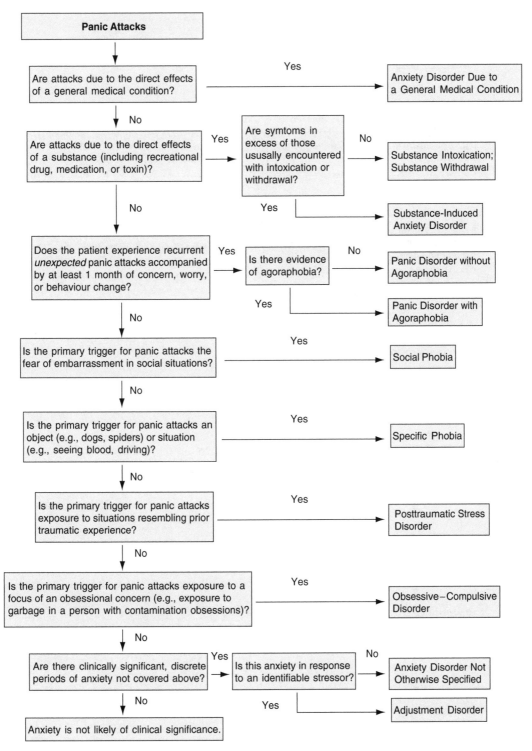

Figure 29-2 *A decision tree for assessment of patients presenting with panic attacks.*

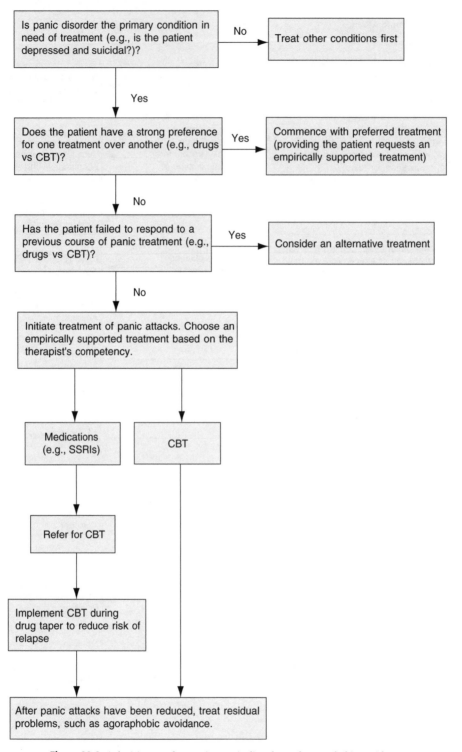

Figure 29-3 *A decision tree for treating panic disorder and agoraphobic avoidance.*

Situational exposure involves activities that bring the individual into feared situations such as shopping malls, bridges, or tunnels. In Sandra B.'s case, situational and interoceptive exposure were combined. She was asked to visit a lighting store to spend time inspecting the various fluorescent lamps. Exposure exercises are often framed as "behavioral experiments" to test individuals' beliefs about the catastrophic consequences of arousal-related sensations. Sandra B.'s exposure exercises helped her test the belief that depersonalization leads to permanent insanity. The exercises were also used to help her test the alternative, noncatastrophic belief that depersonalization is an unpleasant but harmless experience.

A common practice in CBT is to encourage individuals to refrain from engaging in safety behaviors. Prior to treatment, Sandra B. typically engaged in distraction whenever she was exposed to depersonalization-inducing stimuli such as fluorescent lights. The CBT therapist encouraged her to refrain from distraction so she could learn that depersonalization is harmless, even when it becomes intense. Evidence suggests that reducing safety behaviors improves treatment efficacy. Despite the advantages of exposure exercises, they are medically contraindicated in some cases. For example, a hyperventilation exercise would not be used in an individual with severe asthma.

A large body of evidence shows that CBT is effective in reducing panic attacks, agoraphobia, and associated symptoms such as depression. However, not all CBT interventions may be necessary. Interoceptive exposure, situational exposure, and cognitive restructuring are the most widely used and supported interventions. Several studies suggest that breathing retraining reduces panic frequency. However, recent research casts doubt about the importance of hyperventilation in producing panic attacks. This suggests that breathing retraining may only be useful for a minority of individuals, for which chest breathing or hyperventilation plays a role in producing panic symptoms. Breathing retraining may be counterproductive if it prevents individuals from learning that their catastrophic beliefs are unfounded. Given these concerns, breathing retraining should be used sparingly in the treatment of panic disorder. If used at all, the clinician should ensure that the individual understands that breathing exercises are used to remove unpleasant but harmless sensations. Interoceptive exposure and cognitive restructuring are important for helping individuals learn that the sensations are not dangerous.

How effective is CBT compared to other therapies? A growing literature suggests that the efficacy of CBT is equal to or greater than that of alprazolam and

imipramine at posttreatment. Preliminary evidence suggests that CBT is effective in treating individuals who have failed to respond to pharmacotherapies. Follow-up studies suggest that CBT is effective in the long term and is likely to be more effective than short-term pharmacological treatment. It is not known whether drug treatments would be as effective as CBT if individuals remained on their medications. Any conclusions about the long-term efficacy of panic treatments are necessarily tentative because individuals sometimes seek additional treatment during the follow-up interval.

Several other approaches have been used in the treatment of panic disorder, including psychodynamic psychotherapies, hypnosis, Eye Movement Desensitization and Reprocessing (EMDR), and mindfulness meditation. Support for these treatments is limited largely to case studies and uncontrolled trials. Controlled studies, although few in number, indicate that hypnosis and EMDR are of limited value in treating panic disorder. Interventions that look more promising are mindfulness meditation and psychodynamic psychotherapies modified to specifically focus on panic symptoms. However, none has been extensively evaluated as a panic treatment and none has been compared with empirically supported treatments such as CBT or SSRIs.

Combined Treatments

Many clinicians believe the optimal treatment consists of drugs combined with some form of psychosocial intervention. This view arose from observations that even the most effective drugs and the most effective psychosocial interventions do not eliminate panic disorder in all cases. It was thought that combination treatments might be a way to improve treatment outcome. The available evidence provides mixed support for this view. Evidence suggests that the efficacy of CBT is not improved when it is combined with either diazepam or alprazolam. In fact, some studies have found that the efficacy of situational exposure is worsened when alprazolam is added.

Several studies have compared CBT to CBT combined with imipramine. These results have also been mixed. Adding imipramine in the range of 150–300 mg/day to either situational exposure or CBT sometimes improves treatment outcome in the short term, provided that individuals are able to tolerate the dose. Any advantage of combined treatment tends to be lost at follow-up. Similarly, studies of combining CBT with SSRIs (fluvoxamine or paroxetine) have produced mixed results, with some studies finding the combination is no better than CBT alone, others finding that the combination is most effective, and yet others finding the combination to be most effective for some symptoms but not others. Methodological limitations of these studies might account for the inconsistent findings.

It remains unclear whether treatment outcome is enhanced by combining CBT with SSRIs. Neuroanatomical models of panic disorder with their dual emphasis on cortical and serotonergic mechanisms suggest that this combined treatment might be superior to CBT alone and to SSRIs alone. On the other hand, pharmacotherapies such as SSRIs might undermine the individual's confidence in implementing CBT, particularly if they attribute their gains to medications rather than to their own efforts at using the skills learned in CBT. Large, well-designed studies are needed to explore these important issues.

A more promising type of combined therapy is a sequential approach, in which individuals are treated with pharmacotherapy during the acute phase, and then are treated with CBT as the medication is phased out. Several studies have shown that adding CBT during the tapering period for alprazolam and clonazepam reduces the relapse rate associated with these drugs.

COMPARISON OF DSM-IV-TR AND ICD-10 DIAGNOSTIC CRITERIA

The ICD-10 Diagnostic Criteria for Research for a panic attack are identical to the DSM-IV-TR criteria set except that ICD-10 includes an additional item (i.e., dry mouth). In contrast to the DSM-IV-TR algorithm, which does not give special weight to any particular symptom, the ICD-10 algorithm requires that at least one of the symptoms be palpitations, sweating, trembling, or dry mouth. Like DSM-IV-TR, ICD-10 requires recurrent panic attacks but, in contrast to DSM-IV-TR, it does not include a criterion requiring that the panic attacks be clinically significant.

The ICD-10 Diagnostic Criteria for Research for Agoraphobia differ markedly from the DSM-IV-TR criteria. The ICD-10 Diagnostic Criteria for Research specify that there be fear or avoidance of at least two of the following situations: crowds, public places, traveling alone, or traveling away from home. Furthermore, ICD-10 requires that at least two symptoms of anxiety (i.e., from the list of 14 panic symptoms) be present together on at least one occasion and that these anxiety symptoms be "restricted to, or predominate in, the feared situations or contemplation of the feared situations." In contrast, DSM-IV-TR Agoraphobia is defined in terms of "anxiety about being in places or situations from which escape might be difficult (or embarrassing) or in which help may not be available in the event of having an unexpected or situationally predisposed panic attack." No specific avoided situations or specific types of anxiety symptoms are required for a diagnosis.

30 • Anxiety Disorders: Social and Specific Phobias

DIAGNOSIS

The experience of fear and the related emotion of anxiety are universal and familiar to everyone. Fear exists in all cultures and appears to exist across species. Presumably, the purpose of fear is to protect an organism from immediate threat and to mobilize the body for quick action to avoid danger. Emotion theorists consider fear to be an alarm response that fires in the presence of imminent threat or danger. The function of the primarily noradrenergic-mediated fear response is to facilitate immediate escape from threat (flight) or attack on the source of threat (fight). Therefore, fear is often referred to as a fight-or-flight response. All the manifestations of fear are consistent with its protective function. For example, heart rate and breathing rate increase to meet the increased oxygen needs of the body, increased perspiration helps to cool the body to facilitate escape, and pupils dilate to enhance visual acuity.

Anxiety, on the other hand, is a future-oriented mood state in which the individual anticipates the possibility of threat and experiences a sense of uncontrollability focused on the upcoming negative event. In the DSM-IV-TR, anxiety is defined as "the apprehensive anticipation of future danger or misfortune accompanied by a feeling of dysphoria or somatic symptoms of tension" (p. 820). If one were to put anxiety into words, one might say, "Something bad might happen soon. I am not sure I can cope with it but I have to be ready to try." Anxiety is primarily mediated by the gamma-aminobutyric acid-benzodiazepine system.

Despite evidence that fear and anxiety are mediated by different brain systems, anxiety and fear are related, which makes sense ethologically. Experiencing anxiety after encountering signals of impending danger seems to lower the threshold for fear that is triggered when danger actually occurs (e.g., being attacked by a mugger or almost being hit by an automobile). Anxiety leads to a shift in attention toward the source of danger so that individuals become more vigilant for relevant threat cues and therefore are more likely to experience fear in the face of perceived immediate threat.

Fear and anxiety are not always adaptive, however. At times, the responses can occur in the absence of any realistic threat or it may be out of proportion to the actual danger. Almost everyone has situations that arouse anxiety and fear despite the fact that the actual risk is minimal. It is not unusual to become anxious before a job interview or a speech. Many individuals feel fearful when exposed to situations such as dental visits, seeing certain animals, or being at certain heights. For some people, these fears reach extreme levels and may cause significant distress or impairment in functioning. It is at this point that what we typically refer to as shyness and fearfulness might meet diagnostic criteria for social phobia or specific phobia, respectively.

In the DSM-IV-TR, social phobia (also known as social anxiety disorder) is defined as a "marked and persistent fear of one or more social or performance situations in which the person is exposed to unfamiliar people or to possible scrutiny of others" (see DSM-IV-TR diagnostic criteria, page 302). Typical situations feared by individuals with social phobia include meeting new people, interacting with others, attending parties or meetings, speaking formally, eating or writing in front of others, dealing with people in authority, and being assertive. Specific phobia is defined as a "marked and persistent fear that is excessive or unreasonable, cued by the presence or anticipation of a specific object or situation (e.g., flying, heights, animals, receiving an injection, seeing blood)" (see DSM-IV-TR diagnostic criteria, page 302).

The diagnostic criteria for specific and social phobias share many features. For both disorders, the phobic situation must almost invariably lead to an anxiety response (immediately, in the case of specific phobias), which may take the form of a panic attack. In addition, the individual must recognize that the fear is excessive or unreasonable (although this feature may be absent in children), avoid the phobic situation or endure it

DSM-IV-TR Diagnostic Criteria

300.23 SOCIAL PHOBIA (SOCIAL ANXIETY DISORDER)

A. A marked and persistent fear of one or more social or performance situations in which the person is exposed to unfamiliar people or to possible scrutiny by others. The individual fears that he or she will act in a way (or show anxiety symptoms) that will be humiliating or embarrassing. **Note:** In children, there must be evidence of the capacity for age-appropriate social relationships with familiar people and the anxiety must occur in peer settings, not just in interactions with adults.

B. Exposure to the feared social situation almost invariably provokes anxiety, which may take the form of a situationally bound or situationally predisposed panic attack. **Note:** In children, the anxiety may be expressed by crying, tantrums, freezing, or shrinking away from social situations with unfamiliar people.

C. The person recognizes that the fear is excessive or unreasonable. **Note:** In children, this feature may be absent.

D. The feared social or performance situations are avoided or else are endured with intense anxiety or distress.

E. The avoidance, anxious anticipation, or distress in the feared social or performance situation(s) interferes significantly with the person's normal routine, occupational (or academic) functioning, or social activities or relationships, or there is marked distress about having the phobia.

F. In individuals under age 18 years, the duration is at least 6 months.

G. The fear or avoidance is not due to the direct physiological effects of a substance (e.g., a drug of abuse, a medication) or a general medical condition and is not better accounted for by another mental disorder (e.g., panic disorder with or without agoraphobia, separation-anxiety disorder, body dysmorphic disorder, a pervasive developmental disorder, or schizoid personality disorder).

H. If a general medical condition or another mental disorder is present, the fear in criterion A is unrelated to it, for example, the fear is not of stuttering, trembling in Parkinson's disease, exhibiting abnormal eating behavior in anorexia nervosa or bulimia nervosa.

Specify if:

Generalized: if the fears include most social situations (also consider the additional diagnosis of avoidant personality disorder)

DSM-IV-TR Diagnostic Criteria

300.29 SPECIFIC PHOBIA

A. Marked and persistent fear that is excessive or unreasonable, cued by the presence or anticipation of a specific object or situation (e.g., flying, heights, animals, receiving an injection, seeing blood).

B. Exposure to the phobic stimulus almost invariably provokes an immediate anxiety response, which may take the form of a situationally bound or situationally predisposed panic attack. **Note:** In children, the anxiety may be expressed by crying, tantrums, freezing, or clinging.

C. The person recognizes that the fear is excessive or unreasonable. **Note:** In children, this feature may be absent.

D. The phobic situation(s) is avoided or else is endured with intense anxiety or distress.

E. The avoidance, anxious anticipation, or distress in the feared situation(s) interferes significantly with the person's normal routine, occupational (or academic) functioning, or social activities or relationships, or there is marked distress about having the phobia.

F. In individuals under age 18 years, the duration is at least 6 months.

G. The anxiety, panic attacks, and phobic avoidance associated with the specific object or situation are not better accounted for by another mental disorder, such as obsessive–compulsive disorder (e.g., fear of dirt in someone with an obsession about contamination), posttraumatic stress disorder (e.g., avoidance of stimuli associated with a severe stressor), separation-anxiety disorder (e.g., avoidance of school), social phobia (e.g., avoidance of social situations because of fear of embarrassment), panic disorder with agoraphobia, or agoraphobia without history of panic disorder.

Specify type:

Animal type

Natural environment type (e.g., heights, storms, water)

Blood–injection–injury type

Situational type (e.g., airplanes, elevators, enclosed places)

Other type (e.g., fear of choking, vomiting, or contracting an illness; in children, fear of loud sounds or costumed characters)

with intense distress, and experience marked distress or functional impairment as a result of the phobia. In the case of social phobia, the fear must not be related to another mental disorder or medical condition. For example, if an individual develops difficulties communicating after suffering a stroke, the fear must be unrelated to having other people notice one's problems in speaking. However, if the clinician judges that social anxiety is substantially in excess of what most individuals with this disability would experience, a diagnosis of anxiety disorder not otherwise specified may be appropriate.

Finally, for both disorders the fear must not be better accounted for by another problem. For example, an individual with obsessive–compulsive disorder who fears contamination from contact with injections would not receive an additional diagnosis of specific phobia unless there were additional concerns about injections that were unrelated to contamination (e.g., fear of fainting during an injection, fear of pain from the needle). Each diagnosis has specifiers and subtypes to allow for the provision of more specific diagnostic information. For social phobia, the clinician can specify whether the phobia is generalized (i.e., includes most social situations). For specific phobias, the clinician can indicate which one of five types best describes the focus of the phobia: animal, natural environment, blood–injection–injury, situational, or other.

These specific phobia types tend to differ on a variety of dimensions including age at onset, sex composition, patterns of covariation among phobias, focus of apprehension, timing and predictability of the phobic response, and type of physiological reaction during exposure to the phobic situation.

Although anxiety about physical sensations and the occurrence of panic is a feature typically associated with panic disorder, several studies have shown that panic-focused and symptom-focused apprehensions are not unique to panic disorder and agoraphobia. Individuals with specific phobias tend to report anxiety about the sensations (e.g., racing heart, breathlessness, dizziness) typically associated with their fear. Also, there is evidence that in addition to fearing danger from the phobic object (e.g., a plane crash, being bitten by a dog), many individuals with specific phobias fear danger as a result of their reaction in the phobic situation (e.g., having a panic attack, losing control, being embarrassed). Also, the few relevant studies that have been conducted suggest that there may be differences in sensation-focused apprehension across specific phobia types.

Data are converging to indicate that individuals with phobias from the situational (e.g., claustrophobia) and blood–injury–injection types may be especially internally focused on their fear. Whereas individuals with situational phobias tend to fear the possible consequences of panic, those with blood-injury-injection phobias seem uniquely concerned about sensations that indicate that fainting is imminent (e.g., lightheadedness, hot flashes).

Specific phobia types may differ with respect to timing and predictability of the phobic response as well. One study based on retrospective self-reports found that individuals with phobias of driving, enclosed places, and blood–injury were more likely to report that their fear was delayed in the phobic situation than were those with animal phobias. This suggests that delayed and unpredictable panic attacks may be more characteristic of situational phobias than of other phobia types, consistent with the argument that situational phobias share more features with agoraphobia than do other specific phobia types.

Perhaps the most consistent difference among specific phobia types is the tendency for individuals with blood–injury–injection phobias to report a history of fainting in the phobic situation. Although all phobia types are associated with panic attacks in the phobic situation, only individuals with blood and injection phobias report fainting. Specifically, individuals with blood–injury–injection phobias experience a diphasic physiological response, which includes an initial increase in arousal followed by a sharp drop in heart rate and blood pressure that can lead to fainting. This response occurs at times in approximately 70% of people with blood phobias and 56% of those with injection phobias and seems to be unique to situations involving blood and medical procedures. In other words, people who faint in these situations still show the usual type of response (i.e., increased arousal) in other situations that they fear. Disgust has been identified as a potential mediator of faintness associated with blood–injury–injection stimuli.

The different responses experienced in different phobias have been explained from an evolutionary perspective. As mentioned earlier, the typical phobic responses of fear and panic are adaptive in that the increased arousal facilitates escape. In contrast, the most adaptive response during serious injury may be a drop in blood pressure to prevent excessive bleeding. It has been suggested that this response is mediated by an overactive sinoaortic baroreflex that is triggered by heightened arousal in situations involving blood or needles. Of course, in people with blood and injection phobias, the response is excessive and unwarranted, as there is typically no danger of excessive blood loss.

Having a phobia of one specific phobia type makes an individual more likely to have additional phobias of the same type than of other types. For example, about 70% of individuals with blood phobias tend to have injection phobias as well. However, the research on the classification of specific phobia types is inconsistent. For example, in several studies, height phobias tend to be associated with situational phobias (e.g., claustrophobia), despite height phobias being listed as an example of the natural environment type in DSM-IV-TR.

Specific phobias tend to co-occur with other specific phobias. One study found that 76% of a sample of 915 individuals with a lifetime history of specific phobias had one or more co-occurring specific phobias, which is consistent with research showing that individuals with specific phobias often report multiple fears on a fear survey. However, other research indicates that comorbid phobias may not be as prevalent and that numbers in previous studies may have been inflated by a lack of discrimination between multiple phobias and fears of multiple situations that are accounted for by a single phobia. A recent methodologically rigorous study found that 15% of individuals with a principal diagnosis of specific phobia also met criteria for another type of specific phobia.

For social phobia, DSM-IV-TR allows the clinician to specify whether it is "generalized," that is, it includes most social situations. In addition, a "discrete or circumscribed" subtype is often used by investigators to describe individuals with only one domain of social anxiety, usually involving performance-related situations (e.g., public speaking). Several studies have examined differences among these subtypes. Specifically, individuals with generalized social phobias tend to be younger, less educated, and less likely to be employed than are individuals with discrete social phobias. In addition, generalized social phobias are associated with more depression, anxiety, general distress, and concerns about negative evaluation from others. Discrete social phobias appear to be associated with greater cardiac reactivity.

As is the case with most disorders, a comprehensive assessment is important in helping the clinician to decide which treatment approach is most appropriate for a given individual. In the case of specific and social phobias, a thorough evaluation should include a structured or semistructured interview, self-report measures, and a behavioral assessment. Each of these measures provides different types of information that may be relevant to later treatment decisions.

During all parts of the initial evaluation, the clinician should be sensitive to several issues. First, for many individuals with phobias, even discussing the phobic object can provoke anxiety. For example, some individuals with spider phobias experience panic attacks when they discuss spiders. Some individuals with blood phobias faint when they discuss surgical procedures. Therefore, the clinician should ask the individual whether discussing the phobic object or situation will provoke anxiety. If the interview is likely to be a source of stress, the clinician should emphasize the importance of the information that is being collected, as well as the potential therapeutic value of discussing the feared object. As described later, exposure to the feared stimulus is an essential component of the treatment of most specific phobias. Of course, the interviewer should use his or her judgment when deciding how much to push the individual in the first session. For treatment to be effective, establishing trust in the clinician early in the course of treatment is essential.

With respect to social phobia, the assessment itself may be considered a phobic stimulus. Because individuals with social phobia fear the evaluation of others, a clinical interview may be especially frightening. Even completing self-report questionnaires in the waiting room may be difficult for individuals who fear writing in front of others. The clinician should be sensitive to this possibility and provide reassurance when appropriate.

Behavioral testing is an important part of any comprehensive evaluation for a phobic disorder. This is particularly the case if behavioral or cognitive–behavioral treatment is used. Because most individuals with phobias avoid the objects and situations that they fear, individuals may find it difficult to describe the subtle cues that affect their fear in the situation. In addition, it is not unusual for individuals to misjudge the amount of fear that they typically experience in the phobic situation. A behavioral approach test can be useful for identifying specific fear triggers as well as for assessing the intensity of the individual's fear in the actual situation.

To conduct a behavioral approach test, individuals should be instructed to enter the phobic situation for several minutes. For example, an individual with a snake phobia should be instructed to stand as close as possible to a live snake and note the specific cues that affect the fear (e.g., size of snake, color, movement) and the intensity of the fear (perhaps rating it on a 0–100 point scale). Individuals should pay special attention to their physical sensations (e.g., palpitations, sweating, blushing), negative thoughts (e.g., "I will fall from this balcony"), and anxious coping strategies (e.g., escape, avoidance, distraction).

Specific phobias tend to be more common among women than men. This finding seems to be strongest for phobias from the animal type, whereas sex differences are smaller for height phobias and blood–injury–injection phobias. In addition, social phobia tends to be slightly more prevalent among women than men, although these differences are relatively small. Whereas men tend to be more fearful than women of urinating in public bathrooms and returning items to a store, women are more likely to be fearful than men of a number of situations including talking to people in authority, public speaking, being the center of attention, expressing disagreement, and throwing a party.

A variety of studies have shown that specific phobias, social phobia, and related conditions exist across cultures. For example, in Japan, a condition exists called *taijin kyôfu* in which individuals have an "obsession of shame." This condition has much overlap with social phobia in that it is often accompanied by fears of blushing, having improper facial expressions in the presence of others, looking at others, shaking, and perspiring in front of others. Interestingly, in some other cultures, the sex ratio for phobias tends to be reversed. For example, in studies from Saudi Arabia and India, up to 80% of individuals reporting for treatment of phobias were male. Similarly, in Japan about 60% of individuals with *taijin kyôfu* are male. In the case of phobias in India, it has been suggested that traditional gender roles may account for the difference in treatment seeking in Indian men and women. Specifically, Indian women are often discouraged from leaving the house alone or conversing with others without the husband's permission. It is difficult to know how cultural expectations affect sex differences in phobias in other cultures.

Clinicians treating individuals from different cultures should be aware of cultural differences in presentation and response to treatment. Many cues that a clinician might use to aid in the diagnosis of social phobia in white Americans may not be useful for diagnosing the condition in other cultures. For example, although many clinicians interpret a lack of eye contact as indicating shyness or a lack of assertiveness, avoidance of eye contact among Japanese and Mexican-Americans is often viewed as a sign of respect. In contrast to white Americans, Japanese are apparently more likely to view smiling as a sign of embarrassment or discomfort. Furthermore, cultural differences in tone and volume of speech may lead mental health professional to misinterpretations. For example, whereas white Americans often are uncomfortable with silence in a conversation, British and Arab individuals may be more likely to use silence for privacy and other cultures use silence to indicate agreement among the parties or as a sign of respect. In addition, Asian individuals have been reported to speak more quietly than white Americans, who in turn speak more quietly than those from Arab countries. Therefore, differences in the volume of speech should not be taken to imply differences in assertiveness or other indicators of social anxiety.

Among children, specific and social fears are common. Because these fears may be transient, DSM-IV-TR has included a provision that social and specific phobias not be assigned in children unless they are present for more than 6 months. In addition, children may be less likely than adults to recognize that their phobia is excessive or unrealistic. The specific objects feared by children are often similar to those feared by adults, although children may be more likely to fear objects and situations that are not easily classified in the four main specific phobia types in DSM-IV-TR (e.g., balloons or costumed characters). In addition, children often report specific and social phobias having to do with school. Children with social phobia tend to avoid changing for gym class in front of others, eating in the cafeteria, or speaking in front of the class.

Phobias are among the most common mental disorders. Findings based on large community samples from five sites in the Epidemiological Catchment Area (ECA) study yielded lifetime prevalence estimates of 11.25% for specific phobias and 2.73% for social phobia. Estimates from the National Comorbidity Survey (NCS) were consistent with previous findings on specific phobias: a lifetime prevalence of 11.30% in a sample of more than 8000 individuals from across the United States. For social phobia, data from the NCS indicate a lifetime prevalence rate of 13.3%, much higher than that in the previously reported ECA study. This difference is likely due to methodological variations across the two studies.

Specific phobias and social phobia tend to run in families. It appears that being a first-degree relative of an individual with a specific phobia puts one at a greater risk for a specific phobia compared with first-degree relatives of never mentally ill controls (31% versus 11%). However, the particular phobia that is transmitted is usually different from that in the relative, although it is often from the same general type (e.g., animal, situational). Furthermore, relatives of people with specific phobias are not at increased risk for other types of anxiety disorders (including social phobia) or subclinical fears. The heritability of blood and injection phobias may be even greater than that for other phobias.

Findings for individuals with social phobia and their families show a similar pattern. In one study, 16% of first-degree relatives of subjects with social phobia had symptoms that met criteria for social phobia, whereas only 5% of first-degree relatives of never mentally ill control subjects had social phobia. Furthermore, there is no increased risk among relatives of people with social phobia to develop other anxiety disorders.

Course

The mean age at onset of social phobia is in the middle teens. The age at onset of specific phobias varies depending on the phobia type, with phobias of animals, blood, storms, and water tending to begin in early childhood, phobias of heights beginning in the teens, and situational phobias beginning in the late teens to middle twenties. Although childhood fears are often transient (e.g., most children outgrow fear of the dark without treatment), fears that persist into adulthood usually have a chronic course unless treated.

Although many phobias begin after a traumatic event, many individuals do not recall the specific onset of their fear, and few empirical data have examined the initial period after the fear onset. Clinically, however, some individuals report a sudden onset of fear, whereas others report a more gradual onset. Studies examining the onset of phobias have tended to assess the onset of the *fear* rather than the onset of the *phobia* (i.e., the point at which the fear creates significant distress or functional impairment). Phobias typically began at an average of 9 years after the fear onset. Anecdotally, the types of factors leading to the transition from fear to phobia included gradual increases in the intensity of fear, additional traumatic events (e.g., panic attacks, car accidents), increased life stress, and changes in living situation (e.g., starting a job that requires exposure to heights). Similarly, it is not unusual for individuals with social phobia to report having been shy as children, although their anxiety may not have reached phobic proportions until later.

Differential Diagnosis

Social anxiety is associated with a variety of DSM-IV-TR disorders. Similarly, several disorders other than specific phobia are associated with fear and avoidance of circumscribed stimuli. Therefore, accurate diagnosis of specific and social phobias depends on a thorough understanding of the DSM-IV-TR criteria and knowledge of how to distinguish these disorders from related conditions. Correct diagnosis depends on being able to evaluate the individual's focus of apprehension, reasons for avoidance, and range of situations feared.

Panic disorder with agoraphobia may easily be misdiagnosed as social phobia or a specific phobia (especially the situational type). For example, many individuals with panic disorder avoid a variety of social situations because of anxiety about having others notice their symptoms. In addition, some individuals with panic disorder may avoid circumscribed situations, such as flying, despite reporting no other significant avoidance. Four variables should be considered in making the differential diagnosis: (1) type and number of panic attacks, (2) focus of apprehension, (3) number of situations avoided, and (4) level of intercurrent anxiety.

Individuals with panic disorder experience unexpected panic attacks and heightened anxiety outside of the phobic situation, whereas those with specific and social phobias typically do not. In addition, individuals with panic disorder are more likely than those with specific and social phobias to report fear and avoidance of a broad range of situations typically associated with agoraphobia (e.g., flying, enclosed places, crowds, being alone, shopping malls). Finally, individuals with panic disorder are typically concerned only about the possibility of panicking in the phobic situation or about the consequences of panicking (e.g., being embarrassed

by one's panic symptoms). In contrast, individuals with specific and social phobias are usually concerned about other aspects of the situation as well (e.g., being hit by another driver, saying something foolish).

Consider two examples in which the differential diagnosis with panic disorder might be especially difficult. First, individuals with claustrophobia are typically extremely concerned about being unable to escape from the phobic situation as well as being unable to breathe in the situation. Therefore, like individuals with panic disorder and agoraphobia, they usually report heightened anxiety about the possibility of panicking. The main variable to consider in such a case is the presence of panic attacks outside of claustrophobic situations. If panic attacks occur exclusively in enclosed places, a diagnosis of specific phobia might best describe the problem. In contrast, if the individual has unexpected or uncued panic attacks as well, a diagnosis of panic disorder might be more appropriate.

A second example is an individual who avoids a broad range of situations including shopping malls, supermarkets, walking on busy streets, and various social situations including parties, meetings, and public speaking. Without more information, this individual's problem might appear to meet criteria for social phobia, panic disorder with agoraphobia, or both diagnoses. As mentioned earlier, individuals with panic disorder often avoid social situations because of anxiety about panicking in public. In addition, individuals with social phobia might avoid situations that are typically avoided by individuals with agoraphobia for fear of seeing someone that they know or of being observed by strangers. To make the diagnosis in this case, it is necessary to assess the reasons for avoidance.

It may be difficult to distinguish among types of specific phobias. For example, is a bridge phobia best considered a situational type (i.e., driving) or a natural environment type (i.e., heights)? This decision should be based on the context of the bridge phobia. If the individual fears falling or fears other high places, a height phobia may be the appropriate diagnosis. In contrast, if bridges are one of many driving-related situations that the person fears, a driving phobia might be more appropriate.

Other diagnoses that should be considered before a diagnosis of specific phobia is assigned include posttraumatic stress disorder (PTSD) (if the fear follows a life-threatening trauma and is accompanied by other PTSD symptoms such as reexperiencing the trauma), obsessive–compulsive disorder (if the fear is related to an obsession, e.g., contamination), hypochondriasis (if the fear is related to a belief that he or she has some serious illness), separation-anxiety disorder (if the fear is of situations that might lead to separation from the family, for example, traveling on an airplane without one's parents), eating disorders (if the fear is of eating certain foods but not related to a fear of choking), and psychotic disorders (if the fear is related to a delusion).

Social phobia should not be diagnosed if the fear is related entirely to another disorder. For example, if an individual with obsessive–compulsive disorder avoids social situations only because of the embarrassment of having others notice her or his excessive hand washing, a diagnosis of social phobia would not be given. Furthermore, individuals with depression, schizoid personality disorder, or a pervasive developmental disorder may avoid social situations because of a lack of interest in spending time with others. To be considered social phobia, an individual must avoid these situations specifically because of anxiety about being evaluated negatively.

In the case of generalized social phobia, the diagnosis of avoidant personality disorder should be considered as well. Individuals with avoidant personality disorder tend to display more interpersonal sensitivity and have poorer social skills than social phobic individuals without avoidant personality disorder. Furthermore, most studies suggest that the differences between avoidant personality disorder and social phobia are more quantitative than qualitative and that the former may simply be a more severe form of the latter. Therefore, most individuals who meet criteria for avoidant personality disorder will meet criteria for social phobia as well.

Finally, social and specific phobias should be distinguished from normal states of fear and anxiety. Many individuals report mild fears of circumscribed situations or mild shyness in certain social situations. Others may report intense fears of public speaking or heights but insist that these situations rarely arise and that they have no interest in being in these situations. For the criteria for a specific or social phobia to be met, the individual must report significant distress about having the fear or must report significant impairment in functioning.

A variety of factors should be considered in deciding whether an individual's fear exceeds the threshold necessary for a diagnosis of specific or social phobia. To make the differential diagnosis between normal fears and clinical phobias, the clinician should consider the extent of the individual's avoidance, the frequency with which the phobic stimulus is encountered, and the degree to which the individual is bothered by having the fear. For example, an individual who fears seeing snakes in the wild but who lives in the city, never encounters snakes, and never even thinks about snakes would probably not be diagnosed with a specific phobia. In contrast, when an individual's fear of snakes leads to avoidance of walking through parks, camping, swimming, and watching certain television programs, despite having an interest in doing these things, a diagnosis of specific phobia would be appropriate.

Similar factors should be considered in deciding at what point normal shyness reaches an intensity that warrants a diagnosis of social phobia. An individual who is somewhat quiet in groups or when meeting new people but does not avoid these situations and is not especially distressed by his or her shyness would probably not receive a diagnosis of social phobia. In contrast, an individual who frequently refuses invitations to socialize because of anxiety, quits a job because of anxiety about having to talk to customers, or is distressed about her or his social anxiety would be likely to receive a diagnosis of social phobia.

Diagnostic decision trees for social and specific phobias are presented in Figures 30-1 and 30-2.

TREATMENT

The main goal of treatment is to decrease fear and phobic avoidance to a level that no longer causes significant distress or functional impairment. In some cases, treatment includes strategies for improving specific skill deficits as well. For example, individuals with social phobia may lack adequate social skills and can sometimes benefit from social skills training. Likewise, some individuals with specific phobias of driving may have poor driving skills if their fear prevented them from learning how to drive properly. Typically, effective treatment for social phobia lasts several months, although treatment of discrete social phobias (e.g., public speaking) may take less time. Specific phobias can usually be treated relatively quickly. In fact, for certain phobias, the vast majority of individuals are able to achieve clinically significant, long-lasting improvement in as little as one session of behavioral treatment.

Effective treatments fall into one of two main categories: pharmacological treatment and cognitive–behavioral therapy (CBT). Pharmacological treatments have been used effectively for treating social phobia, although it is generally accepted that they are of limited utility for treating specific phobias. In contrast, CBT has been used with success for the treatment of specific and social phobias. Despite the existence of effective treatments, fewer than half of those who seek treatment in an anxiety disorders specialty clinic have previously received evidence-based treatments for their social anxiety. Tables 30-1 and 30-2 summarize various

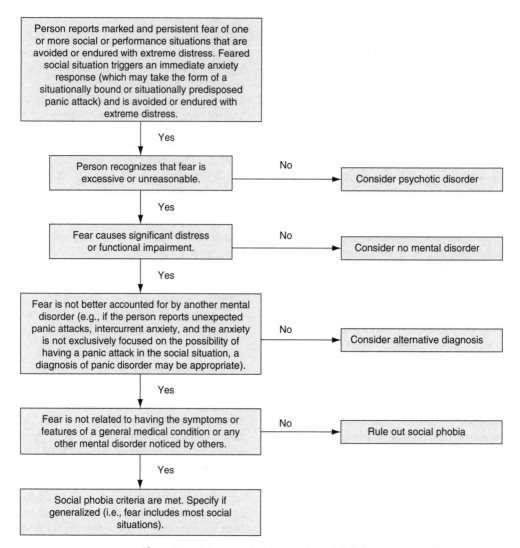

Figure 30-1 *Diagnostic decision tree for social phobia.*

treatments for social and specific phobias. Treatment decision trees for social and specific phobias are presented in Figures 30-3 and 30-4.

Somatic Treatments

Although pharmacotherapy is generally thought to be ineffective for specific phobias, it is not uncommon for phobic individuals occasionally to be prescribed low dosages of benzodiazepines to be taken in the phobic situation (e.g., while flying). Studies have been conducted that have examined the use of benzodiazepines and beta blockers alone or in combination with behavioral treatments for specific phobias and in general have found that drugs do not contribute much to the treatment of specific phobias. However, one problem

with the research to date is that it has not taken into account differences among specific phobia types. For example, claustrophobia and other phobias of the situational type appear to share more features with panic disorder than with the other specific phobia types. Therefore, medications that are effective for panic disorder (e.g., imipramine, alprazolam) may prove to be effective for situational phobias. Although there are few studies examining this hypothesis, some data suggest that benzodiazepines may be helpful in the short term but lead to greater relapse in the long term and possibly interfere with the therapeutic effects of exposure across sessions. For example, one study found that CBT and providing a benzodiazepine both led to fear reduction during dental surgery; however, whereas benzodiazepine treatment was associated with greater

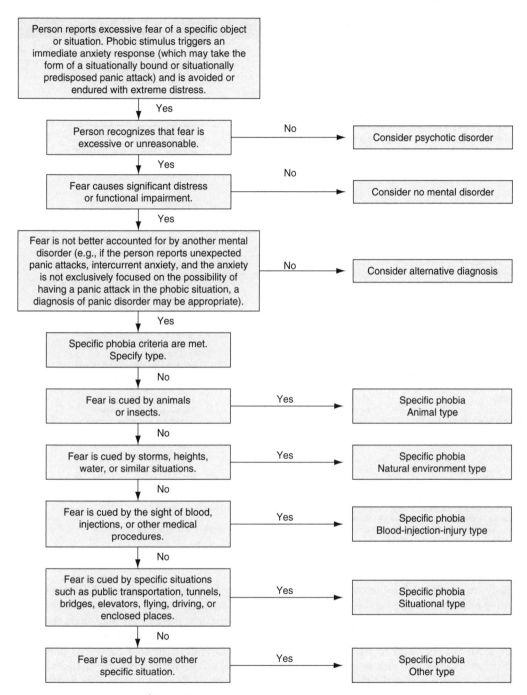

Figure 30-2 *Diagnostic decision tree for specific phobia.*

relapse during follow-up, CBT was associated with further improvements.

In contrast to specific phobias, social phobia has been treated successfully with a variety of pharmacological interventions including SSRIs, benzodiazepines such as clonazepam and alprazolam, traditional MAOIs such as phenelzine, and reversible inhibitors of monoamine oxidase A (RIMA) such as moclobemide and brofaromine. Numerous controlled trials across a range of SSRIs including sertraline, fluvoxamine, and paroxetine have demonstrated their effectiveness in the treatment of social phobia, such that the SSRIs

Table 30-1	Treatments for Social Phobia		
Treatment	**Advantages**	**Disadvantages**	**Rating**
Cognitive–behavioral therapy (CBT) (e.g., exposure, cognitive restructuring, social skills training, education)	Good treatment response Brief course of treatment Treatment gains maintained at follow-up Considered first line.	May lead to temporary increases in discomfort or fear.	++++
SSRIs (e.g., paroxetine, fluvoxamine, sertraline)	Good treatment response Early response, relative to CBT Broad spectrum efficacy for comorbid disorders (i.e., depression) Lack of abuse potential Considered first line	Side effects are common Cost is a factor May be a risk of relapse after discontinuation	+++
Moclobemide	Good treatment response in some studies Fewer side effects than phenelzine Considered second line	Side effects common Does not separate from placebo in some studies Potential exists for relapse after discontinuation	++
Benzodiazepines (e.g., clonazepam, alprazolam)	Good treatment response Considered adjunctive or second line	Side effects and withdrawal occur Potential for abuse Relapse after discontinuation is likely. Does not treat certain comorbid conditions (i.e., depression)	++
MAOIs (e.g., phenelzine)	Good treatment response Early response Considered third line	Relatively high rate of adverse effects Dietary restrictions must be followed Numerous drug interactions Potential exists for relapse after discontinuation	++
Gabapentin	Possibly beneficial Considered third line	Side effects are common More research is needed	++
β-blockers (e.g., atenolol)	Appears to be useful for "stage fright" in actors, musicians, and other performers	Drugs are not effective for generalized social phobia Benefits for discrete social phobias are questionable Side effects occur Potential exists for relapse after discontinuation	+

++++ First treatment of choice. Helpful for most patients, with few side effects. Good long-term benefits.
+++ Helpful for most patients. Potential for relapse after treatment is discontinued.
++ More controlled research needed, although preliminary studies suggest potential benefit OR research has been mixed.
+ Not especially effective for generalized social phobia.

are currently considered the first-line medication treatment. Owing to their tolerability and efficacy, the SSRIs have been referred to as "the new gold standard" in pharmacological treatment for social phobia. Another benefit of SSRIs is their broad spectrum efficacy for common comorbid disorders such as depression and panic disorder. Treatment of social phobia with other antidepressants (e.g., imipramine, venlafaxine) has also been studied in a number of uncontrolled open trials, with positive results.

Research on the use of anxiolytics for the treatment of social phobia have focused on high potency benzodiazepines (e.g., clonazepam, alprazolam) and the nonbenzodiazepine buspirone. Several studies have examined the utility of clonazepam for treating social phobia. For example, one placebo-controlled study found that 78% of individuals responded to clonazepam (mean dosage, 2.4 mg/day), whereas only 20% responded to placebo. Another study comparing clonazepam to cognitive–behavioral group therapy found that individuals in both conditions improved significantly and no differences between treatment conditions were observed aside from greater improvement in the clonazepam group at 12 weeks of treatment. In addition, uncontrolled pilot studies have suggested that alprazolam (mean dosage, 2.9 mg/day) may be effective for social phobia, although more controlled clinical trials are needed. The findings on buspirone are mixed, with a number of controlled trials finding no significant advantage of buspirone over placebo, which is in contrast to previous uncontrolled studies that found some benefit.

Table 30-2	Treatments for Specific Phobias		
Treatment	**Advantages**	**Disadvantages**	**Rating**
In vivo exposure	Highly effective Early response Treatment gains maintained at follow-up	May lead to temporary increases in discomfort or fear	++++
Applied tension	Highly effective for individuals with blood–injection phobias who faint Early response Treatment gains maintained at follow-up	Treatment is relevant for a small percentage of individuals with specific phobias	+++
Applied relaxation	May be effective for some individuals	Treatment has not been extensively researched for specific phobias	++
Cognitive therapy	May help to reduce anxiety about conducting exposure exercises	Treatment has not been extensively researched for specific phobias Treatment is probably not effective alone	++
Benzodiazepines	May reduce anticipatory anxiety before individual enters phobic situation, and may reduce fear, particularly in situational specific phobias	Treatment has not been extensively researched for specific phobias Treatment is probably not effective alone, in many cases Side effects (e.g., sedation) occur Discontinuation of symptoms may undermine benefits of treatment	++
SSRIs	May reduce panic sensations for individuals with situational phobias that are similar to panic disorder (e.g., claustrophobia)	Treatment has not been extensively researched for specific phobias There are a few studies (primarily case reports) with promising results Discontinuation of medication may result in a return of fear	++

++++ Treatment of choice. Effective for almost all individuals.
+++ Very effective for a subset of individuals.
++ May be helpful for some individuals. More research needed.

Owing to the potentially severe side effects of MAOIs as well as the necessity for certain dietary restrictions, they are not recommended as a first-line treatment. The findings from more recent trials involving RIMAs have been less encouraging than initial studies suggested. For example, a fixed-dose study conducted over 12 weeks found that moclobemide did not have a significant benefit over placebo at five dosages ranging from 75 to 900 mg/day. Discontinuation of MAOIs and RIMAs have been associated with a tendency to relapse.

Research on beta blockers indicates that they are no better than placebo for most individuals with generalized social phobia. Although beta blockers have been used to treat individuals from nonpatient samples with heightened performance anxiety (e.g., people with public speaking anxiety, musicians with stage fright), their efficacy for treating individuals with discrete social phobia has not been established. Nevertheless, beta blockers are often prescribed for discrete performance-related social phobias.

Preliminary findings suggest that gabapentin, a medication typically used in the treatment of partial seizures, may be effective in the treatment of social phobia. A placebo-controlled trial found that individuals taking gabapentin had significant reductions in social anxiety compared to the placebo group. However, more research is needed to confirm this finding.

Psychosocial Treatments

Numerous studies have shown that exposure-based treatments are effective for helping individuals to overcome a variety of specific phobias, including fears of blood, injections, dentists, spiders, snakes, rats, enclosed places, thunder and lightning, water, flying, heights, choking, and balloons. Furthermore, the way in which exposure is conducted may make a difference. Exposure-based treatments can vary on a variety of dimensions including the degree of therapist involvement, duration and intensity of exposure, frequency and number of sessions, and the degree to which the feared situation is confronted in imagination versus in real life. In addition, because individuals with certain specific phobias often report a fear of panicking in the feared situation, some investigators have suggested that adding various panic management strategies (e.g., cognitive restructuring, exposure to feared sensations) may help increase the efficacy of behavioral treatments

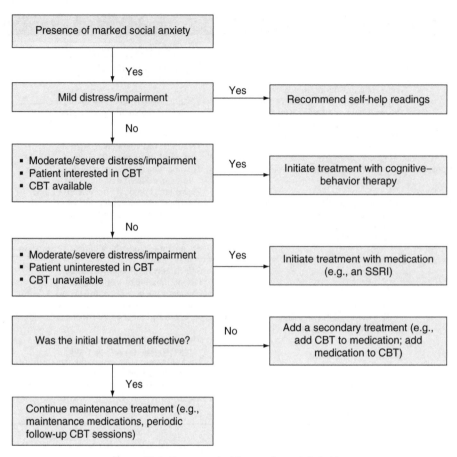

Figure 30-3 *Treatment decision tree for social phobia.*

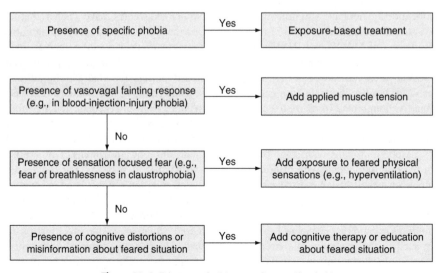

Figure 30-4 *Treatment decision tree for specific phobia.*

for specific phobias. It remains to be shown whether the addition of these strategies will improve the efficacy of treatments that include only exposure.

Several reviews have summarized the effects of the above-mentioned variables on exposure-based treatments. First, exposure seems to work best when sessions are spaced close together. Second, prolonged exposure seems to be more effective than exposure of shorter duration. Third, during exposure sessions, individuals should be discouraged from engaging in subtle avoidance strategies (e.g., distraction) and overreliance on safety signals (e.g., being accompanied by one's spouse during exposure). Fourth, real-life exposure is more effective than exposure in imagination. Fifth, exposure with some degree of therapist involvement seems to be more effective than exposure that is exclusively conducted without the therapist present. Exposure may be conducted gradually or quickly. Both approaches seem to work equally well, although individuals may be more compliant with a gradual approach. Finally, in the case of blood and injection phobias, the technique called applied muscle tension should be considered as an alternative or addition to exposure therapy. Applied muscle tension involves having individuals repeatedly tense their muscles, which leads to a temporary increase in blood pressure and prevents fainting upon exposure to blood or medical procedures.

Cognitive strategies have also been used either alone or in conjunction with exposure for treating specific phobias. The evidence suggests that the addition of cognitive strategies to exposure may provide added benefit for some individuals.

Specific phobias are among the most treatable of the anxiety disorders. For example, in as little as one session of guided exposure lasting 2 to 3 hours, the majority of individuals with animal or injection phobias are judged much improved or completely recovered. Moreover, exposure conducted with a parent present was equally effective as exposure treatment conducted alone. However, despite how straightforward the concept of exposure may seem, many subtle clinical issues can lead to problems in implementing exposure-based treatments. For example, although an individual might be compliant with therapist-assisted exposure practices, he or she may refuse to attempt exposure practices alone between sessions. In such cases, involving a spouse or other family member as a coach during practices at home may help. In addition, gradually increasing the distance between therapist and individual during the therapist-assisted exposures will help the individual to feel comfortable when practicing alone. However, to maintain the individual's trust and to maximize the effectiveness of behavioral interventions, it is important that exposure practices proceed in a predictable way, so that the individual is not surprised by unexpected events. Several self-help books and manuals for treating a range of specific phobias have been published in the past decade and may be helpful for some individuals.

Developments in technology are having an impact on the treatment of specific phobias. Videotapes are commonly used to show feared stimuli to individuals during exposure. Computer-administered treatments have also been used. More recent is the use of virtual reality to expose individuals to simulated situations that are more difficult to replicate *in vivo* such as flying and heights. Although data on the effectiveness of virtual reality is encouraging, other studies indicate that *in vivo* exposure is still superior.

Empirically validated psychosocial interventions for social phobia have primarily come from a cognitive–behavioral perspective and include four main types of treatment: (1) exposure-based strategies, (2) cognitive therapy, (3) social skills training, and (4) applied relaxation. Exposure-based treatments involve repeatedly approaching fear-provoking situations until they no longer elicit fear. Through repeated exposure, individuals learn that their fearful predictions do not come true despite their having confronted the situation. Table 30-3 illustrates an example of an exposure hierarchy that might be used to structure an individual's exposure practices. An exposure hierarchy is a list of feared situations that are rank ordered by difficulty and used to guide exposure practices for phobic disorders including social phobia and specific phobia. The individual and the therapist generate a list of situations that the individual finds anxiety provoking. Items are placed in descending order from most anxiety provoking to least anxiety provoking, and each item is rated with respect to how anxious the individual might be to

Table 30-3	Exposure Hierarchy for Generalized Social Phobia	
Item		**Fear Rating (0–100)**
Have a party and invite everyone from work.		99
Go to work Christmas party for 1 h without drinking		90
Invite Cindy to have dinner and see a movie.		85
Go for a job interview		80
Ask boss for a day off from work		65
Ask questions in a meeting at work		65
Eat lunch with coworkers		60
Talk to a stranger on the bus		50
Talk to cousin on the telephone for 10 min		40
Ask for directions at the gas station.		35

practice the item. Exposure practices are designed to help the individual become more comfortable engaging in the activities from the hierarchy. Cognitive therapy helps individuals identify and change anxious thoughts (e.g., "Others will think I am stupid if I participate in a conversation at work") by teaching them to consider alternative ways of interpreting situations and to examine the evidence for their anxious beliefs. Social skills training is designed to help individuals become more socially competent when they interact with others. Treatment strategies may include modeling, behavioral rehearsal, corrective feedback, social reinforcement, and homework assignments. Finally, applied relaxation involves learning to relax one's muscles during rest, during movement, and eventually in anxiety-provoking social situations.

Although these methods are presented as four distinct treatment approaches, there is often overlap among the various treatments. Social skills training typically requires exposure to the phobic situation so that new skills may be practiced (e.g., behavioral rehearsal). The same may be said of applied relaxation, which includes learning to conduct relaxation exercises in the phobic situation. In fact, most treatments for social phobia involve some type of exposure to anxiety-provoking social interactions and performance-related tasks. Furthermore, many cognitive–behavioral therapists treat individuals using several different strategies delivered in a comprehensive package.

In summary, it seems clear that effective psychosocial treatments and medications for social phobia exist. Although both types of treatments appear to be equally effective, each has advantages and disadvantages. Medication treatments may work more quickly and are less time-consuming for the individual and the therapist. In contrast, improvement after CBT appears to last longer. Owing to medication side effects, CBT may be more appropriate for some individuals. More studies are needed to examine the efficacy of combined medication and psychosocial treatments for social phobia.

Treatment Nonresponse

Several variables may lead to an initially poor treatment response. Anticipating potential difficulties will help increase treatment efficacy. Possible reasons for a worse outcome include poor compliance, poor motivation, and poor understanding of the treatment procedures. In addition, interpersonal issues and other possible conflicts may interfere with the successful treatment of specific and social phobias.

Individuals fail to comply with treatment procedures for a variety of reasons. In the case of pharmacological treatments, individuals may avoid taking medications because of side effects, lack of confidence in efficacy, or preference for an alternative type of treatment. If individuals are not compliant with medications, the clinician should attempt to identify the reasons for poor compliance and to suggest methods of increasing compliance or changing to another type of treatment.

In the case of CBT, common reasons for poor compliance are anxiety about conforming to treatment, lack of time, and lack of motivation to conduct the treatment properly. Because CBT requires individuals to confront the situations they fear most, individuals often feel extreme anxiety about participating in the treatment. Individuals should be reassured that their anxiety is normal and that they will never be forced to do anything that they are unwilling to try. Furthermore, the difficulty of exposure tasks should be increased gradually to maximize treatment compliance. If individuals do not have the time or motivation to conduct treatment as suggested, therapists should be willing to find ways to make the treatment more accessible to the individual. For example, involvement of a friend or relative of the individual as a coach may allow the individual to conduct more practices without the therapist's assistance. The therapist could also explore the possibility that the individual consider beginning treatment later, when more time is available.

Poor motivation can lead to poor compliance with the treatment procedures. If an individual's symptoms are not especially severe, the distress and impairment created by the disorder may not be enough to motivate the individual to take medications regularly or to confront the phobic situation in a systematic way. Furthermore, as an individual improves in treatment, she or he may experience a decrease in motivation. Individuals should be encouraged to continue with treatment assignments even after improvement. More complete improvements may protect against a return of symptoms.

Finally, treatment procedures may be complicated for some individuals. This is especially the case for CBT. Individuals may fail to complete homework assignments (e.g., monitoring anxious cognitions) simply because the treatment rationale and the specifics of how to conduct the treatment procedures were not made clear. Therefore, therapists should continually assess the individual's understanding of the treatment procedures.

COMPARISON OF DSM-IV-TR AND ICD-10 DIAGNOSTIC CRITERIA

The ICD-10 Diagnostic Criteria for Research for Social Phobia specify that at least two symptoms of anxiety (i.e., from the list of 14 panic symptoms) be present together on at least one occasion along with at least one of the following anxiety symptoms: blushing or shaking, fear of vomiting, and urgency or fear of micturition or defecation. Furthermore, these anxiety symptoms must be "restricted to, or predominated in, the feared situations or contemplation of the feared situations." In contrast, the DSM-IV-TR criteria do not specify any particular types of anxiety symptoms nor is any restriction placed on whether anxiety can occur in situations other than social situations.

For specific phobia, the ICD-10 Diagnostic Criteria for Research also specify that the anxiety symptoms be "restricted to, or predominated in, the feared situations or contemplation of the feared situation." DSM-IV-TR again does not impose any such restriction.

Anxiety Disorders: Obsessive–Compulsive Disorder

Obsessive–Compulsive Disorder

DIAGNOSIS

Obsessive–compulsive disorder (OCD) is an intriguing and often debilitating syndrome characterized by the presence of two distinct phenomena: obsessions and compulsions. Obsessions are intrusive, recurrent, unwanted ideas, thoughts, or impulses that are difficult to dismiss, despite their disturbing nature. Compulsions are repetitive behaviors, either observable or mental, that are intended to reduce the anxiety engendered by obsessions. Both obsessions and compulsions have been described in a wide variety of mental and neurological disorders. However, obsessions and compulsions that clearly interfere with the functioning and/or cause significant distress are the hallmark of OCD (see DSM-IV-TR diagnostic criteria, page 317).

OCD's clinical presentation is characterized by phenomenological subtypes based on the content of the obsessions and corresponding compulsions. The list of subtypes in the Yale-Brown Obsessive–Compulsive Scale (Y-BOCS) (Table 31-1) was generated on the basis of clinical interviews with OCD patients in the 1980s. The basic types of obsessions and compulsions seem to be consistent across cultures. The most common obsession is the fear of contamination, followed by pathological doubt, a need for symmetry, and aggressive obsessions. The most common compulsion is checking, which is followed by washing, symmetry, the need to ask or confess, and counting. Children with OCD present most commonly with washing compulsions, which are followed by repeating rituals.

Most individuals with OCD have multiple obsessions and compulsions over time, with a particular fear or concern dominating the clinical picture at any one time. The presence of obsessions without compulsions, or compulsions without obsessions, is unusual. In the DSM-IV OCD field trial of 431 individuals, only 2% had predominantly obsessions and 2% had predominantly compulsions; the remaining 96% endorsed both obsessions and compulsions Individuals who appear to have obsessions without compulsions frequently have unrecognized reassurance rituals or mental compulsions, such as repetitive, ritualized praying, in addition to their obsessions. Pure compulsions are also unusual in adults, although they do occur in children, especially in the young (e.g., 6 to 8 years of age). Most people have both mental and behavioral compulsions; in the DSM-IV field trial, 79.5% reported having both mental and behavioral compulsions, 20.3% had behavioral compulsions only, and 0.2% had only mental compulsions.

Contamination obsessions are the most frequently encountered obsessions in OCD. Such obsessions are usually characterized by a fear of dirt or germs. For example, a 38-year-old computer programmer was excessively preoccupied with the thought that her apartment would become dirty. She had never allowed a visitor into her apartment or worn a coat during the winter, because she feared that she would be unable to protect her apartment from dirt brought inside by either a visitor or a coat. Excessive washing is the compulsion most commonly associated with contamination obsessions. This behavior usually occurs after contact with the feared object; however, proximity to the feared stimulus is often sufficient to engender severe anxiety and washing compulsions, even though the contaminated object has not been touched. Most individuals with washing compulsions perform these rituals in response to a fear of contamination, but these behaviors occasionally occur in response to a drive for perfection or a need for symmetry. Some individuals, for example, repeatedly wash themselves in the shower until they feel "right" or must wash their right arm and then their left arm the same number of times.

Need for symmetry is a term that describes a drive to order or arrange things perfectly or to perform certain behaviors symmetrically or in a balanced way.

DSM-IV-TR Diagnostic Criteria

300.3 OBSESSIVE–COMPULSIVE DISORDER

A. Either obsessions or compulsions:

Obsessions as defined by (1), (2), (3), and (4):

(1) recurrent and persistent thoughts, impulses, or images that are experienced, at some time during the disturbance, as intrusive and inappropriate and that cause marked anxiety or distress
(2) the thoughts, impulses, or images are not simply excessive worries about real-life problems
(3) the person attempts to ignore or suppress such thoughts, impulses, or images, or to neutralize them with some other thought or action
(4) the person recognizes that the obsessional thoughts, impulses, or images are a product of his or her own mind (not imposed from without as in thought insertion)

Compulsions as defined by (1) and (2):

(1) repetitive behaviors (e.g., hand washing, ordering, checking) or mental acts (e.g., praying, counting, repeating words silently) that the person feels driven to perform in response to an obsession, or according to rules that must be applied rigidly
(2) the behaviors or mental acts are aimed at preventing or reducing distress or preventing some dreaded event or situation; however, these behaviors or mental acts either are not connected in a realistic way with what they are designed to neutralize or prevent or are clearly excessive

B. At some point during the course of the disorder, the person has recognized that the obsessions or compulsions are excessive or unreasonable. Note: This does not apply to children.
C. The obsessions or compulsions cause marked distress, are time consuming (take more than 1 hour a day), or significantly interfere with the person's normal routine, occupational (or academic) functioning, or usual social activities or relationships.
D. If another Axis I disorder is present, the content of the obsessions or compulsions is not restricted to it (e.g., preoccupation with food in the presence of an eating disorder; hair pulling in the presence of trichotillomania; concern with appearance in the presence of body dysmorphic disorder (BDD); preoccupation with drugs in the presence of a substance use disorder; preoccupation with having a serious illness in the presence of hypochondriasis; preoccupation with sexual urges or fantasies in the presence of a paraphilia; or guilty ruminations in the presence of major depressive disorder).
E. The disturbance is not due to the direct physiological effects of a substance (e.g., a drug of abuse, a medication) or a general medical condition.

Specify if:

With poor insight: if, for most of the time during the current episode, the person does not recognize that the obsessions and compulsions are excessive or unreasonable

TABLE 31-1	Yale-Brown Obsessive–Compulsive Scale Symptom Checklist

Aggressive obsessions
  Fear might harm others
  Fear might harm self
  Violent or horrific images
  Fear of blurting out obsessions or insults
  Fear of doing something embarrassing
  Fear of acting on other impulses (e.g., robbing a bank, stealing groceries, overeating)
  Fear of being responsible for things going wrong (e.g., others will lose their job because of the patient)
  Fear something terrible might happen (e.g., fire, burglary)
  Other
Contamination obsessions
  Concerns or disgust with bodily waste (e.g., urine, feces, saliva)
  Concern with dirt or germs
  Excessive concern with environmental contaminants (e.g., asbestos, radiation, toxic wastes)
  Excessive concern with household items (e.g., cleansers, solvents, pets)
  Concerned will become ill
  Concerned will become ill (aggressive)
  Other
Sexual obsessions
  Forbidden or perverse sexual thoughts, images, or impulses
  Content involves children
  Content involves animals
  Content involves incest
  Content involves homosexuality
  Sexual behavior toward others (aggressive)
  Other
Hoarding or collecting obsessions
Religious obsessions
Obsession with need for symmetry or exactness
Miscellaneous obsessions
  Need to know or remember
  Fear of saying certain things
  Fear of not saying things just right
  Intrusive (neutral) images
  Intrusive nonsense sounds, words, or music
  Other
Somatic obsession–compulsion
Cleaning or washing compulsions
  Excessive or ritualized hand washing
  Excessive or ritualized showering, bathing, brushing the teeth, or grooming
  Involves cleaning of household items or inanimate objects
  Other measures to prevent contact with contaminants
Counting compulsions
Checking compulsions
  Checking that did not or will not harm others
  Checking that did not or will not harm self
  Checking that nothing terrible did or will happen
  Checking for contaminants
  Other
Repeating rituals
Ordering or arranging compulsions
Miscellaneous compulsions
  Mental rituals (other than checking or counting)
  Need to tell, ask, or confess
  Need to touch
Measures to prevent
  Harm to self
  Harm to others
  Terrible consequences
Other

Individuals describe an urge to repeat motor acts until they achieve a "just right" feeling that the act has been completed perfectly. Individuals with a prominent need for symmetry may have little anxiety but rather describe feeling unsettled or uneasy if they cannot repeat actions or order things to their satisfaction. Individuals with a need for symmetry frequently present with obsessional slowness, taking hours to perform acts such as grooming or brushing their teeth. A 23-year-old cook spent 2 hours a day brushing his teeth in a symmetrical fashion and as a result developed gingival erosion. He reported being exquisitely aware of exactly how the toothbrush touched each surface of each tooth and of how he placed the toothbrush and cup down after finishing. He was unable to describe any obsession or fear about not performing this task adequately but rather felt unable to stop until he had brushed completely, despite warnings from his dentist about the harm he was causing.

Individuals with somatic obsessions are worried about the possibility that they have or will contract an illness or disease. In the past, the most common somatic obsessions consisted of fears of cancer or venereal diseases. However, a fear of developing AIDS has become increasingly common. Checking compulsions consisting of checking and rechecking the body part of concern, as well as reassurance seeking, are commonly associated with this fear. For example, a 29-year-old firefighter spent 3 hours a day examining his throat in the mirror and palpating his lymph nodes to determine whether he had throat cancer.

People with sexual or aggressive obsessions are plagued by fears that they might harm others or commit a sexually unacceptable act such as molestation. Often, they are fearful not only that they will commit a dreadful act in the future but also that they have already committed the act. Individuals are usually horrified by the content of their obsessions and are reluctant to divulge them. It is striking that the content of these obsessions tends to consist of ideas that individuals find particularly abhorrent. A 32-year-old librarian who wanted to be a good mother had intrusive thoughts of stabbing her daughter. Individuals with these highly distressing obsessions frequently have checking and confession or reassurance rituals. They may report themselves to the police or repeatedly seek out priests to confess their imagined crimes. For example, a 29-year-old secretary constantly checked the local news to be certain that she had not murdered someone. An unsolved murder case caused her tremendous anxiety and led to extensive reassurance rituals.

Pathological doubt is a common feature of individuals with OCD who have a variety of different obsessions and compulsions. Individuals with pathological doubt are plagued by the concern that, as a result of their carelessness, they will be responsible for a dire event. They may worry, for example, that they will start a fire because they neglected to turn off the stove before leaving the house. Although many individuals report being fairly certain that they performed the act in question (e.g., locking the door, unplugging the hairdryer, paying the correct amount on a bill), they cannot dismiss the nagging doubt "What if?" Excessive doubt and associated feelings of excessive responsibility frequently lead to checking rituals. For example, individuals may spend several hours checking their home before they leave. As with contamination obsessions, pathological doubt can lead to marked avoidance behavior. Some individuals become housebound to avoid the responsibility of potentially leaving the house unlocked.

There has been considerable interest in the role of insight, or awareness, in OCD. An ability to recognize the senselessness of the obsessions and the ability to resist obsessional ideas have been considered as the fundamental components of OCD. However, research findings during the past decade have demonstrated a continuum of insight in this disorder, which ranges from excellent (i.e., complete awareness of the senselessness of the content of the obsessions), through poor insight, to delusional thinking (i.e., the obsessions are held with delusional conviction). Combining data from a number of studies, 20–25% of individuals with OCD at some point during their illness are fairly convinced that their obsessions are realistic and that consequences other than anxiety would occur if they did not perform their compulsions. Nonetheless, most people with OCD are aware that other people think their symptoms are unrealistic and that the obsessions are caused by a mental disorder. To reflect the fact that many individuals lack insight, DSM-IV-TR includes a specifier "With Poor Insight" that applies to "an individual who, for most of the time in the current episode, does not recognize that the obsessions or compulsions are excessive or unreasonable." DSM-IV-TR also acknowledges that the beliefs that underlie OCD obsessions can be delusional and notes that, in such cases, an additional diagnosis of delusional disorder or psychotic disorder not otherwise specified may be appropriate.

Women appear to develop OCD slightly more frequently than do men. A predominance of males has been observed in child and adolescent OCD populations.

OCD frequently occurs in association with other Axis I disorders. In a study of 100 individuals with primary OCD, 67 had a lifetime history of major depressive disorder and 31 had symptoms that met criteria for current major depressive disorder. Although it may be difficult to distinguish a primary from a secondary diagnosis, some individuals with OCD view their depressive symptoms as occurring secondary to the demoralization and hopelessness accompanying their OCD and report that they would not be depressed if they did not have OCD. However, others view their major depressive symptoms as occurring independently of their OCD symptoms, which may be less severe when they cycle into an episode of major depression, because they feel too apathetic to be as concerned with their obsessions and too fatigued to perform compulsions. Conversely, OCD symptoms may intensify during depressive episodes.

Although findings have varied, the generally accepted frequency of tic disorders in individuals with OCD is far higher than in the general population, with a rate of approximately 5–10% for Tourette's Disorder and 20% for any tic disorder. Conversely, individuals with Tourette's disorder have a high rate of comorbid OCD, with 30–40% reporting obsessive–compulsive symptoms. The likelihood of childhood onset of OCD is greater in this group, and the presence of tics is associated with more severe OCD symptoms in children. There is an increased rate of both OCD and tic disorders in the first-degree relatives of OCD probands with a family lifetime history of tics and an increased frequency of tic disorders in the first-degree relatives of OCD probands compared to controls.

Studies of individuals with schizophrenia or schizoaffective disorder have found rates of OCD ranging from 8% to 46%. This strikingly large range is most likely due to the OCD criteria used (i.e., subclinical OCD symptoms versus OCD symptoms severe enough to cause significant impairment or distress). Regardless, it is clear that a significant number of people with schizophrenia have OCD symptoms that require assessment, and may benefit from treatment.

The relationship between OCD and personality disorders, particularly obsessive–compulsive personality disorder (OCPD), has received considerable attention. Early observations noted the presence of OCPD traits in individuals with OCD. Systematic studies, however, have yielded inconsistent findings.

Until the mid-1980s, OCD was considered extremely rare. This perception was based on studies from the 1950s and 1960s that examined the frequency of mental disorders in inpatient and outpatient settings. The results of a large epidemiological study, the national ECA survey, conducted in the United States in 1984, painted a different picture of OCD's prevalence. This study found that OCD was the fourth most common mental disorder (after the phobias, substance use disorders, and major depressive disorder), with a prevalence of 1.6% over 6 months and a lifetime prevalence of

2.5%. Although the ECA survey has been criticized as overestimating OCD's prevalence, a subsequent study in the United States and several epidemiological studies in other countries have supported its findings.

Course

Age at onset usually refers to the age when OCD symptoms (obsessions and compulsions) reach a severity level, wherein they lead to impaired functioning or significant distress or are time consuming (i.e., meet DSM-IV-TR criteria for the disorder). Reported age at onset is usually during late adolescence. People with OCD, however, usually describe the onset of minor symptoms in childhood, well before the onset of symptoms meeting the full criteria for the disorder.

In several studies, earlier age at onset has been associated with an increased rate of OCD in first-degree relatives. These data suggest that there is a familial type of OCD characterized by early onset. Age at onset of OCD may also be a predictor of course. The vast majority of individuals report a gradual worsening of obsessions and compulsions prior to the onset of full-criteria OCD, which is followed by a chronic course. However, a subtype of OCD that begins before puberty and is characterized by an episodic course with intense exacerbations has been described. Exacerbations of OCD symptoms in this subtype have been linked with Group A beta-hemolytic streptococcal infections, which has led to the subtype designation of pediatric autoimmune neuropsychiatric disorders associated with streptococcal infections (PANDAS). In a study of 50 children with PANDAS, the average age of onset was 7.4 years. Whether the course of illness in individuals with PANDAS continues to be episodic into adulthood, or, as is the case with postpubertal onset, tends to be chronic, is not known.

The course of OCD is usually waxing and waning—that is, once an individual acquires OCD, obsessions or compulsions, or both, are present continuously, with varying degrees of intensity over time. Relatively few individuals have either a progressively deteriorating course or a truly episodic course.

Differential Diagnosis

OCD is sometimes difficult to distinguish from certain other disorders. Obsessions and compulsions may appear in the context of other syndromes, which can raise the question whether the obsessions and compulsions are a symptom of another disorder or whether both OCD and another disorder are present. A general guideline is that if the content of the obsessions is not limited to the focus of concern of another disorder (e.g., an appearance concern, as in body dysmorphic disorder [BDD], or food concerns, as in an eating disorder) and if the obsessions or compulsions are preoccupying as well as distressing or impairing, OCD should generally be diagnosed. Diagnostic dilemmas may also arise when it is unclear whether certain thoughts are obsessions or whether, instead, they are ordinary worries, ruminations, overvalued ideas, or delusions. In a similar vein, questions may develop about whether certain behaviors constitute true compulsions or whether they should instead be conceptualized as impulses, tics, or addictive behaviors.

Both OCD and the other anxiety disorders are characterized by the use of avoidance to manage anxiety. However, OCD is distinguished from these disorders by the presence of compulsions. For individuals with preoccupying fears or worries but no rituals, several other features may be useful in establishing the diagnosis of OCD. In social phobia and specific phobia, fears are circumscribed and related to specific triggers (in specific phobia) or social situations (in social phobia). As many as 60% of people with OCD experience full-blown panic symptoms. However, unlike panic disorder, in which panic attacks occur spontaneously, panic symptoms occur in OCD only during exposure to specific feared triggers such as contaminated objects. The worries that are present in generalized anxiety disorder (GAD) are more egosyntonic and involve an exaggeration of ordinary concerns, whereas the obsessional thinking of OCD is more intrusive, is limited to a specific set of concerns (e.g., contamination, blasphemy), and usually has an irrational, senseless, or unreasonable quality.

One question is how to differentiate OCD from psychotic disorders such as schizophrenia and delusional disorder. Another question is how to distinguish OCD with insight from OCD without insight (delusional OCD). One distinguishing feature between OCD and the psychotic disorders is that the latter are not characterized by prominent ritualistic behaviors. If compulsions are present in an individual with prominent psychotic symptoms, the possibility of a comorbid OCD diagnosis should be considered. Furthermore, although schizophrenia may be characterized by obsessional thinking, other characteristic features of the disorder, such as prominent hallucinations or thought disorder, are also present. With regard to delusional disorder, paranoid and grandiose concerns are generally not considered to fall under the OCD rubric. However, some other types of delusional disorder, such as the somatic and jealous types, seem to bear a close resemblance to OCD and are not always easily distinguished from it.

The second issue noted above—how to distinguish OCD with insight from OCD without insight—is complex. As previously discussed, insight in OCD is increasingly being recognized as spanning a spectrum from good to poor to absent. Both clinical observations and research findings indicate that some individuals hold their obsessional concerns with delusional intensity, and believe that their concerns are reasonable. In DSM-IV-TR, delusional OCD may be double coded as both OCD and delusional disorder or as both OCD and psychotic disorder not otherwise specified; in other words, individuals with delusional OCD would receive both diagnoses. This double coding reflects the fact that it is unclear whether OCD with insight and OCD without insight constitute the same or different disorders. Further research using validated scales to assess insight in OCD is needed to shed light on this question.

Differential diagnosis questions have been raised with regard to kleptomania, trichotillomania, pathological gambling, and other disorders involving impulsive behaviors. Several features have been said to distinguish these disorders from OCD. For example, compulsions—unlike behaviors of the impulse control disorders—generally have no gratifying element, although they do diminish anxiety. In addition, the affective state that drives the behaviors associated with these disorders may differ. In OCD, fear is frequently the underlying drive that leads to compulsions, which, in turn, decrease anxiety. In the impulse control disorders, individuals frequently describe heightened tension, but not fear, preceding an impulsive behavior.

Complex motor tics of Tourette's disorder may be difficult to distinguish from OCD compulsions. Both tics and compulsions are preceded by an intrusive urge and are followed by feelings of relief. However, OCD compulsions are usually preceded by both anxiety and obsessional concerns, whereas, in Tourette's disorder, the urge to perform a tic is not preceded by an obsessional fear. This distinction breaks down to some extent when considering the "just right" perceptions of some individuals with OCD. The "just right" perception refers to the need to perform a certain motor action, such as touching, tapping, checking, ordering, arranging, or counting, until it feels right. Determining when an action has been performed enough or perfectly may depend on tactile, visual, or auditory perceptions. In a study of individuals with Tourette's disorder and OCD symptoms, most individuals could distinguish between the mental urge to do something repeatedly until it felt right and a physical urge to perform a motor tic. However, it is sometimes difficult for mental health professionals to distinguish between complex tics and compulsions, especially when an individual has both disorders.

Fears of illness that occur in OCD, referred to as somatic obsessions, may be difficult to distinguish from hypochondriasis. Usually, however, individuals with somatic obsessions have other current or past classic OCD obsessions unrelated to illness concerns. Individuals with OCD also often engage in classic OCD rituals, such as checking or reassurance seeking, in an attempt to diminish their illness concerns. Unlike individuals with OCD, individuals with hypochondriasis experience somatic and visceral sensations. BDD, a preoccupation with an imagined or slight defect in appearance (e.g., thinning hair, facial scarring, or a large nose), has many similarities to OCD. Individuals with BDD experience obsessional thinking about the supposed defect and usually engage in associated repetitive ritualistic behaviors, such as mirror checking and reassurance seeking. Preliminary evidence suggests that BDD also appears similar to OCD in terms of age of onset, course of illness, and other variables. Nonetheless, emerging data suggest that there are some important differences between the two disorders and they are currently classified separately in DSM-IV-TR. Insight, for example, is more frequently impaired in BDD than in OCD. If the content of a individual's obsessions involves a concern about a supposed defect in appearance, BDD, rather than OCD, is the diagnosis that should be given.

Obsessive–compulsive personality disorder is a lifelong maladaptive personality style characterized by perfectionism, excessive attention to detail, indecisiveness, rigidity, excessive devotion to work, restricted affect, lack of generosity, and hoarding. OCD and OCPD have historically been considered variants of the same disorder on a continuum of severity, with OCD viewed as the more severe manifestation of illness. Contrary to this notion, studies using structured interviews to establish diagnosis have found that not all individuals with OCD also have OCPD. One reason for the perception that these disorders are linked lies in the frequency of several OCPD traits in individuals with OCD. In one study, the majority of 114 individuals with OCD had perfectionism and indecisiveness (82 and 70, respectively). In contrast, other OCPD traits, such as restricted affect, excessive devotion to work, and rigidity, were seen infrequently.

Although perfectionism and indecisiveness are relatively common traits in individuals with OCD, the distinction between OCD and OCPD is important, and several guidelines may be useful in distinguishing them. Unlike OCPD, OCD is characterized by distressing, timeconsuming egodystonic obsessions and repetitive rituals aimed at diminishing the distress engendered by obsessional thinking. One of the hallmarks that has been traditionally used to distinguish OCD from OCPD is that, in contrast, OCPD features are considered egosyntonic. In addition, as previously noted, the traits of restricted affect, excessive devotion to work, and rigidity are generally characteristic of OCPD but not OCD. Although useful, these guidelines are not absolute, and some individuals defy easy categorization. Some individuals, for example, spend hours each day engaged in egosyntonic behaviors such as excessive cleaning; such individuals may seek treatment not because they are disturbed by their behaviors but because the behaviors cause problems in functioning or family friction. It is unclear whether some of these individuals should be diagnosed with OCPD or subthreshold OCD.

TREATMENT

Both pharmacologic and behavioral therapies have proved effective for OCD. The majority of controlled treatment trials have been performed with adults aged 18 to 65 years. However, these therapies have been shown to be effective for individuals of all ages. In general, children and the elderly tolerate most of these medications well. For children, lower doses are indicated because of lower body mass. For instance, the recommended dose for clomipramine in children is up to 150 mg/day (3 mg/kg/day) versus 250 mg/day in adults. Use of lower doses should also be considered in the elderly because their decreased ability to metabolize medications can increase the risk of side effects and toxicity. Behavioral therapy has also been used successfully in all age groups, although when treating children with this modality it is usually advisable to use a parent as a cotherapist. A flowchart that outlines treatment options for OCD is shown in Figure 31-1.

In general, the goals of treatment are to reduce the frequency and intensity of symptoms as much as possible and to minimize the amount of interference the symptoms cause. It should be noted that few individuals experience a cure or complete remission of symptoms. Instead, OCD should be viewed as a chronic illness with a waxing and waning course. Symptoms are often worse during times of psychosocial stress. Even when on medication, individuals with OCD are often upset when they experience even a mild symptom exacerbation, anticipating that their symptoms will revert to their worst, which is rarely the case. Anticipating with the individual that stress may make the symptoms worse can often be helpful in long-term treatment.

Somatic Treatments

The most extensively studied agents for OCD are medications that affect the serotonin system. The principal

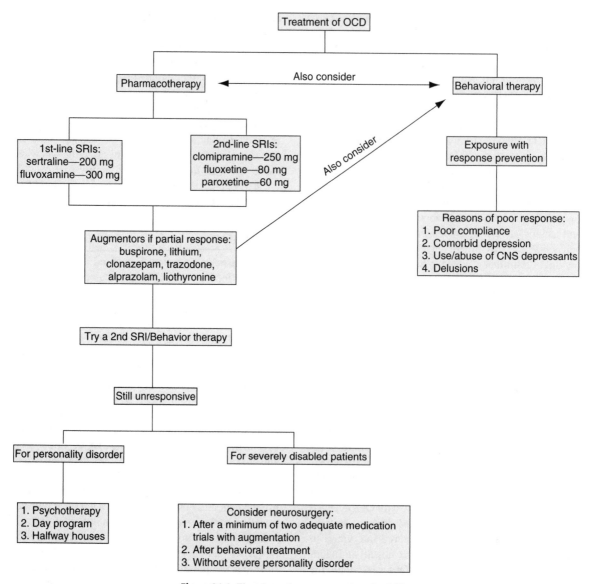

Figure 31-1 *Flowchart of treatment options for OCD.*

pharmacologic agents used to treat OCD are the SRIs, which include clomipramine, fluoxetine, fluvoxamine, sertraline, paroxetine, citalopram, and escitalopram.

The tricyclic antidepressant clomipramine is among the most extensively studied pharmacological agents in OCD. This drug is unique among the antiobsessional agents in that in addition to its potency as an SRI, it has significant affinity for noradrenergic, dopaminergic, muscarinic, and histaminic receptors. The most common side effects were those typical of the tricyclic antidepressants, including dry mouth, dizziness, tremor, fatigue, somnolence, constipation, nausea, increased sweating, headache, mental cloudiness, and sexual dys-

function. Previous data have indicated that at doses of 300 mg/day or more, the risk of seizures is 2.1%, but at doses of 250 mg/day or less, the risk of seizures is low (0.48%) and comparable to that of other tricyclic antidepressants. It is therefore recommended that doses of 250 mg/day or less be used.

Recent studies of IV clomipramine have been particularly promising because it seems to have a quicker onset of action and fewer side effects than the oral form, and it may be effective even in individuals who do not respond to oral clomipramine. Oral clomipramine, like other SRIs, usually takes a minimum of 4 to 6 weeks to produce a clinically significant clinical response, but in at least one study using IV pulse dosing, individuals showed a response within 4.5 days. The reasons for this unique response are not fully understood, but it is postulated that the IV preparation avoids first-pass hepatoenteric metabolism, leading to increased bioavailability of the parent compound clomipramine. This in turn may play a role in rapidly desensitizing serotonergic receptors or initiating changes in postsynaptic serotonergic neurons. Although studies of IV clomipramine for obsessional states date as far back as 1973, this preparation is still not FDA-approved for clinical use in the United States. Cardiac monitoring is recommended during the use of IV clomipramine.

Fluoxetine (as well as fluvoxamine, sertraline, paroxetine, citalopram and escitalopram) is often referred to as a selective serotonin reuptake inhibitor (SSRI) because it has a far more potent effect on serotonergic than on noradrenergic or other neurotransmitter systems. Despite their different chemical structures, all of the SSRIs appear to have similar efficacy in treating OCD. Fluoxetine and the other SSRIs have fewer side effects than clomipramine, reflecting its more selective mechanism of action. The most common side effects are headache, nausea, insomnia, anorexia, dry mouth, somnolence, nervousness, tremor, and diarrhea. Side effects occur more frequently at higher doses. Most studies of other medications for OCD have consisted of only case reports or small samples. One small trial suggested that venlafaxine, a medication which, like clomipramine, inhibits the reuptake of both serotonin and norepinephrine, may hold some promise.

The efficacy of each SSRI—clomipramine, fluoxetine, fluvoxamine, sertraline, paroxetine, and citalopram—is supported by existing data. During the past 10 years, at least seven head-to-head SRI comparison studies have been done. All of the studies found that the agents studied were equally efficacious, although they may have been underpowered to detect differences among medications. However, several meta-analyses of OCD trials, which compared SRIs across large placebo-controlled multicenter trials, lend some support to the notion that clomipramine might be more effective than the more selective agents. However, like most meta-analyses, these studies are flawed by factors that include variations in the study protocol, sample size, and the number of treatment-resistant and treatment-naïve subjects. The meta-analyses do support a trial of clomipramine in all individuals who do not respond to SRIs, even though clomipramine tends to cause more side effects.

It is worth noting that the SSRIs, via their effect on the liver cytochrome system, can inhibit the metabolism of certain other drugs. Fluoxetine can elevate blood levels of a variety of coadministered drugs, including tricyclic antidepressants (such as clomipramine), carbamazepine, phenytoin, and trazodone. However, the other SSRIs (with the exception of citalopram) can theoretically cause similar elevations, although fewer reports on such interactions are currently available. Some clinicians have taken advantage of these interactions by carefully combining fluvoxamine with clomipramine in order to block clomipramine's metabolism to desmethylclomipramine; this in turn favors serotonin reuptake inhibition provided by the parent compound rather than the norepinephrine reuptake inhibition provided by the metabolite. However, caution should be exercised with this approach since the elevation in clomipramine levels, and perhaps other compounds, can be nonlinear and quickly lead to dangerous toxicity. At the very least, clomipramine levels should be carefully monitored.

All of the SSRIs are generally well tolerated, with a relatively low percentage of individuals experiencing notable side effects or discontinuing them because of side effects. In addition, these compounds are unlikely to be lethal in overdose, except for clomipramine, which can lead to cardiac arrhythmias and death. All these agents can cause sexual side effects, ranging from anorgasmia to difficultly with ejaculatory function. However, such symptoms are not readily volunteered by the individual; thus it is important to ask. Should such symptoms be experienced, conservative measures may include dosage reduction, transient drug holidays for a special weekend or occasion, or switching to another SSRI since individuals may not have the same degree of dysfunction with a different agent. However, if the clinician feels that it is critical to continue with the same agent, various treatments have been reported in the literature. Usually taken within a few hours of sexual activity, no one agent has been shown to work consistently. Among those that have been tried are yohimbine, buspirone, cyproheptadine, ropinirole, buproprion, dextroamphetamine, methylphenidate, amantidine, and nefazodone, to name a few.

If an individual has had only a partial response to an antiobsessional agent of adequate dose and duration, the next question is whether to change the SSRI or add an augmenting agent. Current clinical practice suggests that if there is no response at all to an SSRI, it may be best to change to another SSRI. However, if there has been some response to treatment, an augmentation trial of at least 2 to 8 weeks may be warranted. No augmentation agent has been firmly established as efficacious. Although many augmentation agents appeared promising in open trials, they failed to be effective in more systematic trials although some of the

Table 31-2	Potential Augmenting Agents for Treatment-Resistant Obsessive–Compulsive Disorder
Augmenting Agent	**Suggested Dosage Range***
Lithium	300–600 mg/day[†]
Clonazepam	1–3 mg/day
Tryptophan	2–10 g/day[‡]
Trazodone	100–200 mg/day
Buspirone	15–60 mg/day
Alprazolam	0.5–2 mg/day
Methylphenidate	10–30 mg/day
Haloperidol	2–10 mg/day
Pimozide	2–10 mg/day
Nifedipine	10 mg t.i.d.
Liothyronine sodium	10–25 mg/day
Clonidine	0.1–0.6 mg/day
Fenfluramine	Up to 60 mg/day

*Add these to an ongoing trial of antidepressant medication. It should be noted that most of these dosages have not been tested with rigorous clinical trials but simply represent some of the reported doses tried in the current literature. Some would not recommend augmentation unless the initial treatment showed some response.
[†]*Use with caution*—there have been some reports of elevated lithium levels with ongoing fluoxetine treatment.
[‡]Because the use of l-tryptophan has been implicated in an increased incidence of eosinophilia, the authors advise against the prescribing and use of this agent until the issue is resolved.

Source: Jenike MA (1991) Management of patient with treatment-resistant obsessive–compulsive disorder. In *Current Treatments of Obsessive–Compulsive Disorder*, Pato MT and Zohar J (eds). Copyright, American Psychiatric Press, Washington DC, p. 146.

later studies did not report response to the SRI alone, leaving unanswered the question of whether some augmentation strategies may be effective in partial SSRI responders. Many questions about augmentation remain unanswered, including the optimal duration of augmentation, comparative efficacy of different agents, predictors of response, and mechanism of action. Nonetheless, these agents do help some individuals significantly, and thus their systematic use should be considered (see Table 31-2).

In individuals with severe symptoms or comorbid psychosis or tic disorder, pimozide 1–3 mg/day, haldol 2–10 mg/day, and other neuroleptic agents (risperidone 2–8 mg/day and olanzapine 2.5–10 mg/day) have been used with some success. However, the use of a neuroleptic agent should be considered carefully in light of the risk of extrapyramidal symptoms and side effects such as weight gain, lethargy, and tardive dyskinesia. Thus, when a neuroleptic drug is used, target symptoms should be established before beginning treatment and the medication discontinued within several months if target symptoms do not improve.

The use of lithium (300–600 mg/day) and buspirone (up to 60 mg/day) as augmentation agents has also been explored. Both agents looked promising in open trials but failed to be effective in more systematic trials.

Augmentation with fenfluramine (up to 60 mg/day), clonazepam (up to 5 mg/day), clonidine (0.1–0.6 mg/day), and trazodone (100–200 mg/day), as well as the combination of clomipramine with any of the SSRIs, has had anecdotal success but has not been evaluated in methodologically rigorous studies. Some potential augmenting agents and their dosage ranges are presented in Table 31-2.

Occasionally, even after receiving adequate pharmacotherapy (including augmentation), adequate behavioral therapy, and a combination of behavioral therapy and pharmacotherapy, individuals may still experience intractable OCD symptoms. Such individuals may be candidates for neurosurgery. Although criteria for who should receive neurosurgery vary, it has been suggested that failure to respond to at least 5 years of systematic treatment is a reasonable criterion. The procedures that have been most successful interrupt tracts involved in the serotonin system. The surgical procedures used—anterior capsulotomy, cingulotomy, and limbic leukotomy—all aim to interrupt the connection between the cortex and the basal ganglia and related structures. Current stereotactic surgical techniques involve the creation of precise lesions, which are often only 10 to 20 mm, to specific tracts. These procedures have often been done with radio-frequency heated electrodes and more recently with gamma knife techniques. Postsurgical risks have been minimized, and in some cases cognitive function and personality traits improve along with symptoms of OCD.

Psychosocial Treatments

Behavioral therapy is effective for OCD both as a primary treatment and as an augmentation agent. This form of therapy is based on the principle of exposure and response prevention. The individual is asked to endure, in a graduated manner, the anxiety that a specific obsessional fear provokes while refraining from compulsions that allay that anxiety. The principles behind the efficacy of behavioral treatment are explained to the individual in the following way. Although compulsions, either covert or overt, usually immediately relieve anxiety, this is only a short-term solution; the anxiety will ultimately return, requiring the performance of another compulsion. However, if the individual resists the anxiety and urge to ritualize, the anxiety will eventually decrease on its own (i.e., habituation will occur), and the need to perform the ritual will eventually disappear. Thus, behavioral therapy helps the individual habituate to the anxiety and extinguish the compulsions.

Compulsions, especially overt behaviors like washing rituals, are more successfully treated by behavioral therapy than are obsessions alone or covert rituals like mental checking. This is because covert rituals are harder to physically resist than are rituals like hand washing and checking a door. It has been reported that washing rituals are the most amenable to behavioral treatment, followed by checking rituals and then mental rituals.

For rituals that do not constitute overt behaviors, techniques other than exposure and response prevention have been used in conjunction with exposure and response prevention. These approaches include imaginal flooding and thought stopping. In imaginal flooding, the anxiety provoked by the obsessions is evoked by continually repeating the thought, often with the help of a continuous-loop tape or the reading of a "script" composed by the individual and therapist, until the thought no longer provokes anxiety. In thought stopping, a compulsive mental ritual (e.g., continually repeating a short prayer in one's head) is stopped by simply shouting, making a loud noise, or snapping a rubber band on the wrist in an attempt to interrupt the thought.

In the early stages of treatment, a behavioral assessment is performed. During this assessment, the content, frequency, duration, amount of interference and distress, and attempts to resist or ignore the obsessions and compulsions are catalogued. An attempt is made to clarify the types of symptoms, any triggers that bring on the obsessions and compulsions, and the amount and type of avoidance used to deal with the symptoms. The individual, usually with the help of a therapist, then develops a hierarchy of situations according to the amount of anxiety they provoke. During treatment, individuals gradually engage in the anxiety-provoking situations included in their hierarchy without performing anxiety-reducing rituals.

Despite its efficacy, behavioral therapy has limitations. To begin with, about 15–25% of individuals refuse to engage in behavioral treatment initially or drop out early in treatment because it is so anxiety provoking. Behavioral treatment fails in another 25% of individuals for a variety of other reasons, including concomitant depression; the use of central nervous system depressants, which may inhibit the ability to habituate to anxiety; lack of insight; poor compliance with homework, resulting in inadequate exposure; and poor compliance on the part of the therapist in enforcing the behavioral paradigm. Thus, overall, 50–70% of individuals are helped by this form of therapy.

Behavior therapy can be used as the sole treatment of OCD, particularly with individuals whose contamination fears or somatic obsessions make them resistant to taking medications. Behavioral treatment is also a powerful adjunct to pharmacotherapy. Some research appears to indicate that combined treatment may be more effective than pharmacotherapy or behavioral therapy alone, although these findings are still preliminary. Some studies have even suggested that adding pharmacotherapy to behavior therapy may be particularly helpful in reducing obsessions, while compulsions respond to behavior therapy. From a clinical perspective, it may be useful to have individuals begin treatment with medication to reduce the intensity of their symptoms or comorbid depressive symptoms if present; individuals may then be more amenable to experiencing the anxiety that will be evoked by the behavioral challenges they perform. The data on the discontinuation of behavioral therapy are encouraging. Overall, about 75% of individuals continue to do well at follow-up, but are symptom free.

The use of psychotherapeutic techniques of either a psychoanalytic or a supportive nature has not been proved successful in treating the specific obsessions and compulsions that are a hallmark of OCD. However, the more characterological aspects that are part of OCPD may be helped by a more psychoanalytically oriented approach. The defense mechanisms of reaction formation, isolation, and undoing, as well as a pervasive sense of doubt and need to be in control, are hallmarks of the obsessive–compulsive character. In therapy the individual must be encouraged to take risks and learn to feel comfortable with, or at least less anxious about, making mistakes and to accept anxiety as a natural and normal part of human experience. Techniques for meeting such goals in treatment may include the therapist's being relatively active in therapy to ensure that the individual focuses on the present rather than getting lost in perfectly recounting the past, as well as the therapist's being willing to take risks and present herself or himself as less than perfect.

COMPARISON OF DSM-IV-TR AND ICD-10 DIAGNOSTIC CRITERIA

The ICD-10 Diagnostic Criteria for Research for Obsessive–Compulsive Disorder differentiate between obsessions and compulsions on the basis of whether they are thoughts, ideas, or images (obsessions) or acts (compulsions). In contrast, DSM-IV-TR distinguishes between obsessions and compulsions on the basis of whether the thought, idea, or image causes anxiety or distress or prevents or reduces it. Thus, in DSM-IV-TR, there can be cognitive compulsions that would be considered obsessions in ICD-10. In addition, ICD-10 sets a minimum duration of at least 2 weeks, whereas DSM-IV-TR has no minimum duration.

Posttraumatic Stress Disorder

DIAGNOSIS

Posttraumatic stress disorder (PTSD) is defined in the DSM-IV-TR by six different criteria (see DSM-IV-TR diagnostic criteria, page 327). The diagnosis of PTSD is based on a history of exposure to a traumatic stressor, the simultaneous appearance of three different symptom clusters, a minimal duration, and the existence of functional disturbance. To qualify as traumatic, the event must have involved actual or threatened death or serious injury or a threat to the individual or others, and exposure to this event must arouse an intense affective response characterized by fear, helplessness, or horror. In children, disorganized or agitated behavior can be seen in lieu of an intense affective response. Symptomatically, there must be at least one of five possible intrusive-reexperiencing symptoms. These have the quality of obsessive, recurring, intrusive, and distressing recollections either in the form of imagery or thoughts or in the form of recurrent distressing dreams. Intense psychological distress or physiological reactivity on exposure to either an external reminder or an internal reminder of the trauma can also occur. The flashback experience, or reliving of the event, is less common.

Symptom cluster C in the DSM-IV-TR criteria in actuality embodies two somewhat different psychopathologies—namely, phobic avoidance and numbing or withdrawal. The phobic avoidance is expressed either in (1) efforts to avoid thoughts and feelings and conversations associated with the trauma or (2) in efforts to avoid activities, places, or people that arouse recollections of the trauma. (3) Psychogenic amnesia, a more dissociative symptom, also is in this symptom grouping, followed by (4) markedly diminished interest, (5) feeling detached or estranged, (6) having a restricted range of affect, and (7) having a sense of a foreshortened future. At least three of these seven symptoms must be present.

Hyperarousal symptoms, somewhat similar to those of generalized anxiety disorder, are also present in PTSD and at least one of five of the following symptoms is required: difficulty sleeping, irritability or anger, poor concentration, hypervigilance, and exaggerated startle response.

With regard to the symptoms as a whole, it is evident that they embody features of different psychiatric disorders, including obsessive–compulsive processes, generalized anxiety disorder, panic attacks, phobic avoidance, dissociation, and depression. Finally, it is necessary for symptoms to have lasted at least 1 month and for the disturbance to have caused clinically significant distress or impairment.

Community-based studies conducted in the United States have documented a lifetime prevalence rate for PTSD of approximately 8% of the adult population. General population female-to-male lifetime prevalence ratio is 2 : 1. The highest rates of PTSD occurrence for particular traumatic exposures (occurring in one-third to three-fourths of those exposed) are among survivors of rape, military combat and captivity, graves registration (i.e., registering dead bodies through the morgue), and ethnically or politically motivated interment and genocide.

Epidemiological studies show that PTSD often remains chronic, with a significant number of people remaining symptomatic, several years after the initial event. In support of this view are epidemiological data that show that recovery does not occur frequently. For example, the National Vietnam Veterans Readjustment study found lifetime and current prevalence rates of PTSD to be, respectively, 30.9% and 15.2% in men and 26.9% and 8.5% in women. In a population of rape victims, lifetime prevalence of PTSD was found to be 75.8% with a current prevalence rate of 39.4%. The National Comorbidity Survey, a large epidemiological survey conducted in the United States in the early 1990s, documented that one-third of those diagnosed with PTSD fail to recover even after many years. Therefore,

Clinical Guide to the Diagnosis and Treatment of Mental Disorders. M. B. First and A. Tasman
© 2006 John Wiley & Sons, Ltd.   ISBN 0 470 019158

DSM-IV-TR Diagnostic Criteria

309.81 Posttraumatic Stress Disorder

A. The person has been exposed to a traumatic event in which both of the following were present:

   (1) the person experienced, witnessed, or was confronted with an event or events that involved actual or threatened death or serious injury, or a threat to the physical integrity of self or others
   (2) the person's response involved intense fear, helplessness, or horror. **Note:** In children, this may be expressed instead by disorganized or agitated behavior

B. The traumatic event is persistently reexperienced in one (or more) of the following ways:

   (1) recurrent and intrusive distressing recollections of the event, including images, thoughts, or perceptions. **Note:** In young children, repetitive play may occur in which themes or aspects of the trauma are expressed
   (2) recurrent distressing dreams of the event. **Note:** In children, there may be frightening dreams without recognizable content
   (3) acting or feeling as if the traumatic event were recurring (includes a sense of reliving the experience, illusions, hallucinations, and dissociative flashback episodes, including those that occur on awakening or when intoxicated). **Note:** In young children, trauma-specific reenactment may occur
   (4) intense psychological distress at exposure to internal or external cues that symbolize or resemble an aspect of the traumatic event
   (5) physiological reactivity on exposure to internal or external cues that symbolize or resemble an aspect of the traumatic event

C. Persistent avoidance of stimuli associated with the trauma and numbing of general responsiveness (not present before the trauma), as indicated by three (or more) of the following:

   (1) efforts to avoid thoughts, feelings, or conversations associated with the trauma
   (2) efforts to avoid activities, places, or people that arouse recollections of the trauma
   (3) inability to recall an important aspect of the trauma
   (4) markedly diminished interest or participation in significant activities
   (5) feeling of detachment or estrangement from others
   (6) restricted range of affect (e.g., unable to have loving feelings)
   (7) sense of a foreshortened future (e.g., does not expect to have a career, marriage, children, or a normal life span)

D. Persistent symptoms of increased arousal (not present before the trauma), as indicated by two (or more) of the following:

   (1) difficulty falling or staying asleep
   (2) irritability or outbursts of anger
   (3) difficulty concentrating
   (4) hypervigilance
   (5) exaggerated startle response

E. Duration of the disturbance (symptoms in criteria B, C, and D) is more than 1 month.
F. The disturbance causes clinically significant distress or impairment in social, occupational, or other important areas of functioning.

Specify if:

Acute: if duration of symptoms is less than 3 months

Chronic: if duration of symptoms is 3 months or more

Specify if:

With delayed onset: if onset of symptoms is at least 6 months after the stressor

Reprinted with permission from the *Diagnostic and Statistical Manual of Mental Disorders*, 4th ed., Text Rev. Copyright 2000 American Psychiatric Association.

chronicity of PTSD is not limited to the more severe treatment-seeking samples.

Course

Immediately following traumatic exposure, a high percentage of individuals develop a mixed symptom picture, which includes disorganized behavior, dissociative symptoms, psychomotor change, and sometimes, paranoia. The diagnosis of Acute Stress Disorder accounts for many of these reactions. These reactions are generally short-lived, although by 1 month

the symptom picture often settles into a more classic PTSD presentation. After rape, for example, as many as 90% of individuals may qualify for the diagnosis of PTSD. Approximately 50% of people with PTSD recover, and approximately 50% develop a persistent, chronic form of the illness still present 1 year following the traumatic event.

The longitudinal course of PTSD is variable. Permanent recovery occurs in some people, whereas others show a relatively unchanging course with only mild fluctuation. Still others show a more obvious fluctuation with intermittent periods of well-being and recurrences of major symptoms. In a limited number of cases, the passage of time does not bring a resolution of symptoms, and the individual's condition tends to deteriorate with age. Particular symptoms that have been noted to increase with time in many people include startle response, nightmares, irritability, and depression. Clinicians during World War II also observed that the existence of marked startle response and hypervigilance in the acute aftermath of exposure to combat often represented a comparatively poor prognostic sign. In children, PTSD can be, and often is, chronic and debilitating.

General medical conditions may occur as a direct consequence of the trauma (e.g., head injury, burns). In addition, chronic PTSD may be associated with increased rates of adverse physical outcomes, including musculoskeletal problems and cardiovascular morbidity

Differential Diagnosis

PTSD symptoms may overlap with symptoms of a number of other disorders in the DSM-IV-TR. Both PTSD and adjustment disorder are etiologically related to stress exposure. PTSD may be distinguished from adjustment disorder by assessing whether the traumatic stress meets the severity criteria described earlier. Also, if there are an insufficient number of symptoms to qualify for the diagnosis, a diagnosis of adjustment disorder might be merited.

Specific phobias may arise after traumatic exposure. For example, after an automobile accident, victims may develop phobic avoidance of traveling, but without the intrusive or hyperarousal symptoms. In such cases, a diagnosis of specific phobia should be given instead of a diagnosis of PTSD.

The criteria set for generalized anxiety disorder includes a list of six symptoms of hyperarousal, of which four are common to PTSD: being on edge, poor concentration, irritability, and sleep disturbance. PTSD requires the additional symptoms as described earlier, and the worry in PTSD is focused on concerns about reexperiencing the trauma. In contrast, the worry in generalized anxiety disorder is about a number of different situations and concerns. However, it is possible for the two conditions to coexist.

In obsessive–compulsive disorder, recurring and intrusive thoughts occur, but the individual recognizes these to be inappropriate and unrelated to any particular life experience. Obsessive–compulsive disorder is a common comorbid condition in PTSD and may develop with generalization (e.g., compulsive washing for months after a rape to reduce contamination feelings).

It may also develop by activation of an underlying obsessive–compulsive disorder diathesis.

Autonomic hyperarousal is a cardinal part of panic attack, which may indicate a diagnosis of panic disorder. To distinguish between panic disorder and PTSD, the therapist needs to assess whether panic attacks are related to the trauma or reminders of the same (in which case they would be subsumed under a diagnosis of PTSD) or whether they occur unexpectedly and spontaneously (in which case a diagnosis of panic disorder would be justified).

Depression and PTSD share a significant overlap, including four of the criterion C cluster symptoms and three of the criterion D cluster symptoms. Thus, an individual who presents with reduced interest, estrangement, numbing, impaired concentration, insomnia, irritability, and sense of a foreshortened future may manifest either disorder. PTSD may give rise to depression as well, and it is possible for the two conditions to coexist. In a few instances, an individual with prior depression may be more vulnerable to developing PTSD. Reexperiencing symptoms are present only in PTSD.

Dissociative disorders also overlap with PTSD. In the early aftermath of serious trauma, the clinical picture may be predominantly one of the dissociative states (see the section on Acute Stress Disorder [ASD], page 332). ASD differs from PTSD in that the symptom pattern occurs within the first few days after exposure to the trauma, lasts no longer than 4 weeks, and is typically accompanied by prominent dissociative symptoms.

More rarely, PTSD must be distinguished from other disorders producing perceptual alterations, such as schizophrenia and other psychotic disorders, delirium, substance use disorders, and general medical conditions producing psychosis (e.g., brain tumors).

The differential diagnosis is important but, notwithstanding, PTSD is unlikely to occur in isolation. Psychiatric comorbidity is the rule rather than the exception, and a number of studies have demonstrated that, in both clinical and epidemiological populations, a wide range of disorders is likely to occur at an increased probability. These include major depressive disorder, all of the anxiety disorders, alcohol and substance use disorders, somatization disorder, and schizophrenia and schizophreniform disorder.

TREATMENT

A number of goals are common to all treatments of PTSD and can be summarized as follows: (1) to reduce intrusive symptoms; (2) to reduce avoidance symptoms; (3) to reduce numbing and withdrawal; (4) to dampen hyperarousal; (5) to reduce psychotic symptoms when present; and (6) to improve impulse control when this is a problem. By reducing troublesome symptoms, a number of other important goals can also be accomplished as follows: (1) to develop the capacity to interpret events more realistically with respect to their threat content; (2) to improve interpersonal work and leisure functioning; (3) to promote self-esteem, trust, and feelings of safety; (4) to explore and clarify meanings attributed to the event; (5) to promote access to memories that have been dissociated or repressed when judged to be clinically appropriate; (6) to strengthen social support systems; and (7) to move from identification as a victim to that of a survivor.

The three major treatment approaches, pharmacotherapeutic, cognitive–behavioral, and psychodynamic, all emphasize different aspects of the problem. Pharmacotherapy targets the underlying neurobiological alterations found in PTSD and attempts to control symptoms so that the above treatment goals can be more effectively accomplished. Cognitive–behavioral treatments emphasize the phobic avoidance and counterproductive reenactments that often occur, along with the identification of faulty beliefs that arise owing to the trauma, and replace them with more adaptive beliefs, usually in association with direct therapeutic exposure. The psychodynamic approach emphasizes the associations that arise from the trauma experience and that lead to unconscious and conscious representations. Defense mechanisms that lead to lack of memory, and the contributions from early development, are also brought into play in psychodynamic therapy.

General principles of treating PTSD involve explanation and destigmatization, which can be provided both to the individual and to family members. This often includes a description of the symptoms of PTSD and the way in which it can affect behaviors and relationships. Information can be given about general treatment principles, pointing out that sometimes cure is attainable but that at other times symptom containment is a more realistic treatment goal, particularly in chronic and severe PTSD. Regaining self-esteem and attaining greater control over impulses and affect are also desired in many instances. Information can be provided as to appropriate literature, local support groups and resources, and names and addresses of national advocacy organizations. If the therapist attends to these important issues early in treatment, the individual is able to more readily build trust and also to appreciate that the therapist shows a good understanding both of the condition and of the individual.

PTSD is sometimes comparatively straightforward to treat and at other times it is more complicated. However, treatment by a mental health clinician (rather than a primary care clinician) is almost always indicated. The initial history taking can evoke strong affect to a greater degree than is customarily found in other disorders. In fact, it may take several interviews for the details to emerge. A sensitive yet persistent approach is needed on the part of the interviewer. During treatment, although the mental health care clinician will clearly want to impart a sense of optimism to the individual, it is also a reflection of reality to point out early that recovery may be a slow process and that some symptoms (e.g., phobic avoidance, startle response) may persist. It is important for the mental health care clinician to be comfortable in hearing and tolerating unpleasant affect and often horrifying stories. All these must take place in a noncritical and accepting manner. Specific treatment approaches include the use of pharmacotherapy, psychotherapy, anxiety management, and attention to the general issues described earlier.

A stepwise sequence of approaches may be used in the treatment of PTSD but it must be said that there are no definitive guidelines currently in place. As a result, the particular order in which treatments are considered varies on the basis of individual circumstances. Also, no uniform definition exists as to what constitutes a good or poor response to treatment. In general, some symptoms of chronic PTSD persist, albeit at a considerably reduced level, in people who have undergone treatment.

Somatic Treatments

PTSD may be accompanied by enduring neurochemical and psychophysiological changes and can lead to substantial impairment and distress. Sometimes, the intensity of symptoms is severe enough to preclude the effective use of trauma-focused psychotherapy. In these situations, the use of medication should not be delayed unnecessarily. Initial studies showed benefit for the tricyclic antidepressant and monoamine oxidase inhibitor medications. However, the selective serotonin reuptake inhibitors (SSRIS) have now replaced these as first-line agents, based upon evidence from several placebo-controlled trials. The main groups of medications relevant to the treatment of PTSD along with dose ranges and chief side effects are listed in Table 32-1. A suggested sequencing of treatment is outlined in Table 32-2.

Several placebo-controlled trials have shown positive effects for the SSRI medications, Data support positive effects for SSRI in men and women and in adults who have survived all major classes of trauma (e.g., combat, sexual violence, nonsexual violence, and accident). Each of these medications has broad-spectrum

Table 32-1	Medications in Posttraumatic Stress Disorder: Dose Ranges and Side Effects	
Drug Category	**Dose Range (mg/day)**	**Common or Problematical Side Effects**
Antidepressants		
Selective serotonin reuptake inhibitors		Gastrointestinal disturbance, sexual dysfunction, agitation
Fluoxetine	10–60	
Fluvoxamine	50–300	
Sertraline	50–200	Insomnia
Paroxetine	10–60	Tiredness
Citalopram	20–60	
Tricyclic antidepressants		Anticholinergic effects, cardiovascular symptoms, weight gain
Amitriptyline	50–300	Sexual dysfunction, sedation (for all tricyclic antidepressants)
Imipramine	50–300	
Monoamine oxidase inhibitors		
Phenelzine	15–90	Weight gain, dizziness, sleep disturbance, sexual dysfunction, hypertensive reactions, hyperpyretic states
Anticonvulsants		
Carbamazepine	200–1500	Hematological effects
Valproic acid	125–2000	Gastrointestinal disturbance, sedation
Lamotrigine	50–200	Rash, exfoliative dermatitis, Stevens–Johnson syndrome
Mood stabilizers		
Lithium carbonate	300–1200	Gastrointestinal disturbance, polyuria, headache
Antiadrenergic drugs		
Propranolol	20–160	Depression, hypertension, rebound hypertension
Clonidine	0.1–0.4	Memory problems, dizziness, tiredness
Prazosin	2–10	Dizziness, hypotension
Anxiolytics	0.5–6	
Benzodiazepines		
Clonazepam	0.5–6	Sedation, memory problems, incoordination, dependence
Alprazolam	0.25–4	Withdrawal, rebound, disinhibition (for all benzodiazepines)
Diazepam	2–40	
Chlordiazepoxide	5–40	
Others		
Azapirones	5–60	Agitation, gastrointestinal disturbance, headaches
Buspirone		
Neuroleptics		
Thioridazine	25–300	Extrapyramidal symptoms
Haloperidol	0.5–4	Sedation, anticholinergic effects
Others		

Table 32-2	Pharmacotherapy Steps for Posttraumatic Stress Disorder

Step 1
Selective serotonin reuptake inhibitor (SSRI)
Adjunctive medications:
  If prominent hyperarousal: benzodiazepine or buspirone
  If prominent mood liability or explosiveness: anticonvulsant or lithium
  If prominent dissociation: valproic acid
  If persistent insomnia: trazodone
  If psychotic: atypical antipsychotic

Step 2
If no response or intolerance to SSRI:
  Dual action antidepressant, e.g., mirtazapine, venlafaxine
  Adjunctive medications as above

Step 3
If no response to Step 1 or 2:
  Monoamine oxidase inhibitor
  Adjunctive medications as above

Step 4
Other useful drugs:
  Propranolol—hyperarousal
  Clonidine—startle response
  Neuroleptics—psychosis, poor impulse control

properties across the full symptom range of the disorder as well as improving function and, perhaps, resilience or stress coping. They also support the benefit of SSRI in those with and without comorbid major depression.

At this point, the indications for antipsychotic and mood-stabilizing drugs are poorly defined, but clinical experience suggests that they continue to have a role in the pharmacologic treatment of PTSD. Antipsychotic medications can be useful in individuals with poor impulse control or in those who manifest features of borderline personality disorder. Lithium and carbamazepine can also be useful in such individuals but might benefit individuals who are subject to mood swings and angry or explosive outbursts. The appropriate role for the use of benzodiazepines is not well defined. The antiphobic and antiarousal effects of the benzodiazepines should, in theory, be helpful in PTSD. However, withdrawal from short-acting benzodiazepines may also introduce an additional set of problems with intense symptom rebound. In individuals who have a propensity to abuse alcohol and other substances, benzodiazepines are not recommended.

Overall, the antidepressants, mood stabilizers, and anticonvulsants are the medication groups that are generally considered primary for treating PTSD; beta-blockers, alpha-2-agonists, and anxiolytics have a less clearly defined place. Often, individuals need a combination of drugs, but polypharmacy should be utilized in a carefully planned fashion. Also, since the time course of response may be slow, it is advisable to persist with a particular course of action for at least 8 weeks before deciding that it has been unhelpful. It is possible that avoidance and numbing symptoms respond more effectively to SSRI drugs.

Cognitive and Behavioral Therapies

Despite theoretical differences, most schools of psychotherapy recognize that cognitively oriented approaches to the treatment of anxiety must include an element of exposure. Because PTSD involves aberrant and voluntary programs for the avoidance of danger that are conditioned by real experience, correction of these "fear structures" requires exposure to ensure habituation. Prolonged exposure depends on the fact that anxiety will be extinguished in the absence of real threat, given a sufficient duration of exposure *in vivo* or in imagination to traumatic stimuli. In PTSD, the individual retells the traumatic experience as if it were happening again, until doing so becomes a pedestrian exercise and anxiety decreases. Between sessions, individuals perform exposure homework, including listening to tapes of the flooding sessions and limited exposure *in vivo*. However, not every individual may be a candidate for exposure. Owing to the high anxiety and temporarily increased symptoms associated with prolonged exposure, there are individuals who will be reluctant to confront traumatic reminders. Individuals in whom guilt or anger are primary emotional responses to the traumatic event (as opposed to anxiety) may not profit from prolonged exposure.

Anxiety management techniques are designed to reduce anxiety by providing individuals with better skills for controlling worry and fear. Among such techniques are muscle relaxation, thought stopping, control of breathing and diaphragmatic breathing, communication skills, guided self-dialogue, and stress inoculation training (SIT).

Further, cognitive approaches to the treatment of PTSD have also seen shown to be effective. A cognitive approach to treatment includes training individuals in challenging problematic cognitions such as self-blame. In a comparison of cognitive therapy to imaginal exposure in the treatment of chronic PTSD, both treatments were associated with positive improvements at posttreatment and follow-up, with no differences in outcome between treatments. However, individuals who received imaginal exposure were more likely to experience an increase in PTSD symptoms during the treatment course, and those who did were more likely to miss treatment sessions, rate the therapy as less credible, and be rated as less motivated by the therapist. Other approaches have focused on efficaciously treating one aspect of PTSD symptomatology, such as anger, nightmares, or authority problems.

Psychodynamic Therapy

Psychodynamically based approaches emphasize the interpretation of the traumatic event as being a critical determinant of symptoms. Treatment is geared to alter attributions, usually by means of slow exposure and through confrontation and awareness of the negative affects that have been generated by the trauma. Conflictual meanings begin to appear, and it is the task of treatment to reinterpret the experience in a more realistic and adaptive fashion. During such treatment, it is important to ensure that the affect intensity is not overwhelming or disorganizing. Obviously, support needs to be provided throughout, and sometimes other treatment approaches are used adjunctively. Excessive and maladaptive behaviors such as avoidance, use of alcohol or work, or risk taking may occur as a means of coping with the experience and these need to be identified and addressed.

Acute Stress Disorder

DIAGNOSIS

It has long been recognized that clinically significant dissociative states are seen in the immediate aftermath of overwhelming trauma. In addition, many individuals may experience less clinically severe dissociative symptoms or alterations of attention and time sense. Because such syndromes, even when short-lasting, can produce major disruption of everyday activities, they may require clinical attention. During triage situations after a disaster, it can be important to recognize this clinical picture, which may require treatment intervention and which may also be predictive of later PTSD. As a result of these considerations, a decision was made to include in DSM-IV a new entity, acute stress disorder (ASD), grouped together with PTSD in the anxiety disorders section. Essentially, it represents the clinical features of PTSD along with conspicuous

DSM-IV-TR Diagnostic Criteria

308.3 ACUTE STRESS DISORDER

A. The person has been exposed to a traumatic event in which both of the following were present:

 (1) the person experienced, witnessed, or was confronted with an event or events that involved actual or threatened death or serious injury, or a threat to the physical integrity of self or others
 (2) the person's response involved intense fear, helplessness, or horror

B. Either while experiencing or after experiencing the distressing event, the individual has three (or more) of the following dissociative symptoms:

 (1) a subjective sense of numbing, detachment, or absence of emotional responsiveness
 (2) a reduction in awareness of his or her surroundings (e.g., "being in a daze")
 (3) derealization
 (4) depersonalization
 (5) dissociative amnesia (i.e., inability to recall an important aspect of the trauma)

C. The traumatic event is persistently reexperienced in at least one of the following ways: recurrent images, thoughts, dreams, illusions, flashback episodes, or a sense of reliving the experience; or distress on exposure to reminders of the traumatic event.

D. Marked avoidance of stimuli that arouse recollections of the trauma (e.g., thoughts, feelings, conversations, activities, places, people).

E. Marked symptoms of anxiety or increased arousal (e.g., difficulty sleeping, irritability, poor concentration, hypervigilance, exaggerated startle response, motor restlessness).

F. The disturbance causes clinically significant distress or impairment in social, occupational, or other important areas of functioning or impairs the individual's ability to pursue some necessary task, such as obtaining necessary assistance or mobilizing personal resources by telling family members about the traumatic experience.

G. The disturbance lasts for a minimum of 2 days and a maximum of 4 weeks and occurs within 4 weeks of the traumatic event.

H. The disturbance is not due to the direct physiological effects of a substance (e.g., a drug of abuse, a medication) or a general medical condition, is not better accounted for by brief psychotic disorder, and is not merely an exacerbation of a preexisting Axis I or Axis II disorder.

Reprinted with permission from the *Diagnostic and Statistical Manual of Mental Disorders*, 4th ed., Text Rev. Copyright 2000 American Psychiatric Association.

dissociative symptoms, of which at least three must be present. The possible dissociative symptoms in ASD are a subjective sense of numbing; detachment or absence of emotional response; reduced awareness of one's surroundings; derealization; depersonalization; and dissociative amnesia.

Because ASD, by definition, cannot last longer than 1 month, if the clinical picture persists, a diagnosis of PTSD is appropriate. Some increased symptoms are expected in the great majority of subjects after exposure to major stress. These remit in most cases and only reach the level of clinical diagnosis if they are prolonged, exceed a tolerable quality, or interfere with everyday function. Resolution may be more difficult if there has been previous psychiatric morbidity, subsequent stress, and lack of social support.

Little is known about the epidemiology of ASD as defined in DSM-IV-TR, but after events such as rape and criminal assault, the clinical picture of acute PTSD is found in 70 to 90% of individuals, although the frequency of the particular dissociative symptoms is unknown. One problem of most postdisaster surveys is that they evaluate subjects at points several months or years after the event. This makes any meaningful assessment of acute stress syndromes difficult. One exception was the self-report-based assessment of morbidity 2 months after an earthquake in Ecuador, which found a 45% rate of caseness (being a clinical case), with the most prominent symptoms being fear, nervousness, tenseness, worry, insomnia, and fatigue.

Course

Although data do not exist on the course and natural history of ASD as now defined, prior studies have indicated that dissociative and cognitive symptoms, which are so common in the immediate wake of trauma, improve spontaneously with time. However, it was also found that the likelihood of developing PTSD symptoms at 7-month follow-up was more strongly related to the occurrence of dissociative symptoms than to anxiety symptoms immediately after exposure to the trauma.

Differential Diagnosis

ASD may need to be distinguished from several related disorders (Figure 32-1). Brief psychotic disorder may be a more appropriate diagnosis if the predominant symptoms are psychotic. It is possible that a major depressive disorder can develop posttraumatically and that there may be some overlap with ASD, in which case both disorders are appropriately diagnosed. When ASD-like symptoms are caused by direct physiological perturbation, the symptoms may be more appropriately diagnosed with reference to the etiological agent. Thus, an ASD-like picture that develops secondary to head injury is more appropriately diagnosed as mental disorder

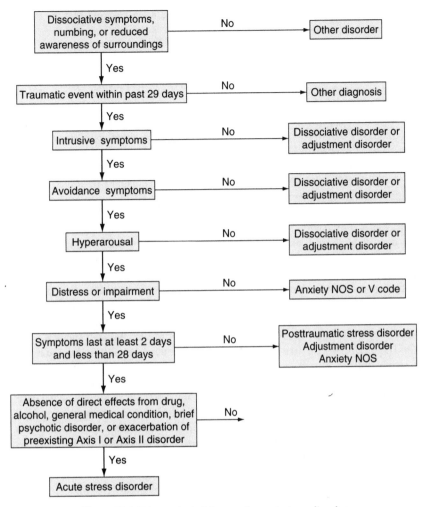

Figure 32-1 *Diagnostic decision tree for acute stress disorder.*

due to a general medical condition, whereas a clinical picture related to substance use (e.g., alcohol intoxication) is appropriately diagnosed as substance-induced disorder. Substance-related ASD is confined to the period of intoxication or withdrawal. Head injury-induced ASD needs substantiating by evidence from the history, physical examination, and laboratory testing that the symptoms are a direct physiological consequence of head trauma.

TREATMENT

There are six general principles involved in administering any treatment immediately after trauma. These include principles of brevity, immediacy, centrality, expectancy, proximity, and simplicity. That is, treatment of acute trauma is generally aimed at being brief, provided immediately after the trauma whenever possible, administered in a centralized and coordinated fashion with the expectation of the person's return to normal function and as proximately as possible to the scene of the trauma, and not directed at any uncovering or explorative procedures but rather at maintaining a superficial, reintegrating approach.

People most highly at risk, and therefore perhaps most in need of treatment, are as follows: survivors with psychiatric disorders; traumatically bereaved people; children, especially when separated from their parents; individuals who are particularly dependent on psychosocial supports, such as the elderly, handicapped, and mentally retarded individuals; and traumatized survivors and body handlers.

Different components of treatment include providing information, psychological support, crisis intervention, and emotional first aid. Providing information about the trauma is important as it can enable the survivor to fully recognize and accept all the details of what happened. Information needs to be given in a way that conveys hope and the possibility that psychological pain and threat of loss may be coped with. Unrealistic hope needs to be balanced by the provision of realistic explanations as to what happened. Psychological support helps to strengthen coping mechanisms and promotes adaptive defenses. The survivor benefits if he or she recognizes the need to take responsibility for a successful outcome and is as actively involved with this as possible. Crisis intervention is often used after disasters and acts of violence or other serious traumas.

There is little investigation as to whether early recognition and effective treatment of acute stress reactions prevent the development of PTSD, although it is safe to assume that they are likely to have beneficial effects in this regard. Nonetheless, as was recognized during World War II, rapid and effective treatment of acute combat stress did not always prevent veterans from developing subsequent chronicity. More recently, an intervention designed to prevent the development of PTSD and administered in the acute phase, critical incident stress debriefing, has been found to be ineffective in preventing the development of PTSD. However, there has been an initial study with motor vehicle accident survivors that suggested exposure therapy, and exposure therapy with anxiety management training may be effective in preventing PTSD.

COMPARISON OF DSM-IV-TR AND ICD-10 DIAGNOSTIC CRITERIA

The ICD-10 Diagnostic Criteria for Research for Posttraumatic Stress Disorder provide a different stressor criterion: a situation or event "of exceptionally threatening or catastrophic nature, which would be likely to cause pervasive distress in almost everyone," which is similar to the DSM-III-R definition of a traumatic stressor. DSM-IV-TR instead defines a traumatic stressor as "an event or events that involved actual or threatened death or serious injury, or a threat to the physical integrity of self or others." Furthermore, the ICD-10 diagnostic algorithm differs from that specified in DSM-IV-TR in that the DSM-IV-TR criterion D (i.e., symptoms of increased arousal) is not required. In contrast to DSM-IV-TR, which requires that the symptoms persist for more than one month, the ICD-10 Diagnostic Criteria for Research do not specify a minimum duration.

For acute stress disorder, the ICD-10 Diagnostic Criteria for Research differ in several ways from the DSM-IV-TR criteria: (1) primarily anxiety symptoms are included; (2) it is required that the onset of the symptoms be within 1 hour of the stressor; and (3) the symptoms must begin to diminish after not more than 8 hours (for transient stressors) or 48 hours (for extended stressors). In contrast to DSM-IV-TR, the ICD-10 Diagnostic Criteria for Research do not require dissociative symptoms or that the event be persistently reexperienced.

CHAPTER

33　　Anxiety Disorders: Generalized
Anxiety Disorder

DIAGNOSIS

Generalized Anxiety Disorder (GAD) is defined as
excessive anxiety and worry (apprehensive expectation) occurring for a majority of days during at least a
6-month period, about a number of events or activities
(such as work or school performance). In individuals
with GAD, the anxiety and worry are accompanied by
at least three of six somatic symptoms (only one accompanying symptom is required in children), which are
restlessness or feeling keyed up or on edge, being easily
fatigued, difficulty concentrating or mind going blank,
irritability, muscle tension, and sleep disturbance. In
addition, the affected individual has difficulty controlling his/her worry, and the anxiety, worry, or somatic
symptoms cause clinically significant distress or impairment in social, occupational, and/or other important areas of functioning. Further, the GAD symptoms
should not be due to the direct physiological effects of
a substance such as drugs or alcohol or a general medical condition, and should not occur exclusively during a
mood disorder, psychotic disorder, or pervasive developmental disorder.

Worry and anxiety are part of normal human behavior and it may be difficult to define a cutoff point
distinguishing normal or trait anxiety (i.e., a relatively stable tendency to perceive various situations
as threatening) from GAD. However, as described in
the DSM-IV-TR definition of GAD, individuals suffering from a *disorder* exhibit significant distress and
impairment in functioning as a result of their anxiety
symptoms.

Individuals with GAD experience chronic anxiety
and tension. They find the worry as being uncontrollable. However, some individuals intentionally initiate
and maintain worry with an almost superstitious assumption that, by doing so, they can avert a negative
event. Individuals tend to worry predominantly about
family, personal finances, work, and illness. They are
also likely to report worrying over minor matters, such

DSM-IV-TR Diagnostic Criteria

300.02 GENERALIZED ANXIETY DISORDER

A. Excessive anxiety and worry (apprehensive expectation), occurring more days than not for at least
6 months, about a number of events or activities (such
as work or school performance).
B. The person finds it difficult to control the worry.
C. The anxiety and worry are associated with three (or
more) of the following six symptoms (with at least some
symptoms present for more days than not for the past
6 months). **Note:** Only one item is required in children.

(1) restlessness or feeling keyed up or on edge
(2) being easily fatigued
(3) difficulty concentrating or mind going blank
(4) irritability
(5) muscle tension
(6) sleep disturbance (difficulty falling or staying
asleep, or restless unsatisfying sleep)

D. The focus of anxiety and worry is not confined to features of an Axis I disorder, for example, the anxiety or
worry is not about having a panic attack (as in panic
disorder), being embarrassed in public (as in social phobia), being contaminated (as in obsessive–compulsive
disorder), being away from home or close relatives (as
in separation anxiety disorder), gaining weight (as in anorexia nervosa), having multiple physical complaints (as
in somatization disorder), or having a serious illness (as
in hypochondriasis), and the anxiety and worry do not
occur exclusively during posttraumatic stress disorder.
E. The anxiety, worry, or physical symptoms cause clinically significant distress or impairment in social, occupational, or other important areas of functioning.
F. The disturbance is not due to the direct physiological
effects of a substance (e.g., a drug of abuse, a medication) or a general medical condition (e.g., hyperthyroidism) and does not occur exclusively during a
mood disorder, a psychotic disorder, or a pervasive
developmental disorder.

Reprinted with permission from the *Diagnostic and Statistical
Manual of Mental Disorders*, 4th ed., Text Rev. Copyright 2000
American Psychiatric Association.

---

as making a slight social *faux pas*. The majority report
being anxious for at least 50% of the time during an
average day. In children and adolescents, the worries
often revolve around the quality of their performance

Clinical Guide to the Diagnosis and Treatment of Mental Disorders. M. B. First and A. Tasman
© 2006 John Wiley & Sons, Ltd.　ISBN 0 470 019158

in school or other competitive area. They may also worry about potential catastrophic events. They are concerned with their own physical or mental imperfections or inadequacies, and typically require excessive reassurance. They often appear shy, overcompliant, perfectionistic, and frequently describe multiple physical complaints. They may have an unusually mature and serious manner and appear older than their actual age. These children are often the eldest in small, competitive, achievement-oriented families.

Individuals with GAD commonly complain of feeling tense, jumpy, and irritable. They have difficulty falling or staying asleep, and tire easily during the day. Particularly distressing to such individuals is the difficulty in concentrating and collecting their thoughts. Cognitions appear to play a central role in GAD, as well as other anxiety disorders. Patterns of cognitions, however, appear to be disorder-specific. When the frequency of anxiety, worry, or panic attacks among individuals with GAD and panic disorder, as well as the severity of anxiety associated with each were examined, 34% of GAD individuals' cognitions were found to center on interpersonal conflict or the issue of acceptance by others, while only 1.4% of panic disorder individuals reported such concerns. While individuals with GAD also had exaggerated worries over relatively minor matters, panic disorder individuals reported a significantly greater frequency of cognitions concerning physical dangers or catastrophes (e.g., accident, injury, death).

Individuals may present with complaints of muscular tension, especially in their neck and shoulders. They may experience headaches, frequently described as frontal and occipital pressure or tension. They complain about sweaty palms, feel shaky and tremulous, complain of dryness of the mouth, and experience palpitations and difficulty in breathing. Individuals may also experience gastrointestinal symptoms such as heartburn and epigastric fullness. Approximately 30% of individuals experience severe gastrointestinal symptoms of irritable bowel syndrome. The physical complaints frequently lead individuals to seek medical attention, and most will initially consult a primary care physician. Although they frequently complain of palpitations and breathing difficulty, studies suggest that individuals with GAD do not differ from normal comparison subjects on measures of respiration and heart rate. Individuals with GAD may also present complaining of chest pain. Although chest pain is more frequently reported by individuals with panic disorder, it has been observed that 34% of individuals with GAD without panic attacks experienced chest pain. They also found that these individuals were predominantly males

and many had undergone extensive cardiac evaluations that revealed no demonstrable cardiac pathology.

Special laboratory and diagnostic evaluation of individuals with GAD may occasionally be required to exclude general medical conditions that mimic symptoms of generalized anxiety (see Differential Diagnosis, page 335). An evaluation to identify these disorders includes a personal and family medical history, review of systems, and a careful physical examination including neurological examination. Laboratory evaluation should include an electrocardiogram, screening for abusable substances, urinalysis, complete blood count, serum electrolytes, liver and thyroid function tests, calcium, phosphorus, and blood urea nitrogen.

An examination of the relative frequencies of various comorbid diagnoses in individuals with GAD obtained from the available studies reveals that other anxiety and mood disorders frequently complicate the course of GAD (see Figure 33-1). Findings from a longitudinal epidemiological study in Zurich, Switzerland showed strong associations between GAD and major depression and between GAD and dysthymia, but found a relatively low association with panic disorder. A high comorbidity of GAD with hypomania was also found. Further, the presence of comorbidity was associated with a high suicide attempt risk. In addition, individuals with comorbid disorders were treated more frequently and endorsed more work impairment than GAD individuals without comorbid disorders.

Alcoholism also complicates the clinical course of GAD for some individuals; however, the available literature suggests that the diagnosis of alcohol abuse is not as prevalent in GAD as in other anxiety disorders, and the pattern of abuse is often a brief and nonpersistent one. GAD onset is usually later than that of the alcohol use disorder. Personality disorders have been observed to co-occur in approximately 50% of individuals with GAD. For example, rates of GAD and personality disorders in clinical populations have ranged from 31%–46%. Cluster C personality disorders, specifically avoidant personality disorder, dependent personality disorder, and obsessive–compulsive personality disorder, are common. Interestingly, Cluster A personality traits, in particular, suspiciousness and mistrust, may be prominent in GAD as well.

Despite the shifting diagnostic criteria affecting the prevalence studies, current data indicate that GAD is probably one of the more common psychiatric disorders. A lifetime prevalence of 45% for GAD was reported according to DSM-III diagnostic criteria. However, when the more stringent criteria outlined in the DSM-III-R, which required a duration of 6 months were used, the prevalence rate dropped dramatically to

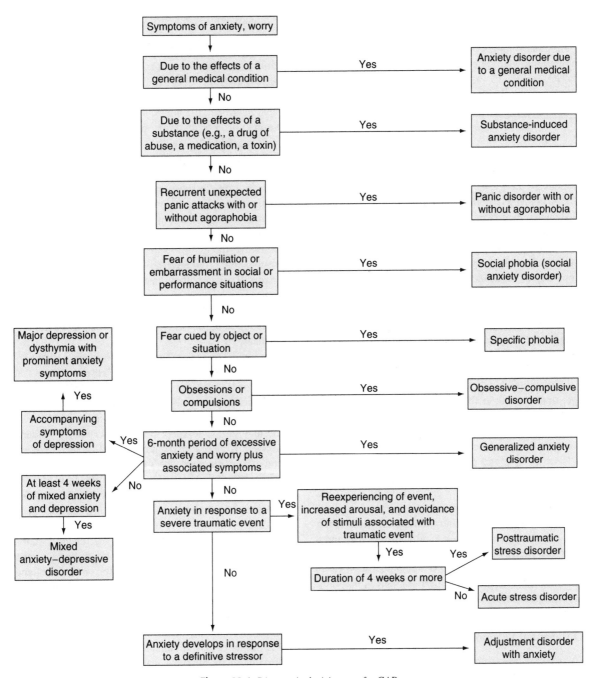

Figure 33-1 *Diagnostic decision tree for GAD.*

9%. The Epidemiologic Catchment Area Study (ECA) a five-center epidemiological study of the prevalence of psychiatric disorders in the United States, reported a lifetime prevalence for DSM-III-defined GAD of 4.1–6.6% in the three sites that assessed for GAD. Prevalence rates of DSM-III-R GAD in the National Comoribidty Study were 1.6% for current GAD (defined as the most recent 6-month period of anxiety), 3.1% for 12-month GAD, and 5.1% for lifetime GAD, with lifetime prevalence higher in females (6.6%) than males (3.6%).

GAD appears at even higher rates in clinical settings, particularly in primary care settings. For example, prevalence rates of GAD, using DSM-III-R criteria, reported by individuals at four primary care centers, were found to be twice as high as those reported in community samples (i.e., 10% versus 5.1%). Similarly, a collaborative study by the World Health Organization (WHO) across 15 international sites reported prevalence rates of GAD at approximately 8% in primary care settings.

Course

GAD individuals frequently report that they have been anxious all their lives. Typically, they were moderately anxious during childhood, later developing full-blown GAD when their stress levels increased through activities such as attending college or starting work. Individuals with early onset of symptoms report experiencing significant anxiety and fears, social isolation, obsessionality, more academic difficulties, and disturbed home environment during their childhood. The social maladjustment and emotional overreactivity persist into adulthood. Epidemiological studies and clinical studies suggest that the onset of GAD typically begins between the late teens and late twenties. However, not all GAD individuals have a lifelong history of excessive anxiety. Some individuals develop their disorder at a later age, that is, in their thirties or later. These individuals frequently report identifiable, precipitating stressful events, specifically unexpected, negative, important events in the year preceding development of GAD.

Retrospective and prospective reports indicate that the typical course of GAD is chronic, nonremitting, and that it often persists for a decade or longer. It has been reported that approximately 80% of subjects with GAD reported substantial interference with their life, a high degree of professional help-seeking, and a high prevalence of taking medications because of their GAD symptoms. The disability associated with GAD has been found to be similar to that found in individuals with panic disorder or major depression.

Differential Diagnosis

Anxiety can be a prominent feature of many psychiatric disorders and a number of disorders should be considered in the differential diagnosis of GAD (Figure 33-1). Several symptom profiles discriminate between major depressive disorder or dysthymic disorder and GAD. Individuals with major depressive disorder exhibit higher rates of dysphoric mood, psychomotor retardation, suicidal ideation, guilt, hopelessness, and helplessness, as well as more work impairment than individuals with GAD. In contrast, individuals with GAD show higher rates of somatic symptoms, specifically, muscle tension

and autonomic symptoms (e.g., respiratory or cardiac complaints) than depressed individuals.

Panic disorder is characterized by the presence of panic attacks; that is, recurrent, discrete episodes of intense anxiety or fear associated with a cluster of somatic symptoms reflecting autonomic hyperactivity such as rapid heartbeat, dizziness, numbness or tingling, trouble breathing or choking, and nausea or vomiting. In contrast, individuals with GAD predominantly experience symptoms of muscle tension and vigilance such as fatigue, muscle soreness, insomnia, difficulty in concentrating, restlessness, and irritability. Anxiety is also a part of the clinical picture of obsessive–compulsive disorder (OCD) and may be a central factor in initiating and maintaining obsessions and compulsions. Obsessive thoughts are described as egodystonic intrusions that often take the form of urges, impulses, or images. They are often senseless and are frequently accompanied by time-consuming compulsions designed to reduce mounting anxiety. In contrast, the worries in GAD are about realistic concerns, such as health and finances.

In phobic disorders, the anxiety is characteristically associated with a specific phobic object or situation that is frequently avoided by the individual. Such is the case with social anxiety disorder as well, in which the individual is afraid of or avoids situations in which he or she may be the focus of potential scrutiny by others. Anxiety is also a characteristic part of the presentation of posttraumatic stress disorder (PTSD) and acute stress disorder (ASD). However, unlike in GAD, the principal symptoms experienced in PTSD and ASD follow exposure to a traumatic event and are characterized by avoidance of reminders of the event and persistent reexperiencing of the traumatic event. Finally, in adjustment disorders, anxiety when present occurs in response to a specific life stressor or stressors and generally does not persist for more than 6 months.

Many general medical conditions may present with prominent anxiety symptoms and must be considered in the differential diagnosis of generalized anxiety (see Table 33-1). Individuals with GAD may complain of palpitations, skipped heartbeats, and chest pain. In addition, many GAD individuals, especially males, fear having an acute myocardial infarction and often present to the emergency room for evaluation. However, most individuals with GAD without a concomitant cardiovascular disease do not experience severe chest pain. Following the controversial evidence suggesting an association between mitral valve prolapse (MVP) and panic disorder, researchers evaluated the prevalence of MVP in individuals with GAD and found no evidence of increased prevalence in individuals with

Table 33-1	Medical Conditions and Drugs that may Cause Anxiety

Endocrine Disorders
Addison's disease
Cushing's syndrome
Hyperparathyroidism
Hyperthyroidism
Hypothyroidism
Carcinoid
Pheochromocytoma

Drug Side Effects
Anticonvulsants
Antidepressants
Antihistamines
Antihypertensive agents
Antiinflammatory agents
Antiparkinsonian agents
Caffeine
Digitalis
Sympathomimetics
Thyroid supplements

Substance Use Related
Cocaine
Hallucinogens
Amphetamines

Withdrawal Syndromes
Alcohol
Narcotics
Sedatives–hypnotics

Gastrointestinal Disorders
Peptic ulcer disease

Infectious Diseases
Miscellaneous viral and bacterial infections

Cardiovascular and Circulatory Disorders
Anemia
Congestive heart failure
Coronary insufficiency
Dysrhythmia, e.g. atrial fibrillation
Hypovolemia
Myocardial infarction

Respiratory Disorders
Asthma
Chronic obstructive pulmonary disease
Pulmonary embolism
Pulmonary edema

Immunological, Collagen, and Vascular Disorders
Systemic lupus erythematosus
Temporal arteritis

Metabolic Conditions
Acidosis
Acute intermittent porphyria
Electrolyte abnormalities
Hypoglycemia

Neurological Disorders
Brain tumors
Cerebral syphilis
Cerebrovascular disorders
Encephalopathies
Epilepsy (especially temporal lobe epilepsy)
Postconcussive syndrome
Vertigo
Akathisia

GAD. Nevertheless, individuals with anxiety symptoms associated with unexplained chest pain should be evaluated for possible cardiovascular disease.

Anxiety is a prominent feature of hyperthyroidism with some overlap in the symptomatology of thyrotoxicosis and GAD. Symptoms such as tachycardia, tremulousness, irritability, weakness, and fatigue are common to both disorders. In GAD, however, the peripheral manifestations of excessive concentrations of circulating thyroid hormones are absent, including symptoms such as weight loss, increased appetite, warm and moist skin, heat intolerance, and dyspnea on effort. Pheochromocytomas, also known as chromaffin tumors, produce, store, and secrete catecholamines. They are derived most often from the adrenal medulla, as well as the sympathetic ganglia, and occasionally from other sites. The clinical features of these tumors, most commonly hypertension and hypertensive paroxysms, are predominantly due to the release of catecholamines. Individuals may also experience diaphoresis, tachycardia, chest pain, flushing, nausea and vomiting, headache, and significant apprehension. Although the clinical presentation frequently mimics spontaneous panic attacks, pheochromocytomas should also be considered in the differential diagnosis of GAD. The diagnosis of pheochromocytoma can be confirmed by increased levels of catecholamines (epinephrine and norepinephrine) or catecholamine metabolites (metanephrines and vanillylmandelic acid) in a 24-hour urine collection.

Menopause is commonly referred to as the period that encompasses the transition between the reproductive years and beyond the last episode of menstrual bleeding. Frequently associated with significant anxiety, menopause should be considered in the differential diagnosis of GAD. However, other associated symptoms such as vasomotor instability, atrophy of urogenital epithelium and skin, and osteoporosis make the diagnosis of menopause probable. Another endocrinologic disorder, hyperparathyroidism, can present with anxiety symptoms, and the initial evaluation of serum calcium levels may be indicated. Finally, certain neurologic conditions such as complex partial seizures, intracranial tumors and strokes, and cerebral ischemic attacks may be associated with symptoms typically observed in anxiety disorders and may require appropriate evaluation.

Anxiety disorders can occur frequently in association with intoxication and withdrawal from several classes of substances (see Table 33-1). Excessive use of caffeine, especially in children and adolescents, may cause significant anxiety. Cocaine intoxication may be associated with anxiety, agitation, and hypervigilance. During cocaine withdrawal, individuals may also present with prominent anxiety, irritability, insomnia, fatigue, depression, and cocaine craving. Adverse reaction to marijuana includes extreme anxiety that usually lasts less than 24 hours. Mild opioid withdrawal presents with symptoms of anxiety and dysphoria. However, accompanying symptoms such as elevated blood pressure, tachycardia, pupilary dilation, rhinorrhea, piloerection, and lacrimation are rare in individuals with GAD.

The clinical phenomenology observed both in alcohol and sedative–hypnotic drug withdrawal and in GAD, although variable, may be highly similar. In both conditions, nervousness, tachycardia, tremulousness, sweating, nausea, and hyperventilation occur prominently. Additionally, the same drugs (i.e., benzodiazepines) can be used to treat anxiety symptoms, and some individuals may use alcohol in an attempt to alleviate anxiety. Thus, the symptoms of an underlying anxiety disorder may be difficult to differentiate from the withdrawal symptoms associated with the use of benzodiazepines or alcohol. The use of many commonly prescribed medications may produce side effects manifesting as anxiety (see Table 33-1). Such medications include sympathomimetics or other bronchodilators such as theophylline, anticholinergics, antiparkinsonian preparations, corticosteroids, thyroid supplements, oral contraceptives, antihypertensive and cardiovascular medications such as digitalis, insulin (secondary to hypoglycemia), and antipsychotic and antidepressant medications. Finally, heavy metals and toxins such as organophosphates, paint, and insecticides may also cause anxiety symptoms.

TREATMENT

Since GAD is a chronic, relapsing illness, most treatments do not cure the individual and when treatments are discontinued, symptoms may return. Each case

must be considered individually according to the severity and chronicity of the disorder, the severity of somatic symptoms, the presence of stressors, and the presence of specific personality traits. The clinician may also need to work with the individual to determine how much improvement is sufficient. For example, a reduction in disability may occur without a marked change in symptoms. Symptoms may persist but occur less frequently, or their intensity may be reduced. All these variations have important treatment implications, including decisions regarding the need for long-term treatment. Individuals with milder forms of GAD may respond well to simple psychological interventions, and require no medication treatment. In more severe forms of GAD, it may become necessary to see the individual regularly and to provide both more specific psychological and pharmacological interventions. Figure 33-2 can be used as a guide to the treatment of GAD using, primarily, medications.

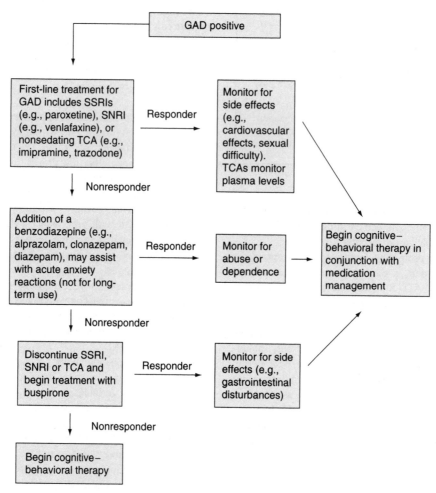

Figure 33-2 *Generalized anxiety disorder treatment flowchart emphasizing pharmacotherapy.*

During the early (acute) phase of treatment, an attempt should be made to control the individual's symptomatology. It may take 3 to 6 months for an optimal response to be achieved. However, there may be a considerable variation in the length of the initial treatment phase. For example, clinical response to benzodiazepines occurs early in treatment. Response to other anxiolytic medications or to cognitive–behavioral or psychodynamic treatment generally requires longer periods of time. During the maintenance phase, treatment gains are consolidated. Unfortunately, studies suggesting how long treatment should be continued are limited. Routinely, pharmacological treatment is continued for a total of 6 to 12 months before attempting to discontinue medications. Some studies indicate that *maintenance* psychotherapeutic treatments such as cognitive–behavioral therapy may be helpful in maintaining treatment gains in individuals with anxiety disorders following the discontinuation of pharmacotherapy. It is clear that many individuals may experience chronic and continuous symptoms that require years of long-term treatment.

The vast majority of individuals with GAD who present for treatment have been ill for many years and frequently have received a variety of treatments. Some individual have been sent to mental health professionals for treatment as a "last resort" in order to learn how to cope with their various ill-defined somatic and emotional complaints. Individuals may feel shame and guilt over their inability to control symptoms. They are often demoralized and angry, and feel that their symptoms are not taken seriously. Thus, it is important to help the individual understand his or her illness and to conceptualize it as a health problem rather than a *personal weakness*. Once the burden of perceived responsibility is lifted from the individual, and he or she believes that effective treatment is possible, a working alliance with the treating clinician can begin. The treatment plan should be outlined clearly, and the individual cautioned that recovery may have a gradual, variable course. Finally, during the critical early stages of treatment, the clinician should make a special effort to be available in person or by phone to answer questions and provide support.

Somatic Therapies

A number of anxiolytic agents are effective in the treatment of GAD (see Table 33-2). Benzodiazepines are commonly used for the treatment of GAD and are still considered by some clinicians to be the first-line treatment for GAD. Several controlled studies have demonstrated the efficacy of different benzodiazepines such as diazepam, chlordiazepoxide, and alprazolam in the treatment of GAD.

The benzodiazepines have a broad spectrum of effects including sedation, muscle relaxation, anxiety reduction, and decreased physiologic arousal (e.g., palpitations, tremulousness, etc.). Interestingly, available studies indicate that benzodiazepines have the most pronounced effect on hypervigilance and somatic symptoms of GAD, but exhibited fewer effects on psychic symptoms such as dysphoria, interpersonal sensitivity, and obsessionality. The main difference between individual benzodiazepines is potency and elimination half-life. These differences may have important treatment implications. For example, benzodiazepines with relatively short elimination half-lives such as alprazolam (range of 10–14 hours) may require dosing at least three to four times a day in order to avoid interdose symptom rebound. Conversely, the use of longer-acting compounds such as clonazepam (range of 20–50 hours) may minimize the risk of interdose symptom recurrence.

Benzodiazepines exert their therapeutic effects quickly, often after a single dose. However, concern has emerged over the use of benzodiazepines, particularly, long-term benzodiazepine use. Side effects of benzodiazepines, such as sedation, psychomotor impairment, and memory disruption, have been noted by treating clinicians, and confirmed in research studies. Further, although it was suggested that the use pattern of benzodiazepines by individuals with anxiety disorders may not represent abuse, addiction, or drug dependence as typically understood, the chronic use of benzodiazepines in the treatment of GAD has been increasingly discouraged in recent years.

When initiating treatment with benzodiazepines, it is helpful for individuals to take an initial dose at home in the evening to see how it affects them. Gradual titration to an effective dose allows for limiting unwanted adverse effects. A final daily dosage of alprazolam between 2 and 4 mg/day, 1 and 2 mg/day for clonazepam, or 15 and 20 mg/day of diazepam, is usually sufficient for the majority of individuals. Upon treatment discontinuation, it is important to consider appropriate taper in order to avoid withdrawal symptoms. Possible factors that may contribute to the severity of withdrawal and the ultimate outcome of benzodiazepine taper include the dosage, duration of treatment, the benzodiazepine elimination half-life and potency, and the rate of benzodiazepine taper (gradual versus abrupt). Additionally, individual factors such as premorbid personality features have been implicated. It appears that a taper rate of 25% per week is probably too rapid for many individuals. A slow benzodiazepine taper of at least 4 to 8 weeks, with the final 50% of the taper conducted even

Table 33-2	Anxiolytic Agents		
Drug	**Daily Dosage Range (mg)**	**Advantages**	**Disadvantages**
Selective serotonin reuptake inhibitors			
Paroxetine	20–40	Efficacy with GAD	Gastrointestinal side effects
Fluoxetine	20–60	Efficacy with comorbid depression	Delayed onset
Sertraline	50–200		Sexual side effects
Citalopram	20–40	Favorable side effects profile compared with TCAs	
Fluvoxamine	100–300	Easy dosing schedule	
Serotonergic and noradrenergic reuptake inhibitors			
Venlafaxine extended release (XR)	75–225	Efficacy with GAD	Gastrointestinal side effects
		Efficacy with comorbid depression	Sexual side effects
			Potential for increased blood pressure
Benzodiazepines			
Alprazolam	2–6	Rapid onset of action	Sedation
Clonazepam	1–3	Favorable side effects profile	Multiple doses for shorter acting agents
Lorazepam	4–10		Physical dependence
Diazepam	15–20		Limited antidepressant effects Sexual side effects
Tricyclic antidepressants			
Imipramine	75–300	Once-daily dosage Efficacy with comorbid depression	Delayed onset Need for titration
			Activation Anticholinergic effects Orthostatic hypotension Weight gain Toxicity in overdose Sexual side effects
Atypical antidepressants			
Trazodone	150–600	Once-daily dosage Efficacy with comorbid depression	Delayed onset Orthostatic hypotension
		Low anticholinergic effects	Weight gain Sexual side effects Priapism (rare) Sedation
Azapirones			
Buspirone	30–60	No withdrawal symptoms No physical dependence Favorable side effects profile	Multiple doses

more gradually, is recommended, with the individual decreasing the daily dose of the benzodiazepines during this period by the lowest possible percentage.

Clinical trials conducted in the early 1990s have confirmed that tricyclic antidepressants (TCAs) may also be effective in the treatment of GAD. For example, a placebo-controlled study which compared imipramine, trazodone, and diazepam in GAD individuals without comorbid depression or panic disorder revealed that the efficacy of imipramine and trazodone was comparable to diazepam. It should be noted that diazepam demonstrated greater efficacy than imipramine during the first 2 weeks of treatment with the greatest degree of

response in the somatic and hyperarousal symptoms; however, imipramine and trazodone exhibited higher efficacy after 6 to 8 weeks of treatment with psychic symptoms of tension, apprehension, and worry being more responsive to the antidepressants. Owing, in part, to their side effect profile, need for dose titration, and importantly the emergence of new and effective agents (as described below), the use of TCAs in the treatment of GAD has been reserved for those resistant to these newer agents.

Selective serotonin reuptake inhibitors (SSRIS) are rapidly becoming a key tool in the treatment of GAD. Several controlled double-blind studies have demonstrated the efficacy of paroxetine in the treatment of GAD. The most problematic side effect associated with SSRI use is the interference with sexual function (e.g., delayed orgasm or abnormal ejaculation) in women and men.

The antidepressant venlafaxine extended release (XR) is an inhibitor of both 5-HT and NE reuptake, serotonergic and noradrenergic reuptake inhibitors (SNRI). Several large, placebo-controlled trials have evaluated it in the treatment of individuals with DSM-IV-TR-diagnosed GAD. As a result, venlafaxine XR was the first antidepressant approved by the FDA for the treatment of GAD. The adverse events for GAD individuals treated with venlafaxine XR resembled those in depression trials. The most common adverse events included nausea, somnolence, dry mouth, dizziness, sweating, constipation, and anorexia.

Several other psychotherapeutic agents have been tested in the treatment of individuals with GAD. For example, the alpha-2-adrenoreceptor antagonist mirtazapine, which is also a $5-HT_2$, $5-HT_3$, and H(1) receptor antagonist, has been evaluated as a potential anxiolytic in the treatment of individuals with major depressive disorder and comorbid GAD in an 8-week, open-label study. Results suggest that this antidepressant may be useful in the treatment of anxiety symptoms.

The azapirone group of drugs was introduced in response to concerns over chronic benzodiazepine use in subjects with anxiety symptoms. Buspirone hydrochloride, the only currently marketed azapirone, was the first nonbenzodiazepine anxiolytic agent approved for the treatment of persistent anxiety by the FDA. Results have been mixed about the efficacy of buspirone over placebo and benzodiazepines. For example, in four placebo-controlled studies that compared buspirone to a standard benzodiazepine, two showed no benefit for diazepam and buspirone over placebo, and two showed no benefit for buspirone over placebo. Benzodiazepines may also be slightly more effective than buspirone in the treatment of somatic symptoms of anxiety but no significant differences appear to exist between buspirone and benzodiazepines in measures of psychic anxiety. Buspirone, however, may be more effective in the treatment of anger/hostility symptoms than benzodiazepines.

Side effects most frequently associated with buspirone use included gastrointestinal system-related side effects, such as appetite disturbances and abdominal complaints, and dizziness. Prior use of benzodiazepines may adversely affect the therapeutic response to buspirone It has been reported that a gradual 2-week taper of lorazepam with a simultaneous addition of buspirone for 6 weeks prevents the development of clinically significant rebound anxiety or benzodiazepine withdrawal. This approach was shown to provide clinically significant relief of anxiety symptoms in GAD individuals previously treated with benzodiazepines for 8 to 14 weeks. Perhaps the most significant problem with the use of buspirone has been that experts have advocated too low a dose to produce symptom reduction. In order to achieve optimal response, buspirone dosing in the range of at least 30–60 mg/day is currently recommended.

When faced with treatment resistance, clinician should evaluate whether an adequate treatment trial was completed. An attempt should be made to maintain the individual on medication for at least 6 weeks. Although there are no data suggesting that certain doses may be particularly effective in the treatment of GAD, it is advisable to titrate the medication up to maximally tolerated doses prior to discontinuing the medication for nonresponse. It is important to inquire about the presence of side effects such as sedation, anticholinergic effects, or sexual side effects, which may limit the attainment of a therapeutic dosage and reduce compliance. Additionally, many individuals with GAD fear that they may become *drug dependent* and thus avoid dose increases. Some estimate of the individual's compliance may be helpful in determining whether a treatment was adequate, as indicated by blood plasma levels or pill counts. Drug plasma levels may also be useful to identify individuals who are rapid metabolizers. A careful evaluation for the presence of psychiatric comorbid conditions that may contribute to treatment refractoriness should follow. As mentioned, comorbidity which may reflect more severe loading for psychopathology is often associated with increased severity of illness and poorer response to treatment in comparison to individuals with an uncomplicated (i.e., single) disorder. Thus, treatment strategies in GAD individuals with a concurrent disorder may differ from those in an uncomplicated disorder, often requiring multiple drug therapy. The clinician should also be alert to the presence of underlying general medical conditions such as hyperthyroidism, which may present with refractory anxiety, or conditions/medications that may alter the effects of treatment, such as hepatic disease or medications (e.g., steroids) that affect hepatic clearance.

Psychosocial Therapies

Numerous studies have shown that psychological interventions are beneficial in the comprehensive management of anxiety disorders. However, data suggesting that specific psychotherapeutic techniques yield better results in the treatment of individuals with GAD are inconclusive, and more evidence is needed on the comparative efficacy and long-term effects of different psychological treatments.

In recent years, specific cognitive–behavioral therapy (CBT) interventions for the treatment of individuals with anxiety disorders have been developed. Components of CBT include teaching individuals to identify and label irrational thoughts and to replace them with positive self-statements or modify them by challenging their veracity. The cognitive modification approaches are combined with behavioral treatments such as exposure or relaxation training. There is evidence suggesting that CBT may be more effective in the treatment of GAD than other psychotherapeutic interventions, such as behavioral therapy alone or nonspecific supportive therapy. For example, a study of CBT targeting intolerance of uncertainty, erroneous beliefs about worry, poor problem orientation, and cognitive avoidance demonstrated effectiveness at post-treatment (no change in the delayed treatment control group) 6- and 12-month follow-up, with about three quarters of the treatment group no longer having symptoms meeting criteria for a GAD diagnosis. Cognitive therapy was also compared to analytic psychotherapy, and was found to be significantly more effective Overall, two-thirds in the cognitive therapy group achieved clinically significant improvements, and cognitive therapy was associated with significant reductions in medication usage.

Many individuals with milder forms of GAD will benefit from simple psychological interventions such as supportive psychotherapy. They may experience lessening of anxiety when given the opportunity to discuss their difficulties with a supportive clinician and to become better informed about their illness. Thus, basic supportive techniques such as reassurance, clarification of individual concerns, direct suggestions, and advice are often effective in reducing anxiety symptoms.

Relaxation techniques such as progressive muscle relaxation and biofeedback have also been utilized in the treatment of individuals with anxiety symptoms. Biofeedback has also been found to be effective in the treatment of individuals with GAD. It should be noted that relaxation may be associated with a paradoxical increase in anxiety and tension in individuals with GAD. However, with repeated training, specifically in the context of CBT, this phenomenon may be used to achieve habituation and anxiety extinction.

COMPARISON OF DSM-IV-TR AND ICD-10 DIAGNOSTIC CRITERIA

The ICD-10 Diagnostic Criteria for Research specify that four symptoms from a list of 22 be present. In contrast, DSM-IV-TR requires 3 out of a list of 6 (of which 5 are included among the ICD-10 list of 22).

34 Somatoform Disorders

The somatoform disorders are characterized by physical symptoms suggestive of but not fully explained by a general medical condition or the direct effects of a substance. In this class, symptoms are not intentionally produced and are not attributable to another mental disorder. To warrant a diagnosis, symptoms must be clinically significant in terms of causing distress or impairment in important areas of functioning. The disorders included in this class are somatization disorder, undifferentiated somatoform disorder, conversion disorder, pain disorder, hypochondriasis, body dysmorphic disorder, and somatoform disorder not otherwise specified (NOS). This chapter begins with information about differential diagnosis and treatment as it applies to the diagnostic class as a whole, followed by individual sections covering each of the somatoform disorders.

The somatoform disorders class was created for clinical utility, not on the basis of an assumed common etiology or mechanism. In DSM-IV-TR terms, it was designed to facilitate the differential diagnosis of conditions in which the first diagnostic concern is the need to "exclude occult general medical conditions or substance-induced etiologies for the bodily symptoms." As shown in Figure 34-1, only after such explanations are reasonably excluded should somatoform disorders be considered.

The somatoform disorder concept should be distinguished from traditional concepts of "psychosomatic illness" and "somatization." The psychosomatic illnesses involved structural or physiological changes hypothesized as deriving from psychological factors. In the DSM-III, DSM-III-R, and DSM-IV somatoform disorders, such objective changes are generally not evident. The "classic" psychosomatic illnesses included bronchial asthma, ulcerative colitis, thyrotoxicosis, essential hypertension, rheumatoid arthritis, neurodermatitis, and peptic ulcer. In DSM-IV-TR, most of these illnesses would be diagnosed as a general medical condition on Axis III, and in some cases with an additional designation of psychological factors affecting medical condition on Axis I. By definition, the diagnosis of "psychological factors affecting medical condition" is not a mental disorder, but it is included in DSM-IV-TR in the section for other conditions that may be a focus of clinical attention; it involves the presence of one or more specific psychological or behavioral factors that adversely affect a general medical condition (see Chapter 41 for more information).

Generic Treatment Strategies for Somatoform Disorders

Whereas specific somatoform disorders indicate specific treatment approaches, some general guidelines apply to the somatoform disorders as a whole (Table 34-1). Therapeutic goals in the treatment of somatoform disorders include (1) as an overriding goal, prevention of the adoption of the sick role and chronic invalidism; (2) minimization of unnecessary costs and complications by avoiding unwarranted hospitalizations, diagnostic and treatment procedures, and medications (especially those of an addictive potential); and (3) effective treatment of comorbid mental disorders, such as depressive and anxiety syndromes. General treatment strategies include (1) consistent treatment, generally by the same physician, with careful coordination if multiple physicians are involved; (2) supportive office visits, scheduled at regular intervals rather than in response to symptoms; and (3) a gradual shift in focus from symptoms to an emphasis on personal and interpersonal problems.

Somatization Disorder

DIAGNOSIS

Somatization disorder is a polysymptomatic somatoform disorder characterized by multiple recurring pains and gastrointestinal, sexual, and pseudoneurological symptoms occurring for a period of years with onset before age 30 years (see DSM-IV-TR diagnostic criteria, page 347). The physical complaints are not intentionally produced and are not fully explained by

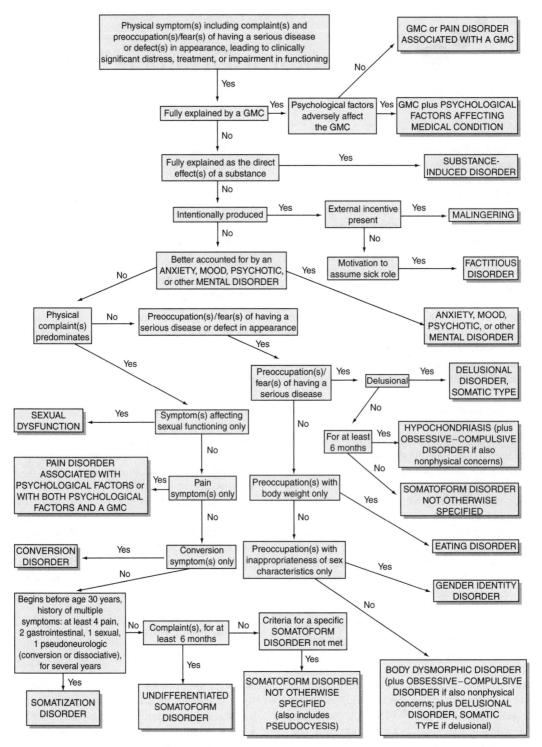

Figure 34-1 *Differential diagnosis of clinically significant physical symptoms. Shadowed boxes represent diagnostic categories; GMC, general medical condition.*

DSM-IV-TR Diagnostic Criteria

300.81 SOMATIZATION DISORDER

A. A history of many physical complaints beginning before age 30 years that occur over a period of several years and result in treatment being sought or significant impairment in social, occupational, or other important areas of functioning.

B. Each of the following criteria must have been met, with individual symptoms occurring at any time during the course of the disturbance:

(1) *four pain symptoms*: a history of pain related to at least four different sites or functions (e.g., head, abdomen, back, joints, extremities, chest, rectum, during menstruation, during sexual intercourse, or during urination)

(2) *two gastrointestinal symptoms*: a history of at least two gastrointestinal symptoms other than pain (e.g., nausea, bloating, vomiting other than during pregnancy, diarrhea, or intolerance of several different foods)

(3) *one sexual symptom*: a history of at least one sexual or reproductive symptom other than pain (e.g., sexual indifference, erectile or ejaculatory dysfunction, irregular menses, excessive menstrual bleeding, vomiting throughout pregnancy)

(4) *one pseudoneurological symptom*: a history of at least one symptom or deficit suggesting a neurological condition not limited to pain (conversion symptoms such as impaired coordination or balance, paralysis or localized weakness, difficulty swallowing or lump in throat, aphonia, urinary retention, hallucinations, loss of touch or pain sensation, double vision, blindness, deafness, seizures; dissociative symptoms such as amnesia; or loss of consciousness other than fainting)

C. Either (1) or (2):

(1) After appropriate investigation, each of the symptoms in criterion B cannot be fully explained by a known general medical condition or the direct effects of a substance (e.g., a drug of abuse, a medication).

(2) When there is a related general medical condition, the physical complaints or resulting social or occupational impairment is in excess of what would be expected from the history, physical examination, or laboratory findings.

D. The symptoms are not intentionally produced or feigned (as in factitious disorder or malingering).

Reprinted with permission from the *Diagnostic and Statistical Manual of Mental Disorders*, 4th ed., Text Rev. Copyright 2000 American Psychiatric Association.

a general medical condition or the direct effects of a substance. To warrant diagnosis, they must result in medical attention or significant impairment in social, occupational, or other important areas of functioning.

Whereas criteria require the onset of symptoms before the age of 30 years, most individuals would have had some symptoms at least by adolescence or early adulthood. Symptoms are often described in a dramatic yet imprecise way and may be reported inconsistently from interview to interview. The medical history is usually complicated, with multiple medical investigations, procedures, and medication trials. If there have been symptoms for at least 6 months but the onset is later than at age 30 years, or if the required number and distribution of symptoms are not evident, undifferentiated somatoform disorder is diagnosed. If the duration has been less than 6 months, a diagnosis of somatoform disorder NOS also applies. In general, the greater the number and diversity of symptoms, and the longer they have been present without development of signs of an underlying general medical condition, the greater can be the confidence that a diagnosis of somatization disorder is correct.

In the US, somatization disorder is found predominantly in women, with a female/male ratio of approximately 10:1 (see Table 34-2). This ratio is not as large in some other cultures (e.g., in Greeks and Puerto Ricans). Thus, gender- and culture-specific rates are more meaningful than generalized figures. The lifetime prevalence of somatization disorder in US women has been estimated to be between 0.2% and 2%. The magnitude of this discrepancy is attributable, at least in part, to methodological differences. The Epidemiological Catchment Area study, the most recent large-scale general population study in the US to include an assessment for somatization disorder, found a lifetime risk of somatization disorder of only 0.2–0.3% in US women. However, this study may have underestimated the prevalence of somatization disorder because non-physician interviewers were used. It is argued that it is difficult for lay interviewers to critically assess whether somatic symptoms are fully explained by physical conditions. As a result, they may more readily accept individuals' general medical explanations of symptoms, resulting in fewer diagnoses of somatization disorder.

Course

Somatization disorder is rare in children younger than 9 years of age (see Table 34-2). Characteristic symptoms of somatization disorder usually begin during adolescence, and the criteria are met by the mid-twenties. Somatization disorder is a chronic illness characterized by fluctuations in the frequency and diversity of symptoms. Full remissions occur rarely, if ever. Whereas the most active symptomatic phase is in early adulthood, aging does not appear to lead to total remission. Longitudinal follow-up studies have confirmed that 80–90% of individuals initially diagnosed with somatization disorder will maintain a consistent clinical picture and

Table 34-1	Treatment of DSM-IV-TR Somatoform Disorders		
Somatoform Disorder	Treatment Goals	Psychotherapy and Psychosocial Strategies and Techniques	Pharmacological and Physical Strategies and Techniques[*]
Somatoform disorders, as a group	1. Prevent adoption of the sick role and chronic invalidism 2. Minimize unnecessary costs and complications by avoiding unwarranted hospitalizations, diagnostic and treatment procedures, and medications 3. Pharmacological control of comorbid syndromes	1. Consistent treatment, generally by same physician, coordinated if multiple 2. Supportive office visits, scheduled at regular intervals 3. Focus gradually shifted from symptoms to personal and social problems	1. Only as clearly indicated, or as time-limited empirical trial 2. Avoid drugs with abuse or addictive potential
Somatization disorder	1, 2, and 3; also • Instill, whenever possible, insight regarding temporal association between symptoms and personal, interpersonal, and situational problems	1, 2, and 3; also • Establish firm therapeutic alliance • Educate the individuals with somatization disorder regarding manifestations of somatization disorder (psychoeducative approach) • Consistent reassurance	1 and 2; also • Antianxiety and antidepressant drugs for comorbid anxiety or depressive disorders; if diagnosis unclear, consider empirical trial
Undifferentiated somatoform disorder	1, 2, and 3	1, 2, and 3	1 and 2
Conversion disorder	1, 2, and 3; also • Prompt removal of symptoms	Acute: • Reassurance, suggestion to remove symptom • Consider narcoanalysis (interview after drowsiness from amobarbital or other sedative–hypnotic, sometimes followed by methylphenidate or other stimulant), hypnotherapy, or behavioral therapy Chronic: 1, 2, and 3 • Exploration of various conflict areas, particularly interpersonal relationships • Long-term, intensive, insight-oriented dynamic psychotherapy recommended by some	1 and 2; also • Consider narcoanalysis as an interviewing or psychotherapy adjunct
Pain disorder	1, 2, and 3; also • Acute pain: Relieve symptom • Chronic pain: Maintain function and motility rather than focus on total pain relief	1, 2, and 3; also • Chronic pain: Consider physical and occupational therapy, operant conditioning, cognitive–behavioral therapy	1 and 2: also • Acute: Acetaminophen and NSAIDs alone or as adjuncts to opioids (if necessary) • Chronic: Tricyclic antidepressants, acetaminophen, and NSAIDs; if necessary, milder opioids or pure opioid agonists, but these only if tied to nonpain objectives (such as increasing activity) • Consider acupuncture, transcutaneous electrical nerve stimulation
Hypochondriasis	1, 2, and 3; also • Pharmacological control of central syndrome itself	1, 2, and 3; also • Cognitive–behavioral therapy involving prevention of checking rituals and reassurance seeking	2; also • Attempt to decrease hypochondriacal symptoms with SSRIs at higher than antidepressant doses or clomipramine
Body dysmorphic disorder	1, 2, and 3, especially avoiding corrective surgery; also • Pharmacological control of central syndrome itself	1, 2, and 3; also • Cognitive–behavioral therapy involving prevention of checking rituals and reassurance seeking	2; also • Attempt to decrease hypochondriacal symptoms with SSRIs at higher than antidepressant doses or clomipramine
Somatoform disorder NOS	1, 2, and 3; also • Evaluate carefully for alternative general medical or other mental disorder to which the symptoms can be attributed	1, 2, and 3	1 and 2

[*]NSAIDs, Nonsteroidal antiinflammatory drugs; SSRIs, selective serotonin reuptake inhibitors.

Table 34-2	Epidemiology and Natural History of the Somatoform Disorders		
Somatoform Disorder	**Prevalence and Incidence**	**Age at Onset**	**Course and Progress**
Somatization disorder	US women 0.2–2%; women/men = 10 : 1	First symptoms by adolescence, full criteria met by mid-20s, not after 30 year by definition	Chronic with fluctuations in severity Most active in early adulthood Full remissions rare
Undifferentiated somatoform disorder	"Abridged somatization disorder" type estimated as 11–15% of US adults, 20% in Puerto Rico Preponderance of women in US but not Puerto Rico	Variable	Variable conversion disorder
Conversion disorder	Conversion symptoms common, as high as 25% Treated conversion symptoms: 11–500 per 100,000 5–14% of general hospital admissions 5–24% of psychiatric outpatients 1–3% of psychiatric outpatient referrals 4% of neurological outpatient referrals 1% of neurological admissions	Late childhood to early adulthood, most before age 35 year If onset in middle or late life, neurological or general medical condition more likely	Individual conversion symptoms generally remit within days to weeks Relapse within 1 year in 20–25%
Pain disorder	10–15% of US adults with work disability owing to back pain yearly A predominant symptom in more than half of general hospital admissions Present in as many as 38% of psychiatric admissions, 18% of psychiatric outpatients	Any age	Good if less than 6 months in duration Unemployment, personality disorder, potential for compensation, and habituation to addictive drugs associated with poorer prognosis
Hypochondriasis	Perhaps 4–9% in general medical settings, but unclear whether full syndrome criteria are met Equal in both sexes	Early adulthood typical	10% recovery, two-thirds a chronic but fluctuating course, 25% do poorly Better prognosis if acute onset, absence of personality disorder, absence of secondary gain
Body dysmorphic disorder	Not routinely screened for in psychiatric or general population studies Perhaps 2% of patients seeking corrective cosmetic surgery	Adolescence or early adulthood Perhaps in women at menopause	Generally chronic, fluctuating severity In a lifetime, multiple defects perceived Incapacitating: one-third house-bound
Somatoform disorder NOS	Unknown	Variable	Variable

be rediagnosed similarly after 6 to 8 years. Women with somatization disorder seen in mental health treatment settings are at increased risk for attempted suicide, although such attempts are usually unsuccessful and may reflect manipulative gestures more than intent to die. It is not clear whether such risk is true for individuals with somatization disorder seen only in general medical settings.

Differential Diagnosis

As defined in DSM-IV-TR, somatization disorder is characterized by multiple recurring physical symptoms and, as will be described, often multiple psychiatric complaints. Thus, it is not surprising that somatization

disorder may present in a manner suggestive of multiple general medical and, although too often forgotten, psychiatric disorders (see Table 34-3). Indeed, it can be said that an essential aspect of somatization disorder is its simulation of other syndromes. Somatization disorder is fundamentally a syndrome of apparent syndromes (see Table 34-3). Thus, the first task in the diagnosis of somatization disorder is the exclusion of other suggested medical and psychiatric conditions.

To help in this, three features have been identified that generally characterize somatization disorder but rarely general medical disorders. Slightly restated, these are (1) involvement of multiple organ systems, (2) early onset and chronic course without development of physical signs or structural abnormalities, and (3)

Table 34-3 Somatoform Disorders: A Syndrome of Simulated Syndromes

Symptom Examples	Examples of Simulated Neurological Conditions	Examples of Simulated Nonneurological General Medical Conditions	Examples of Simulated Psychiatric Conditions
Symptoms* of somatization disorder			
Pain			
Headache	Migraine	Temporal arteritis	Pain disorder
Abdomen	"Abdominal epilepsy"	Peptic ulcer disease	Pain disorder
Back	Lumbosacral radiculopathy	Ruptured disk	Pain disorder
Joints or extremities		Fibromyalgia	Pain disorder
Chest		Angina	Panic disorder
Menstruation, intercourse		Endometriosis	Dyspareunia, vaginismus
Urination	Neurogenic bladder	Urinary tract infection	
Gastrointestinal (nonpain)			
Difficulty swallowing	Myasthenia gravis	Esophageal motility disorder	Eating disorder
Nausea	Raised intracranial pressure	Ménière's disease	Eating disorder
Bloating		Galactase deficiency	Eating disorder
Vomiting (nonpregnancy)		Raised intracranial pressure	Eating disorder
Diarrhea		Irritable bowel syndrome	Eating disorder
Intolerance to several foods		Food allergy	Eating disorder
Sexual (nonpain)			
Loss of interest			Major depressive episode
Erectile–ejaculatory dysfunction	Diabetic neuropathy	Antihypertensive drug effect	
Menorrhagia		Leiomyofibroma	
Vomiting throughout pregnancy		Preeclampsia, eclampsia	
Pseudoneurological			
Conversion			
Sensory	Stroke (hemianesthesia)		Schizophrenia/(hallucinations)
Motor	Huntington's disease	Myopathy	Catatonia
Seizures	Epilepsy	Electrolyte imbalance	Catatonia
Mixed	Multiple sclerosis	Electrolyte imbalance	Catatonia
Dissociative			
Amnesia	Amnestic disorder	Anticholinergic drug effects	Dissociative identity disorder
Loss of consciousness (nonfainting)	Coma	Metabolic encephalopathy	Catatonia
Symptoms* often associated with somatization disorder			
Anxiety, panic		Pheochromocytoma	Generalized anxiety and panic disorders
Dysphoria, affective lability	Frontal lobe syndrome	Endocrinopathy	Major mood disorders
Cluster B personality features	Frontal lobe syndrome	Acute intermittent porphyria	Brief psychotic disorder

*All of these symptoms may be reported by individuals with somatization disorder, without the clinical consistency and pathological findings to support the diagnosis of neurological, general medical, or psychiatric conditions separate from somatization disorder.

Developed in conjunction with Sheldon H. Preskorn.

absence of laboratory abnormalities characteristic of the suggested physical disorders (Table 34-4). Another way of characterizing the distinction is the "reverse funnel effect." With most general medical conditions, the process of investigation "funnels down" to fewer and fewer specific diagnostic possibilities; in somatization disorder, the more extensive the investigation, the greater the number of suggested disorders.

Several general medical conditions may also fit this pattern and may be confused with somatization disorder. These include multiple sclerosis, other neuropathies, systemic lupus erythematosus, acute intermittent porphyria, other hepatic and hematopoietic porphyrias, hypercalcemia, certain chronic systemic infections such as brucellosis and trypanosomiasis, myopathies, and vasculitides. In general, such conditions begin with disseminated, nonspecific subjective symptoms and transient or equivocal physical signs or laboratory abnormalities.

Somatization disorder is characterized by excessive psychiatric as well as physical complaints. Thus, other mental disorders, including anxiety and mood disorders and schizophrenia, may be suggested. Although no specific exclusion criteria regarding other mental disorders are given, one must be careful in accepting "comorbidity" and critically evaluate whether suggested syndromes are truly additional syndromes or simply manifestations of somatization disorder.

Table 34-4	Discrimination of Somatization Disorder from General Medical Conditions
Features Suggesting Somatization Disorder	**Features Suggesting a General Medical Condition**
Involvement of multiple organ systems	Involvement of single or few organ systems
Early onset and chronic course without development of physical signs or structural abnormalities	If early onset and chronic course, development of physical signs and structural abnormalities
Absence of laboratory abnormalities characteristic of the suggested general medical condition	Laboratory abnormalities evident

Source: Martin RL and Yutzy SH (1994) Somatoform disorders. In *The American Psychiatric Press Textbook of Psychiatry*, 2nd ed., Hales RE, Yudofsky SC, and Talbott JA (eds). American Psychiatric Press, Washington, DC, p. 600.

The overlap between somatization disorder and anxiety disorders may be a particular problem. Individuals with somatization disorder frequently complain of many of the same somatic symptoms as individuals with anxiety disorders, such as increased muscle tension, features of autonomic hyperactivity, and even discrete panic attacks. Likewise, individuals with anxiety disorder may report irrational disease concerns and such somatic complaints as those involving gastrointestinal function that are commonly seen in somatization disorder. However, individuals with anxiety disorders neither typically report sexual and menstrual complaints or conversion or dissociative symptoms as in somatization disorder, nor do they have the associated histrionic presentation and personal, marital, and social maladjustment common in individuals with somatization disorder.

Mood disorders (in particular, depression) frequently present with multiple somatic complaints, especially in certain cultures such as in India, where somatic but not mental complaints are acceptable. A longitudinal history identifying age at onset and course of illness may facilitate discrimination of a mood disorder from somatization disorder. In mood disorders, the age at onset of the somatic symptoms is generally later than in somatization disorder; their first appearance generally correlates with the onset of mood symptoms, and a lengthy pattern of multiple recurring somatic complaints is not seen. Also, resolution of the underlying mood disorder will generally result in disappearance of the somatic complaints.

From the other perspective, individuals with somatization disorder often present with depressive complaints. In somatization disorder, a thorough investigation will reveal a multitude of somatic as well as "depressive"

symptoms. Interestingly, somatization disorder individuals complaining of depression have been found to proffer greater depressive symptoms than individuals with major depression. As in anxiety disorders, major depressive episodes may occur in individuals with somatization disorder and must be differentiated from the tendency to have multiple complaints, which is characteristic of somatization disorder. As with anxiety disorders, in considering comorbidity with a depressive disorder, the individual's reports should be corroborated by collateral information or by direct observation. Thus, the veracity of the self-report of overwhelming depression and suicidal ideation should be doubted if the individual appears cheerful and charming, at least at times, when interviewed, or if the individual is reported to be actively involved in social activities on an inpatient psychiatric service.

Schizophrenia may present with generally single but occasionally multiple unexplained somatic complaints. The assessment interview usually uncovers psychotic symptoms such as delusions, hallucinations, or disorganized thought. In some cases, the underlying psychosis cannot be identified initially, but in time, schizophrenia will become manifest. Hallucinations are included as examples of conversion symptoms in DSM-IV-TR which may lead to diagnostic problems. As discussed in the conversion disorder section, careful analysis of this symptom is warranted so that a misdiagnosis is not made, relegating an individual to long-term neuroleptic treatment on the basis of conversion hallucinations.

Individuals with histrionic, borderline, and antisocial personality disorders frequently have an excess of somatic complaints, at times presenting with somatization disorder. Antisocial personality disorder and somatization disorder appear to cluster in individuals and within families and may share common causes. Dissociative phenomena, in particular dissociative identity disorder, are commonly associated with somatization disorder. Because dissociative symptoms are included in the diagnostic criteria for somatization, a separate diagnosis of a dissociative disorder is not made if such symptoms occur only in the course of somatization disorder.

Unlike that in hypochondriasis and body dysmorphic disorder, in which preoccupations and fears concerning the interpretation of symptoms predominate, the focus in somatization disorder is on the physical complaints themselves. Unlike that in pain disorder and conversion disorder, multiple complaints of different types are reported; by definition, in DSM-IV-TR, the history is of pain in at least four sites or functions (e.g., pain with intercourse, pain in swallowing), at least two nonpain gastrointestinal symptoms, at least one nonpain sexual or reproductive symptom, and at least one conversion or dissociative (i.e., pseudoneurological) symptom.

TREATMENT

First, a "management" rather than a "curative" strategy is recommended for somatization disorder. With the current absence of an identified definitive treatment, a modest, practical, empirical approach should be taken. This should include efforts to minimize distress and functional impairments associated with the multiple somatic complaints; to avoid unwarranted diagnostic and therapeutic procedures and medications; and to prevent potential complications including chronic invalidism and drug dependence.

The individual should be encouraged to see a single physician with an understanding of and, preferably, experience in treating somatization disorder. This helps limit the number of unnecessary evaluations and treatments. Routine, brief, supportive office visits scheduled at regular intervals to provide reassurance and prevent individuals from "needing to develop" symptoms to obtain care and attention have been advocated. This "medical" management can well be provided by a primary care physician, perhaps in consultation with a mental health professional. Studies have demonstrated that such a regimen led to markedly decreased health care costs, with no apparent decrements in health or satisfaction of individuals.

Three interrelated components have been proposed for the treatment of somatization disorder: (1) establishment of a strong relationship or bond between the clinician and the individual; (2) education of the individual regarding the nature of somatization disorder; and (3) provision of support and reassurance.

The first component, establishing a strong therapeutic bond, is especially important in the treatment of somatization disorder. Without it, it will be difficult for the individual to overcome skepticism deriving from past experience with many physicians and other therapists who "never seemed to help." In addition, trust must be strong enough to withstand the stress of withholding unwarranted diagnostic and therapeutic procedures that the individual may feel are indicated. The cornerstone of establishing a therapeutic relationship is laid when the clinician indicates an understanding of the individual's pain and suffering, legitimizing the symptoms as real. This demonstrates a willingness to provide direct compassionate assistance. A full investigation of the medical and psychosocial histories, including extensive record review, will illustrate to individuals the willingness of the clinician to gain the fullest understanding of them and their plight. This also provides another opportunity to evaluate for the presence of an underlying

general medical condition and to obtain a fuller picture of psychosocial difficulties that may relate temporally to somatic symptoms.

Only after the diagnosis has been clearly established and the therapeutic alliance is firmly in place can the clinician confidently limit diagnostic evaluations and therapies to those performed on the basis of objective findings as opposed to merely subjective complaints. Of course, the clinician should remain aware that individuals with somatization disorder are still at risk for development of general medical illnesses so that a vigilant perspective should always be maintained.

The second component is education. This involves advising individuals that they suffer from a "medically sanctioned illness," that is, a condition recognized by the medical community and one about which a good deal is known. Ultimately, it may be possible to introduce the concept of somatization disorder, which can be described in a positive light (i.e., the individual does not have a progressive, deteriorating, or potentially fatal medical disorder, and the individual is not "going crazy" but has a condition by which many symptoms will be experienced). A realistic discussion of prognosis and treatment options can then follow.

The third component is reassurance. Individuals with somatization disorder often have control and insecurity issues, which often come to the forefront when they perceive that a particular physical complaint is not being adequately addressed. Explicit reassurance should be given that the appropriate inquiries and investigations are being performed and that the possibility of an underlying physical disorder as the explanation for symptoms is being reasonably considered.

In time, it may be appropriate to gradually shift emphasis away from somatic symptoms to consideration of personal and interpersonal issues. In some individuals, it may be appropriate to posit a causal theory between somatic symptoms and "stress," that is, that there may be a temporal association between symptoms and personal, interpersonal, and even occupational problems. In individuals for whom such "insight" is difficult, behavioral techniques may be useful.

Even following such therapeutic guidelines, individuals with somatization disorder are often difficult to treat. Attention-seeking behavior, demands, and manipulation are common, necessitating firm limits and careful attention to boundary issues. This, again, is a management rather than a curative approach. Thus, such behaviors should generally be dealt with directly rather than interpreted to the individual.

No effective somatic treatments for somatization disorder itself have been identified. Individuals with somatization disorder may complain of anxiety and depression, suggesting readily treatable comorbid mental disorders. As previously discussed, it is often difficult to distinguish actual comorbid conditions from aspects of somatoform disorder itself. Pharmacological interventions are likely to be helpful in the former but not in the latter. At times, such discrimination will be impossible, and an empirical trial of such treatments may be indicated. Individuals with somatization disorder are often inconsistent and erratic in their use of medications. They will often report unusual side effects that may not be explained pharmacologically. This makes evaluation of treatment response difficult. In addition, drug dependence and suicide gestures and attempts are not uncommon.

Undifferentiated Somatoform Disorder

DIAGNOSIS

As defined in DSM-IV-TR, this category includes disturbances of at least 6 months' duration, with one or more unintentional, clinically significant, medically unexplained physical complaints. In a sense, it is a residual category, subsuming syndromes with somatic complaints that do not meet criteria for any of the "differentiated" somatoform disorders, yet are not better accounted for by any other mental disorder. On the

---

DSM-IV-TR Diagnostic Criteria

300.81 UNDIFFERENTIATED SOMATOFORM DISORDER

A. One or more physical complaints (e.g., fatigue, loss of appetite, gastrointestinal or urinary complaints).
B. Either (1) or (2):
  (1) After appropriate investigation, the symptoms cannot be fully explained by a known general medical condition or the direct effects of a substance (e.g., a drug of abuse, a medication).
  (2) When there is a related general medical condition, the physical complaints or resulting social or occupational impairment is in excess of what would be expected from the history, physical examination, or laboratory findings.
C. The symptoms cause clinically significant distress or impairment in social, occupational, or other important areas of functioning.
D. Duration of the disturbance is at least 6 months.
E. The disturbance is not better accounted for by another mental disorder (e.g., another somatoform disorder, sexual dysfunction, mood disorder, anxiety disorder, sleep disorder, or psychotic disorder).
F. The symptom is not intentionally produced or feigned (as in factitious disorder or malingering).

Reprinted with permission from the *Diagnostic and Statistical Manual of Mental Disorders*, 4th ed., Text Rev. Copyright 2000 American Psychiatric Association.

---

other hand, it is a less residual category than somatoform disorder NOS, in that the disturbance must last at least 6 months (see Figure 34-1). Virtually any unintentional, medically unexplained physical symptoms causing clinically significant distress or impairment can be considered. In effect, this category serves to capture syndromes that resemble somatization disorder but do not meet full criteria.

The term undifferentiated somatoform disorder was introduced in 1987 with DSM-III-R, replacing the atypical somatoform disorder of DSM-III. However, the category has not been well used, not only by mental health professionals but also by primary care physicians for whom identification of such a syndrome could be useful. Terms that have been used in a similar manner include *subsyndromal, forme fruste*, or *abridged* somatization disorder.

In addition to the range of symptoms specified in the other somatoform disorders, individuals with undifferentiated somatoform disorder, complaining primarily of fatigue (chronic fatigue syndrome), bowel problems (irritable bowel syndrome), or multiple muscle aches/weakness (fibromyalgia), can be considered for undifferentiated somatoform disorder. Substantial controversy exists regarding the etiology of such syndromes. Even if an explanation on the basis of a known pathophysiological mechanism cannot be established, many argue that the syndromes should be considered general medical conditions. However, for the time being, these syndromes could be considered in a highly tentative manner under the undifferentiated somatoform disorder rubric. Careful reconsideration of the undifferentiated somatoform label should be undertaken at regular intervals if the symptoms persist. The clinician should remain ever vigilant to the emergence of another general medical condition or mental disorder. When individuals are diagnosed with chronic fatigue syndrome, careful evaluation procedures should be followed.

Some have argued that undifferentiated somatoform disorder is the most common somatoform disorder. A 1991 study using an abridged somatization disorder construct requiring six somatic symptoms for women and four for men, reported that 11% of non-Hispanic US whites and Hispanics, 15% of US blacks, and 20% of Puerto Ricans in Puerto Rico fulfilled criteria. A preponderance of women was evident in all groups except the Puerto Rican sample (see Table 34-2).

Course

As shown in Table 34-2, it appears that the course and prognosis of undifferentiated somatoform disorder are highly variable. This is not surprising, because the definition of this disorder allows a great deal of heterogeneity.

Differential Diagnosis

In comparison to the situation when the full criteria for the well-validated somatization disorder are met, exclusion of an as-yet-undiscovered general medical or substance-induced explanation for physical symptoms is far less certain when the less stringent criteria for undifferentiated somatoform disorder are met. Thus, the diagnosis of undifferentiated somatoform disorder should remain tentative, and new symptoms should be carefully investigated.

Because undifferentiated somatoform disorder represents a somewhat residual category, the major diagnostic process, once occult general medical conditions and substance-induced explanations have been considered, is one of exclusion. As shown in Figure 34-1, whether the somatic symptoms are intentionally produced as in malingering and factitious disorder must be addressed. Here, motivation for external rewards (for malingering) and a pervasive intent to assume the sick role (for factitious disorder) must be assessed. The next consideration is whether the somatic symptoms are the manifestation of another mental disorder. Anxiety and mood disorders commonly present with somatic symptoms; high rates of anxiety and major depressive disorders are reported in individuals with somatic complaints attending family medicine clinics. Of course, undifferentiated somatoform disorder could be diagnosed in addition to one of these disorders, so long as the symptoms are not accounted for by the other mental disorder. Crucial in this determination is whether the symptoms are present during periods in which the anxiety or mood disorders are not actively present.

Next, other somatoform disorders must be considered. In general, undifferentiated somatoform disorders are characterized by unexplained somatic complaints, the most common being female reproductive symptoms, excessive gas, abdominal pain, chest pain, joint pain, palpitations, and fainting, rather than preoccupations or fears as in hypochondriasis or body dysmorphic disorder. However, an individual with some manifestations of these two disorders but not meeting full criteria could conceivably receive a diagnosis of undifferentiated somatoform disorder. An example is an individual with recurrent yet shifting hypochondriacal concerns that do respond to medical reassurance. If symptoms are restricted to those affecting the domains of sexual dysfunction, pain, or

pseudoneurological symptoms, and the specific criteria for a sexual dysfunction, pain disorder, and/or conversion disorder are met, the specific disorder or disorders should be diagnosed. If other types of symptoms or symptoms of more than one of these disorders have been present for at least 6 months, yet criteria for somatization disorder are not met, undifferentiated somatoform disorder should be diagnosed. By definition, undifferentiated somatoform disorder requires a duration of 6 months. If this criterion is not met, a diagnosis of somatoform disorder NOS should be considered.

Individuals with an apparent undifferentiated somatoform disorder should be carefully evaluated for somatization disorder. Typically, individuals with somatization disorder are inconsistent historians, at one evaluation reporting a large number of symptoms fulfilling criteria for the full syndrome and at another time endorsing fewer symptoms. In addition, with follow-up, additional symptoms may become evident, and criteria for somatization disorder will be satisfied. Individuals with multiple somatic complaints not diagnosed with somatization disorder because of a reported onset later than 30 years of age may be inaccurately reporting a later age at onset. If the late age at onset is accurate, the individual should be carefully scrutinized for an occult general medical condition.

TREATMENT

In view of the broad inclusion and minimal exclusion criteria for undifferentiated somatoform disorder, it is difficult to make treatment recommendations beyond the generic strategies discussed in the beginning of this chapter. A substantial proportion of individuals with undifferentiated somatoform disorders improve or recover with no formal therapy. However, appropriate psychotherapy and pharmacological intervention may accelerate the process.

Recommendations have been proposed for individuals with symptoms of headache, fibromyalgia, and chronic fatigue syndrome, conditions that some would include under undifferentiated somatoform disorder. Generally recommended are brief psychotherapy of a supportive and educative nature. As with somatization disorder, the physician–patient relationship is of great importance. Judicious use of pharmacotherapy may be of benefit also, particularly if the somatoform syndrome is intertwined with an anxiety or depressive syndrome. Here, usual antianxiety and antidepressant medications are recommended. Individuals with unexplained pains may benefit from pain management strategies as outlined in the pain disorder section.

Conversion Disorder

DIAGNOSIS

As defined in DSM-IV-TR, conversion disorders are characterized by symptoms or deficits affecting voluntary motor or sensory function that are suggestive of, yet are not fully explained by, a neurological or other general medical condition or the direct effects of a substance. The diagnosis is not made if the presentation is explained as a culturally sanctioned behavior or experience, such as bizarre behaviors resembling a seizure during a religious ceremony. Symptoms are not intentionally produced or feigned, that is, the person does not consciously contrive a symptom for external rewards, as in malingering, or for the intrapsychic rewards of assuming the sick role, as in factitious disorder.

Four subtypes with specific examples of symptoms are defined: with motor symptom or deficit (e.g.,

---

DSM-IV-TR Diagnostic Criteria

300.11 CONVERSION DISORDER

A. One or more symptoms or deficits affecting voluntary motor or sensory function that suggest a neurological or other general medical condition.
B. Psychological factors are judged to be associated with the symptom or deficit because the initiation or exacerbation of the symptom or deficit is preceded by conflicts or other stressors.
C. The symptom or deficit is not intentionally produced or feigned (as in factitious disorder or malingering).
D. The symptom or deficit cannot, after appropriate investigation, be fully explained by a general medical condition, or by the direct effects of a substance, or as a culturally sanctioned behavior or experience.
E. The symptom or deficit causes clinically significant distress or impairment in social, occupational, or other important areas of functioning or warrants medical evaluation.
F. The symptom or deficit is not limited to pain or sexual dysfunction, does not occur exclusively during the course of somatization disorder, and is not better accounted for by another mental disorder.

Specify type of symptom or deficit:

With motor symptom or deficit (e.g., impaired coordination or balance, paralysis or localized weakness, difficulty swallowing or lump in throat, aphonia, and urinary retention)
With sensory symptom or deficit (e.g., loss of touch or pain sensation, double vision, blindness, deafness, and hallucinations)
With seizures or convulsions (includes seizures or convulsions with voluntary sensory components)
With mixed presentation (if symptoms of more than one category are evident).

---

impaired coordination or balance, paralysis or localized weakness, difficulty swallowing or lump in throat, aphonia, and urinary retention); with sensory symptom or deficit (e.g., loss of touch or pain sensation, double vision, blindness, deafness, and hallucinations); with seizures or convulsions; and with mixed presentation (i.e., has symptoms of more than one of the other subtypes). The list of examples is also contained among the pseudoneurological symptoms listed in the diagnostic criteria for somatization disorder. Although determination is highly subjective and of questionable reliability and validity, association with psychological factors is required.

The relationship of conversion disorder to the dissociative disorders warrants comment. Long recognized as related, they were subsumed as subtypes of hysterical neurosis in DSM-II: conversion involving voluntary motor and sensory functioning, and dissociation affecting memory and identity. They are unified in one category in ICD-10: dissociative (conversion) disorders. Although DSM-IV-TR classifies conversion disorder with the somatoform disorders; the DSM-IV-TR text acknowledges the symptomatic, epidemiological, and probable pathogenetic similarities between conversion and dissociative symptoms. Such symptoms have been attributed to similar psychological mechanisms, and they often occur in the same individual, sometimes during the same episode of illness. DSM-IV-TR does suggest that individuals with conversion disorder be carefully scrutinized for dissociative symptoms.

Hallucinations are included among the sensory nervous symptoms in DSM-IV-TR. Inclusion of hallucinations as a conversion symptom is supported by the DSM-IV somatization disorder field trial, in which one third of a large sample of nonpsychotic women with evidence of unexplained somatic complaints reported a history of hallucinations. Among the 40% who had symptoms that met criteria for somatization disorder, more than half reported hallucinations. Women with other conversion symptoms were more likely to report hallucinations than were those with no other conversion symptoms.

In general, conversion hallucinations (referred to by some as pseudohallucinations) differ in several ways from those in psychotic conditions. Conversion hallucinations typically occur in the absence of other psychotic symptoms, insight that the hallucinations are not real may be retained, and they often involve more than one sensory modality, whereas hallucinations in psychoses generally involve a single sensory modality, usually auditory. Conversion hallucinations also often have a naive, fantastic, or childish content, as if they are part of a fairy tale, and are described eagerly, sometimes even provocatively, as an interesting story (e.g., "I was driving downtown and a flying saucer flew over my car and I saw you [the psychiatrist] in a window and I heard your voice calling to me"). They often bear some understandable psychological purpose, although the individual may not be aware of intent. In the example given, the "sighting" was reported at the time that no further sessions were scheduled.

Conversion symptoms themselves may be common; it has been reported that 25% of normal postpartum and medically ill women had a history of conversion symptoms at some time during their life, yet in some instances, there may have been no resulting clinically significant distress or impairment. Lifetime prevalence rates of treated conversion symptoms in general populations are much more modest, ranging from 11 to 500 per 100,000 (see Table 34-2). About 5–24% of psychiatric outpatients, 5–14% of general hospital patients, and 1–3% of outpatient psychiatric referrals reported a history of conversion symptoms, although their current treatment was not necessarily for conversion symptoms. A rate of nearly 4% of outpatient neurological referrals and 1% of neurological admissions have involved conversion disorder. In virtually all studies, an excess (to the extent of 2:1 to 10:1) of women reported conversion symptoms relative to men. In part, this may relate to the simple fact that women seek medical evaluation more often than men do, but it is unlikely that this fully accounts for the sex difference. There is a predilection for lower socioeconomic status; less educated, less psychologically sophisticated, and rural populations are overrepresented. Consistent with this, higher rates (nearly 10%) of outpatient psychiatric referrals are for conversion symptoms in "developing" countries. As countries develop, there may be a declining incidence in time, which may relate to increasing levels of education, and medical and psychological sophistication.

Course

Age at onset is typically from late childhood to early adulthood. Onset is rare before the age of 10 and after 35, but cases with an onset as late as the ninth decade have been reported. The likelihood of a neurological or other medical condition is increased when the age at onset is in middle or late life. Development is generally acute, but symptoms may develop gradually as well. The course of individual conversion symptoms is generally short; half to nearly all symptoms remit by the time of hospital discharge. However, symptoms relapse within one year in one-fifth to one-fourth of individuals. Typically, one symptom is present in a single episode, but multiple symptoms are generally involved

longitudinally. Factors associated with good prognosis include acute onset, clearly identifiable precipitants, a short interval between onset and institution of treatment, and good intelligence. Conversion blindness, aphonia, and paralysis are associated with relatively good prognosis, whereas individuals with seizures and tremor do more poorly. Some individuals diagnosed initially with conversion disorder will have a presentation that meets the criteria for somatization disorder when they are observed longitudinally.

Individual conversion symptoms are generally self-limited and do not lead to physical changes or disabilities. Rarely, physical sequelae such as atrophy may occur. Marital and occupational problems are not as frequent in individuals with conversion disorder as they are in those with somatization disorder.

Differential Diagnosis

As shown in Figure 34-1, the first consideration is whether the conversion symptoms are explained on the basis of a general medical condition. Because conversion symptoms by definition affect voluntary motor or sensory function (thus pseudoneurological), neurological conditions are usually suggested, but other general medical conditions may be implicated as well. Neurologists are generally first consulted by primary care physicians for conversion symptoms; mental health clinicians become involved only after neurological or general medical conditions have been reasonably excluded. Nonetheless, the mental health clinician should have a good appreciation of the process of making such exclusions. More than one eighth of actual neurological cases are diagnosed as functional before the elucidation of a neurological illness. Even after referral, vigilance for an emerging general medical condition should continue. A significant percentage–21% to 50%—of individuals diagnosed with conversion symptoms are found to have neurological illness on follow-up.

Apparent conversion symptoms mandate a thorough evaluation for possible underlying physical explanation. This evaluation must include a thorough medical history, physical (especially neurological) examination, and radiographical, blood, urine, and other tests as clinically indicated. Reliance should not be placed on determination of whether psychological factors explain the symptom. Such determinations are unreliable except, perhaps, in cases in which there is a clear and immediate temporal relationship between a psychosocial stressor and the symptom, or in cases in which similar situations led to conversion symptoms in the past. A history of previous conversion or other unexplained symptoms, particularly if somatization disorder is diagnosable, lessens the probability that an occult medical condition will be identified. Although conversion symptoms may occur at any age, symptoms are most often first manifested in late adolescence or early adulthood. Conversion symptoms first occurring in middle age or later should increase suspicion of an occult physical illness.

Symptoms of many neurological illnesses may appear inconsistent with known neurophysiological or neuropathological processes, suggesting conversion and posing diagnostic problems. These illnesses include multiple sclerosis, in which blindness due to optic neuritis may initially present with normal fundi, myasthenia gravis, periodic paralysis, myoglobinuric myopathy, polymyositis, and other acquired myopathies, in which marked weakness in the presence of normal deep tendon reflexes may occur, and Guillain–Barré syndrome, in which early extremity weakness may be inconsistent.

Complicating diagnosis is the fact that physical illness and conversion or other apparent psychiatric overlay are not mutually exclusive. Individuals with physical illnesses that are incapacitating and frightening may appear to be exaggerating symptoms. Also, individuals with actual neurological illness will also have "pseudo" symptoms. For example, individuals with actual seizures may have pseudoseizures as well. Considering these observations, mental health clinicians should avoid a rash and hasty diagnosis of conversion disorder when faced with symptoms that are difficult to interpret.

As with the other somatoform disorders, symptoms of conversion disorder are not intentionally produced, in distinction to malingering or factitious disorder. To a large part, this determination is based on assessment of the motivation for external rewards (as in malingering) or for the assumption of the sick role (as in factitious disorder). The setting is often an important consideration. For example, conversion-like symptoms are frequent in military or forensic settings, in which obvious potential rewards make malingering a serious consideration.

A diagnosis of conversion disorder should not be made if a conversion symptom is fully accounted for by a mood disorder or by schizophrenia (e.g., disordered motility as part of a catatonic syndrome of a psychotic mood disorder or schizophrenia). If the symptom is a hallucination, it must be remembered that the descriptors differentiating conversion from psychotic hallucinations should be seen only as rules of thumb. Differentiation should be based on a comprehensive assessment of the illness. In the case of hallucinations, posttraumatic stress disorder and dissociative identity disorder (multiple personality disorder) must also be excluded. If the conversion symptom cannot be fully accounted for by the other mental disorders, conversion disorder should be diagnosed in addition to the other disorder if it meets criteria (e.g., an episode of unexplained blindness in an individual with a major depressive episode). In hypochondriasis, neurological illness may be feared ("I have strange feelings in my head; it must be a brain tumor"), but the focus here is on preoccupation with fear of having the illness rather than on the symptom itself as in conversion disorder.

By definition, if symptoms are limited to sexual dysfunction or pain, conversion disorder is not diagnosed. Criteria for somatization disorder require multiple symptoms in multiple organ systems and functions, including symptoms affecting motor or sensory function (conversion symptoms) or memory or identity (dissociative symptoms). Thus, it would be superfluous to make an additional diagnosis of conversion disorder in the context of a somatization disorder.

A last consideration is whether the symptom is a culturally sanctioned behavior or experience. Conversion disorder should not be diagnosed if symptoms are clearly sanctioned or even expected, are appropriate to the sociocultural context, and are not associated with distress or impairment. Seizure-like episodes, such as those that occur in conjunction with certain religious ceremonies, and culturally expected responses, such as women "swooning" in response to excitement in Victorian times, qualify as examples of these symptoms.

TREATMENT

Reports of the treatment of conversion disorder date from those of Charcot, which generally involved symptom removal by suggestion or hypnosis. Breuer and Freud, using such psychoanalytic techniques as free association and abreaction of repressed affects, had more ambitious objectives in their treatment of Anna O., including the resolution of unconscious conflicts. To date, whereas some recommend long-term, intensive, insight-oriented psychodynamic psychotherapy in pursuit of such goals, most mental health clinicians advocate a more pragmatic approach, especially for acute cases.

Therapeutic approaches vary according to whether the conversion symptom is acute or chronic. Whichever the case, direct confrontation is not recommended. Such a communication may cause an individual to feel even more isolated. An undiscovered physical illness may also underlie the presentation.

In acute cases, the most frequent initial aim is removal of the symptom. The pressure behind accomplishing this depends on the distress and disability associated with the symptom. If the individual is not in great distress and the need to regain function is not immediate, a conservative approach of reassurance, relaxation, and suggestion is recommended. With this technique, the individual is reassured that on the basis of evaluation the symptom will disappear completely and, in fact, is already beginning to do so. The individual can then be encouraged to ventilate about recent events and feelings, without any causal relationships being suggested. This is in contrast to attempts at abreaction, by which repressed material, particularly regarding a painful experience or a conflict, is brought back to consciousness.

If symptoms do not resolve with such conservative approaches, a number of other techniques for symptom resolution may be instituted. It does appear that prompt resolution of conversion symptoms is important because the duration of conversion symptoms is associated with a greater risk of recurrence and chronic disability. The other techniques include narcoanalysis (e.g., amobarbital interview), hypnosis, and behavioral therapy. In narcoanalysis, amobarbital or another sedative–hypnotic medication such as lorazepam is given intravenously to the point of drowsiness. Sometimes this is followed by administration of a stimulant medication, such as methamphetamine. The individual is then encouraged to discuss stressors and conflicts. This technique may be effective acutely, leading to at least temporary symptom relief as well as expansion of the information known about the individual. This technique has not been shown to be especially effective with more chronic conversion symptoms. In hypnotherapy, symptoms may be removed with the suggestion that the symptoms will gradually improve posthypnotically. Information regarding stressors and conflicts may be explored as well. Formal behavioral therapy, including relaxation training and even aversive therapy, has been proposed and reported by some to be effective. In addition, simply manipulating the environment to interrupt reinforcement of the conversion symptom is recommended.

Anecdotally, somatic treatments including phenothiazines, lithium, and electroconvulsive therapy have been reported effective. However, in many cases, this may be attributable to simple suggestion. In other cases, resolution of another psychiatric disorder, such as a psychotic disorder or a mood disorder, may have led to the symptom's removal. It is also likely that in various rituals, such as exorcism and other religious ceremonies, immediate "cures" are based on suggestion. Suggestion seems to play a major role in the resolution of "mass hysteria," in which a group of individuals who believe that they have been exposed to some noxious

influence such as a "toxin" or even a "spell," experience similar symptoms that do not appear to have any organic basis. Often, the epidemic can be contained if affected individuals are segregated. Simple announcements that no such factor has been identified and that symptoms experienced by the group have been linked to mass hysteria have been effective.

Thus far, this discussion has centered on acute treatment primarily for symptom removal. Longer-term approaches include strategies previously discussed for somatization disorder—a pragmatic, conservative approach involving support and exploration of various conflict areas, particularly of interpersonal relationships. A certain degree of insight may be attained, at least in terms of appreciating relationships between various conflicts and stressors and the development of symptoms. Others advocate long-term, intensive, insight-oriented, dynamic psychotherapy.

Pain Disorder

DIAGNOSIS

As defined in DSM-IV-TR, the essential feature of pain disorder is pain with which psychological factors "have an important role in the onset, severity, exacerbation, or maintenance" (see Table 34-2 and DSM-IV-TR diagnostic criteria, page 359). Pain disorder is subtyped as pain disorder associated with psychological factors and pain disorder associated with both psychological factors and a general medical condition. The third possibility, pain disorder associated with a general medical condition, is not considered to be a mental disorder, because the requirement is not met that psychological factors play an important role. It should be noted that the focus of the Pain Disorder diagnosis in DSM-IV-TR is placed on the presence of psychological factors rather than the exasperating determination of whether the pain is attributable to organic disease.

A diagnosis of pain disorder requires that the pain be of sufficient severity to warrant clinical attention, that is, it causes clinically significant distress or impairment. A number of instruments have been developed to assess the degree of distress associated with the pain, including the McGill Pain Questionnaire, and the West Haven–Yale Multidimensional Pain Inventory.

DSM-IV-TR includes a number of exclusionary conventions. By definition, if pain is restricted to pain with sexual intercourse, the sexual disorder, dyspareunia, not pain disorder, is diagnosed. If pain occurs in the context of a mood, anxiety, or psychotic disorder, pain disorder is diagnosed only if it is an independent focus

DSM-IV-TR Diagnostic Criteria

307.xx PAIN DISORDER

A. Pain in one or more anatomical sites is the predominant focus of the clinical presentation and is of sufficient severity to warrant clinical attention.
B. The pain causes clinically significant distress or impairment in social, occupational, or other important areas of functioning.
C. Psychological factors are judged to have an important role in the onset, severity, exacerbation, or maintenance of the pain.
D. The symptom or deficit is not intentionally produced or feigned (as in factitious disorder or malingering).
E. The pain is not better accounted for by a mood, anxiety, or psychotic disorder and does not meet criteria for dyspareunia.

Code as follows:

307.80 Pain Disorder Associated with Psychological Factors: Psychological factors are judged to have the major role in the onset, severity, exacerbation, or maintenance of the pain. (If a general medical condition is present, it does not have a major role in the onset, severity, exacerbation, or maintenance of the pain.) This type of pain disorder is not diagnosed if criteria are also met for somatization disorder.

Specify if:

Acute: Duration of less than 6 months
Chronic: Duration of 6 months or longer
307.89 Pain Disorder Associated with both Psychological Factors and a General Medical Condition: Both psychological factors and a general medical condition are judged to have important roles in the onset, severity, exacerbation, or maintenance of the pain. The associated general medical condition or anatomical site of the pain (see below) is coded on Axis III.

Specify if:

Acute: Duration of less than 6 months
Chronic: Duration of 6 months or longer
Note: The following is not considered to be a mental disorder and is included here to facilitate differential diagnosis.
Pain Disorder Associated with a General Medical Condition: A general medical condition has a major role in the onset, severity, exacerbation, or maintenance of the pain. (If psychological factors are present, they are not judged to have a major role in the onset, severity, exacerbation, or maintenance of the pain.) The diagnostic code for the pain is selected based on the associated general medical condition if one has been established or on the anatomical location of the pain if the underlying general medical condition is not yet clearly established—for example, low back (724.2), sciatic (724.3), pelvic (625.9), headache (784.0), facial (784.0), chest (786.50), joint (719.4), bone (733.90), abdominal (789.0), breast (611.71), renal (788.0), ear (388.70), eye (379.91), throat (784.1), tooth (525.9), and urinary (788.0).

Reprinted with permission from the *Diagnostic and Statistical Manual of Mental Disorders*, 4th ed., Text Rev. Copyright 2000 American Psychiatric Association.

of clinical attention and is not better accounted for by the other disorder, a highly subjective judgment.

If pain occurs exclusively during the course of somatization disorder, pain disorder is not diagnosed

because pain symptoms are part of the criteria for somatization disorder and are thereby subsumed under the more comprehensive diagnosis. Because somatization disorder is virtually a lifelong condition, this exclusion generally applies in someone with somatization disorder by history. Important here is that in addition to pain, somatization disorder involves multiple symptoms of the gastrointestinal system, the reproductive system, and the central and peripheral nervous systems, whereas in pain disorder, the focus is on pain symptoms only.

Specification of acute versus chronic pain disorder on the basis of whether the duration is less than or greater than 6 months is an important distinction. Whereas acute pain, in most cases, will be linked with physical disorders, when pain remains unexplained after 6 months, psychological factors are often involved. However, the clinician must remember that a significant minority (in one study 19%) of individuals with chronic pain of no apparent physical origin will ultimately be found to have occult organic disease.

In individuals with unexplained pelvic pain, clinicians should be warned about cavalier conclusions regarding the absence of physical disease. With laparoscopy, a high frequency of occult organic disease has been identified in several studies. Thus, laparoscopy may be indicated in individuals with pelvic pain. Electromyography may be helpful in distinguishing muscle contraction headaches. Failure to show coronary artery spasm with provocative procedures and failure to respond to nitroglycerin may be useful in distinguishing individuals with pain disorder from those in whom the pain is attributable to coronary artery disease.

Given the fact that diagnostic criteria for pain have significantly changed across the various editions of the DSMs, only estimates can be made for the epidemiological parameters of pain disorder. As to pain itself, some empirical studies suggest that it is common. Perhaps as indirect evidence of this is the proliferation of pain clinics nationally. Of course, many individuals attending these clinics fall into the category of pain disorder associated with a general medical condition, but undoubtedly, some also have involvement of psychological factors as required for a diagnosis of pain disorder as a mental disorder. The same would apply to the 10–15% of adults in the United States in any given year who have work disability because of back pain. Pain has been found to be a predominant symptom in 75% of consecutive general medical patients, with 75% of these (thus 50% overall) judged as having no identifiable physical cause. Whereas primary care and other nonpsychiatric physicians probably see most pain patients, up to 40% of psychiatric inpatient admissions and 20% attending a psychiatric outpatient clinic report pain as a significant problem.

Course

Given the heterogeneity of conditions subsumed under the pain disorder rubric, course and prognosis vary widely. The subtyping at 6 months is of significance. The prognosis for total remission is good for pain disorders of less than 6 months' duration. However, for syndromes of greater than 6 months' duration, chronicity is common. The site of the pain may be another factor. Certain anatomically differentiated pain syndromes can be distinguished, and each has its own characteristic pattern. These include syndromes characterized primarily by headache, facial pain, chest pain, abdominal pain, and pelvic pain. In such syndromes, symptoms tend to be recurrent, with relapses occurring in association with stress. A high rate of depression has been observed among individuals with unexplained facial pain. Facial pain is often alleviated by antidepressant medication. This effect has been observed in both individuals with depressive symptoms and those without.

Other factors affecting course and prognosis include associated mental disorders and external reinforcement. Employment at the outset of treatment predicts improvement. Chronicity is more likely in the presence of certain personality diagnoses or traits, such as pronounced passivity and dependency. External reinforcement includes litigation involving potential financial compensation for disability. Continuation of the pain disorder may prove more lucrative than its resolution and return to work. Level of activity, which is generally associated with improvement, is discouraged by fears of losing compensation. Thus, although outright malingering may be rare, pain behaviors are often reinforced and maintained. Habituation with addictive drugs is associated with greater chronicity.

Differential Diagnosis

As shown in Figure 34-1, the differential diagnosis begins with an assessment of whether the presentation is fully explained by a general medical condition. If not, it may be assumed that psychological factors play a major role. If it is judged that psychological factors do not play a major role, a diagnosis of pain disorder associated with a general medical condition may apply. As previously mentioned, this does not have a mental disorder code.

If psychological factors are involved, the first consideration is whether the pain is feigned. If so, either malingering or factitious disorder is diagnosed,

depending on whether external incentives or assumption of the sick role is the motivation. Evidence of malingering includes consideration of external rewards relative to the chronology of the development and maintenance of the pain. In factitious disorder, a pattern of successive hospitalizations and medical evaluations is evident. Inconsistency in presentation, lack of correspondence to known anatomical pathways or disease patterns, and lack of associated sensory or motor function changes suggest malingering or factitious disorder, but pain disorder associated with psychological factors may show this pattern as well. The key question is whether the individual is experiencing rather than feigning the pain.

Determination of the relative contributions of psychological and general medical factors is difficult. Of course, careful assessment of the nature and severity of the potential underlying medical condition and the nature and degree of pain that would be expected should be made. Traditionally, the so-called conversion V or neurotic triad (consisting of elevation of the hypochondriasis and hysteria scales with a lower score on the depression scale) on the Minnesota Multiphasic Personality Inventory has been purported to indicate emotional indifference to the somatic concerns as might be expected if the symptom is attributable to psychological factors rather than organic disease. However, evidence indicates that this configuration may also occur as an adjustment to chronic illness.

TREATMENT

An overriding guideline in the treatment of pain is that the clinician not do anything that will actually perpetuate and even promote "pain-related behavior." Thus, a major goal is to encourage activity. Other guidelines include avoidance of sedative–antianxiety drugs, judicious use of analgesics on a fixed interval schedule so as not to reinforce pain-related behaviors, avoidance of opioids, and consideration of alternative treatment approaches such as relaxation therapy. Depression should be treated with appropriate antidepressant drugs, not sedative–antianxiety medications. The difficulties in managing individuals with pain disorder have resulted in the establishment of many clinics and programs especially designed for pain. Referral to such a service may be indicated. Intervention should best be provided early in the course of the syndrome, before pain-related behaviors become entrenched. Once continuing disability compensation is established, therapeutic efforts become much more difficult.

The preceding general guidelines apply whether or not a general medical basis for the pain is involved. Of course, if only pain disorder associated with psychological factors is involved, psychological management will be the mainstay. For individuals with pain associated with general medical factors (not a mental disorder) in which psychological factors do not play a major role, efforts should be made to prevent the development of psychological problems in response to the resulting distress, isolation and loss of function, and iatrogenic effects such as exposure to potentially addicting drugs.

In acute pain, the major goal is to relieve the pain. Thus, pharmacological agents generally play a more significant role than in chronic syndromes. Whereas the risk of developing opioid dependence appears to be surprisingly low (4 per 12,000) among individuals without a prior history of dependence, nonopioid agents should be used whenever they can be expected to be effective. These include, in particular, acetaminophen and the nonsteroidal antiinflammatory drugs (NSAIDS), of which aspirin is considered a member. Even if an opioid analgesic is employed, these drugs should be continued as adjuncts; often, they lessen the required dose of the opioid.

It is with the chronic syndromes that proper management is crucial to ease distress and prevent the development of additional problems. The overriding goal is to maintain function, because total relief of the pain may not be possible. Physical and occupational therapy may play a major role. There may be resistance to the involvement of a mental health professional as an indication that the pain is not seen as real. Such issues must first be resolved. An attempt should be made to ascertain the roles that psychological and general medical factors play in the maintenance of the pain.

A large variety of psychotherapies including individual, group, and family strategies have been employed. Two techniques that warrant special attention are operant conditioning and cognitive–behavioral therapy. In operant conditioning, the pattern of reinforcement of pain behavior by medication, attention, and excuse from responsibilities is to be interrupted and reinforcement shifted to usual daily activities. To assess the role of operant conditioning, it may be necessary to have individuals keep a diary and to interview family members to identify any conditioning patterns. In cognitive–behavioral therapies, the goal is the identification and correction of attitudes, beliefs, and expectations. Biofeedback and relaxation techniques may be used to minimize muscle tension that may aggravate if not cause pain. Hypnosis may also be used to achieve muscle relaxation and to help the individual "dissociate" from the pain.

Pharmacological intervention may also be useful in chronic syndromes. Effort should be made to avoid opioids if possible. Agents to be tried first include antidepressants, acetaminophen, NSAIDs (including aspirin), and anticonvulsants such as carbamazepine. Antidepressants seem particularly useful for neuropathic pain, headache, facial pain, fibrositis, and arthritis (including rheumatoid arthritis). Analgesic action seems to be independent of antidepressant effects. Most work has been done with the tricyclic antidepressants; other classes, such as the monoamine oxidase inhibitors (MAOIS) and the selective serotonin reuptake inhibitors (SSRIS), may be effective as well. Although it was thought that the action is mediated by serotoninergic effects, agents such as desipramine with predominantly noradrenergic activity seem to be effective as well. NSAIDs, of which aspirin, ibuprofen, naproxen, and piroxicam are commonly used examples, may alleviate pain through inhibition of prostaglandin synthesis. Unfortunately, this effect may also contribute to side effects, such as aggravation of peptic or duodenal ulcers and interference with renal function. For individuals unable to tolerate NSAIDs, acetaminophen should be tried.

If opioid analgesics are used, it is recommended that use be tied to objectives such as increasing level of activity rather than simply pain alleviation. Milder opioids, such as codeine, oxycodone, and hydrocodone, should be implemented first. The once widely used propoxyphene has less analgesic effect than these drugs; it is not devoid of abuse potential as once thought and is not recommended. Pure opioid agonists such as morphine, methadone, and hydromorphone should be tried next. Meperidine, also in this class, is contraindicated for prolonged use because accumulation of the toxic metabolite, normeperidine, a cerebral irritant, may result in anxiety, psychosis, or seizures. Meperidine may also have a lethal interaction with MAOIs. There are no advantages to mixed opioid agonist–antagonists. The commonly used pentazocine should be avoided because it has abuse potential and psychotomimetic effects in some individuals. It remains to be seen whether newer agents (buprenorphine, butonphanol, and nalbuphine) have lower abuse potential as claimed. Above all, clinicians should be judicious in the use of opioid analgesics, considering not only their abuse potential but their large number of side effects including constipation, nausea and vomiting, excessive sedation, and, in higher doses, respiratory depression that may be fatal.

In addition to pharmacotherapy, a number of other "physical" techniques have been used, such as acupuncture and transcutaneous electrical nerve stimulation. These carry little risk of adverse effects or aggravation of the pain disorder. Other procedures such as trigger point injections, nerve blocks, and surgical ablation may be recommended if specifically indicated by an underlying general medical disorder.

Hypochondriasis

DIAGNOSIS

As defined in DSM-IV-TR, the essential feature in hypochondriasis is preoccupation with fears or the idea of having a serious disease based on the "misinterpretation of bodily symptoms". This is in contrast to somatization disorder, conversion disorder, and pain disorder, in which the symptoms themselves are the predominant focus (see Table 34-2). Bodily symptoms may be interpreted broadly to include misinterpretation of normal body functions. In hypochondriasis, the preoccupation persists despite reassurance from physicians and the accumulation of evidence to the contrary. As in the other somatoform disorders, symptoms must result in clinically significant distress or impairment in important areas of functioning. The duration must be at least 6 months. Hypochondriasis is not diagnosed if the hypochondriacal concerns are better accounted for by another mental disorder, such as major depressive episodes or various psychotic disorders with somatic delusions.

DSM-IV-TR Diagnostic Criteria

300.7 HYPOCHONDRIASIS

A. Preoccupation with fears of having, or the idea that one has, a serious disease based on the person's misinterpretation of bodily symptoms.
B. The preoccupation persists despite appropriate medical evaluation and reassurance.
C. The belief in criterion A is not of delusional intensity (as in delusional disorder, somatic type) and is not restricted to a circumscribed concern about appearance (as in body dysmorphic disorder).
D. The preoccupation causes clinically significant distress or impairment in social, occupational, or other important areas of functioning.
E. The duration of the disturbance is at least 6 months.
F. The preoccupation is not better accounted for by generalized anxiety disorder, obsessive–compulsive disorder, panic disorder, a major depressive episode, separation anxiety, or another somatoform disorder.

Specify if:

With poor insight: If, for most of the time during the current episode, the person does not recognize that the concern about having a serious illness is excessive or unreasonable

Reprinted with permission from the *Diagnostic and Statistical Manual of Mental Disorders*, 4th ed., Text Rev. Copyright 2000 American Psychiatric Association.

Some degree of preoccupation with disease is apparently common. In a 1991 study, 10–20% of "normal" and 45% of "neurotic" persons were reported to have intermittent unfounded worries about illness, with 9% of individuals doubting reassurances given by physicians. Many individuals manifest some hypochondriacal symptoms as part of other mental disorders, and others have transient hypochondriacal symptoms in response to stresses such as serious physical illness yet never fulfill the inclusion criteria for DSM-IV-TR hypochondriasis. Assessment of the incidence and prevalence of hypochondriasis undoubtedly requires study of general or primary care rather than psychiatric populations, because individuals with hypochondriasis are convinced that they suffer from some physical illness. To date, study of such populations suggests that 4–9% of individuals in general medical settings suffer from hypochondriasis.

It does appear that hypochondriasis is equally common in males and females. Data concerning socioeconomic class are conflicting.

Course

Data are conflicting, but it appears that the most common age at onset is in early adulthood. Available data suggest that approximately 25% of individuals with a diagnosis of hypochondriasis do poorly, 65% show a chronic but fluctuating course, and 10% recover. This pertains to the full syndrome. A much more variable course is seen in individuals with just some hypochondriacal concerns. It appears that acute onset, absence of a personality disorder, and absence of secondary gain are favorable prognostically.

Differential Diagnosis

As shown in Figure 34-1, the first step in approaching individuals with distressing or impairing preoccupation with or fears of having a serious disease is to exclude the possibility of explanation on the basis of a general medical condition. Fears that may seem excessive may also occur in individuals with general medical conditions with vague and subjective symptoms early in their disease course. These include neurological diseases, such as myasthenia gravis and multiple sclerosis, endocrine diseases, systemic diseases that affect several organ systems, such as systemic lupus erythematosus, and occult malignant neoplasms. The disease conviction of hypochondriasis may actually be less amenable to medical reassurance than the fears of individuals with general medical illnesses, who may at least temporally accept such encouragement. Hypochondriacal complaints are not often intentionally produced such that differentiation from malingering and factitious disorder is seldom a problem.

Exclusion is made if the preoccupation is better accounted for by another mental disorder. DSM-IV-TR lists generalized anxiety disorder, obsessive–compulsive disorder, panic disorder, a major depressive episode, separation anxiety, or another somatoform disorder as candidates. Chronology will be of utmost importance in such discriminations. Hypochondriacal concerns occurring exclusively during episodes of another disturbance, such as an anxiety or depressive disorder, do not warrant an additional diagnosis of hypochondriasis. The presence of symptoms of another mental disorder will also be helpful. For example, an individual with hypochondriacal complaints as part of a major depressive episode will show other symptoms of depression, such as sleep and appetite disturbance, feelings of worthlessness, and self-reproach, although depressed elderly individuals may deny sadness or other expressions of depressed mood. A confounding factor is that individuals with hypochondriasis often have comorbid anxiety or depressive syndromes. Again, characterizing the symptoms by chronology will be useful. Treatment trials may also have diagnostic significance. Depressed individuals who are hypochondriacal may respond to non-SSRI antidepressant medications or electroconvulsive therapy (often necessary to reverse a depressive state of sufficient severity to lead to such profound symptoms), with resolution of the hypochondriacal as well as the depressive symptoms.

Hypochondriasis is differentiated from other somatoform disorders such as pain, conversion, and somatization disorders by its predominant feature of preoccupation with and fears of having an underlying illness based on the misinterpretation of body symptoms, rather than the physical symptoms themselves. Individuals with these other somatoform disorders at times are concerned with the possibility of underlying illness, but this will generally be overshadowed by a focus on the symptoms themselves.

The next consideration is whether the belief is of delusional proportions. Individuals with hypochondriasis, although preoccupied, generally acknowledge the possibility that their concerns are unfounded. Delusional individuals do not. Somatic delusions of serious illness are seen in some cases of schizophrenia and in delusional disorder, somatic type. In general, individuals with schizophrenia who have such delusions also show other signs of schizophrenia, such as disorganized speech, peculiarities of thought and behavior, hallucinations, and other delusions. Belief that an underlying illness is being caused by some bizarre process may

also be seen (e.g., "I'm trying not to defecate because it will cause my brain to turn to jelly"). Schizophrenic individuals may also show improvement with neuroleptic treatment, at least in the "active" symptoms of their illness, under which somatic delusions are included.

Differentiation from delusional disorder, somatic type, may be more difficult. It is often a thin line between preoccupation and fear that is a conviction and that which is a delusion. Often, the distinction is made on the basis of whether the individual can consider the possibility that the conviction is erroneous. Yet, individuals with hypochondriasis vary in the extent to which they can do this. DSM-IV-TR acknowledges this by its inclusion of the specifier "with poor insight." In the past, some argued that differentiation could be made on the basis of response to neuroleptics, especially pimozide; individuals with delusional disorder, but not hypochondriasis, respond. Interestingly, there is at least one report of successful treatment of a syndrome corresponding to delusional disorder, somatic type, in a nondepressed individual with the SSRI paroxetine. As with hypochondriasis, response was obtained only when the dose was raised beyond an antidepressant dose (to 60 mg/day).

If it is concluded that the preoccupations are not delusional, the next consideration is whether the duration requirement of 6 months has been met (see Figure 34-1). Syndromes of less than 6 months' duration are diagnosed under either somatoform disorder NOS or adjustment disorder if the symptoms are an abnormal response to a stressful life event. The reason to make such a distinction is to distinguish hypochondriasis from transient syndromes, the longitudinal course of which have been shown to be more variable, suggesting heterogeneity.

Other diagnostic considerations include whether the preoccupations or fears are restricted to preoccupations with being overweight, as in anorexia nervosa; with the inappropriateness of one's sex characteristics, as in a gender identity disorder; or with defects in appearance, as in body dysmorphic disorder. The preoccupations of hypochondriasis resemble the obsessions, and the health checking and efforts to obtain reassurance resemble the compulsions of obsessive–compulsive disorder. However, if such manifestations are health centered only, obsessive–compulsive disorder is not diagnosed. If, on the other hand, nonhealth related obsessions and compulsions are present, obsessive–compulsive disorder may be diagnosed in addition to hypochondriasis.

TREATMENT

Individuals with hypochondriasis generally present initially to nonpsychiatric physicians and are often reluctant to see a mental health clinician. Referral should be done sensitively, with the referring physician stressing to the individual that his or her distress is real and that psychiatric evaluation will be a supplement to, not a replacement for, continued medical care.

Initially, the generic strategies outlined for somatoform disorders (see page 353) should be followed. However, it has not been demonstrated that a specific psychotherapy for hypochondriasis is particularly effective. Dynamic psychotherapy appears to be of minimal effectiveness; supportive–educative psychotherapy is only somewhat helpful and primarily for those with syndromes of less than 3 years' duration; and cognitive–behavioral therapy, especially response prevention of checking rituals and reassurance seeking, is of only moderate effectiveness at best. All of these techniques seem to lack definitive effects on hypochondriasis itself.

Until recently, this could be said of pharmacological approaches also. Pharmacotherapy of comorbid depressive or anxiety syndromes was often effective, and control of such syndromes aided in general management, yet hypochondriasis itself was not ameliorated. Although controlled trials are lacking, anecdotal and open-label studies suggest that serotoninergic agents such as clomipramine and the SSRI fluoxetine may be effective in ameliorating hypochondriasis. Similar effects are expected from the other SSRIs. Response to fluoxetine has been reported with doses recommended for obsessive–compulsive disorder, rather than usual antidepressant doses (i.e., 60–80 mg rather than 20–40 mg/day). Such pharmacotherapy is best combined with the generic psychotherapy recommendations for somatoform disorders, as well as with cognitive–behavioral techniques to disrupt the counterproductive checking and reassurance-seeking behaviors.

Body Dysmorphic Disorder

DIAGNOSIS

As defined in DSM-IV-TR, the essential feature of this disorder is preoccupation with an imagined defect in appearance or a markedly excessive concern with a minor anomaly. In body dysmorphic disorder, a person can be preoccupied with an imagined defect while she or he actually has some other anomaly and is not appearing normal. To exclude conditions with trivial or minor symptoms, the preoccupation must cause clinically significant distress or impairment. By definition, body dysmorphic disorder is not diagnosed if symp-

> **DSM-IV-TR Diagnostic Criteria**
>
> **300.7 BODY DYSMORPHIC DISORDER**
>
> A. Preoccupation with an imagined defect in appearance. If a slight physical anomaly is present, the person's concern is markedly excessive.
> B. The preoccupation causes clinically significant distress or impairment in social, occupational, or other important areas of functioning.
> C. The preoccupation is not better accounted for by another mental disorder (e.g., dissatisfaction with body shape and size in anorexia nervosa).
>
> Reprinted with permission from the *Diagnostic and Statistical Manual of Mental Disorders*, 4th ed., Text Rev. Copyright 2000 American Psychiatric Association.

toms are limited to preoccupation with body weight, as in anorexia nervosa or bulimia nervosa, or to perceived inappropriateness of sex characteristics, as in gender identity disorder.

Preoccupations most often involve the nose, ears, face, or sexual organs. Common complaints include a diversity of imagined flaws of the face or head, including defects in the hair (e.g., too much or too little), skin (e.g., blemishes), and shape or symmetry of the face or facial features (e.g., nose is too large and deformed). However, any body part may be the focus, including genitals, breasts, buttocks, extremities, shoulders, and even overall body size.

In terms of its relationship to the psychotic disorders, a continuum exists from clearly nondelusional preoccupations to unequivocal delusions such that defining a discrete boundary between the two ends of the spectrum would be artificial. Furthermore, some individuals seem to move back and forth along this continuum. Perhaps as a reflection of the state of knowledge at this point, both body dysmorphic disorder and delusional disorder, somatic type, can be diagnosed on the basis of the same symptoms, in the same individual, at the same time. Thus, the definition of body dysmorphic disorder differs from hypochondriasis, which is not diagnosed if hypochondriacal concerns are determined to be delusional.

Individuals with body dysmorphic disorder generally first present to nonpsychiatric physicians such as plastic surgeons, dermatologists, and internists because of the nature of their complaints and are not seen psychiatrically until they are referred. Many resist or refuse referral because they do not see their problem as psychiatric; thus, study of psychiatric clinic populations may underestimate the prevalence of the disorder. It has been estimated that 2% of individuals seeking corrective cosmetic surgery suffer from this disorder. Although women outnumber men in this population, it is not known whether this sex distribution holds true in the general population.

Course

Age at onset appears to peak in adolescence or early adulthood. Body dysmorphic disorder is generally a chronic condition, with a waxing and waning of intensity but rarely full remission. In a lifetime, multiple preoccupations are typical; in one study, the average was four. In some, the same preoccupation remains unchanged. In others, new perceived defects are added to the original ones. In still others, symptoms remit, only to be replaced by others. The disorder is often highly incapacitating, with many individuals showing marked impairment in social and occupational activities. Perhaps a third becomes housebound. Most attribute their limitations to embarrassment concerning their perceived defect, but the attention and time-consuming nature of the preoccupations and attempts to investigate and rectify defects also contribute. The extent to which individuals with body dysmorphic disorder receive surgery or medical treatments is unknown. Superimposed depressive episodes are common, as are suicidal ideation and suicide attempts. Actual suicide risk is unknown.

In view of the nature of the defects with which individuals are preoccupied, it is not surprising that they are found most commonly among individuals seeking cosmetic surgery. Preoccupations persist despite reassurance that there is no defect to surgically correct. Surgery or other corrective procedures rarely if ever lead to satisfaction and may even lead to greater distress with the perception of new defects attributed to the surgery.

Differential Diagnosis

The preoccupations of body dysmorphic disorder must first be differentiated from usual concerns with grooming and appearance. Attention to appearance and grooming is universal and socially sanctioned. However, diagnosis of body dysmorphic disorder requires that the preoccupation cause clinically significant distress or impairment. In addition, in body dysmorphic disorder, concerns focus on an imaginary or exaggerated defect, often of something, such as a small blemish, that would warrant scant attention even if it were present. Persons with histrionic personality disorder may be vain and excessively concerned with appearance. However, the focus in this disorder is on maintaining a good or even exceptional appearance, rather than preoccupation with a defect. Such concerns are probably unrelated to body dysmorphic disorder. In addition, by nature, the preoccupations in body dysmorphic disorder are essentially

unamenable to reassurance from friends or family or consultation with physicians, cosmetologists, or other professionals.

Next, the possibility of an explanation by a general medical condition must be considered (see Figure 34-1). As mentioned, individuals with this disorder often first present to plastic surgeons, oral surgeons, and others, seeking correction of defects. By the time a mental health professional is consulted, it has generally been ascertained that there is no physical basis for the degree of concern. As with other syndromes involving somatic preoccupations (or delusions), such as olfactory reference syndrome and delusional parasitosis (both included under delusional disorder, somatic type), occult medical disorders, such as an endocrine disturbance or a brain tumor, must be excluded.

In terms of explanation on the basis of another mental disorder, there is little likelihood that symptoms of body dysmorphic disorder will be intentionally produced as in malingering or factitious disorder. Unlike in other somatoform disorders, such as pain, conversion, and somatization disorders, preoccupation with appearance predominates. Somatic preoccupations may occur as part of an anxiety or mood disorder. However, these preoccupations are generally not the predominant focus and lack the specificity of dysmorphic symptoms. Because individuals with body dysmorphic disorder often become isolative, social phobia may be suspected. However, in social phobia, the person may feel self-conscious generally but will not focus on a specific imagined defect. Indeed, the two conditions may coexist, warranting both diagnoses. Diagnostic problems may present with the mood-congruent ruminations of major depression, which sometimes involve concern with an unattractive appearance in association with poor self-esteem. Such preoccupations generally lack the focus on a particular body part that is seen in body dysmorphic disorder. On the other hand, individuals with body dysmorphic disorder commonly have dysphoric affects described by them variously as anxiety or depression. In some cases, these affects can be subsumed under body dysmorphic disorder; but in other instances, comorbid diagnoses of anxiety or mood disorders are warranted.

Differentiation from schizophrenia must also be made. At times, a dysmorphic concern will seem so unusual that such a psychosis may be considered. Furthermore, individuals with this disorder may show ideas of reference in regard to defects in their appearance, which may lead to the consideration of schizophrenia. However, other bizarre delusions, particularly of persecution or grandiosity, and prominent hallucinations are not seen in body dysmorphic disorder. From the other perspective, schizophrenia with somatic delusions generally lacks the focus on a particular body part and defect. Also in schizophrenia, bizarre interpretations and explanations for symptoms are often present, such as "this blemish was a sign from Jesus that I am to protect the world from Satan." Other signs of schizophrenia, such as hallucinations and disorganization of thought, are also absent in body dysmorphic disorder. As previously mentioned, the preoccupations in body dysmorphic disorder appear to be on a continuum from full insight to delusional intensity whereby the individual cannot even consider the possibility that the preoccupation is groundless. In such instances, both body dysmorphic disorder and delusional disorder, somatic type, are to be diagnosed.

Body dysmorphic disorder is not to be diagnosed if the concern with appearance is better accounted for by another mental disorder. Anorexia nervosa, in which there is dissatisfaction with body shape and size, is specifically mentioned in the criteria as an example of such an exclusion. Although not specifically mentioned in DSM-IV-TR, if a preoccupation is limited to discomfort or a sense of inappropriateness of one's primary and secondary sex characteristics, coupled with a strong and persistent cross-gender identification, body dysmorphic disorder is not diagnosed.

The preoccupations of body dysmorphic disorder may resemble obsessions and ruminations as seen in obsessive–compulsive disorder. Unlike the obsessions of obsessive–compulsive disorder, the preoccupations of body dysmorphic disorder focus on concerns with appearance. Compulsions are limited to checking and investigating the perceived physical defect and attempting to obtain reassurance from others regarding it. Still, the phenomenology is similar, and the two disorders are often comorbid. If additional obsessions and compulsions not related to the defect are present, obsessive–compulsive disorder can be diagnosed in addition to body dysmorphic disorder.

TREATMENT

First, the generic treatment strategies outlined for the somatoform disorders overall (see page 353) should be instituted. These are beneficial in interrupting an unending procession of repeated evaluations and the possibility of needless surgery, which may lead to additional perceptions that surgery has resulted in further disfigurement.

Traditional insight-oriented therapies have not generally proved to be effective. Results with traditional behavioral techniques, such as systematic desensitization and exposure therapy, have been mixed. At least without amelioration with effective pharmacotherapy,

the preoccupations do not extinguish as would be expected with phobias. A cognitive–behavioral approach similar to what was recommended for hypochondriasis may be more effective. This includes response prevention techniques whereby the individual is not permitted to repetitively check the perceived defect in mirrors. In addition, individuals are advised not to seek reassurance from family and friends, and these persons are instructed not to respond to such inquiries. Some individuals adopt such behaviors spontaneously, avoiding mirrors and other reflecting surfaces, refusing even to allude to their perceived defects to others. Such "self-techniques" may be encouraged and refined.

Biological treatments have long been used but until recently were of limited benefit to individuals with body dysmorphic disorder. Approaches have included electroconvulsive therapy, tricyclic and MAOI antidepressants, and neuroleptics (particularly pimozide). In most reports of positive response to tricyclic or MAOI antidepressant drugs, it is unclear whether response was truly in terms of the dysmorphic syndrome or simply represented improvement in comorbid depressive or anxiety syndromes. Response to neuroleptic treatment has been suggested as a diagnostic test to distinguish body dysmorphic disorder from delusional disorder, somatic type. The delusional syndromes often respond to neuroleptics; body dysmorphic disorders, even when the body preoccupations are psychotic, generally do not. Pimozide has been singled out as a neuroleptic with specific effectiveness for somatic delusions, but this specificity does not appear to apply to body dysmorphic disorder.

An exception to this uninspiring picture is the observation of a possible preferential response to antidepressant drugs with serotonin reuptake blocking effects, such as clomipramine, or SSRIs, such as fluoxetine and fluvoxamine. It has been reported that more than 50% of individuals with body dysmorphic disorder showed a partial or complete remission with either clomipramine or fluoxetine, a response not predicted on the basis of coexisting major depressive or obsessive–compulsive disorder. As with hypochondriasis, effectiveness is generally achieved at levels recommended for obsessive–compulsive disorder rather than for depression (e.g., 60–80 mg rather than 20–40 mg/day of fluoxetine). The SSRIs appear to ameliorate delusional as well as nondelusional dysmorphic preoccupations. Successful augmentation of clomipramine or SSRI therapy has been suggested with buspirone, another drug with serotoninergic effects. Neuroleptics, particularly pimozide, may also be helpful adjuncts, particularly if delusions of reference are present. Little seems to be gained with the addition of anticonvulsants or benzodiazepines to the SSRI therapy.

Somatoform Disorder Not Otherwise Specified

Somatoform disorder NOS is the true residual category for this diagnostic class. By definition, disorders considered under this category are characterized by somatic symptoms, but criteria for any of the specific somatoform disorders are not met. Several examples are given, but syndromes potentially included under this category are not limited to these. Unlike for undifferentiated somatoform disorder, no minimal duration is required. DSM-IV-TR lists as examples pseudocyesis, disorders involving hypochondriacal complaints but of less than 6 months' duration, and disorders involving unexplained physical complaints, such as fatigue or body weakness not due to another mental disorder and again of less than 6 months' duration. This last syndrome would seem to resemble neurasthenia of short duration, a syndrome with a long historical tradition with inclusion in DSM-II, ICD-9, and ICD-10. Neurasthenia was considered for inclusion as a separate DSM-IV somatoform disorder but was not included because of difficulties in delineating it from depressive and anxiety disorders and from other somatoform disorders. If included, neurasthenia could have become a clinical "wastebasket" that could facilitate premature closure of diagnostic inquiry, such that underlying general medical conditions as well as other mental disorders would more likely be overlooked.

Inclusion of pseudocyesis as an example of Somatoform Disorder NOS deserves special mention. This syndrome was included in DSM-III and DSM-III-R as an example of a conversion symptom under the broadened definition of conversion, on the basis that it represented a somatic expression of a psychological conflict or need, in this case involving ambivalence toward pregnancy. The resulting conflict was resolved somatically as a false pregnancy, lessening anxiety (primary gain) and leading to unconsciously needed environmental support (secondary gain). With the restriction of conversion in DSM-IV to include only symptoms affecting voluntary motor and sensory function, pseudocyesis was excluded from the conversion disorder definition. In a sense, it is placed in the somatoform disorder NOS category for lack of a more appropriate place. It could also be described as a psychophysiological endocrine disorder since, in many cases, a neuroendocrine change accompanies and at times may antedate the false belief of pregnancy. However, in most instances, a discrete general medical condition (such as a hormone-secreting tumor) cannot be identified.

COMPARISON OF DSM-IV-TR AND ICD-10 DIAGNOSTIC CRITERIA

The ICD-10 Diagnostic Criteria for Research for Somatization Disorder have both a different item set and algorithm. Six symptoms are required out of a list of fourteen symptoms, which are broken down into the following groups: six gastrointestinal symptoms, two cardiovascular symptoms, three genitourinary symptoms, and three "skin and pain" symptoms. It is specified that the symptoms occur in at least two groups. In contrast, DSM-IV-TR requires four pain symptoms, two gastrointestinal symptoms, one sexual symptom, and one pseudoneurological symptom. Furthermore, the ICD-10 Diagnostic Criteria for Research specify that there must be "persistent refusal to accept medical reassurance that there is no adequate physical cause for the physical symptoms." DSM-IV-TR only requires that the symptoms result in treatment being sought or significant impairment in social, occupational, or other important areas of functioning and that the symptoms cannot be fully explained by a known general medical condition or substance. For Undifferentiated Somatoform Disorder, the ICD-10 Diagnostic Criteria for Research and the DSM-IV-TR criteria are almost identical.

Regarding conversion disorder, ICD-10 considers conversion a type of dissociative disorder and includes separate criteria sets for dissociative motor disorders, dissociative convulsions, and dissociative anesthesia and sensory loss in a section that also includes dissociative amnesia and dissociative fugue.

For pain disorder, the ICD-10 Diagnostic Criteria for Research require that the pain last at least 6 months and that it not be "explained adequately by evidence of a physiological process or a physical disorder." In contrast, DSM-IV-TR does not force the clinician to make this inherently impossible judgment and instead requires the contribution of psychological factors. Furthermore, DSM-IV-TR includes both acute (duration less than 6 months) and chronic pain (more than 6 months). This disorder is referred to in ICD-10 as "Persistent Somatoform Pain Disorder."

ICD-10 provides a single criteria set that applies to both the DSM-IV-TR categories of hypochondriasis and body dysmorphic disorder. The ICD-10 Diagnostic Criteria for Research for Hypochondriasis specify that the belief is of a "maximum of two serious physical diseases" and requires that at least one be specifically named by the individual with the disorder. The DSM-IV-TR has no such requirement.

35   Factitious Disorders

DIAGNOSIS

An individual with a factitious disorder consciously induces or feigns illness in order to obtain a psychological benefit by being in the sick role. It is the conscious awareness of the production of symptoms that differentiates factitious disorder from the somatoform disorders in which the individual unconsciously produces symptoms for an unconscious psychological benefit. It is the underlying motivation to produce symptoms that separates factitious disorders from malingering. Individuals who malinger consciously feign or induce illness in order to obtain some external benefit such as money, narcotics, or excuse from duties. While the distinctions among these disorders appear satisfyingly clear, in practice, individuals often blur the boundaries. Individuals with somatoform disorders will sometimes consciously exaggerate symptoms that they have unconsciously produced, and it is a rare individual who consciously creates illness and yet receives no external gain at all, be it disability benefits, excuse from work, or even food and shelter.

Individuals with factitious disorders seek, often desperately, the sick role. They usually have little insight into the motivations of their behaviors but are still powerfully driven to appear ill to others. In many cases, they endanger their own health and life in search of this role. Individuals with this disorder will often induce serious illness or undergo numerous unnecessary, invasive procedures. As most people avoid sickness, the actions of these individuals appear to run counter to human nature. Also, since entry into the "sick role" requires that the sick person should try to get better, individuals with factitious disorders must conceal the voluntary origin of their symptoms. The inexplicability of their actions combined with their deceptive behavior stir up both intense interest and intense (usually negative) countertransference in health care providers.

While physicians have known about the feigning of illness since the time of ancient Greece, it is likely that Richard Asher's 1951 article in *Lancet* brought the concept of factitious illness into general medical knowledge. Asher coined the term *Munchausen's syndrome*

referring to the Baron von Munchausen, a character in German literature who was known for greatly exaggerating the tales of his exploits. Asher described Munchausen's syndrome as a severe, chronic factitious disorder combined with antisocial behavior including wandering from hospital to hospital (peregrination). However, his memorable term has often been used interchangeably with "factitious disorder" and incorrectly applied to individuals with less severe forms of the disease.

Individuals have been known to create or feign numerous illnesses, both acute and chronic, in all of the medical specialties. These illnesses can be either physical or psychological. It appears that the only limit is the creativity and knowledge of a given individual. Individuals with a factitious disorder are often quite medically sophisticated. Even though acquired immune deficiency syndrome was not described until the early 1980s, the first factitious cases followed shortly thereafter, at least as early as 1986.

For a diagnosis of factitious disorder (see DSM-IV-TR diagnostic criteria, page 369) to be justified, a person must be intentionally producing an illness; his or her motivation is to occupy the sick role, and there must not be external incentives for the behavior. The diagnosis is further subclassified, depending on whether the factitious symptoms are predominantly physical, psychological, or a combination of both. Individuals who readily admit to inducing symptoms, such as self-mutilating individuals, are not diagnosed with factitious disorder as they are not using their symptoms to occupy the sick role.

Individuals with Factitious Disorder with Predominantly Physical Signs and Symptoms present with physical signs and symptoms. The three main methods that individuals use to create illness are (1) giving a false history, (2) faking clinical and laboratory findings, and (3) inducing illness (e.g., by surreptitious medication use, inducing infection, or preventing wound healing). There are reports of factitious illnesses in all of the medical specialties. Particularly common presentations include fever, self-induced infection, gastrointestinal symptoms, impaired wound healing, cancer, renal disease (especially hematuria and nephrolithiasis), endocrine diseases, anemia, bleeding disorders, and epilepsy. True Munchausen's syndrome fits within this subclass and is the most severe form of the illness. According to the DSM-IV-TR, individuals with Munchausen's syndrome have a chronic factitious disorder with physical signs and symptoms, and in addition, have a history of recurrent hospitalization, peregrination, and *pseudologia fantastica*—dramatic, untrue, and extremely improbable tales of their past experiences.

Another subtype of factitious disorder includes individuals who present feigning psychological illness. They both report and mimic psychiatric symptoms. These individuals can be particularly difficult to diagnose as psychiatric diagnosis depends greatly on the individual's report. There are reports of factitious psychosis, posttraumatic stress disorder, and bereavement. In addition, there are reports of psychological distress due to false claims of being a victim of stalking, rape, or sexual harassment, and these cases are often diagnosed with a factitious psychological disorder such as posttraumatic stress disorder. While individuals with factitious psychological symptoms feign psychiatric illness, they also often suffer from true comorbid psychiatric disorders, particularly Axis II disorders and substance abuse. Case reports suggest that individuals with psychological factitious disorder have a high rate of suicide and a poor prognosis. While Munchausen's syndrome is considered a subset of physical factitious disorder, there are case reports of individuals presenting with

psychological symptoms who also have some of the key features of Munchausen's (pathological lying, wandering, and recurrent hospitalizations).

Numerous reports in the literature describe two different subclasses of factitious individuals. The first type fits with the classic Munchausen's syndrome diagnosis: they have chronic factitious symptoms associated with antisocial traits, pathological lying, minimal social supports, wandering from hospital to hospital, and very poor work and relationship functioning. They are often very familiar with hospital procedure and use this knowledge to present dramatically during off-hours or at house-officer transition times when the factitious nature of their symptoms is least likely to be discovered. Males comprise the majority of these cases. Individuals with Munchausen's syndrome appear to have an extremely poor prognosis. Fortunately, this most severe class of individuals makes up the minority of factitious individuals, probably fewer than 10%.

The second, and more typical, type of individual does not display pathological lying or wandering. Their recurrent presentations are usually within the same community, and they become well-known within the local health care system. They often have stable social supports and employment, and a history of a medically related job. This larger class of factitious individuals is mostly made up of women, and is more likely to accept psychiatric treatment and to show improvement. Finally, there are individuals who may have an episode of factitious disorder in reaction to a life stressor, but may return to premorbid functioning after the stressor is resolved.

All types of factitious disease show a strong association with substance abuse, as well as borderline and narcissistic personality disorders. Factitious individuals span a broad age range. Reports in the literature show individuals ranging from 4 to 85 years.

The diagnosis of factitious disorder is made in several ways (see Figure 35-1). Factitious disorder is occasionally diagnosed accidentally when the individual is discovered in the act of creating symptoms. A history of inconsistent or unexplainable signs and symptoms or failure to respond to appropriate treatment can prompt health care providers to probe for evidence of the disorder, as can evidence of peregrination or pathological lying. In some cases, it is a diagnosis of exclusion in an otherwise inexplicable case.

If there is suspicion of a factitious disorder, confirmation can be difficult. Laboratory examination can confirm some factitious diagnoses such as exogenous insulin or thyroid hormone administration. Collateral information from family members or previous health care providers can also be extremely helpful. Factitious disorder with psychological signs and symptoms can be

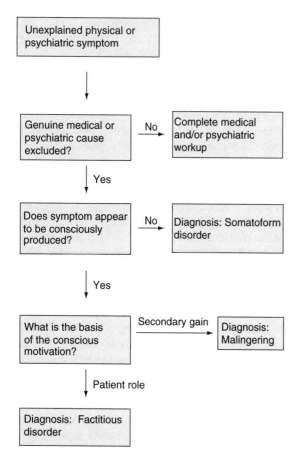

Figure 35-1 *Diagnostic decision tree for factitious disorder.*

particularly difficult to diagnose, as so much of psychiatric diagnosis relies on the individual's report.

The course of untreated factitious disorder is variable. While individuals with factitious disorder commonly suffer a great deal of morbidity, fatal cases appear to be less common. One survey of 41 cases noted only one fatality, though many of the other cases were life-threatening. However, individuals with psychological signs and symptoms are reported to have a high rate of suicide and a poor prognosis.

In factitious disorder by proxy, one person creates or feigns illness in another person, usually a child, though occasionally the victim is an elder or developmentally delayed adult. The veterinary literature even reports cases of factitious disorder by proxy in which the victim is a pet. Factitious disorder by proxy is not defined as a specific disorder in DSM-IV-TR, but instead is listed under the "not otherwise specified" heading with research criteria included. While rare instances of fathers perpetrating factitious disorder by proxy have been reported, the perpetrator is usually the mother.

Usually, the victim is a preverbal child. While numerous symptoms have been reported, common presentations include apnea, seizures, and gastrointestinal problems. The mothers appear extremely caring and attentive when observed, but appear indifferent to the child when they are not aware of being observed.

The diagnosis of factitious disorder by proxy is usually made by having an index of suspicion in a child with unexplained illnesses. The diagnosis is supported if symptoms occur only in the parent's presence and resolve with separation. Covert video surveillance has been used to diagnose this condition, though it raises questions of invasion of privacy. In general, it has been felt that the welfare of the child overrides the parent's right to privacy.

As counterintuitive as it is to comprehend why anyone would induce illness in oneself, it can be even more difficult to understand inducing illness in one's own child. The perpetrator in factitious disorder by proxy appears to seek not the "sick role" but the "parent to the sick child" role. This role is similar to the sick role in that it provides structure, attention from others, caring, and relief from usual responsibilities. The parent also receives some psychological benefit from inducing illness in his or her child. On the basis of case reports, the parent often has a comorbid personality disorder and a history of family dysfunction.

The nature of factitious disorder makes it difficult to determine how common it is within the population. Individuals attempt to conceal themselves, thereby artificially lowering the prevalence. The tendency of individuals to present themselves several times at different facilities, however, may artificially raise the prevalence. Most estimates of the prevalence of the disease, therefore, rely on the number of factitious individuals within a given inpatient population. Such attempts have generated estimates that 0.5–3% of medical and psychiatric inpatients suffer from factitious disorder. There are few data about the prevalence of factitious disorder in an outpatient population. Because factitious individuals do not readily identify themselves in large community surveys, it is not currently possible to determine the prevalence of the disorder in the general population. As in factitious disorder, the exact prevalence of factitious disorder by proxy is unknown. Factitious disorder by proxy appears to have a much higher mortality rate than self-inflicted factitious disorder.

Differential Diagnosis

The differential diagnosis of factitious disorder includes rare or complex physical illness, somatoform disorders, malingering, other psychiatric disorders, and substance abuse. It is especially important to rule out genuine physical illness since individuals with a factitious disorder often induce real physical illness. Furthermore, it is always important to remember that individuals with factitious disorders are certainly not immune to the physical illnesses that plague the general population.

TREATMENT

The goals in treating individuals with a factitious disorder are twofold; first to minimize the damage done by the disorder to both the individual's own health and the health care system. The second goal is to help individuals recover, at least partially, from the disorder. These goals are furthered by treating comorbid medical illnesses, avoiding unnecessary procedures, encouraging individuals to seek psychiatric treatment, and providing support for health care clinicians. Because the literature is based exclusively on case reports and series, determining treatment effectiveness is difficult. As mentioned before, individuals with true Munchausen's syndrome (including antisocial traits, pathological lying, wandering, and poor social support) are felt to be refractory to treatment. While factitious disorder is extremely difficult to cure, effective techniques exist to minimize morbidity, and some individuals are able to benefit greatly from psychiatric intervention.

Soon after Asher's 1951 article was published, many individuals with a factitious disorder were vigorously confronted once the nature of their illness was discovered. Unfortunately, most individuals would deny their involvement and seek another clinician who was unaware of their diagnosis. In addition, the idea of "blacklists" was proposed in order to aid detection of these individuals. However, issues regarding an individual's confidentiality as well as concerns about cursory medical evaluations that might miss genuine physical illness prevented this idea from being adopted. Although aggressive confrontation is usually unsuccessful, supportive, nonpunitive confrontation may be helpful for some. In one case series, 33 individuals were confronted with the factitious nature of their illness. While only 13 admitted feigning illness, most of the individuals' illnesses subsequently improved, at least in the short term.

Three alternatives to confrontation have been found to be effective. First is inexact interpretation, in which the clinician interprets the psychodynamics thought to be underlying the individual's behavior without explicitly identifying the factitious behavior. For example, a consultant suggested to an individual suspected of having factitious disorder who developed septicemia after

her boyfriend proposed marriage that she might feel a need to punish herself when good things happened to her. She agreed, and soon after, admitted that she had injected a contaminant intravenously. The second technique is the therapeutic double-bind. The clinician presents the individual with a new medical intervention to treat his or her illness. The individual is told that one possibility is that the individual's illness has a factitious origin, and that, if so, the treatment would not be expected to work while, if the illness is biological, the treatment will work and the individual will improve. The individual must decide to give up the factitious illness or admit it. A third technique is to provide the individual with a face-saving way, such as hypnosis or biofeedback, of giving up his or her symptoms without admitting that they are not genuine. In emergent situations, however, there may not be time for nonconfrontational techniques, and more directly confrontational means may be necessary.

Another important component in the treatment of individuals with factitious disorder is the coordination of health care among all clinicians. This allows for fewer unnecessary interventions, minimizes splitting among the health care team, and allows the health care team to vent and process the strong emotions that arise when caring for factitious individuals. This decreases both the negative impact on the clinicians and the chance that anger will be acted out on the individual.

While many individuals with factitious disorder are hesitant to pursue mental health treatment, there are numerous case reports of successful treatment of the disorder with long-term psychotherapy. In many of these cases, the therapy lasted several years, including one individual who received treatment while imprisoned for over 10 years. These case reports support the idea that treatment of individuals with factitious disorder is not impossible, and these individuals can improve. However, expectations must be realistic as improvement in the disorder itself can take several years. Techniques that target short-term reduction in the production of factitious symptoms can be effective more quickly. See Figure 35-2 for a treatment flowchart for factitious disorder.

Treating individuals with factitious disorder often raises ethical questions including those regarding confidentiality, privacy, and medical decision-making, and it is important to be alert to these issues. Often, individuals with factious disorder will want to keep their diagnosis confidential, even when to do so may harm the individual or others. For example, although a consulting clinician may diagnose an individual with factitious disorder, the individual may refuse consent to reveal this information to the referring physician. If the

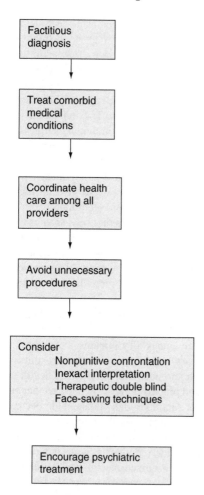

Figure 35-2 *Treatment flowchart for factitious disorder.*

regarding the individual's privacy also arise with factitious individuals. For example, hospital room searches could often help clarify the diagnosis or remove materials the individual is using to harm himself, but these searches also violate the individual's privacy. Dilemmas surrounding medical decision-making can arise when an individual with factitious disorder refuses treatment or requests potentially harmful treatments. It can often be difficult to resolve these ethical dilemmas. In general, even though the factitious individual is deceptive within the relationship between the clinician and the individual, the clinician is not released from his or her responsibilities within that relationship, and the individual retains his or her rights of confidentiality, privacy, and autonomy. As with all such individuals, emergency situations require different ethical guidelines. Often, an ethics consultation can be very helpful in sorting through the difficult issues of care of the individual in the setting of factitious disorder.

Owing to the high morbidity and mortality, treatment of Factitious Disorder By Proxy requires at least temporary separation from the parent and notification of local child protective agencies. The perpetrators often face criminal charges of child abuse. There is high psychiatric morbidity in the children—many go on to develop factitious disorder or other psychiatric illnesses themselves. Psychiatric intervention is necessary to ameliorate this morbidity as much as possible in these children. In this disorder, there are some case reports of successful psychotherapeutic treatments of the parents.

consultant does inform the referring physician, she has violated the individual's confidentiality, but if she does not, the referring physician is likely to continue to treat the individual for the incorrect diagnosis. Dilemmas

COMPARISON OF DSM-IV AND ICD-10 DIAGNOSTIC CRITERIA

The ICD-10 Diagnostic Criteria for Research and the DSM-IV-TR criteria sets are almost identical.

36 Dissociative Disorders

Dissociative phenomena are best understood through the term *désagrégation* (disaggregation) originally given by Janet in 1920. Events normally experienced as connected to one another on a smooth continuum are isolated from the other mental processes with which they would ordinarily be associated. The dissociative disorders are a disturbance in the organization of identity, memory, perception, or consciousness. When memories are separated from access to consciousness, the disorder is dissociative amnesia. Fragmentation of identity results in dissociative fugue or dissociative identity disorder (DID; formerly multiple personality disorder). Disintegrated perception is characteristic of depersonalization disorder. Dissociation of aspects of consciousness produces acute stress disorder and various dissociative trance and possession states. Numbing and amnesia are diagnostic components of posttraumatic stress disorder (PTSD), both of which are described in Chapter 32. These dissociative and related disorders are more a disturbance in the organization or structure of mental contents than in the contents themselves. Memories in dissociative amnesia are not so much distorted or bizarre as they are segregated from one another. The identities lost in dissociative fugue or fragmented in DID are two-dimensional aspects of an overall personality structure. In this sense, individuals with DID suffer not from having more than one personality but rather from having less than one personality. The problem involves information processing: the failure of integration of elements rather than the contents of the fragments.

Dissociative Amnesia

DIAGNOSIS

This is the classical functional disorder of episodic memory. It does not involve procedural memory or problems in memory storage, as in Wernicke–Korsakoff syndrome. Furthermore, unlike dementing illnesses, dissociative amnesia is reversible, for example, by using hypnosis or narcoanalysis. It has three primary characteristics: first, the memory loss is episodic, with first-person recollection of certain events, rather than knowledge of procedures, being lost. Second, the memory loss is for one or more discrete time periods, ranging from minutes to years. It is not vagueness or inefficient retrieval of memories but rather a dense unavailability of memories that were encoded and stored. Unlike the situation in amnestic disorders, for example, resulting from damage to the medial temporal lobe in surgery there is usually no difficulty in learning new episodic information. Thus, the amnesia of dissociative disorders is typically retrograde rather than anterograde. Third, the memory loss is usually for events of a traumatic or stressful nature. Although the majority of cases involved child abuse (60%) in one study, disavowed behaviors such as marital problems, sexual activity, suicide attempts, criminal activity, and the death of a relative have also been reported as precipitants.

Dissociative amnesia most frequently occurs after an episode of trauma, and its onset may be gradual or sudden. It occurs most often in the third and fourth decades of life. Although it usually involves one episode, multiple periods of lost memory are not uncommon.

Individuals with dissociative amnesia may not initially be aware of the memory loss; that is, they do not remember that they do not remember. They often report being told that they have done or said things that they cannot remember. Some individuals do suffer from episodes of selective amnesia, usually for specific traumatic incidents, which may be interwoven with periods of intact memory. In these cases, the amnesia is for a type of material remembered rather than for a discrete time period.

Although information is kept out of consciousness in dissociative amnesia, it may well exert an influence on consciousness: out of sight does not mean out of mind. For example, a rape victim with no conscious recollection of an assault nonetheless behaves like someone who has been sexually victimized. Such individuals often suffer detachment and demoralization, are unable to enjoy intimate relationships, and show hyperarousal to stimuli reminiscent of the trauma.

Individuals with dissociative amnesia generally do not suffer disturbances of identity, except to the extent that their identity is influenced by the warded-off memory. It is not uncommon for such individuals to develop depressive symptoms as well, especially when the amnesia occurs in the wake of a traumatic stressor. Comorbidity with conversion disorder, bulimia nervosa, and alcohol abuse are also common, and Axis II diagnoses of histrionic, dependent, or borderline personality disorders occur in a substantial minority of such individuals.

TREATMENT

Often, individuals suffering from dissociative amnesia experience spontaneous recovery when they are removed from the stressful or threatening situation, when they feel safe, and/or when exposed to personal cues from their past (i.e., home, pets, family members). For cases in which exposure to a safe environment is not enough to restore normal memory functioning, pharmacologically facilitated interviews may prove useful.

Most individuals with dissociative disorders are highly hypnotizable on formal testing and are therefore easily able to make use of hypnotic techniques such as age regression. Hypnosis can enable such individuals to reorient temporally and therefore achieve access to otherwise dissociated and unavailable memories.

If there is traumatic content to the warded-off memory, individuals may abreact, that is, express strong emotion as these memories are elicited. Such abreactions are rarely damaging in themselves but are not intrinsically therapeutic either. They may be experienced by the individual as a reinflicting of the traumatic stressor. Such individuals need psychotherapeutic help in integrating these warded-off memories and the associated affect into consciousness, thereby gaining a sense of mastery over them.

One technique that can help bring such memories into consciousness while modulating the affective response to them is a projective technique known as "the screen technique." While using hypnosis, such individuals are taught to recall the traumatic event as if they were watching it on an imaginary movie or television screen. This technique is often helpful for individuals who are unable to remember the event as if it were occurring in the present, either because for some highly hypnotizable individuals that approach is too emotionally taxing or because others are not sufficiently hypnotizable to be able to engage in such hypnotic age regression.

The screen can be employed to facilitate cognitive restructuring of the traumatic memory, for example, by picturing on the left side of the screen some component of the traumatic experience, and on the right side something they did to protect themselves or someone else during it. This makes the memory both more complex and more bearable.

A particularly useful feature of this technique is that it allows for the recollection of traumatic events without triggering an uncontrolled reliving of the trauma, as is the case of traumatic flashbacks. The screen technique provides a "controlled dissociation" between the psychological and somatic aspects of memory retrieval. Individuals can be put into self-hypnosis and instructed to get their body into a state of floating comfort and safety. They can do this by imagining that they are somewhere safe and comfortable: "Imagine that you are floating in a bath, a lake, a hot tub, or just floating in space." They are reminded that no matter what they see on the screen their bodies are safe and comfortable: "Do the work on your imaginary screen, not in your body." In this way, the tendency for physiological arousal to accompany and intensify the working through of traumatic memories can be controlled, facilitating the psychotherapeutic work.

The psychotherapy of dissociative amnesia involves accessing the dissociated memories, working through affectively loaded aspects of these memories, and supporting the individual through the process of integrating these memories into consciousness.

Dissociative Fugue

DIAGNOSIS

Dissociative fugue combines failure of integration of certain aspects of personal memory with loss of customary identity and automatisms of motor behavior. It involves one or more episodes of sudden, unexpected, purposeful travel away from home, coupled with an inability to recall portions or all of one's past, and a loss of identity or the assumption of a new identity. The onset is usually sudden, and it frequently occurs after a traumatic experience or bereavement. A single episode is not uncommon, and spontaneous remission of symptoms can occur without treatment. It was originally thought that the assumption of a new identity was typical of dissociative fugue. However, in the majority of cases there is loss of personal identity but no clear assumption of a new identity.

Many cases of dissociative fugue remit spontaneously. Again, hypnosis can be useful in accessing dissociated material. Not infrequently, fugue episodes represent dissociated but purposeful activity.

TREATMENT

Hypnosis can be helpful in treating dissociative fugue by accessing otherwise unavailable components of memory and identity. The approach used is similar to that for dissociative amnesia. Hypnotic age regression can be used as the framework for accessing information available at a previous time. Demonstrating to individuals that such information can be made available to consciousness enhances their sense of control over this material and facilitates therapeutic working through of emotionally laden aspects of it.

Once reorientation is established and the overt identity and memory loss of the fugue have been resolved, it is important to work through interpersonal or intrapsychic issues that underlie the dissociative defenses. Such individuals are often relatively unaware of their reactions to stress because they can so effectively dissociate them. Thus, effective psychotherapy is anticipatory, helping individuals to recognize and modify their tendency to set aside their own feelings in favor of those of others. Individuals with dissociative fugue may be helped with a psychotherapeutic approach that facilitates conscious integration of dissociated memories and motivations for behavior previously experienced as automatic and unwilled. It is often helpful to address current psychosocial stressors, such as marital conflict, with the involved individuals. To the extent that current psychosocial stress triggers fugue, resolution of that stress can help resolve it and reduce the likelihood of recurrence. Highly hypnotizable individuals prone to these extreme dissociative symptoms often have great difficulty in asserting their own point of view in a personal relationship. Rather, they interact with others as though they were undergoing a spontaneous trance experience. One such individual described herself as a "disciple in search of a teacher." Psychotherapy can help such individuals recognize and modify their tendency to unthinking compliance with others, and extreme sensitivity to rejection and disapproval.

In the past, medication-facilitated interviews were used to reverse dissociative amnesia or fugue. However, such techniques offer no advantage over hypnosis and are not especially effective. Not infrequently, the ceremony of injecting the drug elicits spontaneous hypnotic phenomena before the pharmacological effect is felt, and sedation, respiratory depression, and other side effects can be troublesome. It also promotes dependency on the therapist. On the contrary, when hyp-

nosis is used, individuals are trained on self-hypnotic techniques, promoting the use of hypnosis instead of spontaneous dissociation. This enhances the individuals' level of control while enhancing a sense of mastery and self-control.

Depersonalization Disorder

DIAGNOSIS

This dissociative disorder involves lack of integration of one or more components of perception. The essential feature of depersonalization disorder is the occurrence of persistent feelings of unreality, detachment, or estrangement from oneself or one's body, usually with the feeling that one is an outside observer of one's own mental processes. Individuals suffering depersonalization are distressed by it. They are aware of some distortion in their perceptual experience and therefore are not hallucinating or delusional. Affected individuals often fear that they are "going crazy." The symptom is not infrequently transient.

Derealization, in which affected individuals notice an altered perception of their surroundings, resulting in the world seeming unreal or dream-like, frequently occurs as well. Such individuals often ruminate anxiously about this symptom and are preoccupied with their own somatic and mental functioning.

Depersonalization frequently co-occurs with a variety of other symptoms, especially anxiety, panic, or phobic symptoms. It is often a symptom of PTSD and also occurs as a symptom of alcohol and drug abuse, as

---

DSM-IV-TR Diagnostic Criteria

300.6 DEPERSONALIZATION DISORDER

A. Persistent or recurrent experiences of feeling detached from, and as if one is an outside observer of, one's mental processes or body (e.g., feeling like one is in a dream).

B. During the depersonalization experience, reality testing remains intact.

C. The depersonalization causes clinically significant distress or impairment in social, occupational, or other important areas of functioning.

D. The depersonalization experience does not occur exclusively during the course of another mental disorder, such as schizophrenia, panic disorder, acute stress disorder, or another dissociative disorder, and is not due to the direct physiological effects of a substance (e.g., a drug of abuse, a medication) or a general medical condition (e.g., temporal lobe epilepsy).

Reprinted with permission from the *Diagnostic and Statistical Manual of Mental Disorders*, 4th ed., Text Rev. Copyright 2000 American Psychiatric Association.

a side effect of the use of prescription medication, and during stress and sensory deprivation. The symptom of depersonalization is also commonly seen in the course of a number of other neurological and psychiatric disorders. It is considered a disorder when it is a persistent and predominant symptom. The phenomenology of the disorder involves both the initial symptoms themselves and the reactive anxiety caused by them.

TREATMENT

Depersonalization is most often transient and may remit without formal treatment. Recurrent or persistent depersonalization should be thought of both as a symptom in itself and as a component of other syndromes requiring treatment, such as anxiety disorders and schizophrenia.

The symptom itself may respond to training in self-hypnosis. Paradoxically, induction or deliberate worsening of symptoms may provide relief by teaching a method of controlling them. For example, a hypnotic induction may induce transient depersonalization symptoms, such as a sense of detachment from part of the body, in such individuals. This is a useful exercise, in that by having a structure for inducing the symptoms, one provides the individual with a context for understanding and controlling them. They are presented as a spontaneous form of hypnotic dissociation that can be modified. Such individuals can be taught to induce a pleasant sense of floating lightness or heaviness in place of the anxiety-related somatic detachment. The use of an imaginary screen to picture problems in a way that detaches them from the typical somatic response is also helpful. Other relaxation techniques such as systematic desensitization, progressive muscle relaxation, and biofeedback may also be of help. Psychotherapy aimed at working through emotional responses to any traumatic or other stressors that tend to elicit the depersonalization is also helpful.

Pharmacological approaches involve balancing therapeutic benefit and risk. Antianxiety medications are most commonly used and may be helpful in reducing the amplification of depersonalization caused by anxiety. However, depersonalization and derealization are also side effects of antianxiety drugs, so their use should be carefully monitored. Increasing dosage, a standard technique when there is lack of therapeutic response, may also increase symptoms, leading to a spiral of increasing symptoms and drug dosage but without therapeutic benefit.

However, appropriate pharmacological treatment for comorbid disorders is an important part of treatment. Use of antianxiety medications for generalized anxiety or phobic disorders or of antipsychotic medications for psychotic disorders is often beneficial in conditions in which there is contributory comorbidity.

Dissociative Identity Disorder (Multiple Personality Disorder)

DIAGNOSIS

Dissociative identity disorder (DID) is a rare but real disorder that is the most widely discussed of the dissociative disorders. It involves the presence of two or more distinct identities or personality states (each with its own relatively enduring pattern of perceiving, relating to, and thinking about the environment and self). The diagnostic criteria also require that "At least two of these identities or personality states recurrently take control of the person's behavior" and that there be amnesia (i.e., "Inability to recall important personal information that is too extensive to be explained by ordinary forgetfulness"). It is a failure of integration of various aspects of identity and personality structure. Often different relationship styles (dependent versus assertive/aggressive) and mood states (depressed versus hostile) segregate with different identities and personal memories. Such individuals may be mystified by events that occurred in another "state," or by responses of others to them for behavior that occurred in a different "state." This fragmentation of personality often occurs in response to trauma in childhood, and is perceived by the individual as protective, allowing him or her to tolerate and par-

---

DSM-IV-TR Diagnostic Criteria

308.14 DISSOCIATIVE IDENTITY DISORDER

A. The presence of two or more distinct identities or personality states (each with its own relatively enduring pattern of perceiving, relating to, and thinking about the environment and self).
B. At least two of these identities or personality states recurrently take control of the person's behavior.
C. Inability to recall important personal information that is too extensive to be explained by ordinary forgetfulness.
D. The disturbance is not due to the direct physiological effects of a substance (e.g., blackouts or chaotic behavior during alcohol intoxication) or a general medical condition (e.g., complex partial seizures).

Note: In children, the symptoms are not attributable to imaginary playmates or other fantasy play.

Reprinted with permission from the *Diagnostic and Statistical Manual of Mental Disorders*, 4th ed., Text Rev. Copyright 2000 American Psychiatric Association.

tially evade chronic abuse. These individuals thus view treatment ambivalently as an attempt to deprive them of a defense against attack. They also tend to see others as irrational and unfair, since response to one aspect of their personality frequently reflects experience with other aspects. One DID individual (prior to diagnosis) reported puzzlement about accusations by friends and acquaintances that she had made hostile comments for which she had no memory. She would find people angry at her for no reason. Thus, their personality fragmentation renders them vulnerable to interpersonal problems, yet gives them the belief that they are relatively protected from them.

The diagnosis can be facilitated by psychological testing. Scales of trait dissociation have been developed, and individuals with DID score extremely high on these scales, in contrast to normal populations and other groups of individuals. Those with DID score far higher than normal individuals on standard measures of hypnotizability, whereas schizophrenic individuals tend to have lower than normal scores or the absence of high hypnotizability. Thus, there is comparatively little overlap in the hypnotizability scores of individuals with schizophrenia and those with DID.

DID is more frequently recognized during childhood but typically emerges between adolescence and the third decade of life; it rarely presents as a new disorder after age 40 years, but there is often considerable delay between initial symptom presentation and diagnosis.

Untreated, it is a chronic and recurrent disorder. It rarely remits spontaneously, but the symptoms may not be evident for certain time periods. DID has been called *a disease of hiddenness*. The dissociation itself hampers self-monitoring and accurate reporting of symptoms and history. Many individuals with the disorder are not fully aware of the extent of their dissociative symptoms. They may be reluctant to bring up symptoms because of confusion or shame about the illness or because they encountered previous skepticism. Furthermore, because the majority of individuals report histories of sexual and physical abuse, the shame associated with that and fear of retribution may inhibit reporting of symptoms as well.

There are no convincing studies of the absolute prevalence of DID, although there is widespread agreement that the number of diagnosed cases has increased considerably in the United States and some European countries in the past two decades. Two studies have estimated the prevalence as approximately 1% of psychiatric inpatients. Factors that may account for the increase in the number of true reported cases include (1) more general awareness of the diagnosis among mental health professionals, (2) the availability of specific diagnostic criteria starting with DSM-III, and (3) reduced misdiagnosis of DID as schizophrenia or borderline personality disorder.

Other authors attribute the increase in reported cases to social contagion, hypnotic suggestion, and misdiagnosis. Proponents of this point of view argue that these individuals are highly hypnotizable and therefore quite suggestible. They would therefore be especially vulnerable to direct or implicit hypnotic suggestion. They note that not infrequently a few specialist clinicians make the vast majority of diagnoses. However, it has been observed that the symptoms of individuals diagnosed by specialists in dissociation do not differ from those of individuals diagnosed by psychiatrists, psychologists, and physicians in more general practice who diagnose one or two cases a year. Nonetheless, because these individuals are indeed highly hypnotizable and therefore suggestible, care must be taken in the manner in which the illness is presented to them.

The major comorbid mental disorders are the depressive disorders, substance use disorders, and borderline personality disorder. Sexual, eating, and sleep disorders co-occur less commonly. Such individuals frequently display self-mutilative behavior, impulsiveness, and overvaluing and devaluing of relationships. Indeed, approximately a third of individuals with DID have symptoms that fit criteria for borderline personality disorder as well. Such individuals are also more frequently depressed. Conversely, research shows dissociative symptoms in many individuals with borderline personality disorder, especially those who report histories of physical and sexual abuse. Indeed, the impulsiveness, splitting, hostility, and fear of abandonment, frequently seen in certain personality states, are similar to the presentation of many individuals with borderline personality disorder. Many such individuals also have symptoms that meet criteria for PTSD, with intrusive flashbacks, recurrent dreams of physical and sexual abuse, avoidance of and loss of pleasure in usually pleasurable activities, and symptoms of hyperarousal, especially when exposed to reminders of childhood trauma.

Thus, comorbidity is a complex issue. In addition, these individuals are not infrequently misdiagnosed as having schizophrenia. This diagnostic confusion is understandable in that they have an apparent delusion that their bodies are occupied by more than one person. In addition, they frequently have auditory hallucinations when one personality state speaks to or comments on the activities of another. When misdiagnosed as schizophrenic, individuals with DID are frequently given neuroleptics, which results in a poor therapeutic response and a flattening of affect that tends to confirm the misdiagnosis (since flat affect is characteristic of schizophrenia).

TREATMENT

Psychosocial Treatment

It is possible to help individuals with DID gain control over the dissociative process underlying their symptoms in several ways. The fundamental psychotherapeutic stance should involve meeting persons undergoing treatment halfway, a form of structured empathy in which their experience of themselves as fragmented is acknowledged while the reality that the fundamental problem is a failure of integration of disparate memories and aspects of the self is kept in view. In this sense, such individuals suffer from having less than one personality rather than more than one. Therefore, the goal in therapy is to facilitate integration of disparate elements. This can be done in a variety of ways.

Secrets are frequently a problem with such individuals, who attempt to use the clinician to reinforce a dissociative strategy of withholding relevant information from certain personality states. Such individuals often like to confide in the clinician with the idea that the information is to be kept from other parts of the self, for example, traumatic memories or plans for self-destructive activities.

Clear limit setting and commitment on the part of the clinician to helping all portions of the individual's personality structure learn about warded-off information are important. It is wise to clarify explicitly that the clinician will not become involved in secret collusion. Furthermore, when important agreements are negotiated, such as commitments on the part of individuals to seek medical help before acting on a thought to harm themselves or others, it is useful to discuss with the individuals that this is an "all-points bulletin," requiring attention from all the relevant personality states. The excuse that certain personality states were "not aware" of the agreement should not be accepted.

Hypnosis can be helpful in facilitating psychotherapy as well as establishing the diagnosis. First of all, the simple structure of hypnotic induction may elicit dissociative phenomena. Hypnosis can be particularly helpful in facilitating access to dissociated personalities. They may simply occur spontaneously during hypnotic induction. An alternative strategy is to hypnotize the individual and use age regression to reorient to a time when a different personality state was manifest. An instruction later to change times back to the present usually elicits a return to the other personality state.

This then becomes a means of teaching such an individual how to control the dissociative process.

Alternatively, entering the state of hypnosis may make it possible simply to address and elicit different identities or personality states. Individuals can be taught a simple self-hypnosis exercise for this purpose. For example, the individual can be told to count to herself or himself from one to three. After some formal exercises such as this, it is often possible to ask the individual to speak with a given alter personality, without the formal use of hypnosis. Merely asking to talk with a given identity usually suffices after a while.

Because the loss of memory in DID is complex and chronic, its retrieval is likewise a more extended and integral part of the psychotherapeutic process. The therapy becomes an integrating experience of information sharing among disparate personality elements. Conceptualizing DID as a chronic PTSD, the psychotherapeutic strategy involves a focus on working through traumatic memories in addition to controlling the dissociation.

Controlled access to memories greatly facilitates psychotherapy. As with dissociative amnesia, a variety of strategies can be employed to help individuals with DID break down amnesic barriers. Eliciting various identities or personality states can facilitate access to memories previously unavailable to consciousness. While so-called *pseudomemories* can occur, previously dissociated traumatic memories are often accurate.

Once these memories of earlier traumatic experience have been brought into consciousness, it is crucial to help the individual work through the painful affect, inappropriate self-blame, and other reactions to these memories. It may be useful to have individuals visualize the memories rather than relive them as a means of making their intensity more manageable. It can also be useful to have individuals divide the memories, for example, picturing on one side of an imaginary screen something an abuser did to them and on the other side how they tried to protect themselves from the abuse. Such techniques can help make the traumatic memories more bearable by placing them in a broader perspective, one in which trauma victims can also identify adaptive aspects of their response to the trauma.

This and similar approaches can help these individuals work through traumatic memories, enabling them to bear them in consciousness and therefore reducing the need for dissociation as a means of keeping such memories and associated painful affect out of consciousness. Although these techniques can be helpful and often result in reduced fragmentation and integration, a number of complications can occur in the psychotherapy of these individuals.

The therapeutic process can be thought of as a kind of grief work in which information retrieved from memory is reviewed, traumatic memories are put into perspective, and emotional expression is encouraged and worked through, thereby making it more possible to endure and disseminate the information as widely as possible among various parts of the individual's personality structure. Instructions to other alter personalities to *listen* while a given one is talking and reviewing previously dissociated material can be helpful.

The psychotherapy of DID can be a time-consuming and emotionally taxing process. The rule of thirds is a helpful guideline. Spend the first third of the psychotherapy session assessing the individual's current mental state and life problems and defining a problem area that might benefit from retrieval into conscious memory and working through. Spend the second third of the session accessing and working through this memory. Allow a final third for helping the individual assimilate the information, regulate and modulate emotional responses, and discuss any responses to the clinician and plans for the immediate future. The clinician may resist doing this because the intense abreactive materials are often so compelling and interesting. The individual may also resist sharing information across personalities. Nonetheless, the clinician can be helpful in imposing structure on often chaotic memories and identity states.

Given the intensity of the material that often emerges involving memories of sexual and physical abuse and sudden shifts in mental state accompanied by amnesia, the clinician is called on to take a clear and structured role in managing the psychotherapy. Appropriate limits must be set concerning self-destructive or threatening behavior, agreements must be made regarding physical safety and treatment compliance, and other matters must be presented to the individual in such a way that dissociative ignorance is not an acceptable explanation for failure to live up to the agreements.

Transference applies with special meaning to individuals who have been physically and sexually abused, especially in childhood. They have experienced individuals who are presumed to be caretakers acting instead in an exploitative and sometimes sadistic fashion. They thus expect similar betrayal from mental health clinicians. Although their reality testing is good enough that they can perceive genuine caring, they often unconsciously expect mental health professionals to exploit them. They may experience working through of traumatic memories as a reinflicting of the trauma, with the clinician taking sadistic pleasure in their suffering. They may expect excessive passivity on the part of the clinician, identifying the clinician with some

uncaring family figure who knew that abuse was occurring but did little or nothing to stop it. It is important in managing the therapy to keep these issues in mind and make them frequent topics of discussion. This can diffuse, if not eliminate, such traumatic transference distortions of the therapeutic relationship.

The ultimate goal of psychotherapy is integration of the individual's multiple ego states. It is often the case that one or more of the personality states may exert considerable resistance to the process of integration, particularly early in the process of therapy. Also, individuals may experience efforts of integration as an attempt on the part of the therapist to "kill" personalities. These fears must be worked through and the individual needs to understand that the goal is to learn how to control the episodes of dissociation. This gives individuals a sense of gradually being able to control their dissociative processes in order to work through the traumatic memories. In order to enhance mastery and control, the process of the psychotherapy must help individuals minimize rather than reinforce the content of traumatic memories, which often involves reexperiencing a sense of helplessness in a symbolic reenactment of the trauma.

At the same time, the dissociative defense represents an internalization of the abusive people in the individual's past, a kind of identification with the aggressor, which makes the individual feel powerful rather than helpless. Setting aside the defense also means acknowledging and bearing the helplessness of having been victimized and working through the irrational self-blame that gave such individuals a fantasy of control over events during which they were helpless. Yet, difficult as it is, ultimately the goal of psychotherapy is mastery over the dissociative process, controlled access to dissociative states, integration of warded-off painful memories and material, and a more integrated continuum of identity, memory, and consciousness. The stages of therapy are presented in Table 36-1.

Somatic Treatment

As with other dissociative disorders, there is little evidence that psychoactive drugs are of great help in reversing dissociative symptoms. In the past, short-acting barbiturates such as sodium amobarbital were used intravenously to reverse functional amnesia, but this technique is no longer employed, largely because of poor results. Research data provide no evidence suggesting that any medication regimen has any significant therapeutic effect on the dissociative process manifested by DID individuals. To date, pharmacological treatment

Table 36-1	Stages of Therapy
Stage	**Technique**
Establishing treatment	Education, atmosphere of safety, instill confidence
Preliminary interventions	Confirm diagnosis, set limits, access dissociation with hypnosis
History gathering	Explore components of dissociative structure
Working through trauma	Grief work
Move toward integration	Enhance communication across dissociative states
Integration–resolution	Encourage development of integrated self
Learning coping skills	Help with life decisions and relationships
Solidification of gains	Transference examination
Follow-up	Maintenance

Source: Kluft RP (1991) Multiple personality disorder. In *American Psychiatric Press Review of Psychiatry*, Vol. 10, Tasman A and Goldfinger SM (eds). Copyright, American Psychiatric Press, Washington, DC.

has been limited to symptom control or the management of comorbid conditions (e.g., depression).

Of all available classes of psychotropic agents, antidepressants are the most useful class for the treatment of individuals with DID. That is because individuals suffering from dissociation frequently experience comorbid dysthymic or major depressive disorder. Selective serotonin reuptake inhibitors (SSRIs) are particularly useful, given their high level of effectiveness, low side effect profile, and even lower danger in overdose, compared to tricyclic antidepressants and monoamine oxidase inhibitors. Nevertheless, medication compliance may be a problem with dissociative individuals because dissociated personality states may interfere with medication taking or may take the medication in an overdose attempt.

Benzodiazepines have mostly been used to facilitate recall by controlling secondary anxiety associated with retrieval of traumatic memories (i.e., medication-facilitated interviews). Nevertheless, despite their short-term usefulness, CNS-depressant agents may cause sudden mental state transitions, which may in turn increase rather than decrease amnesic barriers. Therefore, as useful as they could be on a short-term basis (i.e., acute management of a panic attack), the long-term use of these agents may, in fact, contribute to rather than treat dissociative episodes.

There are several uses for anticonvulsant agents. Seizures disorders have a high rate of comorbidity with DID. Thus, anticonvulsant agents may help control the dissociation associated with epileptogenic activity. On the other hand, anticonvulsant agents have proven to be effective in the management of mood disorders, as well

as the impulsiveness associated with personality disorders and brain injury. Also, despite their effectiveness, these agents produce less amnestic side effects than the benzodiazepines and thus may be preferred. On the other hand, the need for closer monitoring due to potential toxicity, particularly in overdoses, makes their use less desirable than the newer SSRIs.

Of all pharmacological agents available, antipsychotics may be the least desirable. First, they are rarely useful in reducing dissociative symptoms. In fact, there have been reports of increased levels of dissociation and an increased incidence of side effects when used in individuals suffering from dissociative disorders.

Dissociative Trance Disorder

DIAGNOSIS

Dissociative-like phenomena have been described in virtually every culture. Yet they appear to be more prevalent in the less-heavily industrialized Second and Third World countries. Studies on the prevalence of dissociative disorders in India have suggested that the 1-year prevalence of dissociative trance disorder is approximately 3.5% of all psychiatric hospitalizations, making it a highly frequent mental disorder. Trance and possession syndromes are by far the most common type of dissociative disorders seen around the world. On the other hand, DID, which is relatively more common in the United States, is virtually never diagnosed in underdeveloped countries. This difference in prevalence and distribution of dissociative disorder across different populations may be mediated by cultural, as well as biological factors. For example, Eastern culture is far more sociocentric than Western culture. Thus, being "possessed" by an outside entity would be more culturally comprehensible and acceptable in the East. On the other hand, an apparent proliferation of individual identities would fit better with the Western preoccupation with individualism. Nonetheless, the underlying dissociative mechanism inhibiting integration of perception, memory, and identity may suggest a common underlying mechanism among these dissociative syndromes.

Trance and possession episodes are usually understood as an idiom of distress and yet they are not viewed as normal. That is, they are not a generally accepted part of cultural and religious practice, which often does involve normal trance phenomena, such as trance dancing in the Balinese Hindu culture. Trance dancers enjoy the remarkable privilege of being the only portion of this socially rigid society able to elevate their social status. The way they are able to do that is by developing the ability to enter trance states. During these altered states of consciousness, which usually occur within the context of a socially acceptable ceremony setting, they dance over hot coals, hold a sword at their throat, or in other ways exhibit supernormal powers of concentration and physical prowess. The mechanism mediating these phenomena is not fully understood, but there is evidence of elevations in plasma noradrenaline, dopamine, and beta-endorphin among Balinese trance dancers during trance states. This form of trance is considered socially normal and even exalted.

By contrast, disordered trance and possession trance are viewed by the local community as an aberrant form of behavior that requires intervention. Such symptoms often arise in the context of family or social distress, for example, discomfort in a new family environment. Thus, cultural informants make it clear that people with dissociative trance disorder are abnormal.

Dissociative trance disorder has been divided into two broad categories, dissociative trance and possession trance. Dissociative trance phenomena are characterized by a sudden alteration in consciousness, not accompanied by distinct alternative identities. In this form, the dissociative symptom involves an alteration in consciousness rather than identity. Also, in dissociative trance, the activities performed are rather simple, usually involving sudden collapse, immobilization, dizziness, shrieking, screaming, or crying. Memory is rarely affected, and if there is amnesia, it is fragmented.

Dissociative trance phenomena frequently involve sudden, extreme changes in sensory and motor control. A classic example is the *ataque de nervios*, prevalent in Latin-American countries. For example, this phenomenon is estimated to have a 12% lifetime prevalence rate in Puerto Rico. A typical episode involves a sudden feeling of anxiety, followed by total body shakes, which may mimic convulsions. This is then followed by hyperventilation, unintelligible screaming, agitation, and often violent bodily movements. Often, this is followed by collapse and probably transient loss of consciousness. After the episode is over, subjects complain of fatigue and having been confused, although this behavior is dramatically different from classic postictal states. Some subjects may experience amnesia at least to some aspects of the event.

In contrast to dissociative trance episodes, possession trance involves the assumption of a distinct alternative identity. The new identity is presumed to be that of a deity, ancestor, or spirit who has transiently taken possession of the subject's mind and body. Different from dissociative trance episodes, which are characterized by rather crude, simplistic, regressive-like behaviors, possession trance victims often exhibit rather complex behavior. During these episodes, subjects may, for example, express otherwise forbidden thoughts or needs, engage in unusual and uncharacteristic aggressive behavior (e.g., verbal or physical expressions of aggression), or may attempt to negotiate for change in family or social status. Also, in contrast to dissociative trance episodes, possession trance episodes are often followed by dense amnesia for a large portion of the episode during which the spirit identity was in control of the subject's behavior.

TREATMENT

Treatment of these disorders varies from culture to culture. Rubbing the body with special potions, negotiating to change the affected person's social circumstances, and physical restraint are often used. Ceremonies to remove or appease the invading spirit are also employed.

COMPARISON OF DSM-IV-TR AND ICD-10 DIAGNOSTIC CRITERIA

The ICD-10 Diagnostic Criteria for Research for dissociative amnesia specify that there be a "convincing association in time between the onset of symptoms of the disorder and stressful events, problems, or needs." In DSM-IV-TR, the criteria set notes that the forgotten information is usually of a stressful or traumatic nature.

For dissociative fugue, in contrast to DSM-IV-TR, the ICD-10 Diagnostic Criteria for Research specify "amnesia for the journey." Furthermore, in contrast to DSM-IV-TR, the ICD-10 Diagnostic Criteria for Research do not indicate that there be an inability to recall one's past during the fugue or that there be confusion about personal identity.

Dissociative identity disorder is included in ICD-10 as an example of an "other dissociative (conversion) disorder" under the rubric "multiple personality disorder." The ICD-10 Diagnostic Criteria for Research and the DSM-IV-TR criteria are almost identical.

Finally, ICD-10 has a single category "depersonalization–derealization syndrome" for presentations characterized by either depersonalization or derealization. In contrast, the DSM-IV-TR category includes only depersonalization and mentions derealization as an associated feature. Furthermore, unlike DSM-IV-TR, which includes this category in the dissociative disorders section, ICD-10 includes the category within the "other neurotic disorders" grouping.

CHAPTER

37 Sexual Disorders

An adult's sexuality has seven components—gender identity, orientation, intention (what one wants to do with a partner's body and have done with one's body during sexual behavior), desire, arousal, orgasm, and emotional satisfaction. The first three components constitute our sexual identity. The second three comprise our sexual function. The seventh, emotional satisfaction, is based on our personal reflections on the first six. The DSM-IV-TR designates impairments of five of these components as pathologies. Variations in orientation and the failure to find ordinary sexual experience emotionally satisfying, although problems for some, are not designated as *disorders* (see Figure 37-1 for a diagnostic decision tree covering the sexual disorders).

Sexual Dysfunctions

DSM-IV-TR specifies three criteria for each sexual dysfunction. The first criterion describes the psychophysiologic impairment—for example, absence of sexual desire, arousal, or orgasm. The second and third criteria are the same for each impairment: the dysfunction causes marked distress or interpersonal difficulty and the dysfunction is not better accounted for by another Axis I diagnosis or not due exclusively to the direct physiological effects of a substance (e.g., a drug of abuse, a medication) or a general medical condition. Table 37-1 lists the first criterion of each of the 12 sexual dysfunction diagnoses. DSM-IV-TR gives the clinician additional latitude for deciding when a person who meets the first criterion qualifies for a disorder. The clinician is asked to consider the effects of the individual's age, experience, ethnicity and cultural background, the degree of subjective distress, adequacy of sexual stimulation, and symptom frequency. No instructions are provided about how to exercise this judgment. In this way, DSM-IV-TR makes it clear that understanding sexual life requires more than counting symptoms; it requires judgment.

Numerous attempts to describe the prevalence of sexual dysfunction have been made in the past 25 years. These range from attempts to define the frequency of

a particular dysfunction, for instance male erectile disorder, to attempts to estimate the prevalence of a series of separate dysfunction—for example, desire, arousal, and orgasmic disorders of women. All such efforts quickly confront methodological influences of sampling, means of obtaining the information, definition of each dysfunction, purpose of the study, and perspective of its authors. These data not surprisingly, therefore, demonstrate a range of prevalence depending on the problem studied. Gender identity disorders are relatively rare (<1–2%). Lifelong sexual desire disorders among women may involve 15% but are less frequent among men. Acquired desire disorders among older individuals are probably three times as common. Perhaps more than half of women at age 55 years have recognized a deterioration in their sexual function. Perhaps 25% of women in their twenties have difficulty having orgasm and 33% of men less than age 40 claim to ejaculate too rapidly. The majority of men by age 70 years are likely to be having erection problems. A careful epidemiologic study from 1994, designed by sociologists, successfully generated a representative sample of the US. They interviewed men and women between age 18 and 59 years and found that sexual dysfunction is common, particularly among young women and older men. This is noteworthy for psychiatrists because our studies of sexual dysfunction caused by medications or acquired psychiatric disorders tend to assume that individuals are generally functionally intact prior to becoming ill or taking medications. This assumption is not tenable on the basis of a generation of epidemiologic studies.

Problems of Sexual Desire

DIAGNOSIS

Sexual desire manifestations are diverse: erotic fantasies, sexual dreams, initiation of sexual behavior, receptivity to partner-initiated sexual behavior, masturbation, genital sensations, heightened responsivity to erotic environmental cues, and sincere statements

---

Clinical Guide to the Diagnosis and Treatment of Mental Disorders. M. B. First and A. Tasman
© 2006 John Wiley & Sons, Ltd.   ISBN 0 470 019158

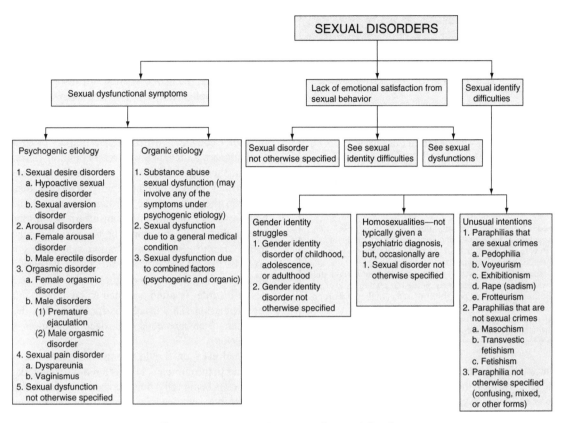

Figure 37-1 *Diagnostic decision tree for sexual disorders.*

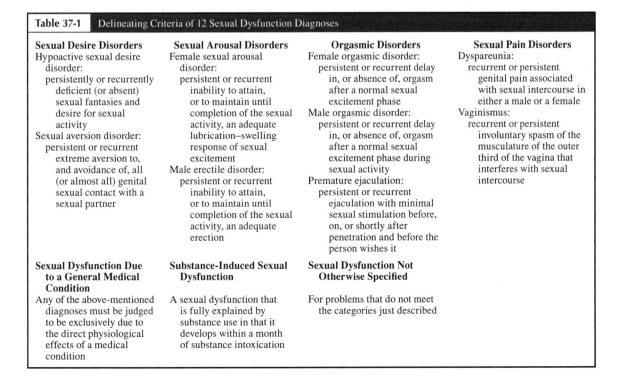

Table 37-1	Delineating Criteria of 12 Sexual Dysfunction Diagnoses		
Sexual Desire Disorders	**Sexual Arousal Disorders**	**Orgasmic Disorders**	**Sexual Pain Disorders**
Hypoactive sexual desire disorder: persistently or recurrently deficient (or absent) sexual fantasies and desire for sexual activity	Female sexual arousal disorder: persistent or recurrent inability to attain, or to maintain until completion of the sexual activity, an adequate lubrication–swelling response of sexual excitement	Female orgasmic disorder: persistent or recurrent delay in, or absence of, orgasm after a normal sexual excitement phase	Dyspareunia: recurrent or persistent genital pain associated with sexual intercourse in either a male or a female
Sexual aversion disorder: persistent or recurrent extreme aversion to, and avoidance of, all (or almost all) genital sexual contact with a sexual partner	Male erectile disorder: persistent or recurrent inability to attain, or to maintain until completion of the sexual activity, an adequate erection	Male orgasmic disorder: persistent or recurrent delay in, or absence of, orgasm after a normal sexual excitement phase during sexual activity	Vaginismus: recurrent or persistent involuntary spasm of the musculature of the outer third of the vagina that interferes with sexual intercourse
		Premature ejaculation: persistent or recurrent ejaculation with minimal sexual stimulation before, on, or shortly after penetration and before the person wishes it	
Sexual Dysfunction Due to a General Medical Condition	**Substance-Induced Sexual Dysfunction**	**Sexual Dysfunction Not Otherwise Specified**	
Any of the above-mentioned diagnoses must be judged to be exclusively due to the direct physiological effects of a medical condition	A sexual dysfunction that is fully explained by substance use in that it develops within a month of substance intoxication	For problems that do not meet the categories just described	

Table 37-2	Three Interactive Components of Sexual Desire

Sexual Drive—Biological Component
Evolves over time, decreasing with increasing age
Diminished by many psychotropic and antihypertensive medications
Manifested by the internally stimulated genital sensations and thoughts of sexual behavior that occur within a person's privacy

Sexual Motivation—Psychological Component
Highly contextual in terms of relationship status
The most socially and psychologically responsive of the three components
Evolves over time but not predictably
Manifested by a person's willingness to bring his or her body to a specific person for sexual behavior

Sexual Wish—Social Component
Expectations for sexual behavior based on membership in various subcultural groups such as family, religion, gender, region, and nation
These expectations begin as cognitions of what is right and wrong and what a person is entitled to sexually and are influenced by what people think others in their cohort are experiencing
Often clinically difficult to distinguish from motivation, which wishes influence

about wanting to behave sexually. For most of the twentieth century, these have been referred to as manifestations of libido. Psychiatrists spoke of libido as if it was a homogeneous instinctive force. Clinicians will find it far more useful to conceptualize that the diverse and changeable desire manifestations are produced by the intersection of three mental forces: drive (biology), motive (psychology), and wish (culture).

The appearance and disappearance of sexual desire is often enigmatic to an individual, but its ebb and flow result from the ever-changing intensities of its components, biological *drive*, psychological *motive*, and socially acquired concepts, *wish* (Table 37-2).

Two diagnoses are given to men and women whose desires for partner sexual behavior are deficient: hypoactive sexual desire disorder (HSDD) and sexual aversion disorder (SAD). The differences between the two revolve around the emotional intensity with which the individual avoids sexual behavior. When visceral anxiety, fear, or disgust is routinely felt as sexual behavior becomes a possibility, sexual aversion is diagnosed. HSDD is far more frequently encountered. It is present in at least twice as many women than men; female to male ratio for aversion is far higher. Like all sexual dysfunctions, the desire diagnoses may be lifelong or may have been acquired after a period of ordinary fluctuations of sexual desire. Acquired disorders may be partner specific (*situational*) or may occur with all subsequent partners (*generalized*).

When the clinician concludes that the individual's acquired generalized HSDD is either due to a medical condition, a medication, or a substance of abuse, the diagnosis is further elaborated to sexual dysfunction due to general medical condition (for instance, HSDD due to multiple sclerosis). The frequency of the specific etiologies are heavily dependent on the clinical setting. In oncology settings, medical causes occur in high frequency; in drug rehabilitation programs, methadone maintenance will be a common cause. In marital therapy clinics, anger and loss of respect for the partner, hidden incompatibility of sexual identity between the self and the partner because of covert homosexuality or paraphilia, an affair, or childhood sexual abuse will commonly be the basis. In general mental health settings, medication side effects will often be the top layer of several causes. When a major depression disorder is diagnosed, for instance, the desire disorder is often assumed to be a symptom of the depression. This usually is incorrect. The desire disorder often preceded the decompensation into depression.

Sexual aversion should strongly suggest three possibilities to the clinician: (1) that a remote traumatic experience is being relived by the partner's expression of interest in sexual behavior; (2) that without the symptom the individual feels powerless to say "no" to sexual advances; or (3) that the individual feels guilty about her own sexual behavior with another person.

The clinician's attention should focus on the individual's sexual development as a child, adolescent, and young adult when the aversion is lifelong, whereas when it is *acquired*, the focus of the history should be on the period immediately prior to the onset of the symptom.

Desire disorders require the clinician to think both in terms of development and personal meanings of sex to the individuals under their care (Table 37-3). Because all explanations are speculative, they should at least make compelling sense of the individuals' life experiences.

TREATMENT

Most sexual desire disorders are difficult to quickly overcome. Brief treatment generally should not be undertaken. Serious individual or couple issues frequently underlie these diagnoses. They have to be afforded time to emerge and to be worked through. However, clinicians need not be pessimistic about all of these conditions. For example, helping a couple resolve a marital dispute may return them to their usual normal sexual desire manifestations. For many

Table 37-3	Obstacles to Discovering the Psychological Contributants to a Sexual Desire Disorder

Obstacles that Reside in the patient

The patient may not tell the psychiatrist the truth about life circumstances

The patient may have strong defenses against knowing the truth

The patient may be unable to tell the truth in front of the partner

The patient may not actually know what is occurring in the partner's life, although she or he is reactive to it

Obstacles that Reside in the Psychiatrist

The psychiatrist may not realize the psychological factors that usually cause these problems

The psychiatrist may not believe that developmental influences can organize an adult sexual function such as sexual motivation

The psychiatrist may not like to deal with the murky complexity of nonbiological developmental and interpersonal issues when thinking about etiology

individuals and couples, therapy assists the couple to more calmly accept the profound implications of continuing marital discord, infidelity, homosexuality, or other contributing factors. Some treatment failures lead to divorce and the creation of a relationship with a new partner. There is then no further sign of the desire problem. Problems rooted in early developmental experiences are particularly difficult to overcome. While DSM-IV-TR asks the clinician to make many distinctions among the desire disorders, no follow-up study has been published in which either the subtypes (lifelong, acquired, situational, and generalized) or etiologic organizers (relationship deterioration with and without extramarital affairs, sexual identity incompatibilities, parental, and medical) are separated into good and poor prognosis categories.

Developmental and identity matters are typically approached in long-term individual psychotherapy. In these sessions, women often discuss the development of their femininity from adolescence to young womanhood, focusing on issues of body image, beauty, social worth to others, moral sensibilities, social awkwardness, and whether they consider themselves deserving of personal physical pleasure. Men often discuss similar issues in terms of masculinity.

Anger, loss of respect, marital discord, and extramarital affairs may be approached in either individual or conjoint formats. In either setting, individuals often formulate the etiology as having fallen out of love with the partner. Those whose cultural backgrounds limit their ease in being a sexual person are often encouraged in educational and cultural experiences that might help them outgrow their earliest notions about what is proper sexual behavior.

Problems with Arousal

DIAGNOSIS

Female Sexual Arousal Disorder

Female sexual arousal disorder implies that drive and motivation are relatively intact although arousal is difficult. The disorder is usually an *acquired* diagnosis. Premenopausal women who have this disorder focus on the lack of moisture in the vagina or their failure to be excited by the behaviors that previously reliably brought pleasure. They have drive and motive and wish, but enigmatically are unable to sustain arousal. Some mental factor arises to distract them from their excitement during lovemaking. Therapy is focused, therefore, on the meaning of what preoccupies them. This often involves the dynamics of their current individual or partnered life or the influence of their past relationships on their present. With therapy, the diagnosis often is changed to an HSDD.

In peri- and postmenopausal women, arousal problems are more often focused on the body as a whole rather than just genital moisture deficiencies. Skin insensitivity, often a euphemism for decreased pleasure in response to oral and manual nipple, breast, and vulvar stimulation, is often initially treated as a symptom of "estrogen" deficiency. Early in the menopause, a small minority of women have an increase in drive due to changing testosterone–estrogen ratios. Yet, they may still subjectively experience arousal as different than it used to be. Therapy often focuses on the women's concerns about estrogen replacement and the consequences of menopause in terms of body image, attractiveness, fears of partner infidelity, loss of health and vigor, and aging.

Male Erectile Disorder

The mechanisms of erection–the sequestering and maintaining of arterial blood within the corpora cavernosa–are being elucidated by urological research. This research has led to a diminishing emphasis on "psychogenic impotence" diagnosis. Urologists may refer to male erectile disorders (ED) of a psychogenic origin as "adrenergic" ED, a reference to the preponderance of sympathetic tone on the corporal mechanisms that maintain flaccidity. Adrenergic dominance of the penile arterial tone is created by a mind that perceives the sexual context as dangerous, frightening, or unwanted.

At every age, *selectivity* of erectile failure is the single most important diagnostic feature of primary erectile dysfunction. Clinicians should inquire about the relative firmness and duration of erections under each of these circumstances: masturbation, sex other than intercourse, sex with other female or male partners, upon stimulation with explicit media materials, in the middle of the night, and upon awakening. If under some circumstances the erection is firm and lasting, the clinician can usually assume that the man's neural, endocrine, and vascular physiology is sufficiently normal and that the problem is psychogenic in origin. This is true even for men in their fifties and older. Clinicians often feel more certain about this diagnosis when no diseases thought to lead to erectile dysfunction are present.

TREATMENT

Lifelong male ED typically is psychogenic and involves either a sexual identity dilemma—such as transvestism, gender identity disorder, a homoerotic orientation, a paraphilia, or another diagnosis that expresses the individual's fear of being sexually close to a partner. Sexual identity problems are often initially denied unless the clinician is nonjudgmental and thorough during the inquiry. However, obsessive–compulsive disorder, schizoid personality, a psychotic disorder, or severe character disorders may be present. Occasionally, a reasonably normal young man with an unusually persistent fear of sexual intercourse seeks attention. These good prognosis cases are sometimes informally referred to as anxious beginners (Table 37-4). With that exception, men with lifelong male arousal disorder (MAD), when taken into individual therapy, are usually perceived as having a strong motive to avoid sexual behavior and while dysfunctional with a partner during much of their therapy, might equally be diagnosed as having HSDD with normal drive but a motive to avoid partner sex. The prognosis with older men with lifelong erectile dysfunction is poor even with modern erectogenic agents. Long-term therapy, even if it does not enable regular intercourse, may enable more emotional and sexual closeness to a partner. Some reasonably masculine-appearing men with mild gender identity problems can quickly become potent if they can reveal their need during sexual relationship to cross-dress (use a fetish article of clothing) to a partner who calmly accepts his requirement. However, most of these men have inordinate fears of sexually bonding to any woman, and, in therapy, become preoccupied with basic developmental issues. Some of them marry and form companionate relationships that are rarely or never consummated.

In dramatic contrast, men with long-established good potency who have recently lost their erectile capacities with their partner—acquired psychogenic ED—have a far better prognosis (Table 37-5). They may be treated in individual or couples format, depending on the precipitants of the sexual problem and the status of their

Table 37-4	What the Clinician Should Expect to Encounter Among Men Who Have Never Been Able to Have Intercourse with a Woman

Unconventional Sexual Identity
Gender identity problem
  Wish to be a woman
  A history of cross-dressing in women's clothing in private and/or public
  Suspected by psychiatrist but information initially withheld
Homoeroticism
  Without sexual behavior with men
  With sexual behavior with men but not known to the female partner
  With sexual behavior with men and known to the female partner
Paraphilia
  One or more of a wide range of paraphilic patterns
  Preference for prepubertal or young adolescents often initially denied unless thoroughly, systematically, and nonjudgmentally questioned
  Compulsivity with or without obvious paraphilic imagery confined to masturbation with the help of pornographic images for stimulation

Serious Character Disorders (Men Have Strong Fear of Closeness to Women)
Obsessive–compulsive
Schizotypal
Schizoid
Avoidant
Past history of psychotic decompensation

Anxious Beginners
Psychiatrically normal young men with inordinate anxiety and shyness that quickly respond to psychiatrist's encouragement and optimism and partner warmth and patience

relationship with their partner. Many of these therapies become focused on resentments that have not been identified, discussed, and worked through by the couple. Such distressed couples are most efficiently helped

Table 37-5	Apparent Precipitants of Recently Acquired Psychogenic Erectile Disorder and Their Associated Private Emotions*

Deterioration of marital relationship: anger, guilt, disdain, sadness
Divorce: abandonment, anger, guilt, sadness, shame
Deterioration of personal or spousal health: sadness, anxiety, anger, shame
Death of spouse (*widower's impotence*): sadness, longing, guilt
Threat of or actual unemployment: anxiety, worthlessness, guilt, anger, shame
Financial reversal: shame, guilt, anxiety
Surreptitious extramarital affair: guilt
Reunited marriage after extramarital affair: shame, anxiety

*These short lists of simple emotions are a mere introduction to what transpires within the man's mind as a result of the meanings that the sexual behavior has for him. Although incomplete and oversimplified, they are listed to remind the psychiatrist that what the man feels about his life competes with sexual arousal during sexual behavior to generate the psychogenic erectile dysfunction.

in a conjoint format. When extramarital affairs are part of the relationship deterioration and cannot be discussed, most clinicians simply work with one spouse. Potency is frequently lost following a separation or divorce. Impaired potency after a spouse's death is either about unresolved grief or problems that existed prior to the wife's terminal illness. Men also often get worried about their potency when their financial or vocational lives crumble, when they have a serious new physical illness such as a myocardial infarction or stroke, or when their wives become seriously ill. The esthetics of lovemaking require a context of reasonable physical health; when one spouse becomes chronically ill or disfigured by illness or surgery, either one of the couple may lose their willingness to be sexual. This may be reflected in impaired erections or sexual avoidance.

Regardless of the precipitating factors, men with arousal disorders have performance anxiety. They anticipate erectile failure before sex begins and vigilantly monitor their state of tumescence during sex. Performance anxiety is present in almost all impotent men. Performance anxiety is efficiently therapeutically addressed by identifying it to the individual and asking him to make love without trying intercourse on several occasions to demonstrate to himself how different lovemaking can feel for him when he is not risking failure. This enables many to relax, concentrate on sensation, and return to previous states of sensual abandon during lovemaking. This technique is known as *sensate focus*.

The psychological treatment of acquired arousal disorders is often highly satisfying for the professional because many of the men are anxious for help. Motivation to behave sexually is often present, fear can be allayed, and men can learn to appreciate the emotional complexity of their lives. They can be shown how their minds prevented intercourse until they could acknowledge what has been transpiring within and around them. Many recently separated men, for example, are grieving, angry, guilty, uncertain, and worried about their finances. Yet, they may propel themselves into a new relationship. Two characteristics seem to predispose to erectile problems at key life transitions: (1) the pursuit of the masculine standard that men ought to be able to perform intercourse with anyone, anywhere, under any circumstances; (2) the inability to readily grasp the nature and significance of his inner experiences.

The introduction of phosphodiesterase-5 (PDE5) inhibitors in 1998 revolutionized the treatment of erectile dysfunction. Sildenafil (Viagra) was introduced first, followed by Vardenafil (Levitra) and Tadalafil (Cialis). When a man gets sexually stimulated, a chain reaction occurs in the tissue of the penis that results in elevated levels of a substance called cyclic guanosine monophosphate (cGMP) and that is the key to getting and sustaining an erection for intercourse. All three medications block the enzyme PDE5, which is responsible for the neutralization of cGMP. PDE5 blockers generally will not cause erections at inappropriate times because they only block degradation of cGMP produced in reaction to sexual stimulation. In the absence of sexual stimulation, there is no cGMP to protect, so the drugs remains in the background. The three medications differ primarily in terms of duration of action: Cialis lasts from 30 to 100 hours, Levitra lasts up to 24 hours, and Viagra lasts from 4-6 hours. These drugs must not be used when any organic nitrate is being taken because it dangerously potentiates the hypotensive effect of the nitrates, risking brain and myocardial infarction. Because the PDE5 inhibitors' rate of improving erections is significantly higher than the restoration of a mutually satisfactory sexual equilibrium (approximately 44%), psychological ED that persists after medication should be treated by a mental health professional.

Problems With Orgasm

Female Orgasmic Disorder

DIAGNOSIS

The attainment of reasonably regular orgasms with a partner is a crucial personal developmental step for young women. This task of adult sexual development rests upon a subtle interplay of physiology, individual psychology, and culture. Orgasm is the reflexive culmination of arousal. It is manifested by rhythmic vaginal wall contractions and the release of muscular tension and pelvic vasocongestion, accompanied by varying degrees of pleasurable body sensations. Its accomplishment requires: (1) the physiologic apparatus to augment and sustain arousal; (2) the psychological willingness to be swept away by excitement; and (3) tenacious focus on the required physical work of augmenting arousal. The diagnosis of female orgasmic disorder (FOD) is made when the woman's psychology persistently interferes with her body's natural progression through arousal.

While assessing for the presence of this disorder, the doctor should determine the answers to the following questions. Does the individual have orgasms under any of the following sexual circumstances: solitary masturbation, partner manual genital stimulation, oral–genital stimulation, vibratory stimulation, any other means? Does she have orgasms with a partner different than her significant other? How are they stimulated? Does a particular fantasy make orgasmic attainment easier or possible? Under what conditions has she ever been orgasmic? Has she had an orgasm during her sleep?

The lifelong *generalized* variety of the disorder is recognized when a woman has never been able to attain orgasm alone or with a partner by any means, although she regularly is aroused. When a woman can only readily attain orgasm during masturbation, she is diagnosed as having a lifelong *situational* type. Women with any form of lifelong FOD more clearly have conflicts about personal sexual expression due to fear, guilt, ignorance, or obedience to tradition than those with the acquired variety. Women who can masturbate to orgasm often feel fear and embarrassment about sharing their private arousal with any other person.

The acquired varieties of this disorder are more common and are characterized by both complete anorgasmia, too-infrequent orgasms, and too-difficult orgasmic attainment. The most common cause of this problem are serotonergic compounds. Prospective studies of various antidepressants have demonstrated up to 70% incidence of this disorder among those treated with serotonergic antidepressants. Bupropion and nefazodone do not cause this problem. When medications are not the cause of an acquired FOD, the clinician needs to carefully assess the meaning of the changes in her life prior to the onset of the disorder.

TREATMENT

The ideal era to begin treatment is young adulthood. Four formats are known to be of help. Individual therapy is the most commonly employed. In lifelong varieties of the disorder, therapy focuses on the cultural sources of sexual inhibition and how and when they impacted upon the individual. In the situational varieties, the therapist focuses on the meaning of the life changes that preceded the onset of the disorder. Group therapy is highly effective in helping women reliably masturbate to orgasm and be moderately effective in overcoming partner inhibition. It is typically done with college and graduate students in campus settings, not older women. Couple therapy may be useful to assist the couple with the subtleties of their sexual equilibrium. The personal and interpersonal dimensions of orgasmic attainment can be stressed. Often, other issues then come to the fore that initially seemed to have little to do with orgasmic attainment. The most cost-effective treatment is bibliotherapy. Female orgasmic attainment has been widely written about in the popular press for several decades. It is widely believed that these articles and books, which strongly encourage knowledge of her genital anatomy, masturbation, and active pursuit of orgasm, have enabled many women to grow more comfortable and competent in sexual expression.

Male Orgasmic Disorder

When a man can readily attain a lasting erection with a partner, yet is consistently unable to attain orgasm in the body of the partner, he is diagnosed with male orgasmic disorder (MOD). The disorder has three levels of severity: (1) the most common form is characterized by the *ability* to attain orgasm with a partner outside of her or his body, either through oral, manual, or personal masturbation; (2) the more severe form is characterized by the man's inability to ejaculate in his partner's presence; and (3) the rarest form is characterized by the inability to ejaculate when awake. The disorder is usually lifelong and not partner specific. Some of these men get better with psychotherapy, others improve spontaneously with time, and, for others, the dysfunction leads to the cessation of the aspiration for sex with a partner. One controlled study of individuals with numerous sexual dysfunctions suggested that bupropion 300–450 mg/day may improve the capacity to ejaculate in a minority of individuals.

Premature Ejaculation

DIAGNOSIS

Premature ejaculation is a high-prevalence (25–40%) disorder seen primarily in heterosexuals characterized by a very low threshold for the reflex sequence of orgasm. The problem, a physiological *efficiency* of sperm delivery, causes social and psychological distress. The range of intravaginal containment times among self-diagnosed individuals extends from immediately before or upon vaginal entry (rare), to less than a minute (usual), to less than the man and his partner desire (not infrequent). Time alone is a misleading indicator, however. The essence of the self-diagnosis is an emotionally unsatisfying sexual equilibrium apparently due to the man's inability to temper his arousal. Most men sometimes ejaculate before they wish to, but not persistently.

The history should clarify the answers to following questions: why is he seeking therapy now? Is the individual a sexual beginner or a beginner with a particular partner? Does he have inordinately high expectations for intravaginal containment time for a man his age and experience? Is he desperate about losing the partner because of the rapid ejaculation? Is the relationship in jeopardy for another reason? Does his partner have a sexual dysfunction? Does she have orgasms with him other than through intercourse? Is he requesting help in order to cover his infidelity? Is his partner now blaming the man's sexual inadequacy for her infidelity? Is his new symptom a reflection of his fear about having a serious physical problem during sex such as angina, a stroke, or another myocardial infarction? The answers will enable the clinician to classify the rapid ejaculation into an acquired or lifelong and specific or general pattern, to sense the larger context in which his sexual behavior is conducted, and to plan treatment.

TREATMENT

There are three efficient approaches to this dysfunction. The first is simply to refuse to confirm the individual's self-diagnosis. Some anxious beginners, men with reasonable intravaginal containment times of 2 or more minutes, and those with exaggerated notions of sexual performance can be reassured with a few visits. When they no longer think of themselves as dysfunctional, their intravaginal containment times improve. The second is the use of serotonergic medications. Numerous reports testify to the fact that various serotonergic reuptake inhibitors can significantly lengthen the duration of intercourse. Clinicians need to determine with each individual whether the medication can be taken within hours or days of anticipated intercourse. Improvement is not sustained after medication is stopped. Serotonergic medications are the most common treatment of rapid ejaculation because they are so quickly effective in over 90% of men. The third approach is behaviorally oriented sex therapy that trains the man to focus his attention on his penile sensations during vaginal containment and to signal his partner to cease movement or to apply a firm squeeze of the glans/shaft area to interrupt the escalation of arousal. This requires an increase in communication and full cooperation of the partner, which in themselves can go a long way in improving their sexual equilibrium.

The advantages of costlier couple psychotherapy are to allow the man and his partner to understand their lives better, to address both of their sexual anxieties, and to deal with other important nonsexual issues in their relationship. Effective psychotherapy allows the man to become positioned to continue the usual biological evolution that occurs during the life cycle from rapid ejaculation, which is true for many young men, to occasional difficulty in ejaculating, which is true for many men in their sixties.

Sexual Pain Disorders

The clinician needs to consider a series of questions when dealing with a woman who reports painful intercourse. Does she have a known gynecologic abnormality that is generally associated with pain? Is there anything about her complaint of pain that indicates a remarkably low pain threshold? Does she now have an aversion to sexual intercourse? At what level of physical discomfort did she develop the aversion? Does her private view of her current relationship affect her willingness to be sexual and her experience of pain? Does her partner's sexual style cause her physical or mental discomfort—for example, is he overly aggressive or does he stimulate memories of former abuse? What has been the partner's response to her pain? What role does her anticipation of pain play in her experience of pain?

These clinical questions are typical biopsychosocial ones. Sex-limiting pain often is the result of the subtle interplay of personal and relational, cognitive and affective, and fundamental biological processes that are inherent in other human sexual struggles that operate to produce these confusing disorders.

The DSM-IV-TR presents dyspareunia and vaginismus as distinct entities. However, they have been viewed as inextricably connected in much of the modern sexuality literature—vaginismus is known to create dyspareunia and dyspareunia has been known to create vaginismus.

Dyspareunia

DIAGNOSIS

Recurrent uncomfortable or painful intercourse in either gender is known as dyspareunia. Women's dyspareunia varies from discomfort at intromission, to severe unsparing pain during penile thrusting, to vaginal irritation following intercourse. In both sexes, recurring coital pain leads to inhibited arousal and sexual avoidance. *Dyspareunia* is used as both a symptom and a diagnosis. When coital pain is caused solely by defined physical pathology, dyspareunia due to a medical condition is diagnosed. When coital pain is due to vaginismus, insufficient lubrication, or other presumably psychogenic factors, dyspareunia not due to a medical condition diagnosis is made.

Because the *symptom* dyspareunia is produced by numerous organic conditions, the clinician should be certain that the individual has had a pelvic examination by a person equipped to assess a broad range of regional pathology. Vulvovestibulitis is diagnosed by pain in response to cotton swab touching in a normal appearing vulvar vestibule. In these individuals and some others, the pain cannot be classified with certainty as a *symptom* or a *disorder*. Pain upon penile or digital insertion may be due to an intact hymen or remnants of the hymenal ring, vaginitis, cervicitis, episiotomy scars, endometriosis, fibroids, ovarian cysts, and so on. Postcoital dyspareunia often begins at orgasm when uterine contractions occur. Fibroids, endometriosis, and pelvic inflammatory disease should be considered. Postmenopausal pain, particularly if the woman has had many years without intercourse, is often a result of thinning of the vaginal mucosa, loss of elasticity of the labia and vaginal outlet, and decreased lubrication. Normal menopause, however, is often associated with mild pain due to inadequate lubrication (in both partners).

Dyspareunia in men is usually due to a medical condition. Herpes, gonorrhea, prostatitis, and Peyronie's disease cause pain during intercourse. Remote trauma to the penis may cause penile chordee or bowing which makes intercourse mechanically difficult and sometimes painful. Pain experienced upon ejaculation can be a side effect of trazodone.

Vaginismus

DIAGNOSIS

Vaginismus is an involuntary spasm of the musculature of the outer third layer of the vagina, which makes penile penetration difficult or impossible. The diagnosis is not made if an organic cause is known. Although a woman with vaginismus may wish to have intercourse, her symptom prevents the penis from entering her body. In lifelong vaginismus, the anticipation of pain at the first intercourse causes muscle spasm. Pain reinforces the fear and on occasion, the partner's response gives her good reason to dread a second opportunity to have intercourse. Early episodic vaginismus may be common among women, but most of the cases that are brought to medical attention are chronic. Lifelong vaginismus is relatively rare. The clinician needs to focus attention on what may have made the idea of intercourse so overwhelming to her: parental intrusiveness, sexual trauma, childhood genital injury, illnesses whose therapy involved orifice penetration, and surgery.

The woman with lifelong vaginismus not only has a history of unsuccessful attempts at penetration but displays an avoidance of finger and tampon penetration. The most dramatic aspect of her history, however, is her inability to endure a speculum examination of her vagina. Vaginismus is a phobia of vaginal entrance.

TREATMENT OF DYSPAREUNIA AND VAGINISMUS

While vaginismus has the reputation of being readily treatable by gynecologists by pairing relaxation techniques with progressively larger vaginal dilators, the mental health professional typically approaches the problem differently. The psychological approach to both vaginismus and dyspareunia is attuned to the role that her symptom plays in her life. The therapy, therefore, does not begin with a one dimensional attempt to remove the symptom, which only frightens some individuals. Rather, it begins with a patient exploration of the developmental and interpersonal meanings of the need for the symptom. "I wonder how this problem originally got started? Can you tell me a bit more about your life?" In the course of assisting women with these problems, a variety of techniques may be utilized including relaxation techniques, sensate focus, dilatation, marital therapy, and medication. Short-term therapies should not be expected to have lasting good results because once the symptom is relieved, other problematic aspects of the individual's sexual equilibrium and nonsexual relationship often come into focus. Clinicians have developed an impression that women with a diagnosis of dyspareunia are particularly difficult to help permanently. This, however, is a largely unstudied topic.

Sexual Dysfunction Due to a General Medical Condition

Many general medical conditions can cause sexual dysfunction, including neurological conditions (e.g., multiple sclerosis, spinal cord lesions, neuropathy, temporal lobe lesions), endocrine conditions (e.g., diabetes mellitus, hypothyroidism, hyper- and hypoadrenocorticism, hyperprolactinemia, hypogonadal states, pituitary dysfunction), vascular conditions, and genitourinary conditions (e.g., testicular disease, Peyronie's disease, urethral infections, postprostatectomy complications, genital injury, atrophic vaginitis, infections of the vagina and external genitalia, postsurgical complications such as episiotomy scars, shortened vagina, cystitis, endometriosis, uterine prolapse, pelvic infections, neoplasms).

The diagnosis of Sexual Dysfunction due to a General Medical Condition applies when the sexual dysfunction is judged to be exclusively due to the direct physiological effects of the general medical condition. This determination is based on history (e.g., impaired erectile functioning during masturbation), physical examination (e.g., evidence of neuropathy), and laboratory findings (e.g., nocturnal penile tumescence, pulse wave assessments, ultrasound studies, intracorporeal pharmacological testing or angiography). If both a primary sexual dysfunction and a general medical condition are present, then the primary diagnosis with the subtype "With Combined Factors" should be used (e.g., Male Erectile Dysfunction With Combined Factors).

Substance-Induced Sexual Dysfunction

The diagnosis of Substance-Induced Sexual Dysfunction applies when a clinically significant sexual dysfunction is judged to be exclusively due to the direct physiological effects of a medication or drug of abuse. Sexual dysfunctions can occur in association with intoxication with the following classes of substances: alcohol, amphetamines and related substances, cocaine, opioids, sedatives, hypnotics, and anxiolytics. Acute intoxication with or chronic abuse of substances of abuse has been reported to decrease sexual interest and cause arousal problems in both sexes. A decrease in sexual interest, arousal disorders, and orgasmic disorders may also be caused by prescribed medications, including antihypertensives, histamine H_2 receptor antagonists, antidepressants, neuroleptics, anxiolytics, anabolic steroids, and antiepileptics. Painful orgasm has been reported with the use of fluphenazine, thioridazine, and amoxapine. Priapism has been reported with use of chlorpromazine, trazodone, closapine, and following penile injections of papaverine or prostaglandin. Serotonin reuptake inhibitors may cause decreased sexual desire, arousal, or orgasmic disorders.

Sexual Dysfunction Not Otherwise Specified (NOS)

This diagnosis is reserved for circumstances that leave the clinician uncertain as to how to diagnose the individual. This may occur when the individual has too many fluctuating dysfunctional symptoms without a clear pattern of prominence of anyone of them. Sometimes, the clinician is unable to determine whether the dysfunction is the basic complaint or whether the sexual complaints are secondary to marital dysfunction. At other times the etiology is the uncertain: psychogenic, due to a general medical condition, or substance induced. When the individual does not emphasize the dysfunction as the problem but emphasizes instead the lack of emotional satisfaction from sex, the psychiatrist may temporarily provide this not otherwise specified (NOS) diagnosis. It is usually possible to find a better dysfunction diagnosis after therapy begins.

Gender Identity Disorder

The organization of a stable gender identity is the first component of sexual identity to emerge during childhood. The processes that enable this accomplishment are so subtle that when a daughter consistently acts as though she realizes that "I am a girl and that is all right," or when a son's behavior announces that "I am a boy and that is all right," families rarely even remember their children's confusion and behaviors to the contrary. Adolescent and adult gender problems are not rare. They are, however, commonly hidden from social view, sometimes long enough to developmentally evolve into other less dramatic forms of sexual identity.

Early Forms: Extremely Feminine Young Boys

Although occasionally the parents of a feminine son have a convincing anecdote about persistent feminine interests dating from early in the second year of life, boyhood femininity is more typically only apparent by the third year. By the fourth year, playmate preferences become obvious. Same-sex playmate preference is a typical characteristic of young children. Cross-gender-identified children consistently demonstrate the opposite sex playmate preference. The avoidance of other boys has serious consequences in terms of social rejection and loneliness throughout the school years. The peer problems of feminine boys cause some of their behavioral and emotional problems, which are in evidence by middle-to-late childhood. However, psychometric studies support clinical impressions that feminine boys have emotional problems even before peer relationships become a factor—that is, something more basic about being cross-gender-identified creates problems. Young feminine boys have been shown to be depressed and have difficulties with separation anxiety.

Early Forms: Masculine Girls (Tomboys)

The masculinity of girls may become apparent as early as age 2 years. The number of girls brought to clinical attention for cross-gendered behaviors, self-statements, and aspirations is consistently less than boys by a factor of 1:5 at any age of childhood in most Western countries. It is not known whether this reflects a genuine difference in incidence of childhood gender disorders, cultural perceptions of femininity as a negative in boys versus the neutral-to-positive perception of boy-like behaviors in girls, the broader range of cross-gender expression permitted to girls but not to boys, or an intuitive understanding that cross-gender identity more accurately predicts homosexuality in boys than girls.

The distinction between tomboys and gender-disordered girls is often difficult to make. Tomboys are thought of as not as deeply unhappy about their femaleness, not as impossible to occasionally dress in stereotypic female clothing, and not thought to have a profound aversion to their girlish and future womanly physiologic transformations. Tomboys are able to enjoy some feminine activities along with their obvious pleasures in masculine-identified toys and games and the company of boys. Girls who are diagnosed as gender-disordered generally seem to have a relentless intensity about their masculine preoccupations and an insistence about their future. The onset of their cross-gendered identifications is early in life. Although most lesbians have a history of tomboyish behaviors, most tomboys develop a heterosexual orientation.

DIAGNOSIS

Adults who permanently change their bodies to deal with their gender dilemmas represent the far end of the spectrum of adaptations to gender problems. Even the lives of those who reject bodily change, however, have considerable pain because the images of a better gendered self may recur throughout life, becoming more powerful whenever life becomes strained or disappointing.

The diagnosis of the extreme end of the gender identity disorder spectrum is clinically obvious. The challenging diagnostic task for clinicians is to suspect a gender problem and inquire about gender identity and its evolution in those whose manner suggests a unisexed or cross-gendered appearance, those with dissociative gender identity disorder (GID), severe forms of character pathology, and those who seem unusual in some undefinable manner.

DSM-IV-TR provides the clinician with two Axis I gender diagnoses: Gender Identity Disorder, and Gender Identity Disorder Not Otherwise Specified (GIDNOS). To qualify for GID, an individual of any age must meet four criteria.

Children, teenagers, and adults exist who rue the day they were born to their biological sex and who long for the opportunity to simply live their lives in a manner befitting the other gender. They repudiate the possibility of finding happiness within the broad framework of roles given to members of their sex by their society. Their repudiation is not motivated by an intellectual attack on sexism, homophobia, or any other injustice imbedded in cultural mores. A gender-disordered person literally repudiates his or

DSM-IV-TR Diagnostic Criteria

GENDER IDENTITY DISORDER

A. A strong and persistent cross-gender identification (not merely a desire for any perceived cultural advantages of being the other sex). In children, the disturbance is manifested by four (or more) of the following:

(1) repeatedly stated desire to be, or insistence that he or she is, the other sex
(2) in boys, preference for cross-dressing or simulating female attire; in girls, insistence on wearing only stereotypical masculine clothing
(3) strong and persistent preferences for cross-sex roles in make-believe play or persistent fantasies of being the other sex
(4) intense desire to participate in the stereotypical games and pastimes of the other sex
(5) strong preference for playmates of the other sex

In adolescents and adults, the disturbance is manifested by symptoms such as a stated desire to be the other sex, frequent passing as the other sex, desire to live or be treated as the other sex, or the conviction that he or she has the typical feelings and reactions of the other sex. Persistent discomfort with his or her sex or sense of inappropriateness in the gender role of that sex.

In children, the disturbance is manifested by any of the following: in boys, assertion that his penis or testes are disgusting or will disappear or assertion that it would be better not to have a penis, or aversion toward rough-and-tumble play and rejection of male stereotypical toys, games, and activities; in girls, rejection of urinating in a sitting position, assertion that she has or will grow a penis, or assertion that she does not want to grow breasts or menstruate, or marked aversion toward normative feminine clothing.

B. In adolescents and adults, the disturbance is manifested by symptoms such as preoccupation with getting rid of primary and secondary sex characteristics (e.g., request for hormones, surgery, or other procedures to physically alter sexual characteristics to simulate the other sex) or belief that he or she was born the wrong sex.

C. The disturbance is not concurrent with a physical intersex condition.

D. The disturbance causes clinically significant distress or impairment in social, occupational, or other important areas of functioning.

Code based on current age:

302.6 Gender identity disorder in children
302.85 Gender identity disorder in adolescents or adults

Specify (for sexually mature individuals):

Sexually attracted to males
Sexually attracted to females
Sexually attracted to both
Sexually attracted to neither

Reprinted with permission from the *Diagnostic and Statistical Manual of Mental Disorders*, 4th ed., Text Rev. Copyright 2000 American Psychiatric Association.

her body, repudiates the self in that body, and rejects performing roles expected of people with that body. It is a subtle, usually self-contained rebellion against the need of others to designate them in terms of their biological sex.

By mid-adolescence, the extremely gender-disordered have often envisioned the solution for their paralyzing self-consciousness: to live as a member of the opposite gender, to transform their bodies to the extent possible by modern medicine, and to be accepted by all others as the opposite sex. Most people with these cross-gender preoccupations, however, do not go beyond the fantasy or private cross-dressing. Those that do, may often come to psychiatric attention. When a clinician is called in, the family has one set of hopes, the individual another. The clinician has many tasks, one of which is to mediate between the ambitions of the gender-disordered person and society and see what can be done to help the individual.

The usual clarity of distinctions between heterosexual, bisexual, and homosexual orientations rests upon the assumption that the biological sex and psychological gender of the person and the partner are known. A woman who designates herself as a lesbian is understood to mean she is erotically attracted to other women. *Lesbian* loses its meaning if the woman says she feels she *is* a man and lives as one. She insists, "I am a heterosexual man; men are attracted to women as am I!" DSM-IV-TR suggests that adults with GIDs should be subgrouped according to which sex the individual is currently sexually attracted: males, females, both, or neither. This makes sense for most individuals with GID because it is their gender identity that is most important to them. Some are rigid about the sex of those to whom they are attracted because it supports their idea about their gender, others are bierotic and are not too concerned with their orientation, still others have not had enough experiences to overcome their uncertainty about their orientation.

If an accurate community-based study of the gender impaired could be conducted, most cases would be diagnosed as Gender Identity Disorder Not Otherwise Specified (GIDNOS). The diagnostician needs to understand that gender identity development is a dynamic evolutionary process and clinicians get to see people at crisis points in their lives. At any given time, although it is clear that the individual has some form of GID, it may not be that which is described in DSM-IV-TR as GID.

GIDNOS is a large category designed to be inclusive of those with unusual genders who do not clearly fit the criteria of GID. There is no implication that if an individual is labeled GIDNOS that his or her label cannot change in the future. GIDNOS would contain the many forms of transvestism—masculine-appearing boys and teenagers with persistent cross-dressing

(former fetishistic transvestites) who are evolving toward GID, socially isolated men who want to become a woman shortly after their wives or mothers die (secondary transvestites) but express considerable ambivalence about the very matter they passionately desired at their last visit, extremely feminized homosexuals including those with careers as "drag queens" who seem to want to change their sex when depressed, and so on. GIDNOS would also capture men who want to be rid of their genitals without being feminized, unisexual females who imagine themselves as males but who are terrified of any social expression of their masculine gender identity, hypermasculine lesbians in periodic turmoil over their gender, and those women who strongly identify with both male and female who lately want mastectomies. In using gender identity diagnoses, clinicians need to remember that extremely masculine women or extremely feminine men are not to be dismissed as homosexual. "Lesbian" or "gay" is only a description of orientation. They are more aptly described as also cross-gendered.

TREATMENT

The treatment of these conditions, although not as well based on scientific evidence as some psychiatric disorders, has been carefully scrutinized by multidisciplinary committees of specialists within the Harry Benjamin International Gender Dysphoria Association for over 20 years. The treatment of any GID begins after a careful evaluation, including parents, other family members, spouses, psychometric testing, and occasionally physical and laboratory examination. The details will depend on the age of the individual. It is possible, of course, to have a GID as well as mental retardation, a psychosis, dysthymia, severe character pathology, or any other psychiatric diagnosis (Table 37-6).

Psychotherapy

No one knows how to "cure" an adult's gender problem. People who have long lived with profound cross-gender identifications do not get insight—either behaviorally modified or medicated—and find that they subsequently have a conventional gender identity. Psychotherapy is useful, nonetheless. If the individual is able to trust a therapist, there can be much to talk about—family relationships are often painful, barriers to relationship intimacy are profound, work poses many difficult issues, and the individual has to make monumental decisions. The central one is, "How am I going to live my life? Should I go through with cross-gender living, hormone therapy, mastectomy, or genital surgery?" The therapist

Table 37-6	Steps in Evaluation of the Profoundly Gender Disordered

Formal evaluation and diagnosis—gender identity disorder or gender identity disorder NOS. Can the patient be referred to a gender program? Is another treatable psychiatric or physical disorder present?

Individual psychotherapy within the gender program or with an interested professional. Do the diagnoses remain the same? If yes, does the patient consistently want to:

    Discuss his (or her) situation but make no changes?

    Increase cross-dressing toward crossliving?

    Prepare the family for the real-life test?

    Obtain permission to proceed with hormones?

Approval for hormones from a gender committee or on written recommendation from the psychiatrist to an endocrinologist. Individual or group psychotherapy should continue.

Real-life test of living and working full time in the aspired-to gender role for at least 1 year.

    Does the patient want to continue to surgery?

Gender committee approval for surgery. Many patients have cosmetic surgery other than that listed with only ordinary patient–surgeon consent. This most often involves breast augmentation but may include numerous other attempts to improve ability to pass as opposite sex and be attractive.

    Men—genital reconstruction

    Women—mastectomy, hysterectomy, genital reconstruction; Most patients will not complete all of these steps.

can help the individual recognize the drawbacks and advantages of the various available options and to respect the initially unrecognized or unstated ambivalence. Completion of the gender transformation process usually takes longer than the individual desires, and the therapist can be an important source of support during and after these changes.

Group Therapy

Group therapy for gender-disordered people has the advantages of allowing individuals to know others with gender problems, of decreasing their social isolation, and of being among people who do not experience their cross-gender aspirations and their past behaviors as weird. Group members can provide help with grooming and more convincing public appearances. The success of these groups depends on the therapist's skills in selection of the individuals and using the group process. Groups are generally only available in a few specialized treatment programs.

Hormone Therapy

Ideally, hormones should be administered by endocrinologists who have a working relationship with a mental health team dealing with gender problems. The effects of administration of estrogen to a biological male are breast development, testicular atrophy, decreased sexual drive, decreased semen volume and fertility, softening of skin, fat redistribution in a female pattern, and decrease in spontaneous erections. Breast development is often the highest concern to the individual. Because hair growth is not affected by estrogens, electrolysis is often used to remove beard growth. Side effects within recommended doses are minimal but hypertension, hyperglycemia, lipid abnormalities, thrombophlebitis, and hepatic dysfunction have been described. The most dramatic effect of hormones is on the sense of well-being. Individuals report feeling calmer and happier knowing that their bodies are being demasculinized and feminized. All results derive from open-labeled studies.

The administration of androgen to females results in an increased sexual drive, clitoral tingling and growth, weight gain, and amenorrhea and hoarseness. An increase in muscle mass may be apparent if weight training is undertaken simultaneously. Hair growth depends on the individual's genetic potential. Androgens are administrated intramuscularly 200–300 mg/month and are generally safe. It is prudent, however, to periodically monitor hepatic, lipid, and thyroid functioning. Most individuals are delighted with their bodily changes, although some are disappointed that they remain short, wide-hipped, relatively hairless men with breasts that do not significantly regress.

Surgical Therapy

Surgical intervention is the final and obviously irreversible external step. It should not occur without a mental health professional's input, even when the individual provides a heartfelt convincing set of reasons to bypass the real-life test, hormones, and therapeutic relationship. Genital surgery is expensive, time consuming, at times painful, and has frequent anatomic complications and functional disappointments. Surgery can be expected to add further improvements in the lives of some individuals—more social activities with friends and family, more activity in sports, more partner sexual activity, and improved vocational status.

The Paraphilias

DIAGNOSIS

A paraphilia is a disorder of intention, the final component of sexual identity to develop in children and adolescents. Intention refers to what individuals want to do with a sexual partner and what they want the partner to do with them during sexual behavior. Normally, the images and the behaviors of intention fall within ranges of peaceable mutuality. The disorders of intention are recognized by unusual eroticism (images) and often socially destructive behaviors such as sex with children, rape, exhibitionism, voyeurism, masochism, obscene phone calling, or sexual touching of strangers. While 5% of the diagnoses of paraphilia are given to women, most etiologic speculations refer to male sexual identity development gone awry. This raises the important question about what happens to girls who have the same developmental misfortunes that are speculated to create male paraphilia.

Now it is apparent that paraphilias occur among individuals of all orientations and among those with conventional and unconventional gender identities. A homosexual sadist is paraphilic only on the basis of sexual cruelty. A transsexual who desires to be beaten during arousal is paraphilic only on the basis of masochism.

Erotic intentions that are *not* longstanding, unusual, and highly arousing may be problematic in some way but they are not clearly paraphilic. The *sine qua non* of the diagnosis of paraphilia is unusual, often hostile, dehumanized eroticism that has preoccupied the individual for most of his adolescent and adult life. The paraphilic fantasy is often associated with this preoccupying arousal when it occurs in daydreams and masturbation reveries or is encountered in explicit films or magazines. The specific imagery varies from one paraphilic individual to the next, but both the imagined behavior and its implied relationship to the partner are unusual in that they are preoccupied with aggression. Images of rape, obscene phone calling, exhibitionism, and touching of strangers, for example, are rehearsals of victimization. In masochistic images, the aggression is directed at the self—for instance, autoerotic strangulation, slavery, torture, and spanking. In others, the aggression is well disguised as *love* of children or teenagers. In some, such as simple clothing fetishism, the aggression may be absent. Aggression is so apparent in most paraphilic content, however, that when none seems to exist, the clinician needs to wonder whether it is actually absent or being hidden from the doctor. Paraphilic fantasies often rely heavily upon the image of a partner who does not possess "personhood." Some imagery in fact has no pretense of a human partner at all; clothing, animals, or excretory products are the focus. Other themes, such as preoccupation with feet or hair, combine both human and inanimate interests.

Paraphilic images are usually devoid of any pretense of caring or human attachment. The hatred, anger, fear, vengeance, or worthlessness expressed in them require no familiarity with the partner. Paraphilic images are conscious—clearly known to the individual. They should not be confused with speculations about "unconscious" aggression or sadomasochism that some assume are part of all sexual behavior. Clinicians should expect to occasionally see paraphilic individuals whose preoccupations are not hostile to others.

An individual's paraphilic themes often change in intensity or seem to change in content from time to time. The stimuli for these changes often remain unclear. In most instances, it is reasonable to consider that paraphilia is a basic developmental disorder in which particular erotic and sexual manifestations are shaped by the individuality of the person's history. To make a diagnosis of paraphilia, the individual must evidence at least 6 months of the unusual erotic preoccupation. Duration is usually not in question, even among adolescents, however.

To be paraphilic means that the erotic imagery exerts a pressure to play out the often imagined scene. In its milder forms, the pressure results merely in a preoccupation with a behavior. For instance, a man who prefers to be spoken to harshly and dominated by his wife during sex thinks about his masochistic images primarily around their sexual behaviors. He does not spend hours daydreaming of his erotic preferences. In their more intense forms, paraphilias create a *drivenness* to act out the fantasy in sexual behavior—usually in masturbation. Frequent masturbation, often more than once daily, continues long after adolescence. In the most severe situations, the need to attend to the fantasy and masturbate is so overpowering that life's ordinary activities cannot efficiently occur. Masturbation and sometimes partner-seeking behavior is experienced as driven. The individual reports either that he cannot control his behavior or he controls it with such great effort that his work, study, parenting, and relationships are disrupted.

Two other conditions, compulsive sexual behavior and sexual addiction, not part of the DSM-IV-TR, are informally and synonymously used to refer to heterosexual and homosexual men and women who display an intense drivenness to behave sexually without paraphilic imagery. The personal, interpersonal, and medical consequences of paraphilic and nonparaphilic sexual compulsivity seem indistinguishable as do their usual psychiatric comorbidities: depression, anxiety disorders, substance abuse, and attention deficit disorders.

Criminal Sex-Offending Behaviors

Exhibitionism

Exhibitionism generally involves teenagers and men displaying their penises so that the witness will be shocked or (in the paraphilic's fantasy) sexually interested. They may or may not masturbate during or immediately following this act of victimization. This diagnosis is not usually made when a man is arrested for "public indecency" and his penile exposures are motivated to arrange homosexual contact in a public place generally unseen by heterosexuals. Penile display in parks is one way to make anonymous contact. The presence or absence of exhibitionistic imagery allows the clinician to make the distinction between paraphilia and homosexual courting.

Pedophilia

Pedophilia is the most widely and intensely socially repudiated of the paraphilias. Pedophiles are men who erotically and romantically prefer children or young adolescents. They are grouped into categories depending upon their erotic preferences for boys or girls and for infant, young, or pubertal children. Some pedophiles have highly age- and sex-specific tastes, others are less discriminating. Since the diagnosis of pedophilia requires, over a period of at least 6 months, recurrent, intense sexually arousing fantasies, sexual urges, or behaviors involving sexual activity with a prepubescent child or children the disorder should not be expected to be present in every person who is guilty of child molestation. Some intrafamilial child abuse occurs over a shorter time interval and results from combinations of deteriorated marriages, sexual deprivation, sociopathy, and substance abuse. Child molestation, whether paraphilic or not, is a crime, however. Child molesters show several patterns of erectile responses to visual stimulation in the laboratory. Some have their largest arousal to children of a specific age and others respond to both children and adults. Others respond with their greatest arousal to aggressive cues.

Voyeurism

Men whose sexual life consists of watching homosexual or heterosexual videos in sexual book stores occasionally come to psychiatric attention after being charged with a crime following a police raid. They may or may not qualify for this diagnosis. The voyeurs who are more problematic for society are those who watch women through windows or break into their dwellings

for this purpose. Some of these crimes result in rape or nonsexual violence, but many are motivated by pure voyeuristic intent (which is subtly aggressive).

Sexual Sadism

While rape is an extreme variety of sadism, paraphilic sadism is present only in a minority of rapists. It is defined by the rapist's prior use of erotic scripts that involve a partner's fear, pain, humiliation, and suffering. Rapists are highly dangerous men whose antisocial behaviors are generally thought to be unresponsive to ordinary psychiatric methods. Their violence potential often makes psychiatric therapy outside of institutions imprudent. Noncriminal paraphilic sadism—that is, arousal to images of harming another that has not crossed into the behavioral realm—can be treated in outpatient settings.

Frotteurism

Frotteurism, the need to touch and rub against nonconsenting persons, although delineated as a criminal act, is probably better understood as a less malignant form of paraphilic sadism. Frotteurism often occurs in socially isolated men who become sexually driven to act out. They often are unaware of how frightening they can be.

Noncriminal Forms of Paraphilia

Because the individual manifestations of paraphilia depend on the particular individual life history of the affected, over 40 paraphilic categories have been identified, although only a few are listed in the DSM-IV-TR. Most of these are unusual means of attaining arousal during masturbation or consenting partner behaviors. Each of the themes identified below demonstrates a wide range of manifestations from the bizarre to the more "reasonable" and from the common to the unique. They often subtly combine elements of more than one paraphilia.

Fetishism/Transvestic Fetishism

Fetishism, the pairing of arousal with wearing or holding an article of clothing or inanimate object such as an inflatable doll, has a range of manifestations, from infantilism in which a person dresses up in diapers to pretend he is a baby to the far more common use of a female undergarment for arousal purposes. Fetishism when confined to one garment for decades is classified as a paraphilia, but many cases involve more complex varieties of cross-dressing and overlap with gender identity disorders, usually GIDNOS. Fetishistic transvestism is the diagnosis used when it is apparent that the urges to use the clothing of the opposite sex are part of a larger mental preoccupation with that sex.

Sexual Masochism

Sexual masochism is diagnosed over a range of behaviors from the sometimes fatal need to nearly asphyxiate oneself to the request to be spanked by the partner in order to be excited. Masochism may be the most commonly reported or acknowledged form of female paraphilia, although it is more common among men. Sadists and masochists sometimes find one another and work out an arrangement to act out their fantasies and occasionally reverse roles.

Paraphilia Not Otherwise Specified

Paraphilia not otherwise specified is a DSM-IV-TR category for other endpoints of abnormal sexual development that lead to preoccupations with amputated body parts, feces, urine, sexualized enemas, and sex with animals.

TREATMENT

Four general approaches are employed to treat the paraphilias: evaluation only, psychotherapy, medications, and external controls. The treatments are not mutually exclusive; rather, they are often multimodal in application.

Evaluation only is often selected when the evaluator concludes that the paraphilia is benign in terms of society, and the individual will be resistant to the other approaches, and does not suffer greatly in terms of social and vocational functioning in ways that might be improved. Often, these are isolated men with private paraphilic sexual pleasures, such as telephone sex with a masochistic scenario.

What constitutes psychotherapy for paraphilia heavily depends on the therapist training rather than strident declarations of treatment of choice. Little optimism exists that any form of therapy can permanently change the nature of a long-established paraphilic erotic script, even among teenage sex offenders. Individual psychodynamic psychotherapy can be highly useful in diminishing paraphilic intensifications and gradually teaching the individual better management techniques of the situations that have triggered acting

out. Well-described cognitive–behavioral interventions exist for interrupting paraphilic arousal via pairing masturbatory excitement with either aversive imagery or aversive stimuli. Comprehensive behavioral treatment involves social skills training, assertiveness training, and confrontation with the rationalizations that are used to minimize awareness of the victims of sexual crimes, and marital therapy. The self-help movement has created 12-step programs for sexual addictions to which many individuals now belong. Group psychotherapy is offered by trained therapists as well. When the lives of paraphilics are illuminated in various therapies, it becomes apparent that the emotional pain of the individuals is thought to be great; the sexual acting out is often perceived as a defense against recurrent unpleasant emotions from any source. These often, however, involve self-esteem and primitive anxiety.

In the early 1980s, depo-medroxyprogesterone (Provera) was first used to treat those who were constantly masturbating, seeking out personally dangerous sexual outlets, or committing sex crimes. The weekly 400- to 600-mg injections often led to the men being able to work, study, or participate in activities that were previously beyond them because of concentration or attention difficulties. In the late 1980s, the use of oral Provera, 20–120 mg/day led to similar results: the drug enabled these men to leave their former state in which their sexual needs took priority over other life demands—and they did not have depo-Provera's side effect profile: weight gain, hypertension, muscle cramps, and gynecomastia. Today, gonadotrophin-releasing blockers are occasionally used for this purpose. The possible side effects are similar to oral Provera. Despite the fact that the clinical results are among the most powerful effected by any psychopharmacologic treatment, many clinicians cannot overcome their disinclination about giving a "female" hormone to a man or working with individuals who victimize others sexually. Serotonergic agents are now more commonly used as a first line of treatment. While these studies are not as methodologically sophisticated as they need to be, the SSRIs are in widespread use for compulsive sexual behaviors and sexual obsessions. Their efficacy is the source of the speculation that some of the paraphilias may be an obsessive–compulsive spectrum disorder.

Sexual advantage-taking, whether it be by a paraphilic clinician with the individuals under his care, by a pedophilic mentally retarded man in the neighborhood, or of a grandfather who has abused several generations of his offspring, can often be stopped by making it *impossible* for these behaviors to be unknown to most people in his life. The clinician's staff can be told, the neighbors can know, the family can meet to discuss the current crisis and review who has been abused over the years and plan to never allow the grandfather alone with any child in or outside the family. The concept of external control is taken over by the judicial system when sex crimes are highly repugnant or heinous. The offender is removed from society for punishment and the protection of the public. Increasing pressure exists to criminalize sexual advantage-taking by clinicians who are even more susceptible to losing their licenses at least for several years.

Clinicians need to be realistic about the limitations of various therapeutic ventures. Sexual acting out may readily continue during therapy beyond the awareness of the therapist. The more violent and destructive the paraphilic behavior to others, the less the therapist should risk ambulatory treatment. Since paraphilia occurs in individuals with other mental disorders, the clinician needs to remain vigilant that the treatment program is comprehensive and does not lose sight of the paraphilia just because the depressive or compulsive symptoms are improved. Paraphilia may be improved by medications and psychotherapy, but the clinician should expect that the intention disorder is the individual's lasting vulnerability.

Sexual Disorder Not Otherwise Specified

If the clinician is uncertain about how to categorize a person's problem, it is more reasonable to use this diagnosis than one that does not encompass the range of the individual's suffering. Sexual disorder not otherwise specified can be used when the therapist perceives a dramatic interplay between issues of sexual identity and sexual dysfunction, or when "everything" seems to be amiss. DSM-IV-TR, however, encourages the clinician to make multiple sexual diagnoses involving, for instance, a gender identity disorder, a desire disorder, erectile, and orgasmic disorder.

DSM-IV-TR provides two examples when it would be appropriate to use the diagnosis sexual disorder NOS: (1) nonparaphilic compulsive sexual behaviors—that is, relentless pursuit of masturbatory or heterosexual or homosexual partner experiences without evidence of paraphilic imagery; (2) complicated or exaggerated struggles to manage homosexual urges.

COMPARISON OF DSM-IV-TR AND ICD-10 DIAGNOSTIC CRITERIA

For hypoactive sexual desire disorder, the ICD-10 Diagnostic Criteria for Research and the DSM-IV-TR criteria are essentially identical except that ICD-10 specifies a minimum duration of at least 6 months (DSM-IV-TR has no minimum duration).

The ICD-10 Diagnostic Criteria for Research for Sexual Aversion Disorder differ from the DSM-IV-TR criteria in several ways. In contrast to DSM-IV-TR, which restricts the condition to the aversion to, and avoidance of, sexual genital contact, ICD-10 also includes presentations characterized by sexual activity resulting in "strong negative feelings and an inability to experience any pleasure." Furthermore, ICD-10 excludes cases in which the aversion is due to performance anxiety. Finally, ICD-10 specifies a minimum duration of at least 6 month whereas DSM-IV-TR does not specify any minimum duration.

For female sexual arousal disorder and male erectile disorder, the ICD-10 Diagnostic Criteria for Research and the DSM-IV-TR criteria are essentially equivalent except that ICD-10 specifies a minimum duration of at least 6 months. ICD-10 includes a single category ("Failure of Genital Response") with two separate criteria sets by gender. In contrast, DSM-IV-TR includes two separate categories.

For female and male orgasmic disorders, the ICD-10 Diagnostic Criteria for Research and the DSM-IV-TR criteria are essentially equivalent except that ICD-10 specifies a minimum duration of at least 6 months. In contrast to DSM-IV-TR, which has male and female versions defined separately, ICD-10 has a single category that applies to both genders.

For premature ejaculation, the ICD-10 Diagnostic Criteria for Research and the DSM-IV-TR criteria are essentially equivalent except that ICD-10 specifies a minimum duration of at least 6 months. Similarly, the ICD-10 Diagnostic Criteria for Research and the DSM-IV-TR criteria for Dyspareunia and Vaginismus are essentially equivalent except that ICD-10 specifies a minimum duration of at least 6 months. Furthermore, these conditions are referred to in ICD-10 as "Nonorganic Dyspareunia" and "Nonorganic Vaginismus."

The definition of a paraphilia is essentially the same in DSM-IV-TR and ICD-10. However, ICD-10 does not include a separate category for Frotteurism and has a combined "Sadomasochism" category.

For gender identity disorder, ICD-10 defines three separate disorders: "Gender Identity Disorder of Childhood," "Dual-role Transvestism," and "Transsexualism," all of which are included under the single DSM-IV-TR category Gender Identity Disorder.

In the current diagnostic nomenclature DSM-IV-TR, eating disorders consist of two clearly defined syndromes: anorexia nervosa and bulimia nervosa. Many individuals presenting for treatment of an eating disorder fail to meet the formal criteria for either anorexia nervosa or bulimia nervosa, which raises an important theoretical and practical question: what is an eating disorder? Although this topic has received surprisingly little attention, it has been suggested that a working definition of an eating disorder might be "a persistent disturbance of eating behavior or behavior intended to control weight, which significantly impairs physical health or psychosocial functioning." This definition provides a basis for viewing eating disorders as clinically significant problems that do not meet criteria for anorexia nervosa or bulimia nervosa. The term *atypical eating disorder* is often applied to such problems, even though the number of individuals suffering from them may well outnumber those with "typical" eating disorders. One example of an atypical eating disorder is that of women who are overly concerned about their weight, have dieted to a below-normal weight, but have not ceased menstruating and, therefore, do not meet full criteria for anorexia nervosa. Another is that of individuals who binge and vomit regularly, but at less than the twice-a-week frequency required for bulimia nervosa.

An additional example of a clinically important atypical eating disorder is the occurrence of frequent binge-eating that is not followed by the self-induced vomiting or other inappropriate attempts to compensate that are characteristic of bulimia nervosa. This disturbance is a common behavioral pattern among obese individuals who present for treatment at weight-loss clinics.

At present, obesity is not formally considered an eating disorder. Obesity refers to an excess of body fat and is viewed as a general medical, not a psychiatric, condition. At this stage of our knowledge, obesity is conceived as an etiologically heterogeneous condition. Obese individuals are at increased risk for a number of serious medical problems and are subject to significant social stigmatization and its psychological sequelae. The widely held assumption that obesity is the result of a psychiatric disorder in which eating is used as a coping mechanism for depression or anxiety has not been substantiated by empirical research.

Anorexia Nervosa

DIAGNOSIS

The DSM-IV-TR criteria for Anorexia Nervosa require the individual to be significantly underweight for age and height. Although it is not possible to set a single weight-loss standard that applies equally to

---

DSM-IV-TR Diagnostic Criteria

307.1 ANOREXIA NERVOSA

A. Refusal to maintain body weight at or above a minimally normal weight for age and height (e.g., weight loss leading to maintenance of body weight less than 85% of that expected; or failure to make expected weight gain during period of growth, leading to body weight less than 85% of that expected).
B. Intense fear of gaining weight or becoming fat, even though underweight.
C. Disturbance in the way in which one's body weight or shape is experienced, undue influence of body weight or shape on self-evaluation, or denial of the seriousness of the current low body weight.
D. In postmenarcheal females, amenorrhea, i.e., the absence of at least three consecutive menstrual cycles. (A woman is considered to have amenorrhea if her periods occur only following hormone, e.g., estrogen, administration.)

Specify type:

Restricting type: during the current episode of anorexia nervosa, the person has not regularly engaged in binge-eating or purging behavior (i.e., self-induced vomiting or the misuse of laxatives, diuretics, or enemas).
Binge-eating/purging type: during the current episode of anorexia nervosa, the person has regularly engaged in binge-eating or purging behavior (i.e., self-induced vomiting or the misuse of laxatives, diuretics, or enemas).

Reprinted with permission from the *Diagnostic and Statistical Manual of Mental Disorders*, 4th ed., Text Rev. Copyright 2000 American Psychiatric Association.

Clinical Guide to the Diagnosis and Treatment of Mental Disorders. M. B. First and A. Tasman
© 2006 John Wiley & Sons, Ltd. ISBN 0 470 019158

all individuals, DSM-IV-TR provides a benchmark of 85% of the weight considered normal for age and height as a guideline. Despite being of an abnormally low body weight, individuals with anorexia nervosa are intensely afraid of gaining weight and becoming fat, and remarkably, this fear typically intensifies as the weight falls.

DSM-IV-TR criterion C requires a disturbance in the person's judgment about his or her weight or shape. For example, despite being underweight, individuals with anorexia nervosa often view themselves or a part of their body as being too heavy. Typically, they deny the grave medical risks engendered by their semistarvation and place enormous psychological importance on whether they have gained or lost weight. For example, someone with anorexia nervosa may feel intensely distressed if her or his weight increases by half a pound.

DSM-IV-TR suggests that individuals with anorexia nervosa be classed as having one of two variants, either the binge-eating/purging type or the restricting type. Individuals with the restricting type of anorexia nervosa do not engage regularly in either binge-eating or purging, and compared with individuals with the binge-eating/purging form of the disorder, are not as likely to abuse alcohol and other drugs, exhibit less mood lability, and are less active sexually. There are also indications that the two subtypes may differ in their response to pharmacological intervention.

In assessing individuals who may have anorexia nervosa, it is important to obtain a weight history including the individual's highest and lowest weights and the weight he or she would like to be now. For women, it is useful to know the weight at which menstruation last occurred, because it provides an indication of what weight is normal for that individual. Probably the greatest problem in the assessment of individuals with anorexia nervosa is their denial of the illness and their reluctance to participate in an evaluation. A straightforward but supportive and nonconfrontational style is probably the most useful approach, but it is likely that the individual will not acknowledge significant difficulties in eating or with weight and will rationalize unusual eating or exercise habits. It is therefore helpful to obtain information from other sources such as the individual's family.

An impressive array of physical disturbances has been documented in anorexia nervosa, and the physiological bases of many are understood (Table 38-1). Most of these physical disturbances appear to be secondary consequences of starvation, and it is not clear whether or how the physiological disturbances described here contribute to the development and maintenance of the psychological and behavioral abnormalities characteristic of anorexia nervosa. The central nervous system

Table 38-1	Medical Problems Commonly Associated with Anorexia Nervosa

Skin
  Lanugo
Cardiovascular system
  Hypotension
  Bradycardia
  Arrhythmias
Hematopoietic system
  Normochromic, normocytic anemia
  Leukopenia
    Diminished polymorphonuclear leukocytes
Fluid and electrolyte balance
  Elevated blood urea nitrogen and creatinine concentrations
  Hypokalemia
  Hyponatremia
  Hypochloremia
  Alkalosis
Gastrointestinal system
  Elevated serum concentration of liver enzymes
  Delayed gastric emptying
  Constipation
Endocrine system
  Diminished thyroxine level with normal thyroid-stimulating hormone level
  Elevated plasma cortisol level
  Diminished secretion of luteinizing hormone, follicle-stimulating hormone, estrogen, or testosterone
Bone
  Osteoporosis

is clearly affected. Computed tomography has demonstrated that individuals with anorexia nervosa have enlarged ventricles, an abnormality that improves with weight gain. The cerebrospinal fluid concentrations of a variety of neurotransmitters and their metabolites are altered in underweight individuals with anorexia nervosa and tend to normalize as weight is restored.

Some of the most striking physiological alterations in anorexia nervosa are those of the hypothalamic–pituitary–gonadal axis. In women, estrogen secretion from the ovaries is markedly reduced, accounting for the occurrence of amenorrhea. In analogous fashion, testosterone production is diminished in men with anorexia nervosa.

In an adult with anorexia nervosa, the status of the hypothalamic–pituitary–gonadal axis resembles that of a pubertal or prepubertal child–the secretion of estrogen or testosterone, of luteinizing hormone and follicle-stimulating hormone, and of gonadotropin-releasing hormone is reduced.

The functioning of other hormonal systems is also disrupted in anorexia nervosa, although typically not as profoundly as is the reproductive axis. Presumably as part of the metabolic response to semistarvation, the activity of the thyroid gland is reduced. Plasma thyroxine levels are somewhat diminished, but the plasma levels of the pituitary hormone and thyroid-stimulating hormone are not elevated. The activity of the hypothalamic–pituitary–adrenal axis is increased, as indicated by elevated plasma levels of cortisol and by resistance to dexamethasone suppression. The regulation of vasopressin (antidiuretic hormone) secretion from the posterior pituitary is disturbed, contributing to the development of partial diabetes insipidus in some individuals.

Anorexia nervosa is often associated with the development of leukopenia and of a normochromic, normocytic anemia of mild to moderate severity. Surprisingly, leukopenia does not appear to result in a high vulnerability to infectious illnesses. Serum levels of liver enzymes are sometimes elevated, particularly during the early phases of refeeding, but the synthetic function of the liver is rarely seriously impaired so that the serum albumin concentration and the prothrombin time are usually within normal limits. Serum cholesterol levels are sometimes elevated in anorexia nervosa, although the basis of this abnormality remains obscure. In some individuals, self-imposed fluid restriction and excessive exercise produce dehydration and elevations of serum creatinine and blood urea nitrogen. In others, water loading may lead to hyponatremia. The status of serum electrolytes is a reflection of the individual's salt and water intake and the nature and the severity of the purging behavior. A common pattern is hypokalemia, hypochloremia, and mild alkalosis resulting from frequent and persistent self-induced vomiting.

It has become clear that individuals with anorexia nervosa have decreased bone density compared with age- and sex-matched peers and, as a result, are at increased risk for fractures. Low levels of estrogen, high levels of cortisol, and poor nutrition have been cited as risk factors for the development of reduced bone density in anorexia nervosa. Theoretically, estrogen treatment might reduce the risk of osteoporosis in women who are chronically amenorrheic because of anorexia nervosa, but controlled studies indicate that this intervention is of limited, if any, benefit.

Abnormalities of cardiac function include bradycardia and hypotension, which are rarely symptomatic. The pump function of the heart is compromised, and congestive heart failure occasionally develops in individuals during overly rapid refeeding. The electrocardiogram shows sinus bradycardia and a number of nonspecific abnormalities. Arrhythmias may develop, often in association with fluid and electrolyte disturbances. It has been suggested that significant prolongation of the QT interval may be a harbinger of life-threatening arrhythmias in some individuals with anorexia nervosa, but this has not been conclusively demonstrated.

The motility of the gastrointestinal tract is diminished, leading to delayed gastric emptying and contributing to complaints of bloating and constipation. Rare cases of acute gastric dilatation or gastric rupture, which is often fatal, have been reported in individuals with anorexia nervosa who consumed large amounts of food when binge-eating.

Anorexia nervosa is a relatively rare illness. Even among high-risk groups, such as adolescent girls and young women, the prevalence of strictly defined anorexia nervosa is only about 0.5%. The prevalence rates of partial syndromes are substantially higher, however. Despite the infrequent occurrence of anorexia nervosa, most studies suggest that its incidence has increased significantly during the past 50 years, a phenomenon usually attributed to changes in cultural norms regarding desirable body shape and weight.

Anorexia nervosa usually affects women; the ratio of men to women is approximately 1:10 to 1:20. Anorexia nervosa occurs primarily in industrialized and affluent countries and some data suggest that even within those countries, anorexia nervosa is more common among the higher socioeconomic classes. Some occupations, such as ballet dancing and fashion modeling, appear to confer a particularly high risk for the development of anorexia nervosa. Thus, anorexia nervosa appears more likely to develop in an environment in which food is readily available but in which, for women, being thin is somehow equated with higher or special achievement.

Course

Anorexia nervosa often begins innocently. Typically, an adolescent girl or young woman who is of normal weight or, perhaps, a few pounds overweight decides to diet. This decision may be prompted by an important but not extraordinary life event, such as leaving home for camp, attending a new school, or a casual unflattering remark by a friend or family member. Initially, the dieting seems no different from that pursued by many young women, but as weight falls, the dieting intensifies. The restrictions become broader and more rigid; for example, desserts may first be eliminated, then meat, then any food that is thought to contain fat. The person becomes increasingly uncomfortable if she is seen eating and avoids meals with others. Food seems to assume a moral quality so that, for example, vegetables are viewed as "good" and anything with fat is "bad." The individual has idiosyncratic rules about how much exercise she must do, and when, where, and how she can eat.

Food avoidance and weight loss are accompanied by a deep and reassuring sense of accomplishment, and weight gain is viewed as a failure and a sign of weakness. Physical activity, such as running or aerobic exercise, often increases as the dieting and weight loss develop. Inactivity and complaints of weakness usually occur only when emaciation has become extreme. The person becomes more serious and devotes little effort to anything but work, dieting, and exercise. She may become depressed and emotionally labile, socially withdrawn, and secretive, and she may lie about her eating and her weight. Despite the profound disturbances in her view of her weight and of her calorie needs, reality testing in other spheres is intact, and the person may continue to function well in school or at work. Symptoms usually persist for months or years until, typically at the insistence of friends or family, the person reluctantly agrees to see a physician.

Differential Diagnosis

Although depression, schizophrenia, and obsessive–compulsive disorder may be associated with disturbed eating and weight loss, it is rarely difficult to differentiate these disorders from anorexia nervosa. Individuals with major depression may lose significant amounts of weight but do not exhibit the relentless drive for thinness characteristic of anorexia nervosa. In schizophrenia, starvation may occur because of delusions about food, for example, that it is poisoned. Individuals with obsessive–compulsive disorder may describe irrational concerns about food and develop rituals related to meal preparation and eating but do not describe the intense fear of gaining weight and the pervasive wish to be thin that characterize anorexia nervosa.

A wide variety of medical problems cause serious weight loss in young people and may at times be confused with anorexia nervosa. Examples of such problems include gastric outlet obstruction, Crohn's disease, and brain tumors. Individuals whose weight loss is due to a general medical illness generally do not show the drive for thinness, the fear of gaining weight, and the increased physical activity characteristic of anorexia nervosa. However, the clinician is well advised to consider any chronic medical illness associated with weight loss, especially when evaluating individuals with unusual clinical presentations such as late age at onset or prominent physical complaints, for example, pain and gastrointestinal cramping while eating.

TREATMENT

The first goal of treatment is to engage the individual and her or his family. For most individuals with anorexia nervosa, this is challenging. Individuals usually minimize their symptoms and suggest that the concerns of the family and friends, who have often been instrumental in arranging the consultation, are greatly exaggerated. It is helpful to identify a problem that the individual can acknowledge, such as weakness, irritability, difficulty concentrating, or trouble with binge-eating. The clinician may then attempt to educate the individual regarding the pervasive physical and psychological effects of semistarvation and about the need for weight gain if the acknowledged problem is to be successfully addressed.

A second goal of treatment is to assess and address acute medical problems, such as fluid and electrolyte disturbances and cardiac arrhythmias. Depending on the severity of illness, this may require the involvement of a general medical physician. The additional but most difficult and time-consuming goals are the restoration of normal body weight, the normalization of eating, and the resolution of the associated psychological disturbances. The final goal is the prevention of relapse.

As already noted, virtually all of the physiological abnormalities described in individuals with anorexia nervosa are also seen in other forms of starvation, and most improve or disappear as weight returns to normal. Therefore, weight restoration is essential for physiological recovery. Weight restoration also is believed to be essential for psychological recovery as well. Accounts of human starvation amply document the profound impact of starvation on mental health. Starving individuals lose their sense of humor, their interest in friends and family fades, and mood generally becomes depressed. They may develop peculiar behavior similar to that of individuals with anorexia nervosa, such as hoarding food or concocting bizarre food combinations. If starvation disrupts psychological and behavioral functioning in normal individuals, it presumably does so as well in those with anorexia nervosa. Thus, correction of starvation is a prerequisite for the restoration of both physical and psychological health.

A common major impediment to the treatment of individuals with anorexia nervosa is their disagreement with the goals of treatment; many of the features of their illness are simply not viewed by these individuals as a problem. In addition, this may be compounded by a variety of concerns of the individual, such as basic mistrust of relationships, feelings of vulnerability and inferiority, and sensitivity to perceived coercion. Such concerns may be expressed through considerable resistance, defiance, or pseudocompliance with the clinician's interventions, and contribute to the power struggles that often characterize the treatment process. The clinician must try to avoid colluding with the individual's attempts to minimize problems but at the

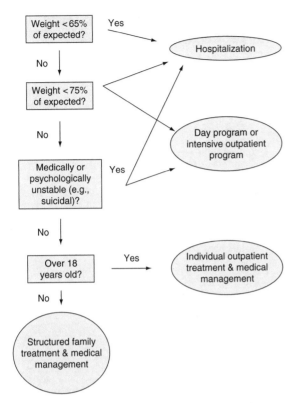

Figure 38-1 *Algorithm for choice of initial treatment of anorexia nervosa.*

same time allow the individual enough independence to maintain the alliance. Dealing with such dilemmas is challenging and requires an active approach on the part of the clinician. In most instances, it is possible to preserve the alliance while nonetheless adhering to established limits and the need for change.

The initial stage of treatment should be aimed at reversing the nutritional and behavioral abnormalities (Figure 38-1). The intensity of the treatment required and the need for partial or full hospitalization should be determined by the current weight, the rapidity of weight loss, and the severity of associated medical and behavioral problems and of other symptoms such as depression. In general, individuals whose weights are less than 75% of the expected weight should be viewed as medically precarious and require intensive treatment, such as hospitalization.

Most inpatient or day treatment units experienced in the care of individuals with anorexia nervosa use a structured treatment approach that relies heavily on supervision of calorie intake by the staff. After the initial medical assessment has been completed and weight has stabilized, calorie intake is gradually increased to an amount necessary to gain 2 to 5 lb/week.

During this phase of treatment, it is necessary to monitor individuals carefully; many will resort to throwing food away or vomiting after meals. Careful supervision is also required to obtain accurate weights; individuals may consume large amounts of fluid before being weighed or hide heavy articles under their clothing.

During the weight restoration phase of treatment, individuals require substantial emotional support. It is probably best to address fears of weight gain with education about the dangers of semistarvation and with the reassurance that individuals will not be allowed to gain "too much" weight. Most eating-disorder units impose behavioral restrictions, such as limits on physical activity, during the early phase of treatment. Some units use an explicit behavior modification regimen in which weight gain is tied to increased privileges and failure to gain weight results in bed rest.

A consistent and structured treatment approach, with or without an explicit behavior modification program, is generally successful in promoting weight recovery but requires substantial energy and coordination to maintain a supportive and nonpunitive treatment environment. In most experienced treatment units, parenteral methods of nutrition, such as nasogastric feeding or intravenous hyperalimentation, are only rarely needed. Nutritional counseling and behavioral approaches can also be effective in helping individuals expand their dietary repertoire to include foods they have been frightened of consuming.

As weight increases, individual, group, and family psychotherapy can begin to address other issues in addition to the distress engendered by gaining weight. For example, it is typically important for individuals to recognize that they have come to base much of their self-esteem on dieting and weight control and are likely to judge themselves according to harsh and unforgiving standards. Similarly, individuals should be helped to see how the eating disorder has interfered with the achievement of personal goals such as education, sports, or making friends.

There is, at present, no general agreement about the most useful type of psychotherapy or the specific topics that need to be addressed. Most eating disorders programs employ a variety of psychotherapeutic interventions. A number of experts recommend the use of individual and group psychotherapy using cognitive–behavioral techniques to modify the irrational overemphasis on weight. Although most authorities see little role for traditional psychoanalytic therapy, individual and group psychodynamic therapy can address such problems as insecure attachment, separation and individuation, sexual relationships, and other interpersonal concerns. There is good evidence supporting the involvement of the family in the treatment of younger individuals with anorexia nervosa. Family therapy can be helpful in addressing family members' fears about the illness; interventions typically emphasize parental cooperation, mutual support and consistency, and establishing boundaries regarding the individual's symptoms and other aspects of his or her life.

Despite the multiple physiological disturbances associated with anorexia nervosa, there is no clearly established role for medication.

A large percentage of individuals with anorexia nervosa remain chronically ill; 30–50% of individuals successfully treated in the hospital require rehospitalization within 1 year of discharge. Therefore, posthospitalization outpatient treatments are recommended to prevent relapse and improve overall short- and long-term functioning. Several studies have attempted to evaluate the efficacy of various outpatient treatments for anorexia nervosa including behavioral, cognitive–behavioral, and supportive psychotherapy, as well as a variety of nutritional counseling interventions. Although most of these treatments seem to be helpful, the clearest findings to date support two interventions. For individuals whose anorexia nervosa started before age 18 years and who have had the disorder for less than 3 years, family therapy is effective, and for adult individuals, cognitive–behavioral therapy reduces the rate of relapse. Preliminary information suggests that fluoxetine treatment may reduce the risk of relapse among individuals with anorexia nervosa who have gained weight, but additional controlled data are required to document the usefulness of this intervention.

Bulimia Nervosa

DIAGNOSIS

The salient behavioral disturbance of bulimia nervosa is the occurrence of episodes of binge-eating. During these episodes, the individual consumes an amount of food that is unusually large considering the circumstances under which it was eaten. Although this is a useful definition and conceptually reasonably clear, it can be operationally difficult to distinguish normal overeating from a small episode of binge-eating. Indeed, the available data do not suggest that there is a sharp dividing line between the size of binge-eating episodes and the size of other meals. On the other hand, while the border between normal and abnormal eating may not be a sharp one, both individual reports and laboratory studies of eating behavior clearly indicate that, when binge-eating, individuals with bulimia ner-

---

DSM-IV-TR Diagnostic Criteria

307.51 Bulimia Nervosa

A. Recurrent episodes of binge-eating. An episode of binge-eating is characterized by both of the following:

  (1) eating, in a discrete period of time (e.g., within any 2-hour period), an amount of food that is definitely larger than most people would eat during a similar period of time and under similar circumstances.

  (2) a sense of lack of control over eating during the episode (e.g., a feeling that one cannot stop eating or control what or how much one is eating).

B. Recurrent inappropriate compensatory behavior in order to prevent weight gain, such as self-induced vomiting; misuse of laxatives, diuretics, enemas, or other medications; fasting; or excessive exercise.

C. The binge-eating and inappropriate compensatory behaviors both occur, on average, at least twice a week for 3 months.

D. Self-evaluation is unduly influenced by body shape and weight.

E. The disturbance does not occur exclusively during episodes of anorexia nervosa.

Specify type:

Purging type: during the current episode of bulimia nervosa, the person has regularly engaged in self-induced vomiting or the misuse of laxatives, diuretics, or enemas.
Nonpurging type: during the current episode of bulimia nervosa, the person has used other inappropriate compensatory behaviors, such as fasting or excessive exercise, but has not regularly engaged in self-induced vomiting or the misuse of laxatives, diuretics, or enemas.

Reprinted with permission from the *Diagnostic and Statistical Manual of Mental Disorders*, 4th ed., Text Rev. Copyright 2000 American Psychiatric Association.

---

vosa do indeed consume larger than normal amounts of food.

Episodes of binge-eating are associated, by definition, with a sense of loss of control. Once the eating has begun, the individual feels unable to stop until an excessive amount has been consumed. This loss of control is only subjective, in that most individuals with bulimia nervosa will abruptly stop eating in the midst of a binge episode if interrupted, for example, by the unexpected arrival of a roommate.

After overeating, individuals with bulimia nervosa engage in some form of inappropriate behavior in an attempt to avoid weight gain. Most individuals who present to eating disorders clinics with this syndrome report self-induced vomiting or the abuse of laxatives. Other methods include misusing diuretics, fasting for long periods, and exercising extensively after eating binges.

In the DSM-IV-TR nomenclature, the diagnosis of bulimia nervosa is not given to individuals with anorexia nervosa. Individuals with anorexia nervosa who recurrently engage in binge-eating or purging behavior should be given the diagnosis of anorexia nervosa, binge-eating/purging subtype, rather than an additional diagnosis of bulimia nervosa.

In DSM-IV-TR, a subtyping scheme was introduced for bulimia nervosa in which individuals are classed as having either the purging or the nonpurging type of bulimia nervosa. This scheme was introduced for several reasons. First, those individuals who purge are at greater risk for the development of fluid and electrolyte disturbances such as hypokalemia. Second, data suggest that individuals with the nonpurging type of bulimia nervosa weigh more and have fewer mental disorders compared with those with the purging type. Finally, most of the published literature on the treatment of bulimia nervosa has been based on studies of individuals with the purging type of this disorder.

Bulimia nervosa typically begins after a young woman who sees herself as somewhat overweight starts a diet and, after some initial success, begins to overeat. Distressed by her lack of control and by her fear of gaining weight, she decides to compensate for the overeating by inducing vomiting or taking laxatives, methods she has heard about from friends or seen in media reports about eating disorders. After discovering that she can successfully purge, the individual may, for a time, feel pleased in that she can eat large amounts of food and not gain weight. However, the episodes of binge-eating usually increase in size and in frequency and occur after a variety of stimuli, such as transient depression or anxiety or a sense that she has begun to overeat. Individuals often describe themselves as "numb" while they are binge-eating, suggesting that the eating may serve to avoid uncomfortable emotional states. Individuals usually feel intensely ashamed of their "disgusting" habit and may become depressed by their lack of control over their eating.

The binge-eating tends to occur in the late afternoon or evening and almost always while the individual is alone. The typical individual presenting to eating disorders clinics has been binge-eating and inducing vomiting 5 to 10 times weekly for 3 to 10 years. Although there is substantial variation, binges tend to contain 1000 or more calories and to consist of sweet, high-fat foods that are normally consumed as dessert, such as ice cream, cookies, and cake. Although individuals complain of "carbohydrate craving," they only rarely binge-eat foods that are pure carbohydrates, such as fruits. Individuals usually induce vomiting or use their characteristic compensatory behavior immediately after the binge and feel substantial relief that the calories are "gone." In reality, it appears that vomiting is the only purging method capable of disposing of a significant

number of ingested calories. The weight loss associated with the misuse of laxatives and diuretics is primarily due to the loss of fluid and electrolytes, not calories.

When not binge-eating, individuals with bulimia nervosa tend to restrict their calorie intake and to avoid the foods usually consumed during episodes of binge-eating. Although there is some phenomenological resemblance between binge-eating and substance abuse, there is no evidence that physiological addiction plays any role in bulimia nervosa.

Among individuals with bulimia nervosa who are seen at eating disorders clinics, there is an increased frequency of anxiety and mood disorders, especially major depressive disorder and dysthymic disorder, of drug and alcohol abuse, and of personality disorders. It is not certain whether this comorbidity is also observed in community samples or whether it is a characteristic of individuals who seek treatment.

In a small fraction of individuals, bulimia nervosa is associated with the development of fluid and electrolyte abnormalities that result from the self-induced vomiting or the misuse of laxatives or diuretics. The most common electrolyte disturbances are hypokalemia, hyponatremia, and hypochloremia. Individuals who lose substantial amounts of stomach acid through vomiting may become slightly alkalotic; those who abuse laxatives may become slightly acidotic.

There is an increased frequency of menstrual disturbances such as oligomenorrhea among women with bulimia nervosa. Several studies suggest that the hypothalamic–pituitary–gonadal axis is subject to the same type of disruption as is seen in anorexia nervosa but that the abnormalities are much less frequent and severe.

Individuals who induce vomiting for many years may develop dental erosion, especially of the upper front teeth. The mechanism appears to be that stomach acid softens the enamel, which in time gradually disappears so that the teeth chip more easily and can become reduced in size. Some individuals develop painless salivary gland enlargement, which is thought to represent hypertrophy resulting from the repeated episodes of binge-eating and vomiting. The serum level of amylase is sometimes mildly elevated in individuals with bulimia nervosa because of increased amounts of salivary amylase.

Most individuals with bulimia nervosa have surprisingly few gastrointestinal abnormalities. Potentially life-threatening complications such as an esophageal tear or gastric rupture occur, but fortunately, rarely. The long-standing use of syrup of ipecac to induce vomiting can lead to absorption of some of the alkaloids and cause permanent damage to nerve and muscle.

Over time, the symptoms of bulimia nervosa tend to improve although a substantial fraction of individuals continue to engage in binge-eating and purging. On the other hand, some controlled clinical trials have reported that structured forms of psychotherapy have the potential to yield substantial and sustained recovery in a significant fraction of individuals who complete treatment. It is not clear what factors are most predictive of good outcome, but those individuals who cease binge-eating and purging completely during treatment are least likely to relapse.

Soon after bulimia nervosa was recognized as a distinct disorder, surveys indicated that many young women reported problems with binge-eating, and it was suggested that the syndrome of bulimia nervosa was occurring in epidemic proportions. Later careful studies have found that although binge-eating is frequent, the full-blown disorder of bulimia nervosa is much less common, probably affecting 1–2% of young women in the United States. Although sufficient research data do not exist to pinpoint specific epidemiological trends in the occurrence of bulimia nervosa, research suggests that women born after 1960 have a higher risk for the illness than those born before 1960.

Bulimia nervosa primarily affects women; the ratio of men to women is approximately 1 : 10. It also occurs more frequently in certain occupations (e.g., modeling) and sports (e.g., wrestling, running).

Differential Diagnosis

Bulimia nervosa is not difficult to recognize if a full history is available. The binge-eating/purging type of anorexia nervosa has much in common with bulimia nervosa, but is distinguished by the characteristic low body weight and, in women, amenorrhea. Some individuals with atypical forms of depression overeat when depressed; if the overeating meets the definition of a binge described previously (i.e., a large amount of food is consumed with a sense of loss of control), and if the binge-eating is followed by inappropriate compensatory behavior, occurs sufficiently frequently, and is associated with overconcern regarding body shape and weight, an additional diagnosis of bulimia nervosa may be warranted. Some individuals become nauseated and vomit when upset; this and similar problems are probably not closely related to bulimia nervosa and should be viewed as a somatoform disorder.

Many individuals who believe they have bulimia nervosa have a symptom pattern that fails to meet full diagnostic criteria because the frequency of their binge-eating is less than twice a week or because what they view as a binge does not contain an abnormally large amount of food. Individuals with these characteristics fall into the broad and heterogeneous category of atypical eating disorders. Binge-eating disorder (see section on Binge-Eating Disorder, page 407), a category currently included in the DSM-IV-TR Appendix B for categories that need additional research, is characterized by recurrent binge-eating similar to that seen in bulimia nervosa but without the regular occurrence of inappropriate compensatory behavior.

TREATMENT

The power struggles that often complicate the treatment process in anorexia nervosa occur much less frequently in the treatment of individuals with bulimia nervosa. This is largely because the critical behavioral disturbances, binge-eating and purging, are less ego-syntonic and are more distressing to these individuals. Most bulimia nervosa individuals who pursue treatment agree with the primary treatment goals, and wish to give up the core behavioral features of their illness.

As with anorexia nervosa, the first treatment consideration is whether the individual is so medically or psychologically unstable so as to require hospitalization or a day treatment program (see Figure 38-2). If the individual is relatively stable, the next decision is whether to choose psychotherapy or medication.

The form of psychotherapy that has been examined most intensively for the treatment of bulimia nervosa is cognitive–behavioral therapy, modeled on the therapy of the same type for depression. Cognitive–behavioral therapy for bulimia nervosa concentrates on the distorted ideas about weight and shape, on the rigid rules regarding food consumption and the pressure to diet, and on the events that trigger episodes of binge-eating. The therapy is focused and highly structured and is usually conducted in 3 to 6 months. Approximately 25–50% of individuals with bulimia nervosa achieve abstinence from binge-eating and purging during a course of cognitive–behavioral therapy, and in most, this improvement appears to be sustained. The most common mode of cognitive–behavioral therapy is individual treatment, although it can be given in either individual or group format. The effect of cognitive–behavioral therapy is greater than that of supportive psychotherapy and of interpersonal therapy, indicating that cognitive–behavioral therapy should be the treatment of choice for bulimia nervosa.

The other commonly used mode of treatment that has been examined in bulimia nervosa is the use of antidepressant medication. This intervention was initially prompted by the high rates of depression among

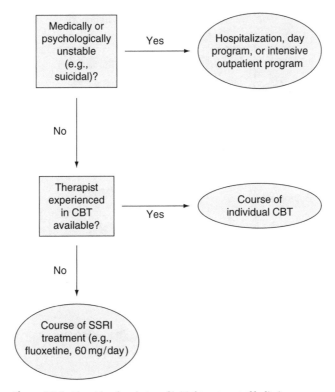

Figure 38-2 *Algorithm for choice of initial treatment of bulimia nervosa.*

individuals with bulimia nervosa and has now been tested in more than a dozen double-blind, placebo-controlled studies using a wide variety of antidepressant medications. Active medication has been consistently found to be superior to placebo, and although there have been no large "head-to-head" comparisons between different antidepressants, most antidepressants appear to possess roughly similar antibulimic potency (Figure 38-3). Fluoxetine at a dose of 60 mg/day is favored by many investigators because it has been studied in several large trials and appears to be at least as effective as, and better tolerated than, most other alternatives. It is notable that it has not been possible to link the effectiveness of antidepressant treatment for bulimia nervosa to the pretreatment level of depression. Depressed and nondepressed individuals with bulimia nervosa respond equally well in terms of their eating behavior to antidepressant medication.

Although antidepressant medication is clearly superior to placebo in the treatment of bulimia nervosa, several studies suggest that a course of a single antidepressant medication is generally inferior to a course of cognitive–behavioral therapy. However, individuals who fail to respond adequately to, or who relapse following a trial of psychotherapy, may still respond to antidepressant medication.

A major factor influencing the treatment of bulimia nervosa is the presence of other significant psychiatric or medical illness. For example, it can be difficult for individuals who are currently abusing drugs or alcohol to use the treatment methods described, and many experts suggest that the substance abuse needs to be addressed before the eating disorder can be effectively treated. Other examples include the treatment of individuals with bulimia nervosa and serious personality disturbance and those with insulin-dependent diabetes mellitus who "purge" by omitting insulin doses. In treating such individuals, the clinician must decide which of the multiple problems must be first addressed, and may elect to tolerate a significant level of eating disorder to confront more pressing disturbances.

Binge-Eating Disorder

DIAGNOSIS

As noted earlier, binge-eating disorder is a proposed diagnostic category related to, but quite distinct from, bulimia nervosa. The phenomenon of binge-eating without purging among the obese was clearly described 20 years before bulimia nervosa was recognized. Yet binge-eating disorder has been the focus of sustained

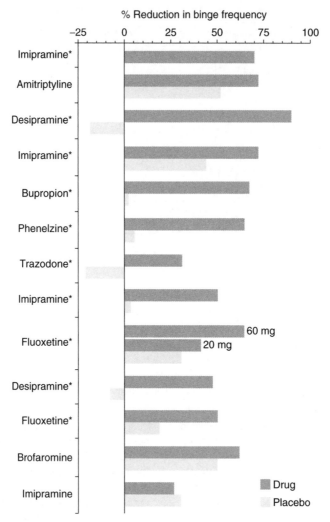

Figure 38-3 *Results of controlled trials of antidepressants in bulimia nervosa. (*indicates a statistically significant difference between the active medication and placebo; Source: Reprinted from Child Adolesc Psychiatr Clin N Am **4**, Walsh BT and Devlin MJ, Eating disorders, 343–357, Copyright 1995 with permission from Elsevier.)*

attention only in the past decade. Suggested diagnostic criteria for binge-eating disorder are included in an appendix of DSM-IV-TR, which provides criteria sets for further study.

In theory, binge-eating disorder should be easy to recognize on the basis of individual self-report: the individual describes the frequent consumption of large amounts of food in a discrete period of time about which he or she feels distressed and unable to control. Difficulties arise, however, because of uncertainty about what precisely constitutes a "large amount of food," especially for an obese individual, and regarding what constitutes a discrete period of time. Many individuals describe eating continuously during the day or evening, thereby consuming a large amount of food,

but it is not clear whether such behavior is best viewed as binge-eating.

Individuals who meet the proposed definition of binge-eating disorder clearly have increased complaints of depression and anxiety compared to individuals of similar weight without binge-eating disorder.

Individuals with binge-eating disorder who are obese should be followed by a primary care physician for assessment and treatment of the complications of obesity. There is no evidence suggesting that the behavioral disturbances characteristic of binge-eating disorder add to the physical risks of obesity. Whether the presence of binge-eating disorder affects the natural history of obesity is an intriguing but unanswered question.

Differential Diagnosis

As noted above, the most difficult issue in the diagnostic assessment of binge-eating disorder is determining whether the eating pattern of concern to the individual meets the proposed definition of binge-eating. There are numerous varieties of unhealthy eating, such as the consumption of high-fat foods, and the nosology of these patterns of eating is poorly worked out. Some individuals with atypical depression binge-eat when depressed; if the individual meets criteria for both binge-eating disorder and an atypical depression, both diagnoses should be made.

TREATMENT

For most individuals with binge-eating disorder, there are three related goals. One is behavioral, to cease binge-eating. A second focuses on improving symptoms of mood and anxiety disturbance, which are frequently associated with binge-eating disorder. The third is weight loss for individuals who are also obese.

Treatment approaches to binge-eating disorder are currently under active study. There is good evidence that psychological (e.g., CBT) and pharmacological (e.g., SSRI) interventions that are effective for bulimia nervosa are also useful in reducing the binge frequency of individuals with binge-eating disorder and in alleviating mood disturbance. However, it is not clear how helpful these approaches are in facilitating weight loss. Standard behavioral weight-loss interventions employing caloric restriction appear useful in helping individuals control binge-eating, but the benefits of such treatment have not been compared to those of more psychologically oriented treatments, such as CBT.

COMPARISON OF DSM-IV-TR AND ICD-10 DIAGNOSTIC CRITERIA

The ICD-10 Diagnostic Criteria for Research and the DSM-IV-TR criteria for anorexia nervosa differ in several ways. ICD-10 specifically requires that the weight loss be self-induced by the avoidance of "fattening foods" and that in men there be a loss of sexual interest and potency (corresponding to the amenorrhea requirement in women). Finally, in contrast to DSM-IV-TR, which gives anorexia nervosa precedence over bulimia nervosa, ICD-10 excludes a diagnosis of anorexia nervosa if regular binge-eating has been present.

For bulimia nervosa, the ICD-10 Diagnostic Criteria for Research and the DSM-IV-TR criteria for bulimia nervosa are similar except that ICD-10 requires a "persistent preoccupation with eating and a strong desire or sense of compulsion to eat." Furthermore, whereas the ICD-10 definition requires a self-perception of being too fat (identical to an item in anorexia nervosa), the DSM-IV-TR criteria set requires instead that "self-evaluation is unduly influenced by body shape and weight."

Both DSM-IV-TR and ICD-10 include categories unique to their systems. DSM-IV-TR has a category for "Binge-Eating Disorder" in its appendix of research categories whereas ICD-10 has categories for "Overeating associated with other psychological disturbances" and "Vomiting associated with other psychological disturbances."

39 Sleep and Sleep–Wake Disorders

Sleep disorders can be divided into four major categories based on the type of sleep disturbance: (1) insomnias, disorders associated with complaints of insufficient, disturbed, or nonrestorative sleep; (2) hypersomnias, disorders of excessive sleepiness; (3) disturbances of the circadian sleep–wake cycle; and (4) parasomnias, abnormal behaviors or abnormal physiological events in sleep. By definition, the DSM-IV-TR limits itself to chronic disorders (at least 1 month in duration). On the other hand, the *International Classification of Sleep Disorders* includes sleep disorders of short-term and intermediate duration, which in fact are more common than chronic disorders.

Sleep disorders can also be categorized according to presumed etiology. According to DSM-IV-TR, primary sleep disorders are presumed to arise from endogenous abnormalities in sleep–wake-generating mechanisms, timing mechanisms, sleep hygiene, or conditioning, rather than occurring secondary to medical or psychiatric disorders. Two types of primary sleep disorders are defined: *dyssomnias* (abnormalities in the amount, quality, or timing of sleep) and *parasomnias* (abnormal behaviors associated with sleep, such as nightmares or sleepwalking). Three other etiologic types of sleep disorders are included in DSM-IV-TR: sleep disorders related to other mental disorders, sleep disorders due to a general medical condition, and substance-induced sleep disorders.

DIAGNOSIS

To assist the individual with a sleep complaint, one needs to have a diagnostic framework with which one can obtain the information needed about both the individual as a person and his or her disorder. Two issues are particularly important: (1) How long has the individual had the sleep complaint? Transient insomnia and short-term insomnia, for example, usually occur in persons undergoing acute stress or other disruptions, such as admission to a hospital, jet lag, bereavement,

or change in medications. Chronic sleep disorders, on the other hand, are often multidetermined and multifaceted. (2) Does the individual suffer from any preexisting or comorbid disorders? Does another condition cause the sleep complaint, modify a sleep complaint, or affect possible treatments? In general, because common sleep disorders are frequently secondary to underlying causes, treatment should be directed at underlying medical, mental, pharmacological, psychosocial, or other disorders.

A detailed history of the complaint and attendant symptoms must be obtained (Table 39-1). Special attention should be given to the timing of sleep and wakefulness; qualitative and quantitative subjective measures of sleep and wakefulness; abnormal sleep-related behaviors; respiratory difficulties; medications or other substances affecting sleep, wakefulness or arousal; expectations, concerns, attitudes about sleep, and efforts used by the individual to control symptoms; and the sleep–wake environment. The clinician must be alert to the possibility that sleep complaints are somatic symptoms, which reflect individual ways of experiencing, expressing, and coping with psychosocial distress, stress, or psychiatric disorders.

Sleep disorders vary with age and gender and, possibly, with culture and social class. As mentioned previously, the circadian timing of rest–activity, duration of sleep at night, and daytime napping and sleepiness vary with age and gender. In addition, parasomnias are most common in boys, Kleine–Levin syndrome in adolescent boys, delayed sleep phase syndrome in adolescents and young adults, insomnia in middle-aged and elderly women, REM sleep behavior disorder and sleep-related breathing disorders in middle-aged men, and advanced sleep phase syndrome in the elderly. Sleep–wake patterns are also influenced by cultural or geographical factors, such as the siesta and late bedtime commonly associated with tropical climates, or the winter hypersomnia and summer hyposomnia said to occur near the arctic circle. Insomnia is more common in lower than

Table 39-1	Office Evaluation of Chronic Sleep Complaints

A detailed history and review of the sleep complaint: predisposing, precipitating, and perpetuating factors

Review of difficulties falling asleep, maintaining sleep, and awakening early

The timing of sleep and wakefulness in the 24-hour day

Evidence of excessive daytime sleepiness and fatigue

Bedtime routines, sleep setting, physical security, preoccupations, anxiety, beliefs about sleep and sleep loss, fears about consequences of sleep loss

Medical and neurological history and examination, routine laboratory examinations: look for obesity, short fat neck, enlarged tonsils, narrow upper oral airway, foreshortened jaw (retrognathia), and hypertension

Psychiatric history and present symptomatology

Use of prescription and nonprescription medications, alcohol, stimulants, toxins, insecticides, and other substances

Evidence of sleep-related breathing disorders: snoring, orthopnea, dyspnea, headaches, falling out of bed, nocturia

Abnormal movements or behaviors associated with sleep disorders: "jerky legs," leg movements, myoclonus, restless legs, leg cramps, cold feet, nightmares, enuresis, sleepwalking, epilepsy, bruxism, sleep paralysis, hypnagogic hallucinations, cataplexy, night sweats, and so on

Social and occupational history, marital status, living conditions, financial and security concerns, physical activity

Sleep–wake diary for 2 weeks

Interview with bed partners or persons who observe individual during sleep

Tape-recording of respiratory sounds during sleep to screen for sleep apnea

in middle and upper socioeconomic classes, perhaps reflecting the stress of poverty, crowding and lack of privacy, poor medical care, drugs and alcohol, lack of physical security, and so forth.

One approach to the differential diagnosis of persistent sleep disorders is suggested in the algorithm in Figure 39-1. First, determine whether the sleep complaint is due to another medical, psychiatric, or substance abuse disorder. Second, consider the role of circadian rhythm disturbances and sleep disorders associated with abnormal events predominantly during sleep. Finally, evaluate in greater detail the complaints of insomnia (difficulty initiating or maintaining sleep) and excessive sleepiness.

Clinicians can usually diagnose most sleep disorders by traditional, simple but systematic clinical methods. Referral to a specialized sleep disorders center, however, should be considered in individuals suspected of having severe intractable insomnia, persistent excessive daytime sleepiness, and sleep disorders due to a general medical condition (such as narcolepsy, REM sleep behavior disorder, sleep apnea, periodic limb movements in sleep [PLMS], or sleep-related epilepsy). Specialists in sleep disorders medicine will evaluate the individual and, if

necessary, arrange for sleep laboratory or ambulatory diagnostic procedures (see Table 39-2 for definitions of terms associated with clinical sleep laboratory studies).

One of the most important and common laboratory examinations is all-night polysomnography, which typically records the EEG activity's eye movements with the electrooculogram, and muscle tone with the electromyogram from the chin (submental) muscles. These measures are used to determine sleep stages visually scored as 20- or 30-second epochs by a sleep technician. To evaluate sleep-related respiration and cardiovascular function, measures are made of nasal and oral air flow with a thermistor; of sounds of breathing and snoring with a small microphone near the mouth; of respiratory movements of the chest and abdominal walls; of heart rate with the electrocardiogram; and of blood-oxygen saturation with finger oximetry. To evaluate PLMS, an electromyogram from the shin (anterior tibial) muscles is obtained. Other more specialized tests include intraesophageal pressures, which increase during the upper airway resistance syndrome if respiration is impeded, nocturnal penile tumescence in the evaluation of impotence, and core body temperature (usually rectal or tympanic membrane).

Daytime sleepiness can be evaluated in the sleep laboratory with the Multiple Sleep Latency Test, which measures sleep latency during opportunities for napping during the day. In addition, subjective sleepiness can be assessed by a questionnaire, the Stanford Sleepiness Scale, in which the subject rates sleepiness on a 7-point scale at set intervals throughout the day.

Dyssomnias

Primary Insomnia

DIAGNOSIS

Primary insomnia is a subjective complaint of poor, insufficient, or nonrestorative sleep lasting more than a month; associated with significant distress or impairment; and without obvious relationships to another sleep, medical or mental disorder, or physiological effects of a substance (see DSM-IV-TR diagnostic criteria, page 413). Primary insomnia is similar to some insomnia diagnoses in the International Classification of Sleep Disorders, including psychophysiological insomnia, which is often ascribed to conditioned arousal factors; sleep state misperception, in which the magnitude of the subjective complaint often exceeds that of the objective abnormality; and idiopathic insomnia, with a childhood onset and lifelong course.

Diagnosis and treatment of chronic insomnia are often challenging and difficult. Both the clinician and

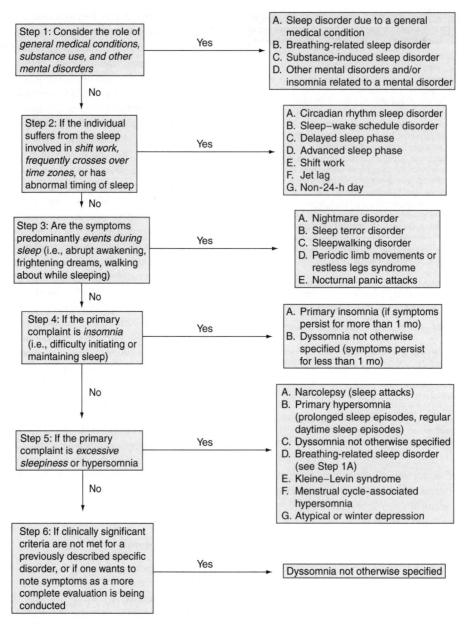

Figure 39-1 *An algorithm for the differential diagnosis of persistent sleep disorder complaints.*

the individual must be forbearing and realistic as they jointly explore the evolution, causes, manifestations, and ramifications of the sleep complaint. In part, the diagnosis of primary insomnia is reached by exclusion after a careful differential diagnosis of other causes. Simple answers and simple solutions are rare. Even if insomnia is initially precipitated by a single event or condition, chronic insomnia is usually maintained by various predisposing and perpetuating factors. For example, a business woman in her early thirties had

insomnia during a period of intense stress in her business, but it continued long after the stress had been satisfactorily resolved. Factors that contributed to chronicity included her lifelong somewhat obsessive, anxious personality structure and after the onset of her insomnia, her gradually escalating concerns about her insomnia; these resulted in advanced sleep phase as she tried to spend more time in bed for "rest" and the use of wine and sleeping pills at bedtime to sleep. If all these factors can be properly sorted out and dealt

Table 39-2	Selected Disorders and Terms Used in Clinical Sleep Disorders Medicine
Term	**Definition**
Apnea index	Number of apneic events per hour of sleep; usually is considered pathological if ≥5.
Cataplexy	Sudden, brief loss of muscle tone in the waking stage, usually triggered by emotional arousal (laughing, anger, surprise), involving either a few muscle groups (i.e., facial) or most of major antigravity muscles of the body; may be related to muscle atonia normally occurring during REM sleep; is associated with narcolepsy.
Hypopnea	50% or more reduction in respiratory depth for 10 seconds or more during sleep.
Multiple sleep latency test	An objective method for determining daytime sleepiness; sleep latency and REM latency are determined for four or five naps (i.e., a 20-min opportunity to sleep every 2 hours between 10 a.m. and 6 p.m.); normal mean values are above 15 minutes.
Periodic limb movements in sleep index	Number of leg kicks per hour of sleep; usually is considered pathological if ≥5.
Polysomnography	Describes detailed, sleep laboratory-based, clinical evaluation of individual with sleep disorder; may include electroencephalographical measures, eye movements, muscle tone at chin and limbs, respiratory movements of chest and abdomen, oxygen saturation, electrocardiogram, nocturnal penile tumescence, esophageal pH, as indicated.
Respiratory disturbance index	Number of apneas and hypopneas per hour of sleep.
Sleep apnea	Sleep-related breathing disorder characterized by at least five episodes of apnea per hour of sleep, each longer than 10 seconds in duration.

DSM-IV-TR Diagnostic Criteria

307.42 PRIMARY INSOMNIA

A. The predominant complaint is difficulty initiating or maintaining sleep, or nonrestorative sleep, for at least 1 month.
B. The sleep disturbance (or associated daytime fatigue) causes clinically significant distress or impairment in social, occupational, or other important areas of functioning.
C. The sleep disturbance does not occur exclusively during the course of narcolepsy, breathing-related sleep disorder, circadian rhythm sleep disorder, or a parasomnia.
D. The disturbance does not occur exclusively during the course of another mental disorder (e.g., major depressive disorder, generalized anxiety disorder, a delirium).
E. The disturbance is not due to the direct physiological effects of a substance (e.g., a drug of abuse, a medication) or a general medical condition.

Reprinted with permission from the *Diagnostic and Statistical Manual of Mental Disorders*, 4th ed., Text Rev. Copyright 2000 American Psychiatric Association.

their apprehensions: "If I don't get to sleep right now, I'll make a bad impression tomorrow." Cognitive–behavioral therapy (CBT) therefore is very effective

Clinical management is often multidimensional, involving psychosocial, behavioral, and pharmacological approaches. The relationship with the treating clinician can often be important since many insomniac individuals are skeptical that they can be helped overtly. They are focused on the symptom rather than the underlying causes, and are not psychologically minded. Behavioral treatments, in combination with addressing sleep hygiene, may be helpful in treating psychophysiological and other insomnias. Relaxation training (progressive relaxation, autogenic training, meditation, deep breathing) can be effective if overtaught to become automatic. Two other behavioral therapies have been shown to be effective for insomnia: stimulus control and sleep restriction therapy.

The aim of stimulus control therapy is to break the negative associations of being in bed unable to sleep (Table 39-3). It is especially helpful for individuals with sleep-onset insomnia and prolonged awakenings. Sleep restriction therapy (Table 39-4) is based on the observation that more time spent in bed leads to more fragmented sleep. Both therapies may take 3 to 4 weeks or longer to be effective.

A wide variety of sedating medications have commonly been used as sleeping pills including benzodiazepines, imidazopyridines (zolpidem), pyrazolopyrimidines (zaleplon), chloral hydrate, antihistamines (diphenhydramine, hydroxyzine, doxylamine), certain

with, both the clinician and the individual will be gratified.

TREATMENT

Treatment of insomnia should, insofar as possible, be directed at identifiable causes, or those factors that perpetuate the disorders, such as temperament and lifestyle, ineffective coping and defense mechanisms, inappropriate use of alcohol or other substances, maladaptive sleep–wake schedules, and excessive worry about poor sleep. The harder these individuals try to sleep, the worse it is. They keep themselves awake by

Table 39-3	Sleep Hygiene and Stimulus Control Rules

Curtail time spent awake while in bed.
Go to bed only when sleepy.
Do not remain in bed for more than 20–30 minutes while awake.
Get up at the same time each day.
Avoid looking at the bedroom clock.
Avoid caffeine, alcohol, and tobacco near bedtime.
Exercise during the morning or afternoon.
Eat a light snack before bed.
Adjust sleeping environment for optimal temperature, sound, and darkness.
Do not worry right before and in bed. Use the bed for sleeping.
Do not nap during the day.

Table 39-4	Sleep Restriction Therapy

Stay in bed for the amount of time you think you sleep each night, plus 15 minutes.
Get up at the same time each day.
Do not nap during the day.
When sleep efficiency is 85% (i.e., sleeping for 85% of the time in bed), go to bed 15 minutes earlier.
Repeat this process until you are sleeping for 8 hours or the desired amount of time.
Example: if you report sleeping only 5 hours a night and you normally get up at 6 a.m., you are allowed to be in bed from 12:45 a.m. until 6 a.m.

antidepressants (amitriptyline, doxepin, trimipramine, and trazodone), barbiturates, and over-the-counter medications. However, they do vary in their pharmacokinetic properties and side effects (Table 39-5). The

Table 39-6	Comparison of Long and Short Half-Life Hypnotics

	Half-Life	
Measure	Short	Long
Sedative hangover effects	+	++++
Accumulation with consecutive nightly use	0	+++
Tolerance	+++	+
Withdrawal insomnia	+++	+
Anxiolytic effects next day	0	+++
Amnesia	+++	++
Full benefits the first night	+++	++

Note: Although zaleplon is short acting, research suggests that it does not have some of the problems of other short-acting hypnotics, such as tolerance or withdrawal insomnia.

ideal sleeping pill would shorten latency to sleep; maintain normal physiological sleep all night without blocking normal behavioral responses to the crying baby or the alarm clock; leave neither hangover nor withdrawal effects the next day; and be devoid of tolerance and side effects such as impairment of breathing, cognition, ambulation, and coordination. Furthermore, sleeping pills should not be habit-forming or addictive. Unfortunately, the ideal sleeping pill has not yet been found. Sleeping pills, if given in appropriate doses, are effective compared to placebo at least from a few days to a few weeks. The duration of action of these medications is important for several reasons (Table 39-6). Drugs with long half-life metabolites may have next-day hangover

Table 39-5	Clinical Characteristics of Sedative–Hypnotics			
Name	Dose (mg)	Absorption	Active Metabolite	Half-Life
Chlordiazepoxide (Librium)	5–10	Intermediate	Yes	2–4 d
Diazepam (Valium)	2–10	Fast	Yes	2–4 d
Estazolam (ProSom)*	0.5–2.0	Intermediate	Yes	17 h
Flurazepam (Dalmane)*	7.5–30	Intermediate to fast	Yes	2–4 d
Clorazepate (Tranxene)	7.5–15	Fast	Yes	2–4 d
Clonazepam (Klonopin)	0.5–1.0	Intermediate	Yes	2–3 d
Quazepam (Doral)*	7.5–15	Intermediate	Yes	2–4 d
Oxazepam (Serax)	10–15	Slow	No	8–12 h
Lorazepam (Ativan)	0.5–4.0	Intermediate	No	10–20 h
Temazepam (Restoril)*	7.5–15	Slow	No	10–20 h
Alprazolam (Xanax)	0.25–2	Intermediate	No	14 h
Zoplicone†	7.5–15	Fast	Yes	4–6.5 h
Triazolam (Halcion)*	0.125–0.5	Intermediate	No	2–5 h
Zolpidem (Ambien)*	5–10	Fast	No	2–5 h
Zaleplon (Sonata)*	5–10	Fast	No	1 h

*Marketed as a sleeping pill in the United States.
†Not yet marketed in the United States.

effects and tend to accumulate with repeated nightly administration, especially in the elderly, who metabolize and excrete the drugs more slowly than the young do. In addition, long half-life metabolites may act addictively or synergistically the next day with alcohol, with drugs with sedative side effects, or during periods of decreased alertness, such as the afternoon dip in arousal levels. Because the elderly are more sensitive to both the benefits and the side effects at a given dose than are younger individuals, a dose for the elderly and debilitated individual should normally be about half of that for young and middle-aged individuals.

Short half-life hypnotics usually produce less daytime sedation than long half-life drugs, but they often result in more rebound insomnia when they are discontinued. Whereas nearly all hypnotics and sedatives can produce amnesia, the problem may be more common with some short half-life drugs, especially for material that is learned during the periods of peak concentrations of drugs, for example, if the subject is awakened during the middle of the night. Administration of zaleplon 4 hours or more before arising in the morning does not appear to be associated with impairment in motor performance.

Individuals should be educated about the anticipated benefits and limitations of sleeping pills, side effects, and appropriate use, and should be followed up by office visits or phone calls regularly if prescriptions are renewed. Although hypnotics are usually prescribed for relatively short periods of time (2–6 weeks at most), about 0.5–1% of the population uses a hypnotic nearly every night for months or years. Whether this practice is good, useless, or bad remains controversial. Treatment of these individuals should focus on the lowest possible effective dose—intermittently if possible—for the treatment of insomnia.

Hypnotics are relatively contraindicated in individuals with sleep-disordered breathing; during pregnancy; in substance abusers, particularly alcohol abusers; and in those individuals who may need to be alert during their sleep period (e.g., physicians on call). In addition, caution should be used in prescribing hypnotics to individuals who snore loudly, to individuals who have renal, hepatic, or pulmonary disease, and to the elderly.

The limited database available suggests that melatonin may eventually have a role in the prevention and treatment of circadian and sleep disturbances. Some evidence suggests that it has intrinsic hypnotic effects. Laboratory studies suggest that people are more likely to sleep during the period of endogenous melatonin secretion than during periods of the day without melatonin secretion. Furthermore, some, but not all, studies suggest that melatonin (0.3–10.0 mg) may induce and

maintain sleep when administered to normal subjects or, in a few studies, to individuals with insomnia, jet lag, or other circadian rhythm disturbances. In addition, it is possible that melatonin administration can shift the phase position of the underlying biological clock. The entraining effects of a dose of 0.5 mg melatonin act like a "dark pulse," that is, the phase–response curve is nearly opposite that of light. Future research is needed to fulfill the promise that melatonin can be used to prevent or treat some forms of insomnia or other sleep disorders, especially in the elderly, or in cases associated with circadian rhythm disorders (jet lag, shift work, the non-24-hour-day syndrome, phase displacement), neurological disorders, or psychiatric disorders.

Melatonin is currently treated by the US Food and Drug Administration as a nutritional supplement rather than a medication. Therefore, purity of the product, safety, efficacy, and claims by manufacturers are not carefully regulated in the United States. Physicians are advised to maintain a watchful eye at this time and to be prudently cautious about recommendations to individuals and the public about the uses and benefits of melatonin.

Primary Hypersomnia

DIAGNOSIS

A specific diagnostic category for primary hypersomnia exists in DSM-IV-TR, defining a disorder characterized by clinically significant excessive sleepiness of at least 1 month's duration, with significant distress or impairment (see DSM-IV-TR diagnostic criteria, page 416).

Previously called non-REM narcolepsy, this relatively rare disorder is represented by perhaps 5–10% of individuals presenting to sleep disorders centers for evaluation of hypersomnia. The diagnosis must be made on the basis of polysomnographic confirmation of hypersomnia; subjective complaints of excessive sleepiness are not adequate. A family history of excessive sleepiness may be present.

Although usually seen as a persistent complaint, primary hypersomnia includes recurrent forms, well defined with periods of excessive sleepiness of at least 3 days' duration occurring several times a year for at least 2 years. Among the recurrent or intermittent hypersomnia disorders are Kleine–Levin syndrome, usually seen in adolescent boys, and menstrual cycle–associated hypersomnia syndrome. In addition to hypersomnia (up to 18 hours per day), individuals with Kleine–Levin syndrome often demonstrate aggressive or inappropriate sexuality, compulsive overeating, and other bizarre behaviors. The rare nature of this

---

DSM-IV-TR Diagnostic Criteria

307.44 PRIMARY HYPERSOMNIA

A. The predominant complaint is excessive sleepiness for at least 1 month (or less if recurrent) as evidenced by either prolonged sleep episodes or daytime sleep episodes that occur almost daily.
B. The excessive sleepiness causes clinically significant distress or impairment in social, occupational, or other important areas of functioning.
C. The excessive sleepiness is not better accounted for by insomnia and does not occur exclusively during the course of another sleep disorder (e.g., narcolepsy, breathing-related sleep disorder, circadian rhythm sleep disorder, or a parasomnia) and cannot be accounted for by an inadequate amount of sleep.
D. The disturbance does not occur exclusively during the course of another mental disorder.
E. The disturbance is not due to the direct physiological effects of a substance (e.g., a drug of abuse, a medication) or a general medical condition.

Specify if:

Recurrent: if there are periods of excessive sleepiness that last at least 3 days occurring several times a year for at least 2 years

Reprinted with permission from the *Diagnostic and Statistical Manual of Mental Disorders*, 4th ed., Text Rev. Copyright 2000 American Psychiatric Association.

---

syndrome and its unusual behaviors may be mistaken for psychosis, malingering, or a personality disorder.

Another syndrome, idiopathic recurring stupor, has been described and may be confused with hypersomnia. Individuals experience attacks of stupor or coma as infrequently as once or twice a year to as often as once a week. The duration of each episode varies from 2 hours to 4 days. Unlike individuals with hypersomnia, these individuals are in a stuporous coma-like state and cannot be easily aroused or awakened.

Aside from associated general medical conditions and mental disorders, the frequency and importance of hypersomnia and daytime sleepiness in otherwise healthy individuals have been increasingly recognized. Sleepiness, for example, as a result of sleep deprivation, disrupted sleep, or circadian dyssynchronization, probably plays a major role in mistakes and accidents in sleepy drivers, interns and medical staff, and industrial workers.

TREATMENT

Clinical management is controversial owing to the lack of controlled studies. As in narcolepsy, the stimulant compounds are the most widely used and most often successful of the treatment options available. However, some individuals are intolerant of stimulants or report

no significant therapeutic effects. For individuals intolerant of, or insensitive to, stimulants, some success has been obtained with the use of stimulating antidepressants, both of the MAOI and the selective serotonin reuptake inhibitor (SSRI) classes. Methysergide, a serotonin receptor antagonist, may be effective in some treatment-resistant cases but must be used with caution in view of the possibility of pleural and retroperitoneal fibrosis with persistent, uninterrupted use. Careful documentation should be maintained of interruption of drug use at regular intervals and of physical examinations that find the absence of obvious side effects of any sort.

Narcolepsy

DIAGNOSIS

Narcolepsy is associated with a pentad of symptoms: (1) excessive daytime sleepiness, characterized by irresistible "attacks" of sleep in inappropriate situations such as driving a car, talking to a supervisor, or social events; (2) cataplexy, which is sudden bilateral loss of muscle tone, usually lasting seconds to minutes, generally precipitated by strong emotions such as laughter, anger, or surprise; (3) poor or disturbed nocturnal sleep; (4) hypnagogic hallucinations, varied dreams at sleep onset; and (5) sleep paralysis, a brief period of paralysis associated with the transitions into, and out of, sleep.

Narcolepsy is lifelong. The first symptom is usually excessive sleepiness, typically developing during the late teens and early twenties. The full syndrome of cataplexy and other symptoms unfolds in several years.

Observers may mistake classic sleepiness in its mild form as withdrawal, poor motivation, negativism, and hostility. The hypnagogic imagery and sleep paralysis symptoms, alone and in combination, may resemble bizarre psychiatric illness. Like many medical disorders, narcolepsy presents a wide range of severity, from mild to cases so severe that employment is functionally impossible. Partial remissions and exacerbations occur. Sleep paralysis and hypnagogic imagery may be seen without cataplexy; cataplexy may present in isolation without other REM-associated phenomena. The presence of REM sleep onset at night or during daytime naps, an important sleep laboratory parameter, remains the most valid and reliable method available for diagnosing narcolepsy. Because of the seriousness of the disorder and likelihood that amphetamine or other stimulants will be used to treat the individual at some time, it is important that the diagnosis of narcolepsy be objectively verified as soon as possible. Furthermore, stimulant abusers have been known to feign symptoms of narcolepsy to obtain prescriptions.

TREATMENT

The major goals of treatment of narcolepsy include (a) to improve quality of life, (b) to reduce excessive daytime sleepiness (EDS), and (c) to prevent cataplectic attacks. The major wake-promoting medications are modafinil, amphetamine, dextroamphetamine, and methylphenidate. Modafinil is preferred on grounds of efficacy, safety, availability, and low risk of abuse and diversion. The pharmacological treatment of cataplexy, sleep paralysis, and hypnagogic hallucinations includes administration of activating SSRIs such as fluoxetine and tricyclic antidepressants such as protriptyline. Another new drug, sodium oxybate xyrem, appears to be well tolerated and beneficial for the treatment of cataplexy, daytime sleepiness, and inadvertent sleep attacks.

Breathing-Related Sleep Disorder

DIAGNOSIS

The essential feature of breathing-related sleep disorder (BRSD) is sleep disruption resulting from sleep apnea or alveolar hypoventilation, leading to complaints of insomnia or, more commonly, excessive sleepiness. The disorder is not accounted for by other medical or psychiatric disorders or by medications or other substances.

Sleep apnea is characterized by repetitive episodes of upper airway obstruction that occur during sleep, resulting in numerous interruptions of sleep continuity, hypoxemia, hypercapnia, bradytachycardia, and pulmonary and systemic hypertension. It may be associated with snoring, morning headaches, dry mouth on awakening, excessive movements during the night, falling out of bed, enuresis, cognitive decline and personality changes, and complaints of either insomnia or, more frequently, hypersomnia and excessive daytime sleepiness. The typical individual with clinical sleep apnea is a middle-aged man who is overweight or who has anatomical conditions narrowing his upper airway.

The most common symptoms of BRSD include excessive daytime sleepiness and snoring. The excessive daytime sleepiness probably results from sleep fragmentation caused by the frequent nocturnal arousals occurring at the end of the apneas, and possibly from hypoxemia. The excessive daytime sleepiness is associated with lethargy, poor concentration, decreased

motivation and performance, and inappropriate and inadvertent attacks of sleep. Sometimes the individuals do not realize they have fallen asleep until they awaken.

The second complaint is loud snoring, sometimes noisy enough to be heard throughout or even outside the house. Often the wife has complained for years about the snoring and has threatened to sleep elsewhere if she has not moved out already. Bed partners describe a characteristic pattern of loud snoring interrupted by periods of silence, which are then terminated by snorting sounds. Snoring results from a partial narrowing of the airway caused by multiple factors, such as inadequate muscle tone, large tonsils and adenoids, long soft palate, flaccid tissue, acromegaly, hypothyroidism, or congenital narrowing of the oral pharynx. Snoring has been implicated not only in sleep apnea but also in angina pectoris, stroke, ischemic heart disease, and cerebral infarction, even in the absence of complete sleep apneas. Because the prevalence of snoring increases with age, especially in women, and because snoring can have serious medical consequences, the psychiatrist must give serious attention to complaints of loud snoring. Snoring is not always a symptom of BRSD. Approximately 25% of men and 15% of women are habitual snorers.

Other symptoms of BRSD include unexplained morning headaches, nocturnal confusion, automatic behavior, dysfunction of the autonomic nervous system, or night sweats. The severity of BRSD will depend on the severity of the cardiac arrhythmias, hypertension, excessive daytime sleepiness, respiratory disturbance index, amount of sleep fragmentation, and amount of oxygen desaturation.

Mild to moderate sleep-related breathing disturbances increase with age, even in elderly subjects without major complaints about their sleep. The frequency is higher in men than in women, at least until the age of menopause, after which the rate in women increases and may approach that of men. With use of the apnea index of 5 or more apneic episodes per hour as a cutoff criterion, prevalence rates range from 27% to 75% for older men and from 0% to 32% for older women. In general, the severity of apnea in these older persons is mild (an average apnea index of about 13) compared with that seen in individuals with clinical sleep apnea. However, older men and women with mild apnea have been reported to fall asleep at inappropriate times significantly more often than older persons without apnea. Furthermore, the frequency of sleep apnea and other BRSDs is higher in individuals with hypertension, congestive heart failure, obesity, dementia, and other medical conditions.

The diagnosis of BRSD must be differentiated from other disorders of excessive sleepiness such as narcolepsy. Individuals with BRSD will not have cataplexy, sleep-onset paralysis, or sleep-onset hallucination. Narcolepsy is not usually associated with loud snoring or sleep apneas. In laboratory recordings, individuals with BRSD do not usually have sleep-onset REM periods either at night or in multiple naps on the Multiple Sleep Latency Test. However, one must be aware that both BRSD and narcolepsy can be found in the same individual. BRSD must also be distinguished from other hypersomnias, such as those related to major depressive disorder or circadian rhythm disturbances.

TREATMENT

Sleep apnea is sometimes alleviated by weight loss, avoidance of sedatives, use of tongue-retaining devices, and breathing air under positive pressure through a face mask (continuous positive airway pressure [CPAP]). Oxygen breathed at night may alleviate insomnia associated with apnea that is not accompanied by impeded inspiration. Surgery may be helpful, for example, to correct enlarged tonsils, a long uvula, a short mandible, or morbid obesity. Pharyngoplasty, which tightens the pharyngeal mucosa and may also reduce the size of the uvula, or the use of a cervical collar to extend the neck, may relieve heavy snoring. Although tricyclic antidepressants are sometimes used in the treatment of clinical sleep apnea in young adults, they may cause considerable toxic effects in older people. The newer shorter-acting nonbenzodiazepine hypnotics seem to be safer in these individuals and may be considered in those individuals who snore.

Circadian Rhythm Sleep Disorder (Sleep–Wake Schedule Disorders)

Circadian rhythm disturbances result from a mismatch between the internal or endogenous circadian sleep–wake system and the external or exogenous demands on the sleep–wake system. The individual's tendency to sleep–wakefulness does not match that of her or his social circumstances or of the light–dark cycle. Although some individuals do not find this mismatch to be a problem, for others the circadian rhythm disturbance interferes with the ability to function properly at times when alertness or sleepiness is desired or required. For those individuals, insomnia, hypersomnia, sleepiness, and fatigue result in significant discomfort and impairment. The circadian rhythm disturbances include delayed sleep phase, advanced sleep phase, shift work, jet lag, and a non-24-hour-day syndrome.

The diagnosis of circadian rhythm sleep disorder is based on a careful review of the history and circadian patterns of sleep–wakefulness, napping, alertness, and behavior. The diagnosis of circadian rhythm sleep disorder requires significant social or occupational impairment or marked distress related to the sleep disturbance. It is often useful for individuals with chronic complaints to keep a sleep–wake diary covering the entire 24-hour day each day for several weeks. If possible, an ambulatory device that measures rest–activity, such as a wrist actigraph, might supplement the sleep–wake diary. Wrist actigraphs record acceleration of the wrist at frequent intervals, such as every minute, and save it for later display. Because the wrist is mostly at rest during sleep, the record of wrist rest–activity provides a fairly accurate estimate of the timing and duration of sleep–wakefulness. In addition, some commercial wrist activity devices have a built-in photometer, which provides a record of ambient light–darkness against which the rest–activity pattern can be compared.

The prevalence of circadian rhythm disturbances has not been established. Approximately two-thirds of shift workers have difficulty with their schedules. Circadian rhythm disturbances must be differentiated from sleep-onset insomnia due to other causes (such as pain, caffeine consumption), early morning insomnia due to depression or alcohol use, and changes in sleep patterns due to lifestyle or lifestyle changes.

Delayed Sleep Phase Type

DIAGNOSIS

In the delayed sleep phase type, there is a delay in the circadian rhythm in the sleep–wake cycle. These individuals are generally not sleepy until several hours after "normal" bedtime (i.e., 2–3 a.m.). If allowed to sleep undisturbed, they will sleep for 7 or 8 hours, which means they awaken around 10 to 11 a.m. People with delayed sleep phase are considered extreme "owls." They may or may not complain of sleep-onset insomnia. They usually enjoy their alertness in the evening and night and have little desire to sleep beginning at 10 p.m. or midnight. Their problem is trying to wake up at normal times (i.e., 6–7 a.m.). In essence, their rhythm is shifted to a later clock time relative to conventional rest–activity patterns.

Individuals with delayed sleep phase often choose careers that allow them to set their own schedules, such as freelance writers. Delayed sleep phase occurs commonly in late adolescence and young adulthood, such as in college students. As many of these individuals age, however, their endogenous sleep–wake rhythm advances and they eventually are able to conform themselves to a normal rest period at night.

For others, however, this phase shift of the endogenous oscillator may lead at a later age to the advanced sleep phase. In this condition, individuals become sleepy earlier in the evening (e.g., 7–8 p.m.). They will also sleep for 7 to 8 hours, but that means they awaken around 2 to 3 a.m. These individuals are "larks," being most alert in the morning. They complain of sleep maintenance insomnia, that is, they cannot stay asleep all night long. This condition is more prevalent in the elderly than in the young.

TREATMENT

Clinical management includes chronobiological strategies to shift the phase position of the endogenous circadian oscillator in the appropriate direction. For example, exposure to bright light in the morning advances the delayed sleep phase, that is, individuals will become sleepy earlier in the evening. On the other hand, administration of bright light in the evening acts to delay the circadian rhythm, that is, individuals will get sleepy later in the evening. Light is usually administered in doses of 2500 lux for a period of 2 hours per day, although the ideal intensity and duration are yet to be determined. For some individuals, spending more time outdoors in bright sunlight may be sufficient to treat the sleep phase. For example, individuals with delayed sleep phase should be encouraged to remove blinds and curtains from their windows, which would allow the sunlight to pour into their bedrooms in the morning when they should arise. In addition, gradual adjustments of the timing of the sleep–wake cycle may be used to readjust the phase position of the circadian oscillator. For example, individuals with delayed phase disorder can be advised to delay the onset of sleep by 2 to 3 hours each day (i.e., from 4 to 7 to 10 a.m., and so on) until the appropriate bedtime. After that, they should maintain regular sleep–wake patterns, with exposure to bright light in the morning.

Shift-Work Type

DIAGNOSIS

Shift-work problems occur when the circadian sleep–wake rhythm is in conflict with the rest–activity cycle imposed by the externally determined work schedule. Rotating work schedules, particularly rapidly shifting schedules, are difficult because constant readjustment

of the endogenous circadian oscillator to the imposed sleep–wake cycle is necessary.

TREATMENT

No totally satisfactory methods currently exist for managing shift-work problems. Because people vary in their ability to adjust to these schedules, self-selection may be involved for those who can find other employment or work schedules. Older individuals appear to be less flexible than younger persons in adjusting to shift work. Some experiments suggest that the principles of chronobiology may be useful in reducing the human costs of shift work. For example, because the endogenous pacemaker has a cycle length (tau) longer than 24 hours, rotating shift workers do better when their schedules move in a clockwise direction (i.e., morning to evening to night) rather than in the other direction. Appropriate exposure to bright lights and darkness may push the circadian pacemaker in the correct direction and help stabilize its phase position, especially in association with the use of dark glasses outside and blackout curtains at home to maintain darkness at the appropriate times for promotion of sleep and shifting of the circadian pacemaker. Naps may also be useful in reducing sleep loss. Modest amounts of coffee may maintain alertness early in the shift but should be avoided near the end of the shift.

Jet Lag Type

DIAGNOSIS

Jet lag occurs when individuals travel across several time zones. Traveling east advances the sleep–wake cycle and is typically more difficult than traveling west (which delays the cycle). Jet lag may be associated with difficulty initiating or maintaining sleep or with daytime sleepiness, impaired performance, and gastrointestinal disturbance after rapid transmeridian flights. Individuals older than 50 years appear to be more vulnerable to jet lag than are younger persons.

TREATMENT

Considerable research and theorizing are under way to better prevent and manage the problems associated with jet lag. Some efforts before departure may be useful to prevent or ameliorate these problems. For persons who plan to readjust their circadian clock to the new location, it may be possible to move the sleep–wake and light–dark schedules appropriately before departure. In addition, good sleep hygiene principles should be respected before, during, and after the trip. For example, many people are sleep deprived or in alcohol withdrawal when they step on the plane because of last-minute preparations or farewell parties. Whereas adequate fluid intake on the plane is necessary to avoid dehydration, alcohol consumption should be avoided or minimized because it causes diuresis and may disrupt sleep maintenance.

On arriving at the destination, it may be preferable to try to maintain a schedule coinciding with actual home time if the trip is going to be short. For example, the individual should try to sleep at times that correspond to the usual bedtime or with the normal midafternoon dip in alertness. If, on the other hand, the trip will be longer and it is desirable to synchronize the biological clock with local time, exposure to appropriate schedules of bright light and darkness may be helpful, at least theoretically. Unfortunately, the exact protocols have not been established in all instances yet and require further research and experimentation. In addition, some of these protocols require avoidance of bright light at certain times, necessitating wearing dark goggles, for example, when traveling.

In addition to synchronizing the clock with the new environment, sleep and rest should be promoted by good sleep hygiene principles, by avoidance of excessive caffeine and alcohol, and, possibly, by administration of short-duration hypnotics. Care should be taken, however, to avoid hangover effects or amnesia associated with hypnotics. Because individual responses to sleeping pills vary considerably from person to person, it is often helpful to develop experience with specific compounds and doses before departure.

Periodic Limb Movements in Sleep

DIAGNOSIS

Periodic limb movements in sleep (PLMS), previously called nocturnal myoclonus, is a disorder in which repetitive, brief, and stereotyped limb movements occur during sleep, usually about every 20 to 40 seconds. Dorsiflexions of the big toe, ankle, knee, and sometimes the hip are involved (Table 39-7)

Questioning of the individual or bed partner often yields reports of restlessness, kicking, unusually cold

Table 39-7	Features of Periodic Limb Movements in Sleep

Leg kicks every 20–40 seconds
Duration of 0.5–5 seconds
Complaints of:
  Insomnia
  Excessive sleepiness
  Restless legs
  Very cold or hot feet
  Uncomfortable sensations in legs

or hot feet, disrupted and torn bedclothes, unrefreshing sleep, insomnia, or excessive daytime sleepiness. Individuals may be unaware of these pathological leg movements or arousals, although their bed partners may be all too aware of the kicking, frequent movements, and restlessness. If these disorders are strongly suspected, the individual should probably be referred to a sleep disorders laboratory for evaluation and an overnight polysomnogram with tibial electromyograms.

A related disturbance, restless legs syndrome, is associated with disagreeable sensations in the lower legs, feet, or thighs that occur in a recumbent or resting position and cause an almost irresistible urge to move the legs. Whereas almost all individuals with restless legs syndrome have PLMS, not all individuals with PLMS have restless legs syndrome. Restless legs syndrome may be frequent in individuals with uremia and rheumatoid arthritis or in pregnant women.

TREATMENT

Because the pathogenesis of PLMS is usually unknown, treatment is often symptomatic (Table 39-8). At the present time, dopaminergic agents such as levodopa (L-dopa), pergolide, or pramipexole generally provide the most effective treatment for both PLMS and restless legs syndrome. Opiates, such as oxycodone and propoxyphene, have also been demonstrated to be effective in the treatment of PLMS and restless legs syndrome. Anticonvulsants, such as carbamazepine and gabapentin, have been shown to be effective in treatment of restless legs syndrome. Clonazepam, a benzodiazepine anticonvulsant, is effective in the treatment of PLMS and possibly for restless legs syndrome. Other benzodiazepines have also been used to treat these conditions, as they will decrease some of the awakenings but may have no effect on the number of leg movements.

Parasomnias

The parasomnias are a group of disorders characterized by disturbances of either physiological processes or behavior associated with sleep, but not necessarily causing disturbances of sleep or wakefulness.

Nightmare Disorder

DIAGNOSIS

The essential feature of this disorder is the repeated occurrence of frightening dreams that lead to full awakenings from sleep. The dreams or awakenings

Table 39-8	Pharmacologic Treatment Options in RLS/PLMS			
Medication	**Dosage Range**	**Side Effects**	**Advantages**	**Disadvantages**
L-dopa/carbidopa	25/100–100/400/D	Dyskinesia	Low cost	Breakthrough restlessness
		Nausea		Loss of efficacy
		Hallucinations		
Pergolide	0.05–1 mg	Dyskinesia	High rate of response	Frequent side effects
		Nausea		
		Rhinitis		
		Dizziness		
Pramipexole	0.25–0.875 mg	Orthostasis	High rate of response	Expense
		Dizziness	Good tolerance	
		Sedation		
Anticonvulsants	Variable	Sedation	Low cost	Variable response
			Sleep promotion	
Opiates	Variable	Nausea	Low cost	Variable response
		Constipation		Abuse potential
Clonazepam	0.5–2 mg	Sedation	Sleep promotion	Variable response
		Dizziness		Abuse potential

cause the individual significant distress or dysfunction. By definition, the disorder is excluded if the nightmare occurs in the course of another mental or medical disorder or as a direct result of a medication or substance

Whereas more than half of the adult population probably experiences an occasional nightmare, nightmares start more commonly in children between the ages of 3 and 6 years. The exact prevalence is unknown.

TREATMENT

The disorder is usually self-limited in children but can be helped sometimes with psychotherapy, desensitization, or rehearsal instructions. Secondary nightmares, as in posttraumatic stress disorder (PTSD), can be difficult to treat.

Sleep Terror Disorder

DIAGNOSIS

This disorder is defined as repeated abrupt awakenings from sleep characterized by intense fear, panicky screams, autonomic arousal (tachycardia, rapid breathing, and sweating), absence of detailed dream recall, amnesia for the episode, and relative unresponsiveness to attempts to comfort the person. Sleep terrors occur primarily during the first third of the night. These episodes may cause distress or impairment, especially for caretakers who witness the event. Sleep terrors may also be called night terrors, *pavor nocturnus*, or incubus.

TREATMENT

Nocturnal administration of benzodiazepines has been reported to be beneficial, perhaps because these drugs suppress delta sleep, the stage of sleep during which sleep terrors typically occur.

Sleepwalking Disorder

DIAGNOSIS

This disorder is characterized by repeated episodes of motor behavior initiated in sleep, usually during delta sleep in the first third of the night. While sleepwalking, the individual has a blank staring face, is relatively unresponsive to others, and may be confused or disoriented initially on being aroused from the episode. Although the person may be alert after several minutes of awakening, complete amnesia for the episode is common the next day. Adult onset of sleepwalking should prompt the search for possible medical, neurological, psychiatric, pharmacological, or other underlying causes, such as nocturnal epilepsy.

TREATMENT

No treatment for sleepwalking is established, but some individuals respond to administration of benzodiazepines or sedating antidepressants at bedtime. The major concern should be the safety of the sleepwalker, who may injure herself or himself or someone else during an episode.

REM Sleep Behavior Disorder

DIAGNOSIS

First described in 1986, this disorder, like sleepwalking, is associated with complicated behaviors during sleep such as walking, running, singing, and talking. In contrast to sleepwalking, which occurs during the first third of the night during delta sleep, REM sleep behavior disorder usually occurs during the second half of the night during REM sleep. Also, in contrast to sleepwalking, memory for the dream content is usually good. Furthermore, the idiopathic form typically occurs in men during the sixth or seventh decade of life. The cause or causes remain unknown. It has been reported in a variety of neurological disorders and during withdrawal from sedatives or alcohol; during treatment with tricyclic antidepressants or biperiden (Akineton); and in various neurological disorders including dementia, subarachnoid hemorrhage, and degenerative neurological disorders.

TREATMENT

Nocturnal administration of clonazepam, 0.5 to 1 mg, is usually remarkably successful in controlling the symptoms of this disorder. Individuals and their families should be educated about the nature of the disorder and warned to take precautions about injuring themselves or others.

Nocturnal Panic Attacks

The typical daytime panic attack, as bizarre and frightening as it may seem to the individual experiencing it, is often fairly obvious to the assessing clinician. When these symptoms occur at night, the task of the assessing clinician is greatly complicated. The individual may assume that the cause is a nightmare or a night terror and may be resistant to the diagnosis of an anxiety disorder, particularly if the symptoms are absent or mild during the daytime. Individuals with panic disorder often have not only disturbed subjective sleep but also panic attacks during sleep. Clinician should remember that panic attacks could occur exclusively during sleep, without daytime symptoms, in some individuals.

Conversely, a report of "awakening in a state of panic" may be associated with a variety of other disorders including obstructive sleep apnea, gastroesophageal reflux, nocturnal angina, orthopnea, nightmares, night terrors, and others.

Sleep-Related Epilepsy

Some forms of epilepsy occur more commonly during sleep than during wakefulness and may be associated with parasomnia disorders. Nocturnal seizures may at times be confused with sleep terror, REM sleep behavior disorder, paroxysmal hypnogenic dystonia, or nocturnal panic attacks. They may take the form of generalized convulsions or may be partial seizures with complex symptoms. Nocturnal seizures are most common at two times: the first 2 hours of sleep, and around 4 to 6 a.m. They are more common in children than in adults. The chief complaint may be only disturbed sleep, torn up bedsheets and blankets, morning drowsiness (a postictal state), and muscle aches. Some individuals never realize that they suffer from nocturnal epilepsy until they share a bedroom or bed with someone who observes a convulsion.

Sleep Disturbances Related to Other Mental Disorders

DIAGNOSIS

Subjective and objective disturbances of sleep are common features of many mental disorders. General abnormalities include dyssomnias (such as insomnia and hypersomnia), parasomnias (such as nightmares, night terrors, and nocturnal panic attacks), and circadian rhythm disturbances (early morning awakening). Before assuming that a significant sleep complaint invariably signals a diagnosis of a mental disorder mental health specialists should go through a careful differential diagnostic procedure to rule out medical, pharmacological, or other causes. Even if the sleep complaint is primarily related to an underlying mental disorder, sleep disorders in the mentally ill may be exacerbated by many other factors, such as increasing age; comorbid mental, sleep, and medical diagnoses; alcohol and substance abuse; effects of psychotropic or other medications; use of caffeinated beverages, nicotine, or other substances; lifestyle; past episodes of psychiatric illness (persisting "scars"); and cognitive, conditioned, and coping characteristics such as anticipatory anxiety about sleep as bedtime nears. Some features of these sleep disorders may persist during periods of clinical remission of the mental disorder and may be influenced by genetic factors. Finally, even if the sleep complaint is precipitated by a nonpsychiatric factor, psychiatric and psychosocial skills may be useful in ferreting out predisposing and perpetuating factors involved in chronic sleep complaints.

Although signs and symptoms of sleep disturbance are common in most mental disorders, an

Table 39-9	Generalized Polygraphic Sleep Features of Individuals with Mental Disorders*						
Disorder	**Total Sleep Time**	**Sleep Efficiency**	**Sleep Latency**	**REM Latency**	**Delta %**	**REM %**	**REM Density**
Depression	↓↓	↓↓	↑↑	↓↓	↓↓	↓↓	↑
Alcoholism	↓	↓/=	↑	=	↓	↑	↑=
Panic disorder	↓/=	↓↓	↑↑	=	=	=	=
Generalized anxiety disorder	=	=	↑	=	=	=	=
Posttraumatic stress disorder	↓↓	↓↓	=	↑/=	=	↓↑	↑/=
Borderline disorder	↓/=	↓/=	↑/=	↓/=	=	=	=
Eating disorders	↓/=	↓/=	=	↓/=	=	=	↓/=
Schizophrenia	↓↓	↓↓	↑↑	↓↓	↓/=	=	↓
Insomnia	↓↓	↓↓	↑↑	=	↓↓	=	=
Narcolepsy	=	↓	↓↓	↓↓	=	=	=

*Two arrows (↑↑ or ↓↓) signify predominance of evidence; one arrow (↑ or ↓) signifies weak evidence, and (−) signifies weak evidence; equal sign (=) means no difference; ↓/= or ↑/= means mixed results.

Reprinted from Dow BM, Kelsoe JRJ, and Gillin JC (1996) Sleep and Dreams in Vietnam and Depression. *Biological Psychiarty* **39**: 42–50, Copyright 1996, Society of Biological Psychiatry.

additional diagnosis of insomnia or hypersomnia related to another mental disorder is made according to DSM-IV-TR criteria only when the sleep disturbance is a predominant complaint and is sufficiently severe to warrant independent clinical attention. Many of the individuals with this type of sleep disorder diagnosis focus on the sleep complaints to the exclusion of other symptoms related to the primary mental disorder. As summarized in Table 39-9, no single measure or constellation of measures has yet been found to be diagnostically pathognomonic for any specific disorder. Most diagnostic disorders are associated with insomnia, characterized by increased sleep latency and reduced total sleep, sleep efficiency, and delta sleep.

TREATMENT

The sleep complaint in the individual with an apparent mental disorder deserves the same careful diagnostic and therapeutic attention that it does in any individual. Just because an individual is depressed does not mean that the complaint of insomnia or hypersomnia can be explained away as a symptom of depression. Too many individuals with depression have been found to have a BRSD; too many individuals with panic disorder to have insomnia secondary to caffeinism. Chronic sleep complaints are multidetermined and multifaceted, even in many individuals with mental disorder. Differential diagnosis remains the first obligation of the clinician before definitive treatment, which should be aimed at the underlying cause or causes.

Sleeping pills should be prescribed reluctantly to individuals who receive adequate doses of antidepressants. Although coadministration of a benzodiazepine may improve sleep during the first week of antidepressant therapy, a low dose of zolpidem, zaleplon, trazodone, or any other sedating antidepressant at night in addition to the antidepressant may be less likely to produce tolerance and may have additive antidepressant benefits. Antipsychotic medications should not be administered as sleeping aids unless the individual is psychotic or otherwise unresponsive to other medications.

Sleep Disorder Due to a General Medical Condition

A sleep disorder due to a general medical condition is defined in DSM-IV-TR as a prominent disturbance in sleep severe enough to warrant independent clinical attention. Subtypes include insomnia, hypersomnia, parasomnia, and mixed types.

As a general rule, any disease or disorder that causes pain, discomfort, or a heightened state of arousal in the waking state is capable of disrupting or interfering with sleep. Examples of this phenomenon include pain syndromes of any sort, arthritic and other rheumatological disorders, prostatism and other causes of urinary frequency or urgency, chronic obstructive lung disease, and other pulmonary conditions. Many of these conditions increase in prevalence with advancing age, suggesting at least one reason that sleep disorders are more likely to be seen in senior populations.

Substance-Induced Sleep Disorder

An important aspect of the evaluation of any individual, particularly those with sleep disorders, is the review of medications and other substances (including prescription, over-the-counter and recreational drugs, as well as alcohol, stimulants, narcotics, coffee and caffeine, and nicotine) and exposure to toxins, or heavy metals. These substances may affect sleep and wakefulness during either ingestion or withdrawal, causing most commonly insomnia, hypersomnia, or, less frequently, parasomnia or mixed types of difficulties. On the basis of DSM-IV-TR criteria, a diagnosis of substance-induced sleep disorder may be made if the disturbance of sleep is sufficiently severe to warrant independent clinical attention and is judged to result from the direct physiological effects of a substance. Substance-induced sleep disorder cannot result from mental disorder or occur during delirium. If appropriate, the context for the development of sleep symptoms may be indicated by specifying with onset during intoxication or with onset during withdrawal.

The recognition of substance-related sleep disturbances usually depends on active searching by the clinician, beginning with a careful history, physical examination, laboratory and toxicological testing, and information (with permission) from former health care providers or friends and relatives. Individuals may not know what prescription medications they are taking or the doses, and may forget to mention over-the-counter medications, coffee, occupational or environmental toxins, and so forth. In the case of alcohol and drugs of abuse, they may deny to themselves and others their use, or quantity, or frequency of use. Substance dependence and abuse is often associated with other psychiatric diagnoses or symptoms. When comorbidity does exist, it is important to establish, if possible, whether the sleep disturbance is primary or secondary; that is, whether the sleep disturbance is substance-induced (secondary) or whether the substance use functions as a form of "self-medication" for sleep disturbance, in which the sleep disturbance would be considered primary. Many individuals with alcoholism experience secondary depression during the first few weeks of withdrawal from alcohol and exhibit short REM latency and other sleep changes similar to those reported in primary depression. This secondary depression usually remits spontaneously. Likewise, about one-third of individuals with unipolar depression and about three-fifths of individuals with bipolar disorder, manic type, have a substance use pattern that meets diagnostic criteria for alcoholism or substance abuse at some point. Prognosis and treatment may be altered in comorbid states, depending on whether the sleep disturbance is primary or secondary. In general, treatment should be aimed at the primary diagnosis after management of any acute withdrawal condition that may exist.

Alcohol, nicotine, amphetamines, caffeine, opiates, sedatives, and anxiolytics can cause or exacerbate sleep problems. Many medications produce sleep disturbance, including those with central or autonomic nervous system effects, like adrenergic agonists and antagonists, dopamine agonists and antagonists, cholinergic agonists and antagonists, antihistamines, and steroids. Among the prescription drugs associated frequently with sleep disorders are the SSRIs, which have been connected with overarousal and insomnia in some individuals and, more commonly, sedation in other individuals. Coadministration of trazodone at night has been shown, to be effective in managing fluoxetine-induced insomnia in depressed individuals. Additional sleep-related disturbances occasionally associated with the SSRIs include sleepwalking, REM sleep behavior disorder, and rapid eye movements during non-REM sleep.

COMPARISON OF DSM-IV-TR AND ICD-10 DIAGNOSTIC CRITERIA

For primary insomnia, the ICD-10 Diagnostic Criteria for Research and the DSM-IV-TR criteria are almost identical except that ICD-10 requires a frequency of at least three times a week for at least a month, whereas DSM-IV-TR does not specify a required frequency. For primary hypersomnia, the ICD-10 Diagnostic Criteria for Research and the DSM-IV-TR criteria are almost identical except that ICD-10 also counts sleep drunkenness as a presenting symptom. Furthermore, ICD-10 requires that the problems occur nearly every day for at least 1 month (or recurrently for shorter periods of time).

Since narcolepsy and breathing-related sleep disorder are included in Chapter VI (Diseases of the Nervous System) in ICD-10, there are no diagnostic criteria provided for these conditions.

For circadian rhythm sleep disorder, the ICD-10 Diagnostic Criteria for Research and the DSM-IV-TR criteria are almost identical except that ICD-10 specifies that the problems occur nearly every day for at least 1 month (or recurrently for shorter periods of time) (DSM-IV-TR has no specified duration). This condition is referred to in ICD-10 as "Nonorganic disorder of the sleep–wake cycle."

The ICD-10 Diagnostic Criteria for Research and the DSM-IV-TR criteria for nightmare disorder and sleepwalking disorder are essentially identical. The ICD-10 Diagnostic Criteria for Research and the DSM-IV-TR criteria sets for sleep terror disorder are almost identical except that ICD-10 explicitly limits the duration of the episode to less than 10 minutes.

40 Impulse Control Disorders

Although dissimilar in behavioral expressions, the disorders in this chapter share the feature of impulse dyscontrol. Individuals who experience such dyscontrol are overwhelmed by the urge to commit certain acts that are often apparently illogical or harmful. The outcome of each of these behaviors is often harmful, either for the afflicted individual (trichotillomania, pathological gambling) or for others (intermittent explosive disorder, pyromania, kleptomania). Trichotillomania, pyromania, and pathological gambling may involve episodes in which a sudden desire to commit the act of hair-pulling, fire-setting, or gambling is followed by rapid expression of the behavior. But in these conditions, the individual may spend considerable amounts of time fighting off the urge, trying not to carry out the impulse. The inability to resist the impulse is the common core of these disorders, rather than the rapid transduction of thought to action.

Because of the limited body of systematically collected data, the following sections largely reflect accumulated clinical experience. Therefore, the practicing psychiatrist should be particularly careful to consider the exigencies of individual subjects in applying treatment recommendations.

Intermittent Explosive Disorder

DIAGNOSIS

Individuals with intermittent explosive disorder have a significant problem with their temper. This definition highlights the centrality of impulsive aggression in intermittent explosive disorder. Impulsive aggression, however, is not specific to intermittent explosive disorder. It is a key feature of several mental disorders and nonpsychiatric conditions, and may emerge during the course of other mental disorders. Therefore, the definition of intermittent explosive disorder as formulated in the DSM-IV-TR is essentially a diagnosis of exclusion. As described in criterion C, a diagnosis of intermittent explosive disorder is made only after other mental disorders that might account for episodes of aggressive

> **DSM-IV-TR Diagnostic Criteria**
>
> **312.34 INTERMITTENT EXPLOSIVE DISORDER**
>
> A. Several discrete episodes of failure to resist aggressive impulses that result in serious assaultive acts or destruction of property.
> B. The degree of aggressiveness expressed during the episodes is grossly out of proportion to any precipitating psychosocial stressors.
> C. The aggressive episodes are not better accounted for by another mental disorder (e.g., antisocial personality disorder, borderline personality disorder, a psychotic disorder, a manic episode, conduct disorder, or attention-deficit/hyperactivity disorder) and are not due to the direct physiological effects of a substance (e.g., a drug of abuse, a medication) or a general medical condition (e.g., head trauma, Alzheimer's disease).
>
> Reprinted with permission from the *Diagnostic and Statistical Manual of Mental Disorders*, 4th ed., Text Rev. Copyright 2000 American Psychiatric Association.

behavior have been ruled out. The individual may describe the aggressive episodes as "spells" or "attacks." The symptoms appear within minutes to hours and, regardless of the duration of the episode, may remit almost as quickly. As in other impulse control disorders, the explosive behavior may be preceded by a sense of tension or arousal and is followed immediately by a sense of relief or release of tension.

Episodes of violent behavior appear in several common psychiatric disorders such as antisocial personality disorder, borderline personality disorder, and substance use disorders and need to be distinguished from the violent episodes of individuals with intermittent explosive disorder, which are apparently rare.

Although not explicitly stated in the DSM-IV-TR definition of intermittent explosive disorder, impulsive aggressive behavior may have many motivations that are not meant to be included within this diagnosis. Intermittent explosive disorder should not be diagnosed when the purpose of the aggression is monetary gain, vengeance, self-defense, social dominance, or expressing a political statement or when it occurs as a part of gang behavior. Typically, the aggressive behavior is egodystonic to individuals with intermittent explosive disorder, who feel genuinely upset, remorseful, regretful, bewildered, or embarrassed about their impulsive aggressive acts.

The physical and laboratory findings relevant to the diagnosis of intermittent explosive disorder and the differential diagnosis of impulsive aggression may be divided into two main groups: those associated with episodic impulsive aggression but not diagnostic of a particular disorder and those that suggest the diagnosis of a psychiatric or medical disorder other than intermittent explosive disorder. No laboratory or physical findings are specific for intermittent explosive disorder.

The first group of findings that are associated with impulsive aggression across a spectrum of disorders includes soft neurological signs such as subtle impairments in hand–eye coordination and minor reflex asymmetries. These signs may be elicited by a comprehensive neurological examination and simple pencil-and-paper tests such as parts A and B of the Trail Making Test. Measures of central serotonergic function such as CSF 5-HIAA levels, the fenfluramine challenge test, and positron emission tomography of prefrontal metabolism also belong to this group. Although these measures advanced our neurobiological understanding of impulsive aggression, their utility in the diagnosis of individual cases of intermittent explosive disorder and other disorders with impulsive aggression is yet to be demonstrated.

The second group of physical and laboratory findings is useful in the diagnosis of causes of impulsive aggression other than intermittent explosive disorder. The smell of alcohol in an individual's breath or a positive alcohol reading with a breathalyzer may help reveal alcohol intoxication. Blood and urine toxicology screens may reveal the use of other substances, and track marks on the forearms may suggest intravenous drug use. Partial complex seizures and focal brain lesions may be evaluated by use of the EEG and brain imaging. In cases without a grossly abnormal neurological examination, magnetic resonance imaging may be more useful than computed tomography of the head. Magnetic resonance imaging can reveal mesiotemporal scarring, which may be the only evidence for a latent seizure disorder, sometimes in the presence of a normal or inconclusive EEG. Diffuse slowing on the EEG is a nonspecific finding that is probably more common in, but not diagnostic of, individuals with impulsive aggression. Hypoglycemia, a rare cause of impulsive aggression, may be detected by blood chemistry screens.

The small literature on the comorbidity of impulsive aggressive episodes suggests that it often occurs with three classes of disorders:

1. Personality disorders, especially antisocial personality disorder and borderline personality disorder. By definition, antisocial personality disorder and borderline personality disorder are chronic and include impulsive aggression as an essential feature. Therefore, their diagnosis effectively excludes the diagnosis of intermittent explosive disorder.
2. A history of substance-use disorders, especially alcohol abuse. A concurrent diagnosis of substance intoxication excludes the diagnosis of intermittent explosive disorder. However, many individuals with intermittent explosive disorder report past or family histories of substance abuse, and in particular alcohol abuse. Therefore, when there is evidence suggesting that alcohol abuse may be present, a systematic evaluation of intermittent explosive disorder is warranted, and vice versa.
3. Neurological disorders, especially severe head trauma, partial complex seizures, dementias, and inborn errors of metabolism. Intermittent explosive disorder is not diagnosed if the aggressive episodes are a direct physiological consequence of a general medical condition. Such cases would be diagnosed as personality change due to a general medical condition, delirium, or dementia.

Some children with Tourette's disorder may be prone to rage attacks. The clinical manifestation of these rage attacks is similar to intermittent explosive disorder (IED) and may be more common among children with Tourette's who have comorbid mood disorders. On the basis of these observations, the rage attacks of these children may flow from an underlying dysregulation of brain function.

Differential Diagnosis

The DSM-IV-TR diagnosis of intermittent explosive disorder is essentially a diagnosis of exclusion, and the clinician should evaluate and carefully rule out more common diagnoses that are associated with impulsive violence. The lifelong nonremitting history of impulsive aggression associated with antisocial personality disorder and borderline personality disorder, together with other features of antisocial behavior (in antisocial personality disorder) or impulsive behaviors in other spheres (in borderline personality disorder) may distinguish them from intermittent explosive disorder, in which baseline behavior and functioning are in marked contrast to the violent outbursts. Other features of borderline personality disorder such as unstable and intense interpersonal relationships, frantic efforts to avoid abandonment, and identity disturbance may also be elicited by a careful history. More than in most psychiatric diagnoses, collateral information from an independent historian may be extremely helpful. This is especially true in forensic settings. Of note, individuals with intermittent explosive disorder are usually genuinely distressed by their impulsive aggressive outbursts and may voluntarily seek psychiatric help to control them. In contrast, individuals with antisocial personality disorder do not feel true remorse for their actions and view them as a problem only insofar as they suffer their consequences, such as incarceration and fines. Although individuals with borderline personality disorder, like individuals with intermittent explosive disorder, are often distressed by their impulsive actions, the rapid development of intense and unstable transference toward the clinician during the evaluation period of individuals with borderline personality disorder may be helpful in distinguishing it from intermittent explosive disorder.

Other causes of episodic impulsive aggression are substance-use disorders, in particular alcohol abuse and intoxication. When the episodic impulsive aggression is associated only with intoxication, intermittent explosive disorder is ruled out. However, as discussed earlier, intermittent explosive disorder and alcohol abuse may be related, and the diagnosis of one should lead the clinician to search for the other.

Neurological conditions such as dementias, focal frontal lesions, partial complex seizures, and postconcussion syndrome after recent head trauma may all present as episodic impulsive aggression and need to be differentiated from intermittent explosive disorder. Other neurological causes of impulsive aggression include encephalitis, brain abscess, normal-pressure hydrocephalus, subarachnoid hemorrhage, and stroke. In these instances, the diagnosis would be personality change due to a general medical condition, aggressive type, and it may be made with a careful history and the characteristic physical and laboratory findings.

Chronic impulsivity and aggression may occur as part of disorders first diagnosed during childhood and adolescence such as conduct disorder, oppositional defiant disorder, attention-deficit/hyperactivity disorder, and mental retardation. In addition, impulsive aggression may appear during the course of a mood disorder, especially during a manic episode, which precludes the diagnosis of intermittent explosive disorder, and during the course of an agitated depressive episode. Impulsive aggression may also be an associated feature of schizophrenia, in which it may occur in response to hallucinations or delusions. Impulsive aggression may also appear in variants of obsessive–compulsive disorder (OCD), which may present with concurrent impulsive and compulsive symptoms.

A special problem in the differential diagnosis of impulsive aggression, which may arise in forensic settings, is that it may represent purposeful behavior. Purposeful behavior is distinguished from intermittent explosive disorder by the presence of motivation and gain in the aggressive act, such as monetary gain, vengeance, or social dominance. Another diagnostic problem in forensic settings is malingering, in which individuals may claim to have intermittent explosive disorder to avoid legal responsibility for their acts.

Common disorders that should be excluded before intermittent explosive disorder is diagnosed and features that may be helpful in the differential diagnosis are summarized in Table 40.1.

TREATMENT

Given the rarity of pure intermittent explosive disorder, it is not surprising that few systematic data are available on its response to treatment and that some of the recommended treatment approaches to intermittent

Table 40-1	Differential Diagnosis of Intermittent Explosive Disorder
Intermittent Explosive Disorder Must Be Differentiated from Aggressive Behavior in	**In Contrast to Intermittent Explosive Disorder, the Other Condition**
Substance intoxication or withdrawal	Is due to the direct physiological effects of a substance
Delirium or dementia (substance induced or due to a general medical condition)	Includes characteristic symptoms (e.g., memory impairment, impaired attention) Requires the presence of an etiological general medical condition or substance use
Personality change due to a general medical condition, aggressive type	Requires presence of an etiological general medical condition
Conduct disorder or antisocial personality disorder	Is characterized by more general pattern of antisocial behavior
Other mental disorders (schizophrenia, manic episode, oppositional defiant disorder, borderline personality disorder)	Includes the characteristic symptoms of the other mental disorder

Source: First M and Frances A (eds) (1995) *DSM-IV Handbook of Differential Diagnosis*. Copyright, American Psychiatric Press, Washington, DC, p. 200.

explosive disorder are based on treatment studies of impulsivity and aggression in the setting of other mental disorders and general medical conditions. Thus, no standard regimen for the treatment of intermittent explosive disorder can be recommended at this time. Both psychological and somatic therapies have been utilized in the treatment of intermittent explosive disorder. A prerequisite for both modalities is the willingness of the individual to acknowledge some responsibility for the behavior and participate in attempts to control it.

Psychosocial Treatments

The major psychotherapeutic task of teaching individuals with intermittent explosive disorder is how to recognize their own feeling states and especially the affective state of rage. Lack of awareness of their own mounting anger is presumed to lead to the buildup of intolerable rage that is then discharged suddenly and inappropriately in a temper outburst. Individuals with intermittent explosive disorder are therefore taught how to first recognize and then verbalize their anger appropriately. In addition, during the course of insight-oriented psychotherapy, they are encouraged to identify and express the fantasies surrounding their rage. Group psychotherapy for temper-prone individuals has also been described. The cognitive–behavioral model of psychological treatment may be usefully applied to problems with anger and rage management.

Somatic Treatments

Several classes of medications have been used to treat intermittent explosive disorder. The same medications have also been used to treat impulsive aggression in the context of other disorders. These included beta-blockers (propranolol and metoprolol), anticonvulsants (carbamazepine and valproic acid), lithium, antidepressants (tricyclic antidepressants and serotonin reuptake inhibitors), and antianxiety agents (lorazepam, alprazolam, and buspirone). Carbamazepine may be more effective in individuals with intermittent explosive disorder and propranolol may be more effective in individuals with attention-deficit/hyperactivity disorder. A substantial body of evidence supports the use of propranolol–often in high doses–for impulsive aggression in individuals with chronic psychotic disorders and mental retardation. Lithium has been shown to have antiaggressive properties and may be used to control temper outbursts. In individuals with comorbid major depressive disorder, OCD, or cluster B and C personality disorders, SSRIs may be useful. Overall, in the absence of more controlled clinical trials,

the best approach may be to tailor the psychopharmacological agent to coexisting psychiatric comorbidity. In the absence of comorbid disorders, carbamazepine, titrated to antiepileptic blood levels, may be used empirically.

Kleptomania

DIAGNOSIS

Kleptomania shares with all other impulse control disorders the recurrent failure to resist impulses, in this case, the impulse to steal. Unfortunately, in the absence of epidemiological studies, little is known about kleptomania. There are no established treatments of choice.

Generally, the diagnosis of kleptomania is not a complicated one to make. However, kleptomania may frequently go undetected because the individual may not mention it spontaneously and the clinician may fail to inquire about it as part of the routine history. The index of suspicion should rise in the presence of commonly associated symptoms such as chronic depression, other impulsive or compulsive behaviors, tumultuous backgrounds, or unexplained legal troubles. It could convincingly be argued that a cursory review of compulsivity and impulsivity, citing multiple examples for the individual, should be a part of any thorough and complete mental health evaluation. In addition, it is important to do a careful differential diagnosis and pay attention to the various exclusion criteria before diagnosing theft as kleptomania. Possible diagnoses of sociopathy, mania, or psychosis should be carefully considered. In this regard, the clinician must inquire about the affective state of the individual during the episodes, the presence

---

DSM-IV-TR Diagnostic Criteria

312.32 KLEPTOMANIA

A. Recurrent failure to resist impulses to steal objects that are not needed for personal use or for their monetary value.
B. Increasing sense of tension immediately before committing the theft.
C. Pleasure, gratification, or relief at the time of committing the theft.
D. The stealing is not committed to express anger or vengeance and is not in response to a delusion or a hallucination.
E. The stealing is not better accounted for by conduct disorder, a manic episode, or antisocial personality disorder.

Reprinted with permission from the *Diagnostic and Statistical Manual of Mental Disorders*, 4th ed., Text Rev. Copyright 2000 American Psychiatric Association.

of delusions or hallucinations associated with the occurrence of the behavior, the motivation behind the stealing, and the fate and subsequent use of the objects.

TREATMENT

The general goal of treatment is the eradication of kleptomanic behavior. Treatment typically occurs in the outpatient setting, unless comorbid conditions such as severe depression, eating disturbances, or more dangerous impulsive behaviors dictate hospitalization. In the acute treatment phase, the aim is to decrease significantly or, ideally, eradicate episodes of stealing during a period of weeks to months. Concurrent conditions may compound the problem and require independently targeted treatment.

The acute treatment of kleptomania has not been, to date, systematically investigated. Recommendations are based on retrospective reviews, case reports, and small case series. Maintenance treatment for kleptomania has not been investigated either, and only anecdotal data exist for individuals who have been followed up for significant periods after initial remission.

No treatments have been systematically shown to be effective for kleptomania. In general, based on case reports and retrospective reviews, it appears that thymoleptic medications and behavioral therapy may be the most efficacious treatments for the short term, whereas long-term psychodynamic psychotherapy may be indicated and have good results for selected individuals.

Pyromania and Fire-Setting Behavior

DIAGNOSIS

The primary characteristics of pyromania are recurrent, deliberate fire-setting, the experience of tension or affective arousal before the fire-setting, an attraction or fascination with fire and its contexts, and a feeling of gratification or relief associated with the setting of a fire or its aftermath.

True pyromania is present in only a small subset of fire-setters. Multiple motivations are cited as causes for fire-setting behavior. These include arson for profit, crime concealment, revenge, vandalism, and political expression. In addition, fire-setting may be associated with other psychiatric diagnoses. Fire-setting behavior may be a focus of clinical attention, even when criteria for pyromania are not present. Because the large majority of fire-setting events are not associated with true pyromania, this section also addresses fire-setting behavior in general.

DSM-IV-TR Diagnostic Criteria

312.33 PYROMANIA

A. Deliberate and purposeful fire-setting on more than one occasion.
B. Tension or affective arousal before the act.
C. Fascination with, interest in, curiosity about, or attraction to fire and its situational contexts (e.g., paraphernalia, uses, consequences).
D. Pleasure, gratification, or relief when setting fires, or when witnessing or participating in their aftermath.
E. The fire-setting is not done for monetary gain, as an expression of sociopathic ideology, to conceal criminal activity, to express anger or vengeance, to improve one's living circumstances, in response to a delusion or hallucination, or as a result of impaired judgment (e.g., in dementia, mental retardation, substance intoxication).
F. The fire-setting is not better accounted for by conduct disorder, a manic episode, or antisocial personality disorder

Reprinted with permission from the *Diagnostic and Statistical Manual of Mental Disorders*, 4th ed., Text Rev. Copyright 2000 American Psychiatric Association.

The diagnosis of pyromania emphasizes the affective arousal, thrill, or tension preceding the act, as well as the feeling of tension relief or pleasure in witnessing the outcome. This is useful in distinguishing between pyromania and fire-setting elicited by other motives (i.e., financial gain, concealment of other crimes, political, arson related to other mental illness, revenge, attention seeking, erotic pleasure, part of conduct disorder).

The onset of pyromania has been reported to occur as early as age 3 years, but the condition may initially present in adulthood. Because of the legal implications of fire-setting, individuals may not admit previous events, which may result in biased perceptions of the common age at onset. Men greatly outnumber women with the disorder.

In children and adolescents, the most common elements are excitation caused by fires, enjoyment produced by fires, relief of frustration by fire-setting, and expression of anger through fire-setting.

Differential Diagnosis

Other causes of fire-setting must be ruled out. Fire-setting behavior may be motivated by circumstances unrelated to mental disorders. Such motivations include profit, crime concealment, revenge, vandalism, and political statement or action. Furthermore, fire-setting may be a part of ritual, cultural, or religious practices in some cultures.

Fire-setting may occur in the presence of other mental disorders. A diagnosis of fire-setting is not made when the behavior occurs as a part of conduct disorder, antisocial personality disorder, or a manic episode or if it occurs in response to a delusion or hallucination. The diagnosis is also not given if the individual suffers from impaired judgment associated with mental retardation, dementia, or substance intoxication.

TREATMENT

Because of the danger inherent in fire-setting behavior, the primary goal is elimination of the behavior. The treatment literature does not distinguish between pyromania and fire-setting behavior of other causes.

Much of the literature is focused on controlling fire-setting behavior in children and adolescents.

Pharmacotherapy

There are no reports of pharmacological treatment of pyromania. Because fire-setting may be frequently embedded in the context of other mental disorders, therapeutic attention may be directed primarily to the underlying disorder.

Psychosocial Treatments

It has been estimated that up to 60% of childhood fire-setting is motivated by curiosity. Such behavior often responds to direct educational efforts. In children and adolescents, focus on interpersonal problems in the family and clarification of events preceding the behavior may help control the behavior. The treatments described as more helpful for fire-setting are largely behavioral or focused on intervening in family or intrapersonal stresses that may precipitate the episode of fire-setting.

Relaxation training may be used (or added to graphing techniques) to assist in the development of alternative modes of dealing with the stress that may precede fire-setting. Principles of cognitive–behavioral therapy have been recently applied to childhood fire-setting.

Pathological Gambling

DIAGNOSIS

Gambling as a behavior is common. Current estimates suggest that approximately 80% of the adult population in the United States gamble. DSM-IV-TR, like DSM-III-R before it, covertly recognized the ubiquity of gambling behavior and the desire to gamble by the careful wording of criterion A for pathological gambling: "Persistent and recurrent maladaptive

gambling behavior as indicated by five (or more) of the following." This definition of pathological gambling differs from some other definitions of impulse control disorders not elsewhere classified, which are worded as "Failure to resist an impulse to." This difference implies that neither gambling behavior nor failure to resist an impulse to engage in it is viewed as pathological in and of itself. Rather, the maladaptive nature of the gambling behavior is the essential feature of pathological gambling and defines it as a disorder.

It is not difficult to diagnose pathological gambling once one has the facts. It is much more of a challenge to elicit the facts, because the vast majority of individuals with pathological gambling view their gambling behavior and gambling impulses as egosyntonic, and may often lie about the extent of their gambling (criterion A7). Individuals with pathological gambling may first seek medical or psychological attention because of comorbid disorders. Given the high prevalence of addictive disorders in pathological gambling and the increased prevalence of pathological gambling in those with alcoholism and other substance abuse, an investigation

---

DSM-IV-TR Diagnostic Criteria

312.31 PATHOLOGICAL GAMBLING

A. Persistent and recurrent maladaptive gambling behavior as indicated by five (or more) of the following:

    (1) is preoccupied with gambling (e.g., preoccupied with reliving past gambling experiences, handicapping or planning the next venture, or thinking of ways to get money with which to gamble)

    (2) needs to gamble with increasing amounts of money in order to achieve the desired excitement

    (3) has repeated unsuccessful efforts to control, cut back, or stop gambling

    (4) is restless or irritable when attempting to cut down or stop gambling

    (5) gambles as a way of escaping from problems or of relieving a dysphoric mood (e.g., feelings of helplessness, guilt, anxiety, depression)

    (6) after losing money gambling, often returns another day to get even ("chasing" one's losses)

    (7) lies to family members, therapist, or others to conceal the extent of involvement with gambling

    (8) has committed illegal acts such as forgery, fraud, theft, or embezzlement to finance gambling

    (9) has jeopardized or lost a significant relationship, job, or educational or career opportunity because of gambling

    (10) relies on others to provide money to relieve a desperate financial situation caused by gambling

B. The gambling behavior is not better accounted for by a manic episode.

of gambling patterns and their consequences is warranted for any individual who presents with a substance abuse problem. Likewise, the high rates of comorbidity with mood disorders suggest the utility of investigating gambling patterns of individuals presenting with an affective episode.

The spouses and the significant others of individuals with pathological gambling deserve special attention. Individuals with pathological gambling usually feel entitled to their behavior and often rely on their families to bail them out (criterion A10). As a consequence, it is often the spouse of the individual with pathological gambling who first realizes the need for treatment and who bears the consequences of the disorder. The spouse may be a valuable and motivated informant who should be questioned about the individual's behavior, and second, spouses should be specifically asked about the effects of the individual's illness on their own well-being and functioning and about suicidal ideation and attempts and the control of their own impulsivity.

Overall, individuals with pathological gambling have high rates of comorbidity with several other psychiatric disorders and conditions. Individuals presenting for clinical treatment of pathological gambling apparently have impressive rates of comorbidity, including alcohol disorders, depression, and bipolar disorder.

Course

Pathological gambling usually begins in adolescence in men and later in life in women. The onset is usually insidious, although some individuals may be "hooked" by their first bet. There may be years of social gambling with minimal or no impairment followed by an abrupt onset of pathological gambling that may be precipitated by greater exposure to gambling or by a psychosocial stressor. The gambling pattern may be regular or episodic, and the course of the disorder tends to be chronic. Over time, there is usually a progression in the frequency of gambling, the amounts wagered, and the preoccupation with gambling and with obtaining money with which to gamble. The urge to gamble and gambling activity generally increase during periods of stress or depression, as an attempted escape or relief (criterion A5).

Without treatment, the prognosis of pathological gambling is poor. It tends to run a chronic course with increasing morbidity and comorbidity, gradual disruption of family and work roles and relationships, depletion of financial reserves, entanglement with criminals and the criminal justice system, and, often, suicide attempts. In the hands of an experienced psychiatrist, treatment is associated with a favorable prognosis.

Differential Diagnosis

The differential diagnosis of pathological gambling is relatively straightforward. Pathological gambling should be differentiated from professional gambling, social gambling, and a manic episode. A diagnosis of pathological gambling should be given only if a history of maladaptive gambling behavior exists at times other than during a manic episode. Problems with gambling may also occur in individuals with antisocial personality disorder. If criteria are met for both disorders, both can be diagnosed.

TREATMENT

The goals of treatment of an individual with pathological gambling are the achievement of abstinence from gambling, rehabilitation of the damaged family and work roles and relationships, treatment of comorbid disorders, and relapse prevention. This approach echoes the goals of treatment of an individual with substance dependence. There are many similarities and several important differences between the treatment of pathological gambling and the treatment of substance dependence. For most individuals without severe acute psychiatric comorbidity, such as major depressive disorder with suicidal ideation or alcohol dependence with a history of delirium tremens, treatment may be given on an outpatient basis. Inpatient treatment in specialized programs may be considered if the gambler is unable to stop gambling, lacks significant family or peer support, or is suicidal, acutely depressed, multiply addicted, or contemplating some dangerous activity.

No standard treatment of pathological gambling has emerged. Despite many reports of behavioral and cognitive interventions for pathological gambling, there are minimal data available from well-designed or clearly detailed treatment studies. Pharmacologic treatments offer promise, but research-guided approaches are still insufficient to offer a standardized approach. Therefore, general approaches, based in clinical experience and available resources (such as Gamblers Anonymous or other support groups) should be considered.

The treatment of pathological gambling may consist of participation in Gamblers Anonymous, individual therapy, family therapy, treatment of comorbid disorders, and medication treatment. As is the case for substance dependence, the gambler needs to be abstinent to be accessible to any or all of these treatment modalities. For many gamblers, participation in Gamblers Anonymous is sufficient, and it is an essential part of most treatment plans. Gamblers Anonymous is a 12-step group built on the same principles as Alcoholics Anonymous. It utilizes empathic confrontation by peers who struggle with the same impulses and a group approach. Gam-Anon is a peer support group for family members of individuals with pathological gambling. Extensive data are lacking, but overall, Gamblers Anonymous appears somewhat less effective than Alcoholics Anonymous in achieving and maintaining abstinence.

The greatest differences between the treatment of pathological gambling and other addictions are in the area of family therapy. Because relapse may be difficult to detect (there is no substance to be smelled on the individual's breath, no dilated or constricted pupils, no slurred speech or staggered gait) and because of a long history of exploitative behavior by the individual, the spouse and the other family members tend to be more suspicious of, and angry at, the individual with pathological gambling compared with families of alcoholic individuals. Frequent family sessions are often essential to offer the gambler an opportunity to make amends, learn communication skills, and deal with preexisting intimacy problems. In addition, the spouse and other family members have often acquired their own psychiatric illnesses during the course of the individual's pathological gambling and need individualized treatment to recover.

Although research reports of the pharmacological treatment of pathological gambling have begun to emerge, there are still as yet insufficient data to come to any conclusions about the utility of medication. The effectiveness of selective serotonin reuptake inhibitors has been examined in a limited number of double-blind trials, but do show promise. The opiate antagonist, naltrexone, has also shown preliminary evidence of efficacy. Doses at the higher end of the usual treatment range should be considered with both these classes of agents. The use of mood stabilizers (lithium and carbamazepine) has been the subject of a limited number of reports. At this time, no clear guidelines for pharmacologic treatment have emerged.

Trichotillomania

DIAGNOSIS

The essential feature of trichotillomania is the recurrent failure to resist impulses to pull out one's own hair. Resulting hair loss may range in severity from mild (hair loss may be negligible) to severe (complete baldness and involving multiple sites on the scalp or body). Individuals with this condition do not want to engage

---

DSM-IV-TR Diagnostic Criteria

312.39 TRICHOTILLOMANIA

A. Recurrent pulling out of one's hair resulting in noticeable hair loss.
B. An increasing sense of tension immediately before pulling out the hair or when attempting to resist the behavior.
C. Pleasure, gratification, or relief when pulling out the hair.
D. The disturbance is not better accounted for by another mental disorder and is not due to a general medical condition (e.g., a dermatological condition).
E. The disturbance causes clinically significant distress or impairment in social, occupational, or other important areas of functioning.

Reprinted with permission from the *Diagnostic and Statistical Manual of Mental Disorders*, 4th ed., Text Rev. Copyright 2000 American Psychiatric Association.

---

in the behavior, but attempts to resist the urge result in great tension. Thus, hair-pulling is motivated by a desire to reduce this dysphoric state. In some cases, the hair-pulling results in a pleasurable sensation, in addition to the relief of tension. Tension may precede the act or may occur when attempting to stop. Distress over the symptom and the resultant hair loss may be severe.

Typically, the person complaining of unwanted hair-pulling is a young adult or the parent of a child who has been seen pulling out hair. Hair-pulling tends to occur in small bursts that may last minutes to hours. Hair-pulling is most commonly limited to the eyebrows and eyelashes. The scalp is the next most frequently afflicted site. However, hairs in any location of the body may be the focus of hair-pulling urges, including facial, axillary, chest, pubic, and even perineal hairs.

Anxiety is almost always associated with the act of hair-pulling. Such anxiety may occur in advance of the hair-pulling behavior. A state of tension may occur spontaneously—driving the person to pull out hair in an attempt to reduce dysphoric feelings. Varying lengths of time must pass before the tension abates. Consequently, the amount of hair that may be extracted in an episode varies from episode to episode and from person to person. Frequently, hair-pulling begins automatically and without conscious awareness. In such circumstances, individuals discover themselves pulling out hairs after some have already been pulled out. In these situations, dysphoric tension is associated with the attempt to stop the behavior.

Circumstances that seem to predispose to episodes of hair-pulling include both states of stress and, paradoxically, moments of particular relaxation. Frequently, hair-pulling occurs when at-risk individuals are engaged in a relaxing activity that promotes distraction and ease (e.g., watching television, reading, talking on the phone).

Patterns of hair-pulling behavior among children are less well described. Usually, the parent observes a child pulling out hair and may note patches of hair loss. Children may sometimes be unaware of the behavior or may, at times, deny it. Childhood trichotillomania has been reported to be frequently associated with thumb sucking or nail biting. It has been suggested that trichotillomania with onset in early childhood may occur frequently with spontaneous remissions. Consequently, some have recommended that trichotillomania in early childhood may be considered a benign habit with a self-limited course. However, many individuals who present with chronic trichotillomania in adulthood report onset in early childhood.

Individuals with trichotillomania have increased risk for mood disorders (major depressive disorder, dysthymic disorder) and anxiety symptoms. The frequency of specific anxiety disorders (such as generalized anxiety disorder and panic disorders as well as OCD) may be increased as well.

In general, the diagnosis of trichotillomania is not complicated. The essential symptom—recurrently pulling out hair in response to unwanted urges—is easily described by the individual. When the individual acknowledges the hair-pulling behavior and areas of patchy hair loss are evident, the diagnosis is not usually in doubt. Problems in diagnosis may arise when the diagnosis is suspected but the individual denies it. Such denial may occur in younger individuals and some adults. When the problem is suspected but denied by the individual, a skin biopsy from the affected area may aid in making the diagnosis.

Despite the hair loss, most individuals with this condition have no overtly unusual appearance on cursory inspection. If the hair loss is not covered by clothing or accessories, artful combing of hair or use of eyeliner and false eyelashes may easily hide it. The ease with which the condition may often be hidden may explain the general underappreciation of its apparent frequency and potential associated distress.

Histological findings are considered characteristic and may aid diagnosis when it is suspected despite denial by the individual. Biopsy samples from involved areas may have the following features. Short and broken hairs are present. The surface of the scalp usually shows no evidence of excoriation. On histological examination, normal and damaged follicles are found in the same area, as well as an increased number of catagen (i.e., nongrowing) hairs. Inflammation is usually minimal or absent. Some hair follicles may show signs of trauma (wrinkling of the outer root sheath). Involved follicles may be empty or contain a deeply pigmented keratinous material. The absence of inflammation distinguishes trichotillomania-induced alopecia from alopecia areata, the principal condition in the differential diagnosis.

Course

The age at onset typically ranges from early childhood to young adulthood. Peak ages at presentation may be bimodal, with an earlier peak about age 5 to 8 years among children in whom it has a self-limited course, whereas among individuals who present to clinicians in adulthood, the mean age at onset is approximately 13 years. Initial onset after young adulthood is apparently uncommon.

Trichotillomania may be one of the earliest occurring conditions in psychiatry. Some parents insist that their child began pulling hair before 1 year of age. When trichotillomania begins before age 6 years, it tends to be a milder condition. It often responds to simple interventions and may be self-limited, with a duration of several weeks to several months, even if not treated. It often occurs in association with thumb sucking. In some cases, it remits spontaneously when therapeutic attention is directed at concurrent, severe thumb sucking. It has been suggested that trichotillomania in childhood may be associated with severe intrapsychic or familial mental disorder. But there is no reliable evidence that supports such a conclusion. Indeed, some have suggested that because it may be common and frequently self-limiting, it should be considered a normal behavior among young children.

Some individuals have continuous symptoms for decades. For others, the disorder may come and go for weeks, months, or years at a time. Sites of hair-pulling may vary over time. Circumscribed periods of hair-pulling (weeks to months) followed by complete remission are reported among children.

Progression of the condition appears to be unpredictable. Waxing and waning of the severity of hair-pulling and number of hair-pulling sites occur in most individuals. It is not known which factors may predict a protracted and unremitting course.

TREATMENT

Treatment of trichotillomania typically occurs in an outpatient setting. Eradication of hair-pulling behavior is the general focus of treatment. Distress, avoidant behaviors, and cosmetic impairment are secondary to the hair-pulling behavior and would be likely to remit if the hair-pulling behavior were controlled. However, if sufficient control of hair-pulling cannot be attained, treatment goals should emphasize these associated problems as well. Even if hair-pulling persists, therapeutic interventions may be targeted at reducing secondary avoidance and diminishing distress.

Treatment may be considered in three phases:

- *Initial Contact.* The diagnosis is made and the individual and clinician agree on a strategy that may incorporate both pharmacological and psychological interventions. If distress is severe, supportive interventions should be immediately considered in anticipation of incomplete treatment response or of a delay of weeks to months before interventions may be beneficial.
- *Acute Treatment.* Even when treatment of hair-pulling behavior is optimally successful, there may be a delay of several weeks to months before adequate control is attained. Therefore, the acute treatment phase may be prolonged.
- *Maintenance.* It is not known how long individuals must maintain active treatment interventions to prevent relapse. It should be anticipated that a substantial number of individuals require ongoing treatment for an extended time. Pharmacological treatments may need to be maintained for open-ended periods. Behavioral or hypnotic intervention may require periodic "booster shots" to support continuation of benefits.

A variety of treatment approaches have been advocated for trichotillomania. However, there have, as yet, been few controlled studies of the efficacy of any treatment approach. A number of investigations of the use of antidepressants with specific inhibition of serotonin reuptake (i.e., fluoxetine and clomipramine) have yielded mixed results A multimodal approach, simultaneously utilizing several complementary treatment options, may turn out to be the most effective approach for most individuals.

While a number of treatment options can be currently offered to individuals with trichotillomania, the durability of long-term outcomes is unclear. Among those who have had a response to treatment, improvements were often lost over time, and persistent treatment and ongoing treatment was common over the course of several years.

Psychosocial Treatments

The most successful technique, habit reversal, is based on designing competitive behaviors that should inhibit the behavior of hair-pulling. For example, if hair-pulling requires raising the arm to the scalp and contracting the muscles of the hand to grasp a hair, the behaviorist may design a behavioral program in which the individual is taught to lower the arm and extend the muscles of the hand. As with behavioral techniques in general, these interventions are most successful when the individual is strongly motivated and compliant. In addition, the treating psychiatrist should be experienced in the use of such techniques. If necessary, a referral should be made to such an experienced individual. Modified behavioral approaches have been described for children and adolescents.

Cognitive–behavioral therapy (CBT) has been developed for, and applied to, individuals with trichotillomania. At this time, the potential for the efficacy of this treatment approach appears good.

Self-help groups for individuals with trichotillomania have appeared. Some are based in the structure of other 12-step programs. Some individuals appear to experience meaningful reduction in hair-pulling symptoms after beginning participation in such a group. Although the efficacy of such groups in reducing symptoms remains to be established, most individuals with trichotillomania can benefit from meeting other individuals with similar symptoms. Because of the lack of general awareness of trichotillomania, these individuals frequently believe that they are "oddball" individuals with a behavior that is unique. Many have experienced parental condemnation for the behavior and have been frequently castigated for a "habit" that may be viewed by others as under their voluntary control. The experience of meeting others with the condition is extremely supportive for such individuals and may help reduce the attendant stress while supporting self-esteem. Where programs specifically oriented toward trichotillomania may not be generally available, these individuals may benefit from groups oriented toward OCD.

COMPARISON OF DSM-IV-TR AND ICD-10 DIAGNOSTIC CRITERIA

The ICD-10 Diagnostic Criteria for Research do not include diagnostic criteria for intermittent explosive disorder. It is included in ICD-10 as an "other habit and Impulse Control Disorder."

The ICD-10 Diagnostic Criteria for Research and the DSM-IV-TR criteria for kleptomania, pyromania, and trichotillomania are essentially equivalent.

Finally, the ICD-10 Diagnostic Criteria for Research for pathological gambling are monothetic (i.e., A plus B plus C plus D are required) whereas the DSM-IV-TR criteria set is polythetic (i.e., 5 out of 10 required) with different items. Furthermore, the ICD-10 criteria specify "two or more episodes of gambling over a period of at least 1 year," whereas DSM-IV-TR does not specify a duration.

41 Adjustment Disorders

DIAGNOSIS

The essential feature of adjustment disorder (AD) is the development of clinically significant emotional or behavioral symptoms in response to an identifiable psychosocial stressor. The symptoms must develop within 3 months after the onset of the stressor (criterion A). The clinical significance of the reaction is indicated either by marked distress that is in excess of what would be expected given the nature of the stressor or by significant impairment in social or occupational (academic) functioning (criterion B). This disorder should not be used if the emotional and cognitive disturbances meet the criteria for *another* specific Axis I disorder (e.g., a specific anxiety or mood disorder) or are merely an exacerbation of a preexisting Axis I or Axis II disorder (criterion C). AD may be diagnosed if other Axis I or II disorders are present, but do not account for the pattern of symptoms that have occurred in response to the stressor. The diagnosis of AD does not apply when the symptoms represent bereavement (criterion D). By definition, AD must resolve within 6 months of the termination of the stressor or its consequences (criterion E). However, the symptoms may persist for a prolonged period (i.e., longer than 6 months) if they occur in response to a chronic stressor (e.g., a chronic, disabling general medical condition) or to a stressor that has enduring consequences (e.g., the financial and emotional difficulties resulting from a divorce).

The symptoms of AD are defined in terms of their being a maladaptive response to a psychosocial stressor. There are, in fact, no specific symptoms of AD; any combination of behavioral or emotional symptoms that occur in association with a stressor may qualify. The nature of the symptomatology is described by a variety of possible "subtypes", including With Depressed Mood, With Mixed Anxiety and Depressed Mood, With Disturbance of Conduct, With Mixed Disturbance of Emotions and Conduct, and Unspecified.

Although this diagnosis lacks rigorous specificity, its treatment is no less challenging or less important. AD's lack of a designated symptom profile results in

---

DSM-IV-TR Diagnostic Criteria

309.xx ADJUSTMENT DISORDERS

A. The development of emotional or behavioral symptoms in response to an identifiable stressor(s) occurring within 3 months of the onset of the stressor(s).
B. These symptoms or behaviors are clinically significant as evidenced by either of the following:

   (1) marked distress that is in excess of what would be expected from exposure to the stressor
   (2) significant impairment in social or occupational (academic) functioning

C. The stress-related disturbance does not meet the criteria for another specific Axis I disorder and is not merely an exacerbation of a preexisting Axis I or Axis II disorder.
D. The symptoms do not represent bereavement.
E. Once the stressor (or its consequences) has terminated, the symptoms do not persist for more than an additional 6 months.

Specify if:

Acute: if the disturbance lasts less than 6 months
Chronic: if the disturbance lasts for 6 months or longer
Adjustment disorders are coded based on the subtype, which is selected according to the predominant symptoms. The specific stressor(s) can be specified on Axis IV.
309.0 With Depressed Mood
309.24 With Anxiety
309.28 With Mixed Anxiety and Depressed Mood
309.3 With Disturbance of Conduct
309.4 With Mixed Disturbance of Emotions and Conduct
309.9 Unspecified

Reprinted with permission from the *Diagnostic and Statistical Manual of Mental Disorders*, 4th ed., Text Rev. Copyright 2000 American Psychiatric Association.

---

this diagnosis having insufficient specificity. However, it is this lack of specificity, which permits the clinician to have a "diagnosis" to use when the individual is presenting with early, vague, nonconcrete symptomatology, which should be noted, identified, and followed. This is similar to the situation with early fever, or fever of unknown origin, which, by the way, may never go on to a specific medical diagnosis, but be at discharge simply diagnosed as a "fever of unknown origin."

Clinical Guide to the Diagnosis and Treatment of Mental Disorders. M. B. First and A. Tasman
© 2006 John Wiley & Sons, Ltd.   ISBN 0 470 019158

According to DSM-IV-TR, even if a specific and presumably causal stressor is identified, if enough symptoms develop so that diagnostic criteria are met for a specific disorder, then that diagnosis should be made instead of a diagnosis of AD. Therefore, the presence of stressors does not automatically signify a diagnosis of AD, and conversely, a diagnosis of a specific disorder (e.g., major depressive or anxiety disorder) does not imply the absence of concomitant or concurrent stressful events.

Although the diagnosis of AD requires evidence of maladaption, it is notable that no specific requirement for functional impairment has been included (e.g., there is no requirement for a certain decrement in the Global Assessment of Functioning Scale score in order to make the diagnosis). The clinician needs to examine the individual's behavior to see whether it is beyond what is expected in a particular situation, and for that individual. In order to do this, the clinician needs to take into account the individual's cultural beliefs and practices, his or her developmental age, and the transient nature of the behavior. If the behavior lasts a few moments or is an impulsive outburst, it would not qualify for a maladaptive response to justify the diagnosis of AD. The behavior in question should be maladaptive for that individual, in his/her culture, and sufficiently persistent to qualify for the maladaptation attribute of the AD diagnosis.

Several studies reported an association of suicidal behavior in adolescents and young adults with AD. One study found that 56% of those hospitalized for suicidal behavior in an urban hospital setting met the DSM-II criteria for transient situational disturbance (an earlier diagnostic label for what came to be called AD). A retrospective review of 325 consecutive hospital admissions for deliberate self-poisoning revealed that 58% of all cases met criteria for AD with depressed mood, the majority of whom were women aged 15 to 24 years. These studies underscore the seriousness of AD in a subset of individuals and suggest that although the diagnosis may be subthreshold, its morbidity can be serious and at times even fatal.

The issue of boundaries between the specific mood and anxiety disorders, depressive disorder or anxiety disorder NOS, and AD remains problematic. The specific mood and anxiety disorders are often associated with, and even precipitated by, stress. Therefore, it is not always possible to say one group of diagnoses is accompanied by stress (the AD) and another (e.g., major depressive disorder) is not. Stress may accompany many of the mental disorders but it is not an essential component to make certain diagnoses (e.g., major depressive disorder). Serial and ongoing observation of the clinical course is required to ascertain whether the AD is a transitory remitting event, the prodromal state of a more serious and developing disorder, or an intermittent chronic state of a low-level mood disorder. There is considerable evidence indicating that major depressive disorder is a highly recurrent, often chronic condition that is frequently associated with low-grade symptoms prior to, and between, major episodes. Thus, the differential diagnoses of depressed mood must be linked to ongoing assessment, not cross-sectional evaluation, which is so often the case; it is essential to maintain a longitudinal view of the subthreshold disorders to know their place in an individual's affective history.

Course

There appear to be important differences in adolescents and adults with regard to prognosis, according to a 5-year follow-up study of adults and adolescents with AD. Although the prognosis was favorable and most adult individuals with AD were symptom free at 5 years (71% were completely well, 8% had an intervening problem, and 21% had a major depressive disorder or alcoholism), adolescents had a far different outcome. A 5-year follow-up study of adolescents indicated that 43% had a major psychiatric disorder (e.g., schizophrenia, schizoaffective disorder, major depressive disorder, substance abuse disorder, and personality disorder); 13% had an intervening mental disorder; and 44% had no mental disorder. In adolescents, behavioral symptoms and the chronicity of the morbidity were the major predictors for psychopathological disorders at the 5-year follow-up. This was not so with the adults in the study, and raises the question of whether these adolescents were diagnosed as having AD as part of a prodrome of another more serious disorder.

TREATMENT

Appropriate and timely treatment is essential for individuals with AD so that their symptoms do not worsen, do not further impair their important relationships, and do not compromise their capacity to work, study, or be active in their interpersonal pursuits. Treatment must attempt to forestall further erosion of the individual's capacity to function that could ultimately have grave and untoward consequences.

There are two approaches to treatment. One is based on the understanding that this disorder emanates from a psychological reaction to a stressor. The stressor needs to be identified, described, and shared with the individual; plans must be made to mitigate it, if possible. The abnormal response may be attenuated if the stressor can be eliminated or reduced. It has been shown that in the medically ill, the most common stressor is the medical illness itself, and the AD may remit when the medical illness improves or a new level of adaptation is reached. The other approach to treatment is to provide intervention for the symptomatic presentation, despite the fact that it does not reach the threshold level for a specific disorder, on the premise that it is associated with impairment and that treatments that are effective for more pronounced presentations of similar pathology are likely to be effective. This may include psychotherapy, pharmacotherapy, or a combination of the two.

Psychosocial Treatments

Psychotherapeutic intervention in AD is intended to reduce the effects of the stressor, enhance coping to the stressor that cannot be reduced or removed, and establish a mental state and support system to maximize adaptation. Psychotherapy can involve any one of several approaches: cognitive–behavioral treatment, interpersonal therapy, psychodynamic efforts, or counseling.

The first goal of these psychotherapies is to analyze the nature of the stressors affecting the individual to see whether they may be avoided or minimized. It is necessary to clarify and interpret the meaning of the stressor for the individual. For example, an amputation of the leg may have devastated an individual's feelings about himself or herself, especially if the individual was a runner. It is necessary to clarify that the individual still has enormous residual capacity; that he or she can engage in much meaningful work, does not have to lose valued relationships, and can still be sexually active; and that it does not necessarily mean that further body parts will be lost. (However, it will also involve redirecting the physical activity to another pastime.) Otherwise, the individual's pernicious fantasies ("all is lost") may take over in response to the stressor (i.e., amputation), make the individual dysfunctional (at work, sex), and precipitate a painful dysphoria or anxiety reaction.

Some stressors may elicit an overreaction (e.g., the individual's attempted suicide or homicide after abandonment by a lover). In such instances of overreaction with feelings, emotions, or behaviors, the therapist would help the individual put his or her feelings and rage into words rather than into destructive actions and gain some perspective. The role of verbalization and the joining of affects and conflicts cannot be overestimated in an attempt to reduce the pressure of the stressor and enhance coping. Drugs and alcohol are to be discouraged.

Psychotherapy, medical crisis counseling, crisis intervention, family therapy, group treatment, cognitive–behavioral treatment, and interpersonal therapy all encourage the individual to express affects, fears, anxiety, rage, helplessness, and hopelessness to the stressors imposed. They also assist the individual to reassess reality in the service of adaptation. Following the example given above, the loss of a leg is not the loss of one's life. But it is a major loss. Brief psychotherapy should attempt to reframe the meaning of the stressor, find ways to minimize it, and diminish the psychological deficit due to its occurrence. The treatment should expose the concerns and conflicts that the individual is experiencing, help the individual gain perspective on the adversity, and encourage the individual to establish relationships and to attend support groups or self-help groups for assistance in the management of the stressor and the self.

Interpersonal psychotherapy was applied to depressed outpatients with human immunodeficiency virus (HIV) infection and was found to be useful. Some of the attributes of interpersonal psychotherapy are psychoeducation regarding the sick role, using a here-and-now framework, formulation of the problems from an interpersonal perspective, exploration of options for changing dysfunctional behavior patterns, and identification of focused interpersonal problem areas.

Support groups have been demonstrated to help individuals adjust and enhance their coping mechanisms, and they may prolong life as well. For example, a 1989 study showed that women with stage IV breast cancer lived longer after ongoing group therapy than those with standard cancer care. However, these findings on group psychological intervention and mortality have not been confirmed in at least two replication trials.

Pharmacological Treatments

Given the potential effectiveness of psychopharmacological interventions for the treatment of minor depression, such measures may also be helpful for other subthreshold disorders. It has been recommended that antidepressant therapy be considered if there is no benefit from 3 months of psychotherapy or other supportive measures. Although psychotherapy is the first choice treatment, psychotherapy combined with benzodiazepines may also be helpful, especially for individuals with severe life stress(es) and a significant anxious component. Tricyclic antidepressants or buspirone are recommended in place of benzodiazepines for individuals with current or past heavy alcohol use because of the greater risk of dependence in these individuals.

Those individuals who do not respond to counseling or the various modes of psychotherapy that have been outlined and to a trial of antidepressant or anxiolytic medications should be regarded as treatment nonresponders. It is essential to reevaluate the individual to ensure that the diagnostic impression has not altered and, in particular, that the individual has not developed a major mental disorder, which would require a more aggressive treatment, often biological. The clinician must also consider that an Axis II disorder might be interfering with the individual's resolution of the AD. Finally, if the stressor continues and cannot be removed (e.g., the continuation of a seriously impairing chronic illness), additional support and management strategies need to be employed to assist the individual in optimally adapting to the stressor.

COMPARISON OF DSM-IV-TR AND ICD-10 DIAGNOSTIC CRITERIA

In contrast to DSM-IV-TR (which requires the onset of symptoms within 3 months of the stressor), the ICD-10 Diagnostic Criteria for Research specify an onset within 1 month. Furthermore, ICD-10 excludes stressors of "unusual or catastrophic type." In contrast, DSM-IV-TR allows extreme stressors so long as the criteria are not met for posttraumatic or acute stress disorder. ICD-10 also provides for several different subtypes, including "brief depressive reaction" (depressive state lasting 1 month or less) and "prolonged depressive reaction" (depressive state lasting up to 2 years).

Personality Disorders

Everybody has a personality, or a characteristic manner of thinking, feeling, behaving, and relating to others. Some persons are typically introverted and withdrawn, others are more extraverted and outgoing. Some persons are invariably conscientious and efficient, whereas other persons might be consistently undependable and negligent. Some persons are characteristically anxious and apprehensive, whereas others are typically relaxed and unconcerned. These personality traits are often felt to be integral to each person's sense of self, as they involve what persons value, what they do, and their innate tendencies and preferences.

It is when personality traits are inflexible and maladaptive and cause significant functional impairment or subjective distress that they constitute a Personality Disorder. The DSM-IV-TR provides the diagnostic criteria for 10 personality disorders. This chapter begins with a discussion of the diagnosis and treatment of personality disorders in general, followed by a discussion of these issues for the 10 individual personality disorders.

Personality Disorder

DIAGNOSIS

A personality disorder is defined in DSM-IV-TR as "an enduring pattern of inner experience and behavior that deviates markedly from the expectations of the individual's culture, is pervasive and inflexible, has an onset in adolescence or early adulthood, is stable over time, and leads to distress or impairment" (page 686).

Personality disorder is the only class of mental disorders in DSM-IV-TR for which an explicit definition and criteria set are provided. A general definition and criteria set can be useful to clinicians because the most common personality disorder diagnosis in clinical practice is often the diagnosis "not otherwise specified" (NOS). Clinicians provide the NOS diagnosis when they determine that a personality disorder is present but the symptomatology fails to meet

---

DSM-IV-TR General Diagnostic Criteria

PERSONALITY DISORDER

A. An enduring pattern of inner experience and behavior that deviates markedly from the expectations of the individual's culture. This pattern is manifested in two (or more) of the following areas:

(1) cognition (i.e., ways of perceiving and interpreting self, other people, and events)
(2) affectivity (i.e., the range, intensity, lability, and appropriateness of emotional response)
(3) interpersonal functioning
(4) impulse control

B. The enduring pattern is inflexible and pervasive across a broad range of personal and social situations.
C. The enduring pattern leads to clinically significant distress or impairment in social, occupational, or other important areas of functioning.
D. The pattern is stable and of long duration and its onset can be traced back at least to adolescence or early adulthood.
E. The enduring pattern is not better accounted for as a manifestation or consequence of another mental disorder.
F. The enduring pattern is not due to the direct physiological effects of a substance (e.g., a drug of abuse, a medication) or a general medical condition (e.g., head trauma).

Reprinted with permission from the *Diagnostic and Statistical Manual of Mental Disorders*, 4th ed., Text Rev. Copyright 2000 American Psychiatric Association.

---

the criteria set for one of the 10 specific personality disorders. A general definition of what is meant by a personality disorder is therefore helpful when determining whether the NOS diagnosis should in fact be provided.

Gender and cultural biases are one potential source of inaccurate personality disorder diagnosis that are worth noting in particular. One of the general diagnostic criteria for personality disorder is that the personality trait must deviate markedly from the expectations of a person's culture. The purpose of this cultural deviation requirement is to compel clinicians to consider the cultural background of the individual. A behavior pattern that appears to be aberrant from the perspective

Clinical Guide to the Diagnosis and Treatment of Mental Disorders. M. B. First and A. Tasman
© 2006 John Wiley & Sons, Ltd.   ISBN 0 470 019158

of one's own culture (e.g., submissiveness or emotionality) could be quite normative and adaptive within another culture. The cultural expectations or norms of the clinician might not be relevant or applicable to an individual from a different cultural background. However, one should not infer from this requirement that a personality disorder is primarily or simply a deviation from a cultural norm. Deviation from the expectations of one's culture is not necessarily maladaptive, nor is conformity to one's culture necessarily healthy. Many of the personality disorders may even represent (in part) extreme or excessive variants of behavior patterns that are valued or encouraged within a particular culture. For example, it is usually adaptive to be confident but not to be arrogant, to be agreeable but not to be submissive, or to be conscientious but not to be perfectionistic. Gender and cultural biases of particular relevance to individual personality disorders will be discussed further in the chapter.

Estimates of the prevalence of personality disorder within clinical settings are typically above 50%. As many as 60% of inpatients within some clinical settings would be diagnosed with borderline personality disorder (BPD) and as many as 50% of inmates within a correctional setting could be diagnosed with antisocial personality disorder (ASPD). Although the comorbid presence of a personality disorder is likely to have an important impact on the course and treatment of an Axis I disorder, the prevalence of personality disorder is generally underestimated in clinical practice owing in part to the failure to provide systematic or comprehensive assessments of personality disorder symptomatology and perhaps as well to the lack of funding for the treatment of personality disorders.

According to the best available estimates, approximately 10–15% of the general population would be diagnosed with one of the 10 DSM-IV-TR personality disorders, excluding personality disorder not otherwise specified (PDNOS). Prevalence rates for individual personality disorders will be discussed later in this chapter.

There is also considerable personality disorder diagnostic co-occurrence. Individuals who meet the DSM-IV-TR diagnostic criteria for one personality disorder are likely to meet the diagnostic criteria for another. DSM-IV-TR instructs clinicians that all diagnoses should be recorded because it can be important to consider, for example, the presence of antisocial traits in someone with a BPD or the presence of paranoid traits in someone with a dependent personality disorder (DPD). However, the extent of diagnostic co-occurrence is at times so extensive that most researchers prefer a more dimensional description of personality.

Diagnostic categories provide clear, vivid descriptions of discrete personality types, but the personality structure of actual individuals might be more accurately described by a constellation of maladaptive personality traits.

Personality disorders must be evident since adolescence or young adulthood and have been relatively chronic and stable throughout adult life (see DSM-IV-TR general diagnostic criteria for personality disorder, page 439). A 75-year-old man can be diagnosed with a DSM-IV-TR DPD, but the symptoms must have been present throughout the duration of his adulthood (e.g., since the age of 18 years), unless the dependent behavior was a direct, explicit expression of a neurochemical disease or lesion.

The requirement that a personality disorder be evident since late adolescence and be relatively chronic thereafter has been a traditional means by which to distinguish a personality disorder from an Axis I disorder. Mood, anxiety, psychotic, sexual, and other mental disorders have traditionally been conceptualized as conditions that arise at some point during a person's life and that are relatively limited or circumscribed in their expression and duration. Personality disorders, in contrast, are conditions that are evident as early as late adolescence (and in some instances prior to that time), are evident in everyday functioning, and are stable throughout adulthood. However, the consistency of this distinction across disorders in the classification has been decreasing with each edition of the DSM, as early-onset and chronic variants of Axis I disorders are being added to the diagnostic manual (e.g., early-onset dysthymia and generalized social phobia).

TREATMENT

One of the mistaken assumptions or expectations of Axis II is that personality disorders are untreatable. In fact, maladaptive personality traits are often the focus of clinical treatment. Personality disorders are among the more difficult of mental disorders to treat as they involve entrenched behavior patterns, some of which will be integral to an individual's self-image. Nevertheless, there is compelling empirical support to indicate that meaningful responsivity to psychosocial and pharmacologic treatment does occur. Treatment of a personality disorder is unlikely to result in the development of a fully healthy or ideal personality structure, but clinically and socially meaningful change to personality structure and functioning does occur. In fact, given the considerable social, occupational, medical, and other costs that are engendered by such personality disorders as the antisocial and borderline, even marginal reductions in symptomatology can represent quite significant and meaningful public health care, social, and clinical benefits.

Specific DSM-IV-TR Personality Disorders

DSM-IV-TR includes 10 individual personality disorder diagnoses that are organized into three clusters: (a) paranoid, schizoid, and schizotypal (placed within an odd–eccentric cluster); (b) antisocial, borderline, histrionic, and narcissistic (dramatic–emotional–erratic cluster); and (c) avoidant, dependent, and obsessive–compulsive (anxious–fearful cluster). Each of these personality disorders will be discussed in turn.

Paranoid Personality Disorder

DIAGNOSIS

Paranoid personality disorder (PPD) involves a pervasive and continuous distrust and suspiciousness of the motives of others, but the disorder is more than just suspiciousness. Persons with this disorder are also hypersensitive to criticism, they respond with anger to threats to their autonomy, they incessantly seek out confirmations of their suspicions, and they tend to be quite rigid in their beliefs and perceptions of others. The presence of PPD is indicated by four or more of the seven diagnostic criteria presented in the DSM-IV-TR criteria for PPD.

Trust versus mistrust is a fundamental personality trait along which all persons vary. Thirteen percent of the adult male population and 6% of the adult female population may be characteristically mistrustful of others. However, only 0.5–2.5% of the population are likely to meet the DSM-IV-TR diagnostic criteria for a PPD. It is suggested in DSM-IV-TR that approximately 10–30% of persons within inpatient settings and 2–10% within outpatient settings have this, but the lower end of these rates may represent the more accurate estimate. It does appear that more males than females have the disorder.

Course

Premorbid traits of PPD may be evident prior to adolescence in the form of social isolation, hypersensitivity, hypervigilance, social anxiety, peculiar thoughts, angry hostility, and idiosyncratic fantasies. As children, individuals may appear odd and peculiar to their peers and they may not have achieved to their capacity in school. Their adjustment as adults is particularly

---

DSM-IV-TR Diagnostic Criteria

301.0 PARANOID PERSONALITY DISORDER

A. A pervasive distrust and suspiciousness of others such that their motives are interpreted as malevolent, beginning by early adulthood, and present in a variety of contexts, as indicated by four (or more) of the following:

(1) suspects, without sufficient basis, that others are exploiting, harming, or deceiving him or her

(2) is preoccupied with unjustified doubts about the loyalty or trustworthiness of friends or associates

(3) is reluctant to confide in others because of unwarranted fear that the information will be used maliciously against him or her

(4) reads hidden demeaning or threatening meanings into benign remarks or events

(5) persistently bears grudges, i.e. is unforgiving of insults, injuries, or slights

(6) perceives attacks on his or her character or reputation that are not apparent to others and is quick to react angrily or to counterattack

(7) has recurrent suspicions, without justification, regarding fidelity of spouse or sexual partner.

B. Does not occur exclusively during the course of schizophrenia, a mood disorder with psychotic features, or another psychotic disorder, and is not due to the direct physiological effects of a general medical condition.

Note: if criteria are met prior to the onset of schizophrenia, add "premorbid," e.g., paranoid personality disorder (premorbid).

Reprinted with permission from the *Diagnostic and Statistical Manual of Mental Disorders*, 4th ed., Text Rev. Copyright 2000 American Psychiatric Association.

---

poor with respect to interpersonal relationships. They may become socially isolated or fanatic members of groups that encourage or at least accept their paranoid ideation. They might maintain a steady employment but are difficult coworkers, as they tend to be rigid, controlling, critical, blaming, and prejudicial. They are likely to become involved in lengthy, acrimonious, and litigious disputes that are difficult, if not impossible, to resolve.

Differential Diagnosis

PPD paranoid ideation is inconsistent with reality and is resistant to contrary evidence, but the ideation is not psychotic, absurd, inconceivable, or bizarre. PPD also lacks other features of psychotic and delusional disorders (e.g., hallucinations) and is evident since early adulthood, whereas a psychotic disorder becomes evident later within a person's life or remits after a much briefer period of time. Persons with PPD can develop psychotic disorders but to diagnose PPD in such cases, the paranoid personality traits must be evident prior to and persist after the psychotic episode. If PPD precedes the onset of schizophrenia, then it should be noted that it is premorbid to the schizophrenia. However, it may not be meaningful to diagnose a person with both PPD and schizophrenia, as the premorbid paranoid traits may in some cases have simply represented a prodromal phase of the schizophrenic pathology.

Paranoid personality traits are evident in other personality disorders. Persons with avoidant personality disorder are socially withdrawn and apprehensive of others; borderline, antisocial, and narcissistic persons may be impatient, irritable, and antagonistic; and schizotypal persons may display paranoid ideation. The diagnosis of PPD often co-occurs with these other personality disorder diagnoses. Persons with PPD are prone to develop a variety of Axis I disorders, including substance-related, obsessive–compulsive, anxiety, agoraphobia, and depressive disorders.

TREATMENT

Persons with PPD rarely seek treatment for their feelings of suspiciousness and distrust. They experience these traits as simply accurate perceptions of a malevolent and dangerous world (i.e., egosyntonic). They may not consider the paranoid attributions to be at all problematic, disruptive, or maladaptive. They are not delusional but they also fail to be reflective, insightful, or self-critical. They may recognize only that they have difficulty controlling their anger and getting along with others. They might be in treatment for an anxiety, mood, or substance-related disorder or for various marital, familial, occupational, or social (or legal) conflicts that are secondary to their personality disorder, but they also externalize the responsibility for their problems and have substantial difficulty recognizing their own contribution to their internal dysphoria and external conflicts. They consider their problems to be due to what others are doing to them, not to how they perceive, react, or relate to others.

The presence of paranoid personality traits complicates the treatment of an Axis I disorder or a relationship problem. Trust is central to the development of an adequate therapeutic alliance, yet it is precisely the absence of trust that is central to this disorder. It can be tempting to be less than forthright and open in the treatment of excessively suspicious persons because they distort, exaggerate, or escalate minor errors, misunderstandings, or inconsistent statements. However, therapists find that they weave an increasingly tangled web as they walk gingerly around the truth. Also, persons with PPD seize upon any kernel of deception to confirm their suspicion that the therapist is not to be trusted. It

is preferable to be especially forthright and precise with paranoid individuals. Details that are inconsequential and of no interest to most individuals can be important to provide to persons with PPD so that they are assured that nothing is being withheld or hidden from them.

Clinicians agree on several general principles in the treatment of paranoid personality traits. It is usually pointless and often harmful to confront (or argue with) the paranoid beliefs. Such efforts may only alienate the individual and confirm his or her suspicions. The therapist should maintain a sincere and consistent respect for the individual's autonomy and for his or her right to make his or her own decisions. However, one should not attempt to ingratiate oneself by being overly acquiescent and compliant. This can appear to be obviously patronizing, insincere, or manipulative. The goal is to develop, in a nonthreatening way, more self-reflection and self-awareness (e.g., recognition of the contribution of the paranoid traits and behaviors to the difficulties he or she has been experiencing). A useful approach can be to communicate a sincere and respectful willingness to explore the implications, logic, and reality of the suspicions. Whenever one appears to be endangering rapport by moving too quickly, one should retreat to a more neutral and accepting position.

One must also be careful to avoid defensive reactions to the inevitable accusations. Any one of the conflicts they have had with others can develop within the therapeutic relationship and persons with PPD have a tendency to be contentious, rigid, accusatory, suspicious, and litigious, which can tax the empathy and patience of the therapist. One must attempt to maintain an empathic concern for their feelings of betrayal, and reassure them in an understanding, forthright manner that is neither patronizing nor disrespectful. Termination of treatment may at times be necessary if continuation would only result in further acrimony.

The suspicions, accusations, and acrimony often makes the person with PPD a poor candidate for group therapies. There is the potential to learn much about themselves within a group, but it is usually very difficult for them to develop the feelings of trust, respect, and security that are necessary for successful group therapy. Their propensity to make unfair hostile accusations alienates them from other group members, and they may quickly become a scapegoat for difficulties and conflicts that develop within the group.

There have been a variety of studies on the pharmacologic treatment of psychotic paranoid ideation and of schizotypal personality disorder (which often includes paranoid personality traits) but little to no research on the pharmacologic responsivity of the nonpsychotic suspiciousness and egosyntonic paranoid ideation of

PPD. Persons with PPD may also perceive the use of a medication to represent an effort to simply suppress or control their accusations and suspicions rather than to respectfully consider and address them. However, they may be receptive and responsive to the benefits of a medication to help control feelings of anxiousness or depression that are secondary to their personality disorder.

Schizoid Personality Disorder

DIAGNOSIS

The schizoid personality disorder (SZPD) is a pervasive pattern of social detachment and restricted emotional expression. Introversion (versus extraversion) is one of the fundamental dimensions of general personality functioning. Facets of introversion include low warmth (e.g., cold, detached, impersonal), low gregariousness (socially isolated, withdrawn), and low positive emotions (reserved, constricted or flat affect, anhedonic), which define well the central symptoms of SZPD. The presence of SZPD is indicated by four or more of the seven diagnostic criteria presented in the DSM-IV-TR criteria for SZPD.

Approximately half of the general population will exhibit an introversion within the normal range of functioning. However, only a small minority of the population would be diagnosed with an SZPD. Estimates of the prevalence of SZPD within the general population have been less than 1%, and SZPD is among the least frequently diagnosed personality disorders within clinical settings. Many of the persons who were diagnosed with SZPD prior to DSM-III are probably now diagnosed with either the avoidant or the schizotypal personality disorders, and prototypic (pure) cases of SZPD are likely to be quite rare within the population.

Course

Persons with SZPD would have been socially isolated and withdrawn as children. They may not have been accepted well by their peers, and may have even borne the brunt of some ostracism. As adults, they have few friendships. The friendships that do occur are likely to be initiated by their peers or colleagues. They have few sexual relationships and may never marry. Relationships fail to the extent to which the other person desires or needs emotional support, warmth, and intimacy. Persons with SZPD may do well and even excel within an occupation, as long as substantial social interaction is not required. They prefer to work in isolation. They may eventually find employment and a relationship

DSM-IV-TR Diagnostic Criteria

301.20 SCHIZOID PERSONALITY DISORDER

A. A pervasive pattern of detachment from social relationships and a restricted range of expression of emotions in interpersonal settings, beginning by early adulthood and present in a variety of contexts, as indicated by four (or more) of the following:

   (1) neither desires nor enjoys close relationships, including being part of a family
   (2) almost always chooses solitary activities
   (3) has little, if any, interest in having sexual experiences with another person
   (4) takes pleasure in few, if any, activities
   (5) lacks close friends or confidants other than first-degree relatives
   (6) appears indifferent to the praise or criticism of others
   (7) emotional coldness, detachment, or flattened affectivity

B. Does not occur exclusively during the course of schizophrenia, a mood disorder with psychotic features, another psychotic disorder, or a pervasive developmental disorder, and is not due to the direct physiological effects of a general medical condition.

Note: if criteria are met prior to the onset of schizophrenia, add "premorbid," e.g., schizoid personality disorder (premorbid).

Reprinted with permission from the *Diagnostic and Statistical Manual of Mental Disorders*, 4th ed., Text Rev. Copyright 2000 American Psychiatric Association.

that is relatively comfortable, but they could also drift from one job to another and remain isolated throughout much of their life. If they do eventually become a parent, they have considerable difficulty providing warmth and emotional support, and they may appear neglectful, detached, and disinterested.

Differential Diagnosis

SZPD can be confused with the schizotypal and avoidant personality disorders as both involve social isolation and withdrawal. Schizotypal personality disorder, however, also includes an intense social anxiety and cognitive–perceptual aberrations. The major distinction with avoidant personality disorder is the absence of an intense desire for intimate social relationships. Avoidant persons will also exhibit substantial insecurity and inhibition, whereas the schizoid person is largely indifferent toward the reactions or opinions of others.

The presence of premorbid schizoid traits can have prognostic significance for the course and treatment of schizophrenia, but more importantly, it might not be meaningful to suggest that a person has an SZPD that is independent of or unrelated to a comorbid schizophrenia. The negative, prodromal, and residual symptoms of schizophrenia resemble closely the features of SZPD. Once a person develops schizophrenia, a diagnosis of SZPD can become rather pointless as all of the schizoid symptoms can then be understood as (prodromal or residual) symptoms of schizophrenia.

TREATMENT

Prototypic cases of SZPD rarely present for treatment, whether it is for their schizoid traits or a concomitant Axis I disorder. They feel little need for treatment, as their isolation is often egosyntonic. Their social isolation is of more concern to their relatives, colleagues, or friends than to themselves. Their disinterest in and withdrawal from intimate or intense interpersonal contact is also a substantial barrier to treatment. They at times appear depressed but one must be careful not to confuse their anhedonic detachment, withdrawal, and flat affect with symptoms of depression.

If persons with SZPD are seen for treatment for a concomitant Axis I disorder (e.g., a sexual arousal disorder or a substance dependence), it is advisable to work within the confines and limitations of the schizoid personality traits. Charismatic, engaging, emotional, or intimate therapists can be very uncomfortable, foreign, and even threatening to persons with SZPD. A more business-like approach can be more successful.

It is also important not to presume that persons with SZPD are simply inhibited, shy, or insecure. Such persons are more appropriately diagnosed with the avoidant personality disorder. Persons with SZPD are perhaps best treated with a supportive psychotherapy that emphasizes education and feedback concerning interpersonal skills and communication. One may not be able to increase the desire for social involvements but one can increase the ability to relate to, communicate with, and get along with others. Persons with SZPD may not want to develop intimate relationships but they will often want to interact and relate more effectively and comfortably with others. The use of role playing and videotaped interactions can at times be useful in this respect. Persons with SZPD can have tremendous difficulty understanding how they are perceived by others or how their behavior is unresponsive to and perceived as rejecting by others.

Group therapy is often useful as a setting in which the individual can gradually develop self-disclosure, experience the interest of others, and practice social interactions with immediate and supportive feedback. However, persons with SZPD are prone to being rejected by a group because of their detachment, flat affect, and indifference to the feelings of others. If the group is patient and accepting, they can benefit from the experience.

There have been many studies on the pharmacologic treatment of the schizotypal PD but no comparable studies on SZPD. The schizotypal and schizoid PDs share many features, but the responsivity of the schizotypal PD to pharmacotherapy will usually reflect schizotypal social anxiety and cognitive–perceptual aberrations that are not seen in prototypic, pure cases of SZPD.

Schizotypal Personality Disorder

DIAGNOSIS

Schizotypal PD (STPD) is a pervasive pattern of interpersonal deficits, cognitive and perceptual aberrations, and eccentricities of behavior. The interpersonal deficits are characterized in large part by an acute discomfort with and reduced capacity for close relationships. The symptomatology of STPD has been differentiated further into components of positive (cognitive, perceptual aberrations) and negative (social aversion and withdrawal) symptoms comparable to the distinctions made for schizophrenia. The presence of STPD is indicated by five or more of the nine diagnostic criteria listed in the DSM-IV-TR criteria for STPD (see page 445).

STPD may occur in as much as 3% of the general population although most studies with semistructured interviews have suggested a somewhat lower percent. STPD might occur somewhat more often in males. STPD co-occurs most often with the schizoid, borderline, avoidant, and paranoid personality disorders. Common Axis I disorders are major depressive disorder, brief psychotic disorder, and generalized social phobia.

Course

STPD is classified within the same diagnostic grouping as schizophrenia in ICD-10 because of its close relationship in phenomenology, etiology, and pathology. However, it is classified as a personality disorder in DSM-IV-TR because its course and phenomenology are more consistent with a disorder of personality (i.e., early onset, evident in everyday functioning, characteristic of long-term functioning, and egosyntonic). Persons with STPD are likely to be rather isolated in childhood. They may have appeared peculiar and odd to their peers, and may have been teased or ostracized. Achievement in school is usually impaired, and they may have been heavily involved in esoteric fantasies and peculiar interests, particularly those that do not involve peers. As adults, they may drift toward esoteric–fringe groups that support their magical thinking and aberrant beliefs. These activities can provide structure for some persons with STPD, but they can also contribute to a further loosening and deterioration if there is an encouragement of aberrant experiences. Only a small proportion of persons with STPD develop schizophrenia. The symptomatology of STPD does not appear to remit with age. The course appears to be relatively stable, with some proportion of schizotypal persons remaining marginally employed, withdrawn, and transient throughout their lives.

Differential Diagnosis

Avoidant personality disorder and STPD share the features of social anxiety and introversion, but the social anxiety of STPD does not diminish with familiarity, whereas the anxiety of avoidant personality disorder (AVPD) is concerned primarily with the initiation of a relationship. STPD is also a more severe disorder that includes a variety of cognitive and perceptual aberrations that are not seen in persons with AVPD.

An initial concern of many clinicians when confronted with a person with STPD is whether the more appropriate diagnosis is schizophrenia. Persons with STPD closely resemble persons within the prodromal or residual phases of schizophrenia. This differentiation is determined largely by the absence of a deterioration in functioning. It is indicated in DSM-IV-TR that one should note that STPD is "premorbid" if the schizotypal symptoms were present prior to the onset of schizophrenia. Premorbid schizotypal traits will have prognostic significance for the course and treatment of schizophrenia and such traits should then be noted. However, as discussed for SZPD, in most of these cases the schizotypal PD symptoms could then be readily understood as prodromal symptoms of schizophrenia.

TREATMENT

Persons with STPD may seek treatment for their feelings of anxiousness, perceptual disturbances, or depression. Treatment of persons with STPD should be cognitive, behavioral, supportive, and/or pharmacologic, as they will often find the intimacy and emotionality of reflective, exploratory psychotherapy to be too stressful and they have the potential for psychotic decompensation.

Persons with STPD will often fail to consider their social isolation and aberrant cognitions and perceptions to be particularly problematic or maladaptive. They may consider themselves to be simply eccentric, creative, or nonconformist. Rapport can be difficult to develop as increasing familiarity and intimacy may only increase their level of discomfort and anxiety. They are unlikely to be responsive to informality or playful humor. The sessions should be well-structured to avoid loose and tangential ideation.

Practical advice is usually helpful and often necessary. The therapist should serve as the individual's counselor, guide, or "auxiliary ego" to more adaptive decisions with respect to everyday problems (e.g., finding an apartment, interviewing for a job, and personal appearance). Persons with STPD should also receive social skills training directed at their awkward and odd behavior, mannerisms, dress, and speech. Specific, concrete discussions on what to expect and do in various social situations (e.g., formal meetings, casual encounters, and dates) should be provided. The rate of progress will tend to be slow, and it is helpful if there remains a continuity in the therapeutic relationship.

Most of the systematic empirical research on the treatment of STPD has been confined to pharmacologic interventions. Low doses of neuroleptic medications (e.g., thiothixene) have shown some effectiveness in the treatment of schizotypal symptoms, particularly the perceptual aberrations and social anxiousness. Group therapy has also been recommended for persons with STPD but only when the group is highly structured and supportive. The emotional intensity and intimacy of unstructured groups will usually be too stressful. Schizotypal individuals with predominant paranoid symptoms may even have difficulty in highly structured groups.

Antisocial Personality Disorder

DIAGNOSIS

Antisocial personality disorder (ASPD) is a pervasive pattern of disregard for and violation of the rights of others. Persons with ASPD will also be irresponsible and exploitative in their sexual relationships, and irresponsible as employees and parents. They may display a lack of empathy, an inflated or arrogant self-appraisal, a callous, cynical, and contemptuous response to the suffering of others, and a glib, superficial charm. This disorder has also been referred to as psychopathy, sociopathy, or dissocial personality disorder. The presence of ASPD is indicated by the occurrence of a conduct disorder prior to age 15 years and by three of the seven adult diagnostic criteria presented in DSM-IV-TR Criteria for ASPD.

Persons with ASPD are at a high risk for developing substance-related and impulse dyscontrol disorders. They are also likely to display borderline, narcissistic, and paranoid personality traits. Females with ASPD will also display histrionic personality traits.

The National Institute of Mental Health Epidemiologic Catchment Area (ECA) study indicated that approximately 3% of males and 1% of females have ASPD. This rate has been replicated in subsequent studies, but it has also been suggested that the ECA finding may have underestimated the prevalence in males because of the failure to consider the full range of ASPD features. Other estimates have been as high as 6% in males. The rate of ASPD within prison and forensic settings has been estimated at 50% but the ASPD criteria may exaggerate the rate within such settings because of the emphasis given to overt acts of criminality, delinquency, and irresponsibility that are common to

DSM-IV-TR Diagnostic Criteria

301.7 ANTISOCIAL PERSONALITY DISORDER

A. There is a pervasive pattern of disregard for and violation of the rights of others (occurring since age 15 years), as indicated by three (or more) of the following:
   (1) failure to conform to social norms with respect to lawful behaviors as indicated by repeatedly performing acts that are grounds for arrest
   (2) deceitfulness, as indicated by repeated lying, use of aliases, or conning others for personal profit or pleasure
   (3) impulsivity or failure to plan ahead
   (4) irritability and aggressiveness, as indicated by repeated physical fights or assaults
   (5) reckless disregard for safety of self or others
   (6) consistent irresponsibility, as indicated by repeated failure to sustain consistent work behavior or honor financial obligations
   (7) lack of remorse, as indicated by being indifferent to or rationalizing having hurt, mistreated, or stolen from another

B. The individual is at least age 18 years.
C. Evidence of conduct disorder with onset before age 15 years.
D. The occurrence of antisocial behavior is not exclusively during the course of schizophrenia or a manic episode.

Reprinted with permission from the *Diagnostic and Statistical Manual of Mental Disorders*, 4th ed., Text Rev. Copyright 2000 American Psychiatric Association.

the persons within these settings. More specific criteria for psychopathy provide a more conservative estimate of 20–30% of male prisoners with ASPD.

ASPD is much more common in males than in females. A sociobiological explanation for the differential sex prevalence is the presence of a genetic advantage for social irresponsibility, infidelity, superficial charm, and deceit in males that contributes to a higher likelihood of developing features of ASPD. It has also been suggested that ASPD and histrionic personality disorder (HPD) share a biogenetic disposition (perhaps towards impulsivity or sensation-seeking) that is mediated by gender-specific biogenetic and sociological factors toward respective gender variants.

Course

ASPD is evident in childhood in the form of a conduct disorder. Evidence of a conduct disorder prior to the age of 15 years is in fact required for a DSM-IV-TR ASPD diagnosis. The continuation into adulthood is particularly likely to occur if multiple delinquent behaviors are evident prior to the age of 10 years. As adults, persons with ASPD are unlikely to maintain steady employment and they may even become impoverished, homeless, or spend years within penal institutions. However, some persons with ASPD characterized by high rather than low levels of conscientiousness may express their psychopathic tendencies within a socially acceptable or at least legitimate profession. They may in fact be quite successful as long as their tendency to bend or violate the norms or rules of their profession and exploit, deceive, and manipulate others, contribute to a career advancement. Their success, however, may at some point unravel when their psychopathic behaviors become problematic or evident to others. The same pattern may also occur within sexual and marital relationships. They may at first appear to be charming, engaging, and sincere, but most relationships will end because of a lack of empathy, responsibility, and fidelity.

There does tend to be a gradual remission of antisocial behaviors, particularly overt criminal acts, as the person ages. Persons with ASPD, however, are more likely than the general population to have died prematurely by violent means (e.g., accidents or homicides) and to engage in quite dangerous, high-risk behavior.

Differential Diagnosis

ASPD will at times be difficult to differentiate from a substance use disorder in young adults because many persons with ASPD develop a substance-related disorder and many persons with substance dependence engage in antisocial acts. The requirement that the ASPD features be evident prior to the age of 15 years will usually assure the onset of ASPD prior to the onset of a substance-related disorder. If both are evident prior to the age of 15 years, then it is likely that both disorders are in fact present and both diagnoses should then be made. ASPD and substance dependence will often interact, exacerbating and escalating each other's development.

Antisocial acts will also be evident in the histrionic and borderline personality disorders, as persons with these disorders will display impulsivity, sensation-seeking, self-centeredness, manipulativeness, and a low frustration tolerance. Females with ASPD are often misdiagnosed with HPD. Prototypic cases of ASPD might be distinguished from other personality disorders by the presence of the childhood history of conduct disorder and the cold, calculated exploitation, abuse, and aggression. Persons with narcissistic personality disorder (NPD) are also characterized by a lack of empathy and may often exploit and use others. In fact, many of the traits of NPD are evident in psychopathy, including

a lack of empathy, glib and superficial charm, and arrogant self-appraisal.

TREATMENT

The presence of ASPD is important to recognize in the treatment of any Axis I disorder, as their tendency to be manipulative, dishonest, exploitative, aggressive, and irresponsible will often disrupt and sabotage treatment. It is also very easy to be seduced by psychopathic charm. Persons with ASPD can be seductive in their engaging friendliness, expressions of remorse, avowed commitment to change, and apparent response to or even fascination with the success, skills, and talents of the therapist, none of which will be sincere or reliable.

The extent to which ASPD is untreatable has at times been overstated and exaggerated. Nevertheless, ASPD is the most difficult personality disorder to treat. Persons with ASPD will often lack a motivation or commitment to change. They might see only the advantages of their antisocial traits and not the costs (e.g., risks of arrest and failure to sustain lasting or meaningful relationships). They are prone to manipulate, abuse, or exploit their fellow individuals and the staff. The immediate motivation for treatment is often provided by an external source, such as a court order or the demands of an employer or relative. Motivation may last only as long as an external pressure remains.

The most effective treatment is likely to be prevention through an identification and intervention early in childhood. In adulthood, the most effective treatment may at times be simply some form of sustained incarceration (e.g., imprisonment), as many antisocial behaviors do tend to dissipate (or burn out) with time. The tendency to rationalize irresponsibility, minimize the consequences of acts, and manipulate others needs to be confronted on a daily and immediate basis. Community residential or wilderness programs that provide a firm structure, close supervision, and intense confrontation by peers have been recommended. The involvement of family members in the treatment has been shown to be helpful, but there are also data to suggest that interventions with little professional input are less successful and are at times counterproductive.

There is some research to suggest that the ability to form a therapeutic alliance is an important indicator of treatment success. Factors to consider are the demographic similarity of the therapist and individual, the quality of the individual's past relationships, and the therapist's positive regard for the individual. Many clinicians may also experience strong feelings of animosity and distaste for antisocial persons who have a history of abusive and exploitative acts. Rational, utilitarian approaches that help the person consider the long-term consequences of behavior can be helpful. This approach does not attempt to develop a sense of conscience, guilt, or even regret for past actions, but focuses instead on the material value and future advantages to be gained by a more prosocial behavior pattern. There are data to suggest the use of pharmacotherapy in the treatment of impulsive aggression but it is unclear whether these findings would generalize to the full spectrum of ASPD psychopathology.

Borderline Personality Disorder

DIAGNOSIS

Borderline personality disorder (BPD) is a pervasive pattern of impulsivity and instability in interpersonal relationships and self-image. A broad domain of general personality functioning is neuroticism (or emotional instability) characterized by facets of angry hostility, anxiousness, depressiveness, impulsivity, and vulnerability; BPD is essentially the most extreme and highly maladaptive variant of emotional instability. This disorder is indicated by the presence of five or more of the nine diagnostic criteria presented in the DSM-IV-TR criteria for BPD.

Axis I disorders are commonly comorbid with BPD. The range of potential Axis I comorbid psychopathology includes mood (major depressive disorder), anxiety (posttraumatic stress disorder), eating (bulimia nervosa), substance (alcohol dependence), dissociative (dissociative identity disorder), and psychotic (brief psychotic) disorders. Persons with BPD also meet DSM-IV-TR criteria for at least one other personality disorder, particularly histrionic, dependent, antisocial, or schizotypal. Researchers and clinicians have at times responded to this extensive co-occurrence by imposing a diagnostic hierarchy whereby other disorders are not diagnosed in the presence of BPD because BPD is generally the most severely dysfunctional disorder. A potential limitation of this approach is that it resolves the complexity of personality by largely ignoring it. This approach may fail to recognize the presence of maladaptive personality traits that could be important for understanding an individual's dysfunctions and for developing an optimal treatment plan.

Approximately 1–2% of the general population would meet the DSM-IV-TR criteria for BPD. BPD is the most prevalent personality disorder within hospital clinical settings. Approximately 15% of all inpatients (51% of inpatients with a personality disorder) and 8% of all outpatients (27% of outpatients with a personality disorder) have a BPD. Approximately

---

DSM-IV-TR Diagnostic Criteria

301.83 BORDERLINE PERSONALITY DISORDER

A. A pervasive pattern of instability of interpersonal relationships, self-image, and affects, and marked impulsivity beginning by early adulthood and present in a variety of contexts, as indicated by five (or more) of the following:

(1) frantic efforts to avoid real or imagined abandonment. **Note:** do not include suicidal or self-mutilating behavior covered in criterion 5

(2) a pattern of unstable and intense interpersonal relationships characterized by alternating between extremes of idealization and devaluation

(3) identity disturbance: markedly and persistently unstable self-image or sense of self

(4) impulsivity in at least two areas that are potentially self-damaging (e.g., spending, sex, substance abuse, reckless driving, binge eating). **Note:** do not include suicidal or self-mutilating behavior covered in criterion 5

(5) recurrent suicidal behavior, gestures, or threats, or self-mutilating behavior

(6) affective instability due to a marked reactivity of mood (e.g., intense episodic dysphoria, irritability, or anxiety usually lasting a few hours and only rarely more than a few days)

(7) chronic feelings of emptiness

(8) inappropriate, intense anger or difficulty controlling anger (e.g., frequent displays of temper, constant anger, recurrent physical fights)

(9) transient, stress-related paranoid ideation or severe dissociative symptoms.

75% of persons with BPD will be female. Persons with BPD often meet DSM-IV-TR criteria for at least one Axis I disorder.

Course

As children, persons with BPD are likely to have been emotionally unstable, impulsive, and angry or hostile. Their chaotic impulsivity and intense affectivity may contribute to involvement within rebellious groups as a child or adolescent, along with a variety of Axis I disorders, including eating, substance use, and mood disorders. BPD is often diagnosed in children and adolescents, but considerable caution should be used when doing so as some of the symptoms of BPD (e.g., identity disturbance and unstable relationships) could be confused with a normal adolescent rebellion or identity crisis. As adults, persons with BPD may require numerous hospitalizations due to their affect and impulse dyscontrol, psychotic-like and dissociative symptomatology, and risk of suicide. Minor problems quickly become crises as the intensity of affect and impulsivity result in disastrous decisions. They are at a high risk for developing depressive, substance-related, bulimic, and posttraumatic stress disorders. The potential for suicide increases with a comorbid mood and substance-related disorder. Approximately 3–10% commit suicide by the age of 30 years. Relationships tend to be very unstable and explosive, and employment history is poor. Affectivity and impulsivity, however, may begin to diminish as the person reaches the age of 30 years, or earlier if the person becomes involved with a supportive and patient sexual partner. Some, however, may obtain stability by abandoning the effort to obtain a relationship, opting instead for a lonelier but less volatile life. The mellowing of the symptomatology, however, can be easily disrupted by the occurrence of a severe stressor (e.g., divorce or death of a significant other) that results in a brief psychotic, dissociative, or mood disorder episode.

Differential Diagnosis

Most persons with BPD develop mood disorders and it is at times difficult to differentiate BPD from a mood disorder if the assessment is confined to the current symptomatology. A diagnosis of BPD requires that the borderline symptomatology be evident since adolescence, which should differentiate BPD from a mood disorder in all cases other than a chronic mood disorder. If there is a chronic mood disorder, then the additional features of transient, stress-related paranoid ideation, dissociative experiences, impulsivity, and anger dyscontrol that are evident in BPD should be emphasized in the diagnosis.

TREATMENT

Persons with BPD often develop intense, dependent, hostile, unstable, and manipulative relationships with their therapists as they do with their peers. At one time they might be very compliant, responsive, and even idealizing, but later angry, accusatory, and devaluing. Their tendency to be manipulatively as well as impulsively self-destructive is often very stressful and difficult to treat.

Persons with BPD are often highly motivated for treatment. Psychotherapeutic approaches tend to be both supportive and exploratory. Therapists should provide a safe, secure environment in which anger can be expressed and actively addressed without destroying the therapeutic relationship. The historical roots of current bitterness, anger, and depression within past familial relationships should eventually be explored, but immediate, current issues and conflicts must also

be explicitly addressed. Suicidal behavior should be confronted and contained, by hospitalization when necessary. Individuals with BPD can be very difficult to treat because the focus of the individual's love and wrath will often be shifted toward the therapist, and the treatment may itself become the individual's latest unstable, intense relationship. Immediate and ongoing consultation with colleagues is often necessary, as it is not unusual for therapists to be unaware of the extent to which they are developing or expressing feelings of anger, attraction, annoyance, or intolerance toward the individual with BPD.

A particular form of cognitive–behavioral therapy, dialectical behavior therapy, has been shown empirically to be effective in the treatment of BPD. Part of the strategy entails keeping individuals focused initially on the priorities of reducing suicidal threats and gestures, behaviors that can disrupt or resist treatment, and behaviors that affect the immediate quality of life (e.g., bulimia, substance abuse, or unemployment). Once these goals are achieved, the focus can then shift to a mastery of new coping skills, management of reactions to stress, and other individualized goals. Individual therapy is augmented by skills-training groups that may be highly structured (e.g., comparable to a classroom format). Individuals are taught skills for coping with identity diffusion, tolerating distress, improving interpersonal relationships, controlling emotions, and resolving interpersonal crises. Individuals are given homework assignments to practice these skills, which are further addressed and reinforced within individual sessions. Negative affect is also addressed through a mindful meditation that contributes to an acceptance and tolerance of past abusive experiences and current stress. The dialectical component of the therapy is that the dialectical therapist helps the individual achieve synthesis of oppositions, rather than focusing on verifying either side of an oppositional argument. An illustrative list of dialectical strategies is presented in Table 42-1.

Dialectical behavior therapy (DBT), however, also includes more general principles of treatment that are important to emphasize in all forms of therapy for BPD, some of which are presented in Table 42-2. For example, exasperated therapists may unjustly experience and even accuse borderline individuals of being unmotivated or unwilling to work. It is important to appreciate that they do want to improve and are doing the best that they can. One should not make the therapy personal, but instead identify the sources of the inhibition or interference to their motivation to change. One should take seriously their complaints that their lives are indeed unbearable but not absolve them of

Table 42-1	Dialectical Behavior Therapy Strategies

Alternate between acceptance and change strategies
Balance nurturing with demands for self-help
Balance persistence and stability with flexibility
Balance capabilities with limitations and deficits
Move with speed, keeping the patient slightly off balance
Take positions whole-heartedly
Look for what is not included in patient's own points of view
Provide developmental descriptions of change
Question intransigence of boundary conditions of the problem
Highlight importance of interrelationships in identity
Advocate a middle path
Highlight paradoxical contradictions in the patient's own behavior, in the therapeutic process, and in life in general
Speak in metaphors and tell parables and stories
Play the devil's advocate
Extend the seriousness or implications of the patient's statements
Add intuitive knowing to emotional experience and logical analysis
Turn problems into assets
Allow natural changes in therapy
Assess the individual, therapist, and process dialectically

Source: Reprinted from *Cognitive–Behavioral Treatment of Borderline Personality Disorder*, Linehan MM, Basic Propositions of BPD Treatment from DBT, 206, Copyright (1993) with permission from Guilford Press.

their responsibility to solve their own problems. They are unlikely to change simply through a passive reception of insight, nurturance, support, and medication. They will need to actively work on changing their lives. Therapists will often be tempted to rescue the individuals under their care, particularly when they are within a crisis. However, it is precisely at such times that there will be the best opportunity to develop and learn new coping strategies. Failures can occur, and it is a failure of the therapy that should be conscientiously and effectively addressed by the therapist. Finally, therapists

Table 42-2	Basic Propositions of BPD Treatment from DBT

1. Patients are doing the best they can.
2. Patients want to improve.
3. Patients need to do better, try harder, and be more motivated to change.
4. Patients may not have caused all of their own problems, but they have to solve them anyway.
5. The lives of suicidal, borderline individuals are unbearable as they are currently being lived.
6. Patients must learn new behaviors in all relevant contexts.
7. Patients cannot fail in therapy.
8. Therapists treating patients with BPD need support.

Source: Reprinted from *Cognitive–Behavioral Treatment of Borderline Personality Disorder*, Linehan MM, Basic Propositions of BPD Treatment from DBT, 106–108, Copyright (1993) with permission from Guilford Press.

need to honestly recognize their own limitations. All therapists have their own flaws and limits, and individuals with BPD invariably strain and overwhelm these limits. Therapists need to be open and receptive to outside support, advice, and criticism.

Pharmacologic treatment of individuals with BPD is varied, as it depends primarily on the predominant Axis I symptomatology. Persons with BPD can display a wide variety of Axis I symptoms, including anxiety, depression, hallucinations, delusions, and dissociations. It is important in their pharmacologic treatment not to be unduly influenced by transient symptoms or by symptoms that are readily addressed through exploratory or supportive techniques. On the other hand, it is equally important to be flexible in the use of medications and not to be unduly resistant to their use. Relying solely upon one's own psychotherapeutic skills can be unnecessary and even irresponsible.

Histrionic Personality Disorder

DIAGNOSIS

Histrionic personality disorder (HPD) is a pervasive pattern of excessive emotionality and attention-seeking. Histrionic persons tend to be emotionally manipulative and intolerant of delayed gratification. HPD is indicated by the presence of five or more of the eight diagnostic criteria presented in DSM-IV-TR criteria for HPD (see page 451).

Approximately 1–3% of the general population may be diagnosed with HPD. A controversial issue is its differential sex prevalence. It is stated in DSM-IV-TR that the sex ratio for HPD is "not significantly different than the sex ratio of females within the respective clinical setting" (p. 712). However, this should not be interpreted as indicating that the prevalence is the same for males and females. It has typically been found that at least two-thirds of persons with HPD are female, although there have been a few exceptions. Whether or not the rate will be significantly higher than the rate of women within a particular clinical setting depends upon many factors that are independent of the differential sex prevalence for HPD.

Course

Little is known about the premorbid behavior pattern of persons with HPD. During adolescence, they are likely to be flamboyant, flirtatious, and attention-seeking. As adults, persons with HPD readily form new relationships but have difficulty sustaining them. They may fall in love quite quickly, but just as rapidly become attracted to another person. They are unlikely to be reliable or responsible. Relationships with persons of the same sexual orientation are often strained because of their competitive sexual flirtatiousness. Employment history is likely to be erratic, and may be complicated by the tendency to become romantically or sexually involved with colleagues, by their affective instability, and by their suggestibility. Persons with HPD may become devoted converts to faddish belief systems. They have a tendency to make impulsive decisions that will have a dramatic (or melodramatic) effect on their lives. The severity of the symptomatology may diminish somewhat as the person ages.

Differential Diagnosis

HPD involves to some extent maladaptive variants of stereotypically feminine traits. The DSM-IV-TR diagnostic criteria for HPD are sufficiently stringent that a normal woman would not meet these criteria, but studies have indicated that clinicians will at times diagnose HPD in females who in fact have antisocial traits. Both of these disorders can involve impulsivity, sensation-seeking, low frustration tolerance, and manipulativeness, and the presence of a female gender may at times contribute to a false presumption of HPD. It is therefore important to adhere closely to the DSM-IV-TR

diagnostic criteria when confronted with histrionic and antisocial symptoms in females.

Persons with HPD will often have borderline, dependent, or narcissistic personality traits. Prototypic cases of HPD can be distinguished from other personality disorders. For example, the prototypic narcissistic person ultimately desires admiration whereas the histrionic person desires whatever attention, interest, or concern can be obtained. As a result, the histrionic person will at times seek attention through melodramatic helplessness and emotional outbursts that could be experienced as denigrating and humiliating to the narcissistic person. However, most cases will not be prototypic and the most accurate description of an individual's constellation of maladaptive personality traits will be the provision of multiple diagnoses.

TREATMENT

Persons with HPD readily develop rapport but it is often superficial and unreliable. Therapists may also fail to appreciate the extent of influence they can have on the highly suggestible individual with HPD. Persons with HPD can readily become converts to whatever the therapist may suggest or encourage. The transformation to the theoretical model or belief system of the clinician is unlikely to be sustained.

A key task in treating the individual with HPD is countering their global and diffuse cognitive style by insisting on attending to structure and detail within sessions and to the practical, immediate problems encountered in daily life. It is also important to explore within treatment the historical source for their needs for attention and involvement. Persons with HPD are prone to superficial and transient insights but they will benefit from a carefully reasoned and documented exploration of their current and past relationships.

Many clinicians recommend the use of group therapy for persons with HPD. It is quite easy for them to become involved within a group, which may then be very useful in helping them recognize and explore their attention-seeking, suggestibility, and manipulation, as well as develop alternative ways to develop more meaningful and sustained relationships. However, it is also important to closely monitor their involvements within the group, as they are prone to dominate and control sessions and they may escalate their attention-seeking to the point of suicidal gestures. The intense affectivity of persons with HPD may also be responsive to antidepressant treatment, particularly those individuals with substantial mood reactivity, hypersomnia, and rejection sensitivity.

Narcissistic Personality Disorder

DIAGNOSIS

Narcissistic personality disorder (NPD) is a pervasive pattern of grandiosity, need for admiration, and lack of empathy. Persons with NPD can be very vulnerable to threats to their self-esteem. They may react defensively with rage, disdain, or indifference but are in fact struggling with feelings of shock, humiliation, and shame. NPD is indicated by the presence of five or more of the nine diagnostic criteria presented in the DSM-IV-TR Criteria for NPD.

Persons with NPD are considered to be prone to mood disorders, as well as anorexia and substance-related disorders, especially cocaine. Persons with NPD are likely to have comorbid antisocial (psychopathic), histrionic, paranoid, and borderline personality traits.

Approximately 18% of males and 6% of females may be characterized as being excessively immodest (i.e., arrogant or conceited), but only a small percent of these persons would be diagnosed with NPD. In fact, the median prevalence rate obtained across 10 community data collections was zero. The absence of any cases within community studies, however, may reflect inadequacies within the diagnostic criteria or limitations of semistructured interview assessments of

DSM-IV-TR Diagnostic Criteria

301.81 NARCISSISTIC PERSONALITY DISORDER

A pervasive pattern of grandiosity (in fantasy or behavior), need for admiration, and lack of empathy, beginning by early adulthood and present in a variety of contexts, as indicated by five (or more) of the following:

A. has a grandiose sense of self-importance (e.g. exaggerates achievements and talents, expects to be recognized as superior without commensurate achievements)
B. is preoccupied with fantasies of unlimited success, power, brilliance, beauty, or ideal love
C. believes that he or she is "special" and unique and can only be understood by, or should associate with, other special or high-status people (or institutions)
D. requires excessive admiration
E. has a sense of entitlement, i.e. unreasonable expectations of especially favorable treatment or automatic compliance with his or her expectations
F. is interpersonally exploitative, i.e., takes advantage of others to achieve his or her own ends
G. lacks empathy: is unwilling to recognize or identify with the feelings and needs of others
H. is often envious of others or believes that others are envious of him or her
I. shows arrogant, haughty behaviors or attitudes.

Reprinted with permission from the *Diagnostic and Statistical Manual of Mental Disorders*, 4th ed., Text Rev. Copyright 2000 American Psychiatric Association.

narcissism. NPD is observed within clinical settings (approximately 2–20% of individuals) although it is also among the least frequently diagnosed personality disorders.

Course

Little is known about the premorbid behavior pattern of NPD, other than through retrospective reports of persons diagnosed when adults. As adolescents, persons with NPD are likely to be self-centered, assertive, gregarious, dominant, and perhaps arrogant. They may have achieved well in school or within some other activity. As adults, many persons with NPD will have experienced high levels of achievement. However, their relationships with colleagues, peers, and staff will eventually become strained as their exploitative use of others and self-centered egotism become evident. Success may also be impaired by their difficulty in acknowledging or resolving criticism, deficits, and setbacks. Interpersonal and sexual relationships are usually easy for them to develop but difficult to sustain owing to their low empathy, self-centeredness, and need for admiration. Persons who are deferential and obsequious, or who share a mutual need for status and recognition, may help sustain a relationship. As parents, persons with NPD may attempt to live through their children, valuing them as long as they are a source of pride. Their personal sense of adjustment may be fine for as long as they continue to experience or anticipate success. Some may not recognize the maladaptivity of their narcissism until middle-age, when the emphasis given to achievement and status may begin to wane.

Differential Diagnosis

Individuals with NPD may often appear relatively high functioning. Exaggerated self-confidence may in fact contribute to success in a variety of professions and narcissistic traits will at times be seen in highly successful persons. A diagnosis of NPD requires the additional presence of interpersonal exploitation, lack of empathy, a sense of entitlement, and other symptoms beyond simply arrogance and grandiosity.

Both narcissistic and antisocial persons may exploit, deceive, and manipulate others for personal gain, and both may demonstrate a lack of empathy or remorse. As indicated above, many of the traits of narcissism, such as arrogance and glib charm, are seen in psychopathic persons. Prototypic cases can be distinguished, as the motivation for the narcissistic person will be for recognition, status, and other signs of success, whereas the prototypic antisocial person would be motivated more for material gain or for the subjugation of others. Antisocial persons will also display an impulsivity, recklessness, and lax irresponsibility that may not be seen in narcissistic persons.

TREATMENT

Persons with narcissistic personality traits seek treatment for feelings of depression, substance-related disorders, and occupational or relational problems that are secondary to their narcissism. Their self-centeredness and lack of empathy are particularly problematic within marital, occupational, and other social relationships, and they usually lack an appreciation of the contribution of their conflicts regarding self-esteem, status, and recognition. It is difficult for them even to admit that they have a psychological problem or that they need help, as this admission is itself an injury to their self-esteem. In addition, one of the characteristics of NPD is the belief that they can only be understood by persons of a comparably high social status or recognition. They may be unable to accept advice or insight from persons they consider less intelligent, talented, or insightful than themselves, which may eventually effectively eliminate most other persons.

When they are involved in treatment, persons with NPD will often require some indication that their therapist is among the best or at least worth their time. They are prone to idealizing their therapists (to affirm that he or she is indeed of sufficient status or quality) or to devalue them (to affirm that they are of greater intelligence, capacity, or quality than their therapist, to reject the insights that they have failed to identify, and to indicate that they warrant or deserve an even better therapist). How best to respond is often unclear. It may at times be preferable to simply accept the praise or criticism, particularly when exploration will likely be unsuccessful, whereas at other times it is preferable to confront and discuss the motivation for the devaluation (or the idealization).

Psychodynamic approaches to the treatment of NPD vary in the extent to which emphasis is given to an interpretation of underlying anger and bitterness, or to the provision of empathy and a reflection (or mirroring) of a positive regard and self-esteem. It does appear to be important to identify the current extent and historical source of the conflicts and sensitivities regarding self-esteem. Active confrontation may at times be useful, particularly when the therapeutic alliance is strong, but at other times the vulnerability of the individual may require a more unconditional support. Cognitive–behavior approaches to NPD emphasize increasing awareness of the impact of narcissistic behaviors and statements on interpersonal relationships. The idealization and devaluation can be responsive to role playing and rational introspection, an intellectual approach that may itself be valued by some persons with NPD. However, therapists must be careful not to become embroiled within intellectual conflicts (or competitions). This approach may not work well with the narcissistic person who is motivated to defeat or humiliate the therapist.

Group therapy can be useful for increasing awareness of the grandiosity, lack of empathy, and devaluation of others. However, these traits not only interfere with the narcissistic person's ability to sustain membership within groups (and within individual therapy) but also may become quite harmful and destructive to the rapport of the entire group. There is no accepted pharmacologic approach to the treatment of narcissism.

Avoidant Personality Disorder

DIAGNOSIS

Avoidant personality disorder (AVPD) is a pervasive pattern of timidity, inhibition, inadequacy, and social hypersensitivity. Persons with AVPD may have a strong desire to develop close, personal relationships but feel too insecure to approach others or to express their feelings. AVPD is indicated by the presence of four or more of the seven diagnostic criteria presented in the DSM criteria for AVPD (see page 454).

Timidity, shyness, and social insecurity are not uncommon problems and AVPD is one of the more prevalent personality disorders within clinical settings, occurring in 5–25% of all individuals presenting with personality disorders. However, AVPD may be diagnosed in only 1–2% of the general population. It appears to occur equally among males and females, with some studies reporting more males and others reporting more females.

Course

Persons with AVPD are shy, timid, and anxious as children. Many are diagnosed with a social phobia during childhood. Adolescence is a particularly difficult developmental period due to the importance at this time of attractiveness, dating, and popularity. Occupational success may not be significantly impaired, as long as there is little demand for public performance. Persons with AVPD may in fact find considerable gratification and esteem through a job or career that they are unable

DSM-IV-TR Diagnostic Criteria

301.82 AVOIDANT PERSONALITY DISORDER

A pervasive pattern of social inhibition, feelings of inadequacy, and hypersensitivity to negative evaluation, beginning by early adulthood and present in a variety of contexts, as indicated by four (or more) of the following:

    A. avoids occupational activities that involve significant interpersonal contact, because of fears of criticism, disapproval, or rejection
    B. is unwilling to get involved with people unless certain of being liked
    C. shows restraint within intimate relationships because of the fear of being shamed or ridiculed
    D. is preoccupied with thoughts of being criticized or rejected in social situations
    E. is inhibited in new interpersonal situations because of feelings of inadequacy
    F. views self as socially inept, personally unappealing, or inferior to others
    G. is unusually reluctant to take personal risks or to engage in any new activities because they may prove embarrassing

Reprinted with permission from the *Diagnostic and Statistical Manual of Mental Disorders*, 4th ed., Text Rev. Copyright 2000 American Psychiatric Association.

to find within their relationships. The job may serve as a distraction from intense feelings of loneliness. Their avoidance of social situations will impair their ability to develop adequate social skills, and this will then further handicap any eventual efforts to develop relationships. As parents, they may be very responsible, empathic, and affectionate, but may unwittingly impart feelings of social anxiousness and awkwardness. Severity of the AVPD symptomatology diminishes as the person becomes older.

Differential Diagnosis

The most difficult differential diagnosis for AVPD is with generalized social phobia. Both involve an avoidance of social situations, social anxiety, and timidity, and both may be evident since late childhood or adolescence. Many persons with AVPD in fact seek treatment for a social phobia. To the extent that the behavior pattern pervades the person's everyday functioning and has been evident since childhood, the diagnosis of a personality disorder would be more descriptive.

Many persons with AVPD may also meet the criteria for DPD. This might at first glance seem unusual, given that AVPD involves social withdrawal whereas DPD involves excessive social attachment. However, once a person with AVPD is able to obtain a relationship, he or she will often cling to this relationship in a dependent manner. Both disorders include feelings of inadequacy, needs for reassurance, and hypersensitivity to criticism and neglect (i.e., abnormally high levels of anxiousness, self-consciousness, and vulnerability). A distinction between AVPD and DPD is best made when the person is seeking a relationship. Avoidant persons tend to be very shy, inhibited, and timid (and are therefore slow to get involved with someone) whereas dependent persons urgently seek another relationship as soon as one ends (i.e., avoidant persons are high in introversion whereas dependent persons are high in extraversion). Avoidant persons may also be reluctant to express their feelings whereas dependent persons can drive others away by continuous expressions of neediness. The differentiation of AVPD from the schizoid, paranoid, and schizotypal personality disorders was discussed in previous sections.

TREATMENT

Persons with AVPD seek treatment for their avoidant personality traits, although many initially seek treatment for symptoms of anxiety, particularly social phobia (generalized subtype). It is important in such cases to recognize that the shyness is not due simply to a dysregulation or dyscontrol of anxiousness. There is instead a more pervasive and fundamental psychopathology, involving feelings of interpersonal insecurity, low self-esteem, and inadequacy.

Social skills training, systematic desensitization, and a graded hierarchy of *in vivo* exposure to feared social situations have been shown to be useful in the treatment of AVPD. However, it is also important to discuss the underlying fears and insecurities regarding attractiveness, desirability, rejection, or intimacy. Persons with AVPD are at times reluctant to discuss such feelings, as they may feel embarrassed, they may fear being ridiculed, or they may not want to "waste the time" of the therapist with such "foolish" insecurities. They may prefer a less revealing or involved form of treatment. It is important to be understanding, patient, and accepting, and to proceed at a pace that is comfortable for the individual. Insecurities and fears can at times be addressed through cognitive techniques as the irrationality is usually readily apparent. It remains useful though to identify the historical source of their development, as this understanding will help the individual appreciate the irrationality or irrelevance of their expectations and perceptions for their current relationships.

Persons with AVPD often find group therapies to be helpful. Exploratory and supportive groups can provide them with an understanding environment in which to discuss their social insecurities, to explore and practice more assertive behaviors, and to develop an increased self-confidence in approaching others and developing relationships outside of the group. Focused and specialized social skills-training groups would be preferable to unstructured groups that might be predominated by much more assertive and extraverted members.

Many persons with AVPD will respond to anxiolytic medications, and at times to antidepressants, particularly monoamine oxidase inhibitors such as phenelzine. Normal and abnormal feelings of anxiousness can be suppressed or diminished through pharmacologic interventions. This approach may in fact be necessary to overcome initial feelings of intense social anxiety that are markedly disruptive to current functioning (e.g., inability to give required presentations at work or to talk to new acquaintances). However, it is also important to monitor closely a reliance on medications. Persons with AVPD could be prone to rely excessively on substances to control their feelings of anxiousness, whereas their more general feelings of insecurity and inadequacy would require a more comprehensive treatment.

Dependent Personality Disorder

DIAGNOSIS

Dependent personality disorder (DPD) involves a pervasive and excessive need to be taken care of, which leads to submissiveness, clinging, and fears of separation. Persons with DPD will also have low self-esteem, and will often be self-critical and self-denigrating. DPD is indicated by the presence of five or more of the eight diagnostic criteria presented in DSM-IV-TR Criteria for DPD.

DPD is among the most prevalent of the personality disorders, occurring in 5–30% of individuals presenting with personality disorders and 2–4% of the general community. A controversial issue is its differential sex prevalence. DPD is diagnosed more frequently in females but there is some concern that there might be a failure to recognize adequately the extent of dependent personality traits within males.

Course

Persons with DPD are likely to have been excessively submissive as children and adolescents, and some may have had a chronic physical illness or a separation anxiety disorder during childhood. Persons with DPD fear intensely a loss of concern, care, and support from others, particularly the person with whom they have an emotional attachment. They are unable

---

DSM-IV-TR Diagnostic Criteria

301.6 DEPENDENT PERSONALITY DISORDER

A pervasive and excessive need to be taken care of that leads to submissive and clinging behavior and fears of separation, beginning by early adulthood and present in a variety of contexts, as indicated by five (or more) of the following:

  A. has difficulty making everyday decisions without an excessive amount of advice and reassurance from others.
  B. needs others to assume responsibility for most major areas of his or her life.
  C. has difficulty expressing disagreement with others because of fear of loss of support or approval (**Note:** Do not include realistic fears of retribution).
  D. has difficulty initiating projects or doing things on his or her own (because of a lack of self-confidence in judgment or abilities rather than to a lack of motivation or energy).
  E. goes to excessive lengths to obtain nurturance and support from others, to the point of volunteering to do things that are unpleasant.
  F. feels uncomfortable or helpless when alone, because of exaggerated fears of being unable to care for himself or herself.
  G. urgently seeks another relationship as a source of care and support when a close relationship ends.
  H. is unrealistically preoccupied with fears of being left to take care of himself or herself.

Reprinted with permission from the *Diagnostic and Statistical Manual of Mental Disorders*, 4th ed., Text Rev. Copyright 2000 American Psychiatric Association.

---

to be by themselves, as their sense of self-worth, value, or meaning is obtained by or through the presence of a relationship. They have few other sources of self-esteem. Along with the need for emotional support are perpetual doubts and insecurities regarding the current source of support. Persons with DPD constantly require reassurance and reaffirmation that any particular relationship will continue, because they anticipate or fear that at some point they may again be alone. Because of their intense fear of being alone, they may become quickly attached to persons who are unreliable, unempathic, and even exploitative or abusive. More desirable or reliable partners are at times driven away by their excessive clinging and continued demands for reassurance. Occupational functioning is impaired to the extent that independent responsibility and initiative are required. Persons with DPD are prone to mood disorders, particularly major depressive disorder and dysthymic disorder, and to anxiety disorders, particularly agoraphobia, social phobia, and perhaps panic disorder. However, the severity of the symptomatology tends to decrease with age, particularly if the person has obtained a reliable, dependable, and empathic partner.

Differential Diagnosis

Excessive dependency will often be seen in persons who have developed debilitating mental and general medical conditions such as agoraphobia, schizophrenia, mental retardation, severe injuries, and dementia. However, a diagnosis of DPD requires the presence of the dependent traits since late childhood or adolescence. One can diagnose the presence of a personality disorder at any age during a person's lifetime, but if, for example, a DPD diagnosis is given to a person at the age of 75 years, this presumes that the dependent behavior was evident since the age of approximately 18 years (i.e., predates the onset of a comorbid mental or physical disorder).

Deference, politeness, and passivity will also vary substantially across cultural groups. It is important not to confuse differences in personality that are due to different cultural norms with the presence of a personality disorder. The diagnosis of DPD requires that the dependent behavior be maladaptive, resulting in clinically significant functional impairment or distress.

Many persons with DPD will also meet the criteria for HPD and BPD. Persons with DPD and HPD may both display strong needs for reassurance, attention, and approval. However, persons with DPD tend to be more self-effacing, docile, and altruistic, whereas persons with HPD tend to be more flamboyant, assertive, and self-centered, and persons with BPD will tend to be much more dysfunctional and emotionally dysregulated.

TREATMENT

Persons with DPD are often in treatment for one or more Axis I disorders, particularly a mood (depressive) or an anxiety disorder. They tend to be very agreeable, compliant, and grateful individuals, at times to excess. An important issue in the treatment of persons with DPD is not letting the relationship with the therapist become an end in itself. Many persons with DPD find the therapeutic relationship satisfying their need for support, concern, and involvement. The therapist can be perceived as a nurturing, caring, and dependable partner who is always available for as long as the individual desires. Successful treatment can in fact be feared because it suggests the termination of the relationship, an outcome that is at times avoided at all costs. As a result, they may be excessively compliant, submissive, agreeable, and cooperative in order to be the individual that the therapist would want to retain. Therapists need to be careful not to unwittingly encourage or exploit this submissiveness, nor to commit

the opposite error of rejecting and abandoning them to be rid of their needy and clinging dependency. Such responses are common in the interpersonal (marital and sexual) history of persons with DPD, and are at times experienced as well within therapeutic relationships. Persons with DPD tend to have unrealistic expectations regarding their therapist. They may attempt to have the therapist take control of their lives, and may make unrealistic requests or demands for their therapist's time, involvement, and availability.

Exploration of the breadth and source of the need for care and support is often an important component of treatment. Persons with DPD often have a history of exploitative, rejecting, and perhaps even abusive relationships that have contributed to their current feelings of insecurity and inadequacy. Cognitive–behavioral techniques are useful in addressing the feelings of inadequacy, incompetence, and helplessness. Social skills, problem-solving, and assertiveness training also makes important contributions.

Persons with DPD may also benefit from group therapy. A supportive group is useful in diffusing the feelings of dependency onto a variety of persons, in providing feedback regarding their manner of relating to others, and in providing practice and role models for more assertive and autonomous interpersonal functioning. There is no known pharmacologic treatment for DPD.

Obsessive–Compulsive Personality Disorder

DIAGNOSIS

Obsessive–compulsive personality disorder (OCPD) includes a preoccupation with orderliness, perfectionism, and mental and interpersonal control. OCPD is indicated by the presence of four or more of the eight diagnostic criteria presented in DSM criteria for OCPD (see page 457).

Conscientiousness is one of the fundamental dimensions of personality, characterized by the tendency to emphasize duty, order, deliberation, discipline, competence, and achievement. Persons who are excessively organized, ordered, deliberate, dutiful, and disciplined would be characterized as having OCPD. Only 1–2% of the general community may meet the diagnostic criteria for the disorder, but this could be an underestimation. Up to 10% of the population has been estimated to be maladaptively stubborn, 4% excessively devoted to work, and 8% excessively perfectionistic. OCPD is one of the less frequently diagnosed personality disorders within inpatient settings, occurring in approximately 3–10% of individuals, but its prevalence may

DSM-IV-TR Diagnostic Criteria

301.4 OBSESSIVE–COMPULSIVE PERSONALITY DISORDER

A pervasive pattern of preoccupation with orderliness, perfectionism, and mental and interpersonal control at the expense of flexibility, openness, and efficiency, beginning by early adulthood and present in a variety of contexts, as indicated by four (or more) of the following:

A. is preoccupied with details, rules, lists, order, organization, or schedules to the extent that the major point of the activity is lost
B. shows perfectionism that interferes with task completion (e.g., is unable to complete a project because his or her own overly strict standards are not met)
C. excessive devotion to work and productivity to the exclusion of leisure activities and friendships (not accounted for by obvious economic necessity)
D. is overconscientious, scrupulous, and inflexible about matters of morality, ethics, or values (not accounted for by cultural or religious identification)
E. is unable to discard worn-out or worthless objects even when they have no sentimental value
F. is reluctant to delegate tasks or to work with others unless they submit to exactly his or her way of doing things
G. adopts a miserly spending style toward both self and others; money is viewed as something to be hoarded for future catastrophes
H. shows rigidity and stubbornness.

Reprinted with permission from the *Diagnostic and Statistical Manual of Mental Disorders*, 4th ed., Text Rev. Copyright 2000 American Psychiatric Association.

be much higher within private practice settings. This disorder does appear to occur more often in males than in females but exceptions to this finding have been reported.

Course

As children, some persons with OCPD may have appeared to be relatively well-behaved, responsible, and conscientious. However, they may have also been overly serious, rigid, and constrained. As adults, many will obtain good to excellent success within a job or career. They can be excellent workers to the point of excess, sacrificing their social and leisure activities, marriage, and family for their job. Relationships with spouse and children are likely to be strained because of their tendency to be detached and uninvolved, yet authoritarian and domineering with respect to decisions. A spouse may complain of a lack of affection, tenderness, and warmth. Relationships with colleagues at work may be equally strained by the excessive perfectionism, domination, indecision, worrying, and anger. Jobs that require flexibility, openness, creativity, or diplomacy may be particularly difficult. Persons with OCPD may be prone to various anxiety and physical disorders that

are secondary to their worrying, indecision, and stress. Those with concomitant traits of angry hostility and competitiveness may be prone to cardiovascular disorders. Mood disorders may not develop until the person recognizes the sacrifices that have been made by their devotion to work and productivity, which may at times not occur until middle age. However, most will experience early employment or career difficulties, or even failures that may result in depression.

Differential Diagnosis

Devotion to work and productivity will vary substantially across cultural groups. One should be careful not to confuse normal cultural variation in conscientiousness with the presence of this personality disorder. A diagnosis of OCPD requires that the devotion to work be maladaptive or to the exclusion of leisure activities and friendships.

OCPD resembles to some extent the obsessive–compulsive disorder (OCD). However, many persons with OCPD fail to develop OCD, and vice versa. OCD involves intrusive obsessions or circumscribed and repetitively performed rituals whose purpose is to reduce or control feelings of anxiety. OCPD, in contrast, involves rigid, inhibited, and authoritarian behavior patterns that are more egosyntonic. If both behavior patterns are present, both diagnoses should be given as these disorders are sufficiently distinct that it is likely that in such cases two different disorders are in fact present.

OCPD may at times resemble narcissistic PD, as both disorders can involve assertiveness, domination, achievement, and a professed perfectionism. However, the emphasis in OCPD will be on work for its own sake, whereas narcissistic persons will work only to achieve status and recognition. Persons with OCPD will also be troubled by doubts, worries, and self-criticism, whereas the narcissistic person will tend to be overly self-assured.

TREATMENT

Persons with OCPD may fail to seek treatment for the OCPD symptomatology. They may seek treatment instead for disorders and problems that are secondary to their OCPD traits, including anxiety disorders, health problems (e.g., cardiovascular disorders), and problems within various relationships (e.g., marital, familial, and occupational). Treatment will be complicated by their inability to appreciate the contribution of their personality to these problems and disorders. It is not unusual for persons with OCPD to perceive themselves as being simply conscientious, dutiful, moral, and responsible, rather than perfectionistic, stubborn, rigid, domineering, and unavailable. Their understanding is complicated further by the contribution of their traits to various achievements and successes (e.g., career advancement) and to the control of negative affect (e.g., ability to control feelings of dysphoria during a crisis). The OCPD traits are not invariably or always maladaptive, and persons with this disorder may not appreciate the disorder's cost to their physical health, psychological well-being, and personal relationships.

Cognitive–behavioral techniques that address the irrationality of excessive conscientiousness, moralism, perfectionism, devotion to work, and stubbornness can be effective in the treatment of OCPD. Persons with OCPD may in fact appreciate the rational approach to treatment provided by cognitive–behavioral therapy. A common difficulty though is the tendency to drift into lengthy and unproductive ruminations and intellectualized speculations. Therapeutic techniques that emphasize the acknowledgment, recognition, and acceptance of feelings will therefore be useful. Gestalt techniques that focus upon and confront feeling states will often feel threatening to persons with OCPD, but precisely for this reason, they can also be quite revealing and useful. Persons with OCPD will attempt to control therapeutic sessions, and techniques that encourage uncontrolled, freely expressed associations to explore historical motivations for control, perfectionism, and workaholism are often helpful.

Persons with OCPD can be problematic in groups. They will tend to be domineering, constricted, and judgmental. There is no accepted pharmacologic treatment for OCPD. Some persons with OCPD will benefit from anxiolytic or antidepressant medications, but this will typically reflect the presence of associated features or comorbid disorders. The core traits of OCPD might not be affected by pharmacologic interventions.

Personality Disorder Not Otherwise Specified

As indicated earlier, DSM-IV-TR includes a diagnostic category, personality disorder not otherwise specified (PDNOS), for persons with a personality disorder who do not meet the diagnostic criteria for any one of the 10 officially recognized diagnoses. PDNOS has in fact been the single most commonly used personality disorder diagnosis in almost every study in which it has been considered. It would not, of course, be possible to discuss the etiology, pathology, course, or treatment of the PDNOS disorder as the diagnosis refers to a wide variety of personality types. However, one usage of PDNOS is for the two personality disorders presented in the appendix to DSM-IV-TR for criterion sets provided for further study, the passive–aggressive and the depressive.

COMPARISON OF DSM-IV-TR AND ICD-10 DIAGNOSTIC CRITERIA

The items sets for paranoid, schizoid, schizotypal, antisocial, histrionic, avoidant, dependent, and obsessive–compulsive personality disorders in the ICD-10 Diagnostic Criteria for Research and the DSM-IV-TR criteria differ but define essentially the same condition. Furthermore, ICD-10 does not consider schizotypal to be a personality disorder and instead includes this condition in the section containing schizophrenia and other psychotic disorders. ICD-10 also refers to several of the DSM-IV-TR disorders by different names: antisocial is called "dissocial," borderline is called "emotionally unstable personality disorder, borderline type," and obsessive–compulsive is called "anankastic."

ICD-10 includes an "emotionally unstable personality disorder" with two subtypes: impulsive type and borderline type; criteria are provided for each subtype but not for emotionally unstable personality disorder. Neither of these subtypes by themselves correspond to the DSM-IV-TR BPD, which includes some items from each of these subtypes. Narcissistic personality disorder in DSM-IV-TR is not included in ICD-10 as a specific personality disorder, although the DSM-IV-TR criteria set is included in Annex I of ICD-10 (i.e., "provisional criteria for selected disorders").

43 Psychological Factors Affecting Medical Condition

DIAGNOSIS

This diagnostic category recognizes the variety of ways in which specific psychological or behavioral factors can adversely affect medical illnesses. Such factors may contribute to the initiation or the exacerbation of the illness, interfere with treatment and rehabilitation, or contribute to morbidity and mortality. Psychological factors may themselves constitute risks for medical diseases, or they may magnify the effects of nonpsychological risk factors. The effects may be mediated directly at a pathophysiological level (e.g., psychological stress inducing myocardial ischemia) or through the individual's behavior (e.g., noncompliance).

The subject of psychological factors affecting medical condition (PFAMC) has become the focus of intense research because of the illumination it may provide of basic disease mechanisms (e.g., psychoneuroimmunology) and because of the deep interest in improving both the outcomes and the efficiency of health care delivery. In epidemiological studies, several mental disorders increase the likelihood of mortality, especially depression, bipolar disorder, schizophrenia, and alcohol abuse or dependence. Psychiatric disorders or symptoms in individuals with medical illness may increase their use of health care services, particularly the length of costly hospital stays. Interest has been further increased by intervention trials aimed at psychological factors or disorders that have demonstrated improvements in medical outcomes and in quality of life in individuals with serious medical disorders.

It should be evident that this diagnosis is not really a discrete diagnostic category but rather a label for the interactive effects of psyche on soma. Mind–body interactions have long been a focus of interest, both in health and in disease. Mental disorder and medical disease frequently coexist. Mental health professionals and investigators of past eras were misled by this frequent comorbidity into premature conclusions that the

DSM-IV-TR Diagnostic Criteria

316. PSYCHOLOGICAL FACTORS AFFECTING MEDICAL CONDITION

A. General medical condition (coded on Axis III) is present.
B. Psychological factors adversely affect the general medical condition in one of the following ways:

  (1) the factors have influenced the course of the general medical condition as shown by a close temporal association between the psychological factors and the development or exacerbation of, or delayed recovery from, the general medical condition
  (2) the factors interfere with the treatment of the general medical condition
  (3) the factors constitute additional health risks for the individual
  (4) stress-related physiological responses precipitate or exacerbate symptoms of the general medical condition.

Choose name based on the nature of the psychological factors (if more than one factor is present, indicate the most prominent):

Mental disorder affecting... [indicate the general medical condition] (e.g., an Axis I disorder such as major depressive disorder delaying recovery from a myocardial infarction)
Psychological symptoms affecting... [indicate the general medical condition] (e.g., depressive symptoms delaying recovery from surgery; anxiety exacerbating asthma)
Personality traits or coping style affecting... [indicate the general medical condition] (e.g., pathological denial of the need for surgery in a patient with cancer; hostile, pressured behavior contributing to cardiovascular disease)
Maladaptive health behaviors affecting... [indicate the general medical condition] (e.g., overeating; lack of exercise; unsafe sex)
Stress-related physiological response affecting... [indicate the general medical condition] (e.g., stress-related exacerbations of ulcer, hypertension, arrhythmia, or tension headache)
Other or unspecified psychological factors affecting... [indicate the general medical condition] (e.g., interpersonal, cultural, or religious factors)

Reprinted with permission from the *Diagnostic and Statistical Manual of Mental Disorders*, 4th ed.,Text Rev. Copyright 2000 American Psychiatric Association.

Clinical Guide to the Diagnosis and Treatment of Mental Disorders. M. B. First and A. Tasman
© 2006 John Wiley & Sons, Ltd.   ISBN 0 470 019158

psychological factors were preeminent in the causation of the medical disorders, and these were designated psychosomatic. A more modern approach has been to recognize that all medical illnesses are potentially affected by many different factors in the biological, psychological, and social realms. The earlier designation of certain disorders as psychosomatic (e.g., peptic ulcer disease) overvalued the contribution of psychological factors to those disorders and undervalued their contribution to other medical disorders (e.g., cancer). Furthermore, whereas labeling medical illnesses as psychosomatic drew attention to the importance of mind–body interactions, it unfortunately and falsely implied to many individuals undergoing treatment and physicians that the illness was basically psychogenic, that the symptoms were not "real," and that the illness was somehow the individual's fault.

The diagnosis of PFAMC focuses attention on one causal direction in the interactions between psyche and soma, that is, the effects of psychological factors on the medical condition (Figure 43-1). This represents a heuristic simplification, highlighting a particular process for further exploration, understanding, and intervention. In most individuals, there are effects in the other direction as well (i.e., the effects of general medical illness on psychological function). Furthermore, both mind and body interact with social and environmental factors, both dramatic (e.g., poverty, racism, war) and more subtle (e.g., employment status, neighborhood), that affect the incidence and outcome of medical illness. Diagnosing PFAMC may help the mental health professional and the individual address an important dimension of care, but the other "arrows" of Figure 43-1 often warrant attention too.

The diagnosis of PFAMC differs from the diagnosis of most other mental disorders in its focus on the interaction between the mental and medical realms. As noted, the criteria require more than that the individual has both a medical illness and contemporaneous psychological factors, because their coexistence does not always include significant interactions between them. To make the diagnosis of PFAMC, either the factors must have influenced the course of the medical condition, interfered with its treatment, contributed to health risks, or physiologically aggravated the medical condition.

Let us consider each of these four ways of making the diagnosis of PFAMC in more detail. The psychological factor's influence on the course of a general medical condition can be inferred from a close temporal relationship between the factor and the development or exacerbation of the medical condition (or delayed recovery). For example, a 45-year-old male executive reports symptoms sounding like typical angina, but occurring only on weekends. Further questioning reveals that he is depressed over deterioration in his marriage. During the week he works late and has limited contact with his family, but he spends the weekend at home. The symptoms began after he and his wife started arguing every weekend. The temporal link between onset and recurrence of angina and marital arguments supports a diagnosis of PFAMC.

PFAMC can also be diagnosed when the psychological factor interferes with treatment, including not seeking medical care, not following up, nonadherence to prescribed drugs or other treatment, or maladaptive modifications in treatment made by the individual or family. The executive with angina rejected his physician's recommendations for further assessment and treatment. He said, "I do get upset at home but I feel just fine at the office, so there couldn't be anything really wrong with me." The individual is able to acknowledge marital discord, but the defense of denial clouds his perception of his physical health and blocks appropriate medical care. This is another form of PFAMC.

PFAMC can also be diagnosed when the psychological factor contributes to health risks, exemplified by the executive increasing his smoking and drinking despite his physician's warnings ("Its the only way I can cope with my wife."). Finally, PFAMC is an appropriate diagnosis when there are stress-related physiological responses precipitating or exacerbating symptoms of the medical condition. The same man observes that angina is most likely to occur after marital arguments during which he becomes irate, yells, slams doors, and throws things.

When a person's medical illness is faring worse than expected and not responding well to standard treatment, clinicians should and often do consider whether a psychological factor may be responsible for the poorer-than-expected outcome. This is a far from trivial task. To ignore the possibility of PFAMC may miss the crucial barrier to the individual's recovery. On

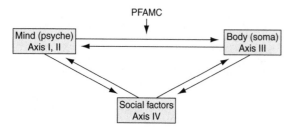

Figure 43-1 *Psychological factors affecting medical condition (PFAMC): interaction between psyche and soma. Social factors warrant attention as well.*

the other hand, premature or facile attribution to psychological factors may lead the clinician to overlook medical or social explanations for "treatment-resistant disease" and unfairly blame the individual, with resultant further deterioration in health outcomes and the clinician–patient relationship.

To illustrate, a common clinical problem is the brittle diabetic adolescent with labile blood glucose levels and frequent episodes of ketoacidosis and hypoglycemia, despite vigorous attempts by the physician to improve diabetic management and glucose control. The considerable difficulty in controlling such persons' diabetes is often attributed to adolescents' dislike of lifestyle restrictions, their tendency to act out and rebel against authority figures, their denial of vulnerability, their ambivalence about their need for nurturance, and their wish to be "normal." There are many adolescent (and some adult) diabetics for whom these psychological issues do play an important role in undermining diabetes management through noncompliance regarding medication, diet, visits to the physician, substance use, and activity limitations. However, psychological factors do not always account for brittleness and are sometimes incorrectly suspected. It has been demonstrated that much of the difficulty in achieving stable glucose control in adolescent diabetics is the result of the dramatically labile patterns of hormone secretion (cortisol, growth hormone) typical of adolescence, independent of psychological status.

PFAMC has descriptive names for subcategories described as follows.

Mental Disorder Affecting a General Medical Condition. If the individual has a mental disorder meeting criteria for an Axis I or Axis II diagnosis, the diagnostic name is mental disorder affecting medical condition, with the particular medical condition specified. In addition to coding PFAMC, the specific mental disorder is also coded on Axis I or Axis II. Examples include major depressive disorder that reduces energy and compliance in an individual with hemodialysis, panic disorder that makes an asthmatic hypersensitive to dyspnea, and schizophrenia in an individual with recurrent ventricular tachycardia who refuses placement of an automatic implantable defibrillator because he fears it will control his mind.

Psychological Symptoms Affecting a General Medical Condition. Individuals who have psychological symptoms that do not meet the threshold for an Axis I diagnosis may still experience important effects on their medical illness, and the diagnosis would be psychological symptoms affecting a medical condition.

Examples include anxiety that aggravates irritable bowel syndrome, depressed mood that hinders recovery from hip replacement surgery, and anger that interferes with rehabilitation after spinal cord injury.

Personality Traits or Coping Style Affecting a General Medical Condition. This may include personality traits or coping styles that do not meet criteria for an Axis II disorder and other patterns of response considered to be maladaptive because they may pose a risk for particular medical illnesses. An example is the competitive hostility component of the type A behavior pattern, and its impact on coronary artery disease. Maladaptive personality traits or coping styles are particularly likely to interfere with the physician–patient relationship as well as the relationships which the individuals have with other caregivers.

Maladaptive Health Behaviors Affecting a General Medical Condition. Many maladaptive health behaviors have significant effects on the course and treatment of many medical conditions. Examples include sedentary lifestyle, smoking, abuse of alcohol or other substances, and unsafe sexual practices. If the maladaptive behaviors can be better accounted for by an Axis I or Axis II disorder, the first subcategory (mental disorder affecting a medical condition) should be used instead.

Stress-Related Physiological Response Affecting a General Medical Condition. Examples of stress-related physiological responses affecting a medical condition include the precipitation by psychological stress of angina, cardiac arrhythmia, migraine, or attack of colitis in medically vulnerable individuals. In such cases, stress is not the cause of the illness or symptoms; the individual has a medical condition that etiologically accounts for the symptoms (e.g., coronary artery disease, migraine, or ulcerative colitis), and the stressor instead represents a precipitating or aggravating factor.

Other or Unspecified Psychological Factors Affecting a General Medical Condition. There are other psychological phenomena that may not fit within one of these subcategories. An interpersonal example is marital dysfunction. A cultural example is the extreme discomfort women from some cultures may experience being alone with a male physician, even while they are fully dressed. A religious example is a Jehovah's Witness who ambivalently refuses blood transfusion. These fall under the residual category of other or unspecified psychological factors affecting a medical condition.

Course

Given the wide range of mental disorders and psychological factors that may affect medical illness and the large number of different general medical conditions that may be influenced, there are no general rules about the course of the PFAMC interaction. Psychological factors may have minor or major effects at a particular point or throughout the course of a medical illness. We do know in general that individuals with general medical conditions who also have significant psychological symptoms have poorer outcomes and higher medical care costs than those individuals with the same general medical conditions but without psychological distress. A number of studies now document that psychological or psychiatric problems (particularly cognitive disorder, depression, and anxiety) in general medical inpatients are associated with significant increases in length of hospital stay. Psychosocial interventions have been able to improve outcomes in medical illness, sometimes with an attendant saving in health care costs.

Differential Diagnosis

As noted before, the close temporal association between psychiatric symptoms and a medical condition does not always reflect PFAMC. If the two are considered merely coincidental, then separate mental disorder and general medical condition diagnoses should be made. In some cases of coincident mental disorders and general medical conditions, the mental symptoms are actually the result of the medical condition (i.e., the causality is in a direction opposite from that of PFAMC). When a medical condition is judged to be pathophysiologically causing the mental disorder (e.g., hypothyroidism causing depression), the correct diagnosis is the appropriate mental disorder due to a general medical condition (e.g., mood disorder due to hypothyroidism, with depressive features). In PFAMC, the psychological or behavioral factors are judged to precipitate or aggravate the medical condition.

Substance use disorders may adversely affect many medical conditions, and this can be described through PFAMC. However, in some individuals, all of the psychiatric and medical symptoms are direct consequences of substance abuse, and it is usually parsimonious to use just the substance-use disorder diagnosis. For example, an individual with delirium tremens after alcohol withdrawal would receive a diagnosis of alcohol withdrawal delirium, not PFAMC, but an individual with alcohol dependence who repeatedly missed hemodialysis treatments because of intoxication would receive diagnoses of alcohol dependence and PFAMC (mental disorder affecting end stage renal disease).

Individuals with somatoform disorders (e.g., somatization disorder, hypochondriasis) present with physical complaints that may mimic a medical illness, but the somatic symptoms are actually accounted for by the psychiatric disorder. In principle, it might seem that somatoform disorders are easily distinguished from PFAMC because PFAMC requires the presence of a diagnosable medical condition. The distinction in practice is sometimes difficult because the individual may have both a somatoform disorder and one or more medical disorders. For example, an individual with seizures regularly precipitated by emotional stress might have true epilepsy aggravated by stress (PFAMC), pseudoseizures (conversion disorder), or both.

TREATMENT

Management of psychological factors affecting the individual's medical condition should be tailored both to the particular psychological factor of relevance and to the medical outcome of concern. Some general guidelines, however, can be helpful. The physician, whether in primary care or a specialty, should not ignore apparent psychiatric illness. Unfortunately, this occurs all too often because of discomfort, stigma, lack of training, or disinterest. Referring the individual to a mental health specialist for evaluation is certainly better than ignoring the psychological problem but should not be regarded as "disposing" of it, because the physician must still attend to its potential impact on the individual's medical illness. Similarly, psychiatrists and other mental health practitioners should not ignore coincident medical disease and should not assume that referral to a nonpsychiatric physician absolves them of all responsibility for the individual's medical problem.

Mental Disorder Affecting a Medical Condition. If the individual has a treatable Axis I disorder, treatment for it should be provided. Whereas this is obviously justified on the basis of providing relief from the Axis I disorder, mental treatment is further supported by the myriad ways in which the mental disorder may currently or in future adversely affect the medical illness. The same psychopharmacological and psychotherapeutic treatments used for Axis I mental disorders are normally appropriate when an affected medical condition is also present. However, even well-established psychiatric treatments supported by randomized controlled trials have seldom been validated in the medically ill, who are typically excluded from the controlled trials. Thus, psychiatric treatments may not always be directly generalizable to, and often must be modified for, the medically ill.

When prescribing psychiatric medications for individuals with significant medical comorbidity, the clinician should keep in mind potential adverse effects on impaired organ systems (e.g., anticholinergic exacerbation of postoperative ileus; tricyclic antidepressant causing completion of heart block), changes in pharmacokinetics (absorption, protein binding, metabolism, and excretion), and drug–drug interactions. Psychotherapy may also require modification in individuals with comorbid medical illness, including greater flexibility regarding the length and frequency of appointments, and deviations from standard therapeutic abstinence and neutrality. Psychotherapists treating individuals with PFAMC should usually be much more active in communicating with other health care professionals caring for the individual (with the individual's consent), than is usually the case in psychotherapy.

If the individual has an Axis II personality disorder or other prominent personality or coping style, the mental health clinician should modify the individual treatment accordingly, which is usually more easily accomplished than trying to change the individual's personality. For example, individuals who tend to be paranoid or mistrustful should receive more careful explanations, particularly before invasive or anxiety-provoking procedures. With narcissistic individuals, the clinician should avoid relating in ways that may seem excessively paternalistic or authoritarian to the individual. With some dependent individuals, it may be advisable to be more directive, without overdoing it and fostering excessive dependency.

Psychological Symptoms Affecting a General Medical Condition. In some instances, psychiatric symptoms not meeting the threshold for an Axis I diagnosis will respond positively to the same treatments used for the analogous Axis I mental disorder, with appropriate modifications as noted before. There is not a great amount of treatment research on subsyndromal psychiatric symptoms, and even less in individuals with comorbid medical illness, so this area of practice remains less evidence-based. Some psychiatric symptoms affecting a medical condition may be amenable to stress management and other behavioral techniques as well as appropriate reassurance.

Any intervention directed by the mental health clinician at a particular individual's psychological symptoms or behavior should be grounded in exploratory discussion with the individual. Interventions without such grounding tend to seem at best superficial and artificial, and at worst are entirely off the mark. For example, if the clinician wrongly presumes to know why a particular individual seems anxious without asking, the individual is likely to feel misunderstood. Facile, nonspecific reassurance can undermine the clinician–patient relationship because the individual is likely to feel that the clinician is out of touch with and not really interested in the individual's experience. It is especially important with depressed individuals that clinicians avoid premature or unrealistic reassurance or an overly cheerful attitude; this tends to alienate depressed individuals, who feel that their clinician is insensitive and either does not understand or does not want to hear about their sadness. Clinicians should provide specific and realistic reassurance, emphasize on a constructive treatment plan, and mobilize the individual's support system.

Personality Traits or Coping Style Affecting a General Medical Condition. As with Axis II disorders affecting a medical condition, clinicians should be aware of the personality style's effects on the therapeutic relationship and modify management to better fit the individual. For example, with type A "time urgent" individuals, clinicians may need to be more sensitive to issues of appointment scheduling and waiting times. Group therapy interventions can enhance active coping with serious medical illnesses like cancer, heart disease, and renal failure but to date have usually been designed to be broadly generalizable rather than targeted to one particular trait or style (with the exception of type A behavior).

Another general guideline is not to attack or interfere with a individual's defensive style unless the defense is having an adverse impact on the medical illness or its management. Clinicians are particularly tempted to intervene when the defense is dramatic, breaks with reality, or makes the clinician uncomfortable.

For example, denial is a defense mechanism that reduces anxiety and conflict by blocking conscious awareness of thoughts, feelings, or facts that an individual cannot face. Denial is common in the medically ill but varies in its timing, strength, and adaptive value. Some individuals are aware of what is wrong with them but consciously suppress this knowledge by avoiding thinking about or discussing it. Others cope with the threat of being overwhelmed by their illness by unconsciously repressing it and thereby remain unaware of their illness. Marked denial, in which the individual emphatically refuses to accept the existence or significance of obvious symptoms and signs of the disease, may be seen by the clinician as an indication that the individual is "crazy" because the individual seems impervious to rational persuasion. In the absence of signs of another major mental disorder (e.g., paranoid delusions), such denial is not often a sign of psychosis but rather represents a defense against overwhelming fear.

The adaptive value of denial may vary, depending on the nature or stage of illness. When an individual's denial does not preclude cooperation with treatment, the clinician should leave it alone. The clinician does have an ethical and professional obligation to ensure that the individual has been informed about the illness and treatment. After that, if the individual accepts treatment but persists with an irrationally optimistic outlook, the clinician should respect the individual's need to use denial to cope. For some, the denial is fragile, and the clinician must decide whether the defense should be supported and strengthened, or if the individual had better give up the denial to discuss fears directly and receive reassurance from the clinician. The clinician should not support denial by giving the individual false information, but rather encourage hope and optimism. When denial is extreme, individuals may refuse vital treatment or threaten to leave against medical advice. Here, the clinician must try to help reduce denial but not by directly assaulting the individual's defenses. Because such desperate denial of reality usually reflects intense underlying anxiety, trying to scare the individual into cooperation will intensify denial and the impulse to flight. A better strategy for the clinician is to avoid directly challenging the individual's claims while simultaneously reinforcing concern for the individual and maximizing the individual's sense of control.

Maladaptive Health Behavior Affecting a General Medical Condition. This is an area of research with many promising approaches. To achieve smoking cessation, bupropion, nicotine replacement, behavioral therapies, and other pharmacological strategies all warrant consideration. Behavioral strategies are also useful in promoting better dietary practices, sleep hygiene, safe sex, and exercise. For some individuals, change can be achieved efficiently through support groups, whereas others change more effectively through a one-to-one relationship with a health care professional.

Stress-Related Physiological Response Affecting a Medical Condition. Biofeedback, relaxation techniques, hypnosis, and other stress management interventions have been helpful in reducing stress-induced exacerbations of medical illness including cardiac, gastrointestinal, headache, and other symptoms. Pharmacological interventions have also been useful (e.g., the widespread practice of prescribing benzodiazepines during acute myocardial infarction to prevent stress-induced increase in myocardial work).

COMPARISON OF DSM-IV-TR AND ICD-10 DIAGNOSTIC CRITERIA

Although the corresponding ICD-10 category ("Psychological and behavioral factors associated with disorders or diseases classified elsewhere") does not have specified diagnostic criteria, it is defined in essentially the same way as DSM-IV-TR.

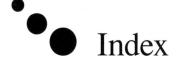

Index

Clinical Guide to the Diagnosis and Treatment of Mental Disorders. M. B. First and A. Tasman
© 2006 John Wiley & Sons, Ltd. ISBN 0 470 019158